Network Pharmacology

Shao Li
Editor

Network Pharmacology

Springer

清華大學出版社
TSINGHUA UNIVERSITY PRESS

Editor
Shao Li
Institute of TCM-X / Department of
Automation
Tsinghua University
Beijing, China

ISBN 978-981-16-0752-3   ISBN 978-981-16-0753-0 (eBook)
https://doi.org/10.1007/978-981-16-0753-0

Jointly published with Tsinghua University Press
The print edition is not for sale in China (Mainland). Customers from China (Mainland) please order the print book from: Tsinghua University Press.

This Springer imprint is published by the registered company Springer Nature Singapore Pte Ltd.
The registered company address is: 152 Beach Road, #21-01/04 Gateway East, Singapore 189721, Singapore

Foreword

With the advancement of medical science, the research on diseases and medicine in Western medicine is changing from "reductionist theory" to "systems theory," and from a single and isolated model to a multi-faceted and systematically researched one. A considerably important development in this transformation involves the use of a biomolecular network to analyze the relationship between disease and drugs, which is a breakthrough in drug research on systems biology and also brings in new changes and challenges to the medical research model.

Conversely, Traditional Chinese Medicine (TCM) has always been based on holistic analysis and treatment of patients, and overall systematic adjustment of the disease is its advantages and characteristics. However, a vital concern for the development of TCM is to surmise how to associate medicine with the complex human body, to carry out qualitative and quantitative analysis. Based on the biomolecular network, network pharmacology analyzes the relationship between diseases and medicine, which is in line with the needs of TCM development, thereby initiating the innovation of TCM research methods.

The biomolecular network is the basis of complex biological systems, and reflects the interrelationships of various biomolecules within organisms, such as the gene regulation network, protein interaction network, signal transduction network, metabolic network, etc. At the same time, it can also describe the associations between medicine, medicine and functions, medicine and diseases at distinct levels, such as TCM component network, phenotype and drug component network, biological function network, etc. It is a link between micro and micro, micro and macro, as well as unit and system. Owing to these features, network pharmacology based on biomolecular networks materialized. Since China possesses thousands of years of TCM theories and practices, and as TCM involves the holistic observation and analysis of people, the country took the lead in the inception of the idea of a relationship between diseases and biological molecular network in the field of network pharmacology. As early as 1999, before the name *network pharmacology* appeared internationally, Professor Shao Li and his research group propounded the hypothesis that TCM syndromes are related to biomolecular networks, and also discovered an interconnection between biomolecular networks and cold and heat syndromes. In 2011, they presented the concept of *network target*, which identifies the relationship between medicine and disease syndromes at the level of biomolecular networks, and in addition elucidated the systemic regulation of medicine on disease syndromes. On this premise, the system analysis method based on network target was proposed, including the construction of biomolecular network, network target analysis method, network target analysis of drug action mechanism, and network target verification. These concepts and methods are highly esteemed by scholars in China and overseas. Thanks to network pharmacology, which is based on the correlation between biological molecular network and disease syndrome, the effect of TCM can be explained by the effect on the human body's biomolecular network. By virtue of the biomolecular network of the human body, the effect of TCM on the human body has changed from qualitative analysis and quantitative testing in the past, to the stage where quantitative analysis can be implemented. This was indubitably a breakthrough in TCM development, in view of the fact that it provided a scientific basis for explaining its principles and mechanisms. This significant progress typically, attracted the attention of the TCM community and was effectuated actively, which allowed network pharmacology develop fervidly in China and led to a succession of gratifying accomplishments. This is a very important and outstanding contribution made by Chinese scholars to the world of network pharmacology.

Contemporarily, with the augmentation of network pharmacology, innovative techniques and applications have come to light, thereby making it imperative to recapitulate and meliorate them eventually to make their development and application more standardized and effective. On the other hand, big data, artificial intelligence, complex system theory, and other technologies are rapidly developing and inevitably playing a role in network pharmacology, resulting in new concepts, models, and methods. Thus, we are able to conduct more in-depth analysis, and create more accurate and effective methods. These aspects also require our timely guidance and progression. For instance, the core of network pharmacology is analysis and inference of drug targets; primarily the analysis of the relationship between nodes of complex networks and disease treatment. In this respect, the understanding and application of "relationship inference" (belonging to the category of artificial intelligence) between nodes of complex networks and treatment of diseases plays a vital role.

Tsinghua University, Beijing, China

Chinese Academy of Sciences
Beijing, China
19 January 2020

Yan-da Li

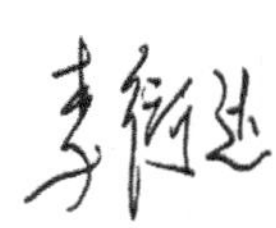

Foreword

Network pharmacology is a discipline which developed on the basis of the theories of systems biology and bioinformatics. After Hopkins's first proposal of the concept in 2007, it has attracted the attention of academic circles around the world and has been applied and developed by pharmacologists and drug researchers and developers in China. In the same year, Professor Shao Li of Tsinghua University proposed the research model and practice of prescriptions based on biological network regulation in the *Journal of Chinese Integrative Medicine*. Since 2008, a large number of research reports have been published in the world, and the application value of network pharmacology in the research of TCM pharmacology and innovative medicine is progressively emerging.

In order to meet the pressing requirements of systematic research methods of TCM, procure development opportunities, and to be completely integrated with TCM, the arrival of the new trend of biomedical systematic research in the era of big data and artificial intelligence has become a frontier and hot spot in the field of TCM research in recent years. With respect to safety, network toxicology proposed by us in 2011 is also based on the "gene–protein–drug–toxicity" interaction network, which helps to explain the mechanism of action of TCM and compound prescriptions, interpret the scientific connotation of contraindications, promote the rational use of medicine in clinical practice, and reduce the occurrence of adverse reactions, and is similar to network pharmacology. In recent years, I proposed the concept of Q-Marker, which has now become a new model of quality control in TCM. Network pharmacology and network toxicology are effective methods in the discovery and confirmation of quality markers of TCM.

In the midst of a new cycle of scientific and technological revolution and industrial transformation, the new generation of information technology represented by the Internet, big data, and artificial intelligence is constantly changing. TCM research must forge ahead with the times, make headway perspicuously, revise and innovate, and promote its modernization and internationalization. Comprehension of the integrated regulation of TCM's "multi-component, multi-channel, and multi-target" approach has always been a challenge. Perception of the complexity of TCM and the material basis and action mechanism of Chinese medicine is a challenging quandary, and the means to establish a scientific evaluation system of effective efficacy and safety of TCM is the key. Therefore, we can say that network pharmacology is another key to understand the value of TCM. Based on the unique TCM theories, such as "Four Qi" and "Five Flavors," "Floating," and "Sinking," the key of science is to inherit the essence, observe innovation, and establish new modes and techniques that are in line with the TCM theories and scientific connotations. Therefore, network pharmacology has also opened another research path for the creation of a unique academic system.

Network pharmacology came into being based on the modern research of TCM. In 1999, Professor Shao Li, the Chief Editor of the book, took the lead in proposing the scientific hypothesis of the correlation between TCM and molecular networks and put forward the core theory of network target for the first time, and created a series of techniques that made outstanding contributions to the exploration and development of network pharmacology. Efficacy, safety, and quality control are the basic attributes of medicine. Network pharmacology has the characteristics of network regulation and integrality. Based on the interaction network of "disease–gene–target–medicine" and in terms of effectiveness, it can more notably interpret the intervention and regulation effect of TCM on the syndrome or disease network at the molecular level of the system, reveal the mystery of the medicine's synergistic action on the human body, and competently predict the effective components and effect targets of the medicine.

Professor Shao Li, the Chief Editor of this book, is a leading figure in network pharmacology. He was the first to systematically discuss the development process of network pharmacology, and the core theory, main research methods, and research results of network target. At the same time, the author also arranged many famous experts in the related fields of network pharmacology to discuss and summarize the methods, application, and practice of network pharmacology in various aspects. The book takes into account the theory and application of network pharmacology, and is well-organized with a plethora of deep insights, which are concurrently substantiated by a great number of established cases.

In my opinion, with the development of modern science and technology, people in the industry will have a more detailed understanding of the vital role of network pharmacology in TCM development, and its application in the systematic research of TCM will definitely make expansive contributions to the modernization of Traditional Chinese Medicine.

I would like to thank the author for his contribution to the development of network pharmacology in China, and I wish the publication of this book will contribute to the development of a new discipline. I trust this book will also be salubrious to its readers.

Drug Evaluation Research Center
Tianjin Institute of Pharmaceutical
Research, Tianjin, China

Chinese Academy of Engineering
Beijing, China
12 April 2020

Changxiao Liu

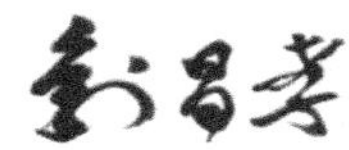

Foreword

The development of Traditional Chinese Medicine is at a critical historical node in our country: how to promote the innovative development of traditional Chinese medicine in modern society and make it better for the people of our country and the world is not only the mission of the times of all traditional Chinese medicine workers, but also is a historical examination placed to the vast number of scientific research and clinical frontline traditional Chinese medicine workers. Therefore, in the front of this book, I have two thoughts to share with you.

First, stick to the origin, inherit the tradition, and dare to innovate. The traditional Chinese medicine has been passed down for thousands of years, and it is an important part of China's excellent traditional culture, and it is also a treasure of the Chinese nation. At all times, we must carry forward and carry forward the cause of traditional Chinese medicine. I have been engaged in clinical and research in Xin'an Medicine for more than 70 years. I put forward the view of "originated from Xin'an, based on clinical practice, based on traditional Chinese culture and moving towards science," and realized that traditional Chinese medicine needs to be inherited, innovated, and developed. We must be aware that, our interpretation of the complex mechanism of action of traditional Chinese medicine is not clear up to now, and this is the root cause of hindering the further innovation and development of traditional Chinese medicine. As an emerging discipline, network pharmacology highlights the new thinking of combining system theory and reduction theory, combining macro and micro, and combining inheritance and development. It combines artificial intelligence, big data, and medical life sciences and is also in line with the characteristics of the holistic view of traditional Chinese medicine. It is undoubtedly an important theoretical breakthrough and method innovation in assisting traditional Chinese medicine workers in interpreting the human body that has been unable to "see through" for thousands of years.

Second, focus on scientific research, ensure accurate data, and return to the clinic. The majority of researchers should pay equal attention to theoretical research and clinical practice. Traditional Chinese medicine has been abolished, but can still be passed down to today, relying on its clinical efficacy. Therefore, when using network pharmacology to analyze the complex mechanism of traditional Chinese medicine, it is necessary to continuously improve the accuracy of research methods and research technologies, continuously explore the thinking characteristics and practical experience of traditional Chinese medicine, and continuously improve the scientificity and effectiveness of traditional Chinese medicine for disease prevention and treatment. Simultaneously, no matter how accurate the data is obtained in the research, the final conclusion must be returned to the clinic for reverification to promote its clinical applications and achieve the goal of better disease prevention and treatment and benefit the people. The so-called benevolence of doctors, humble self-herd, careful beginning, and respecting the end, that is the case.

Back to this book. To enable readers to have a deeper understanding of the overall thinking and methods of network pharmacology research, the editor systematically introduces the core content, research tools and methods, representative achievements, and typical cases of network pharmacology for the first time. I hope that by reading this book, more talents will join the network pharmacology research team. Combine young and modern thinking with the ancient and profound wisdom of the Chinese nation to bring the great cause of traditional Chinese medicine bloom again with dazzling light.

Nowadays, Chinese researchers and international peers are leading the rapid development of the emerging discipline of network pharmacology. This has set up a bridge for the modernization and internationalization of traditional Chinese medicine to communicate ideals and reality, and has an important exemplary role. Future inheritors of traditional Chinese medicine will also shoulder a more important historical mission while continuously learning and inheriting the classic academic ideas and diagnosis experience of traditional Chinese medicine for thousands of years, sharping our minds, and ability to talk to modern technology and the world. In this way, the modern rejuvenation of traditional Chinese medicine will be smoother and the prospects will be brighter.

This is the preface.

The First Affiliated Hospital of Wannan Medical College, Anhui, China

China Academy of Chinese Medical Sciences, Beijing, China

Jiren Li

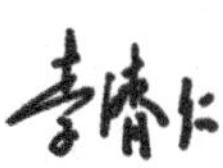

April 5, 2020

Preface

The current research model of "single gene, single target, and single drug" has been created based on the concept of "reductionism." This research model has made great progress and great contribution to the scientification, modernization, and changing of modern medicine and pharmacy. However, this research model faces challenges when it comes to explaining the scientific basis of TCM characterized by its holistic feature, and it is also difficult to systematically open the "black box" of the human body in the process of diagnosis and treatment. At the same time, the incidence of major diseases such as cancer remains high, and unanticipated diseases such as COVID-19 are sweeping the world. It can be seen that in the face of the common enemy—the disease, Chinese and Western medicine are not yet perfect and need to join hands for common development. It is exigent for medical research to explore new ideas and techniques that not only conform to the overall characteristics of TCM, but also adapt to the characteristics of the diagnosis and treatment of complex disease systems. TCM and modern medicine jointly look towards the innovation of research models and research methods.

On the one hand, the holistic characteristics of the treatment process and rich experience in Chinese medicine diagnosis highlight the limitations of the reductionist medicine research model. On the other hand, it has nurtured the emergence of a new generation of research models featuring networks and systems. Among them, an important aspect is to understand the internal mechanism of complex diseases and drug action mechanism from the overall perspective of complex biological network, which provides unprecedented opportunities and challenges for the profound transformation of the medical research model. As a breakthrough point for cross-innovation between Chinese and Western medicine and intelligent information, the study of biological networks is expected to build a new model of intelligent disease prevention and control, and thus network pharmacology emerged in the framework of new science and technology.

Network pharmacology is a new frontier discipline of systematic drug research in the era of artificial intelligence and big data. It is also an original discipline integrating systems biology, bioinformatics, network science, multidirectional pharmacology, systems pharmacology, and other related disciplines. It emphasizes the analysis of molecular association between medicine and their therapeutic objects from the perspective of system level and biological network, reveals the systematic pharmacological mechanism of medicine, and guides the research and development of new medicine and clinical treatment. The so-called network, on the one hand, refers to the description and analysis methods to describe the relationship between elements in the biological system. As a case in point, the theory and method in complex network science are used to promote the research of biological networks. Conversely, it refers to the basis of construction of complex biological systems, which has different biological networks at different levels, including the gene regulation network, protein interaction network, signal transduction network, metabolism network, etc. In a broad sense, there are—biological function networks, cell–cell networks, TCM component networks, compatibility networks of TCM, disease–disease networks, and TCM–disease networks.

In order to systematically reveal the biological basis of TCM and modern medical diagnosis and treatment, we first put forward a new concept of network target, which has become the core theory of network pharmacology. Network target refers to the theory that systematically establishes the mechanism relationship between drugs and diseases at the level of the biological network, and explains the interaction between drugs and diseases through multiple targets and forms the overall regulatory effect. In TCM studies, network target theory can explain how many components of Traditional Chinese Medicine cooperate with each other in the biological network and play an overall regulatory role.

With the development of network pharmacology and the progress of calculational and experimental methods, the progress in this field is expected to provide additional reliable information for the systematic understanding of the interaction between drugs and diseases, and provide key technical support for drug research and development, mechanism interpretation, efficacy evaluation, and precise drug use. It is expected to promote the innovation of research methodology from "reductionism" to "system theory" and provide strong impetus for the popularization and application of "next generation medicine research model."

Network pharmacology has widespread prospects, yet it is paramount to ensure its benign and rapid development. On the one hand, the development of network pharmacology requires the integration of information science, life science, modern medicine, and Traditional Chinese Medicine, and the use of modern technology to promote the objectification and precision of network pharmacology research. In contrast, network pharmacology research also needs to break across the limitations of basic theoretical knowledge from basic information science, life science, medicine, pharmacy, and other disciplines.

This book is devoted to systematically introducing the research progress of the theories, methods, and applications of network pharmacology, and mainly includes four parts: (1) Concepts and Theories Involved in Network Pharmacology (Chap. 1); (2) Common Analysis Methods, Database, and Analysis Software (Chaps. 2, 3, and 4); (3) Typical Cases of TCM Modernization and Modern Medicine Research Based on Network Pharmacology (Chaps. 5 and 6); and (4) Disease-medicine-based

Network Pharmacology Practice Process (Chaps. 7, 8, and 9). The core contents and principal authors of each chapter are as follows:

Chapter	Content	Principal Authors
1	"Network Target" Theory and Network Pharmacology	Shao Li, Qingyang Ding, Xin Wang
2	Application of Network Pharmacology Based on Artificial Intelligence Algorithm in Drug Development	Wenxia Zhou, Xuejun Li, Lu Han, Shengjun Fan
3	Common Network Pharmacology Databases	Haiyu Xu, Yangiong Zhang, Feifei Guo
4	Common Network Pharmacology Software	Xuezhong Zhou, Ning Wang, Xing Zhai
5	Case Study of Network Pharmacology and Modernization of Traditional Chinese Medicine	Shibing Su, Yuanjía Hu, Huali Zuo
6	Network Pharmacology and Modern Drug R&D Cases	Weidong Zhang, Jing Zhao
7	Drug-Based Network Pharmacology Practice Process	Xiaobo Sun, Xiaoyan Xing, Min Wang
8	Disease-Based Network Pharmacology Practice Process	Xiaohui Fan, Xiang Li
9	Drug-Disease-Based Network Pharmacology Practice Process	Weiwei Su, Panlin Li

Finally, I sincerely extend my gratitude to Academician Li Yanda and Academician Liu Changxiao for taking the time out to write the preface for this book; their astute insights were veracious, encouraging and filled with foresight. I would also like to thank Professor Yuanjia Hu, Dr. Kuo Yang and the students (e.g., Wuai Zhou, Siqin Zhang, Ziyi Wang and Lan Wang) for their assistance in compilation of this book, alongside the students who gave affable attention and effervescent support to the writing of this book, and to editor Kai Zhao and Dr. Bo Zhang for their efforts in publishing this book.

In particular, it should be pointed out that the Network Pharmacology Professional Committee of the World Federation of Chinese Medicine Societies, together with Tsinghua University, China Academy of Chinese Medical Sciences, and other institutions, launched the Network Pharmacology Standards of the World Federation of Chinese Medicine Societies (*Guidelines for Evaluation Methods of Network Pharmacology)*, which is also the first international standard in the field of network pharmacology (see Appendix A). This standard specifies the principles, processes, and evaluation indicators for data collection, network analysis, and experimental verification in the process of network pharmacology research and is applicable to researchers and assessors engaged in network pharmacology.

Beijing, China Shao Li
April 2020

Contents

Chapter 1
"Network Target" Theory and Network Pharmacology

Shao Li, Qingyang Ding, and Xin Wang

Guide to This Chapter

In the biomedical big data and artificial intelligence era, pioneering interdisciplinary information science research, life science, and medicine represent a complex biological network which has attracted increasing attention from researchers. Complex biological network includes qualitative and quantitative description of the relationship between tissues, cells, and molecules in an organism. It lays the foundation for constructing complex biological systems, and is also an important bridge connecting information science, life science, and medicine. Network pharmacology has two distinct characteristics regarding current scientific and technological background. Firstly, it promotes the moving from "reductionism" to "system-based theory," which is widely considered as "the next generation medicine research mode." Secondly, the accumulation of modern biomedical big data and the development of artificial intelligence as well as other computing methods provide an important driving force for the development of network pharmacology.

Traditional Chinese Medicine (TCM) plays a key role in the origin and development of network pharmacology. As an integral treasure of China, Chinese medicine offers a holistic approach, puts forth characteristic theories of syndrome differentiation and treatment, and showcases rich experience in clinical practice. Many prescriptions used in long-term TCM clinical practices are the basis for holistic treatment in TCM. Network pharmacology focuses on understanding the internal mechanism and drug action of complex diseases and syndromes (referred to as disease-syndrome) including our biological network, thus conforming to the holistic concept and clinical practice of TCM. Network target is the core theory of network pharmacology. It comes from the modern exploration of TCM. Its hypothesis, practice and concept have existed prior to the concept of network pharmacology.

S. Li (✉) · Q. Ding · X. Wang
Institute of TCM-X/Department of Automation, Tsinghua University, Beijing, China
e-mail: shaoli@tsinghua.edu.cn

S. Li (ed.), *Network Pharmacology*, https://doi.org/10.1007/978-981-16-0753-0_1

Network target aims to establish the relationship between medicine and diseases at the systematic level, and to explain the theory of drug interactions on biological networks through multiple targets and has a holistic regulatory effect overall on the body. Network pharmacology with network targets as the core is an important symbol of the original development of TCM research ideas and methods, and is expected to become a significant and innovative breakthrough of modern times.

This chapter introduces the main content and history of network pharmacology and research based on the core theory of network target.

1.1 Network Pharmacology: Next Generation Medicine Research Mode

With the gradual rise of cross-disciplines such as computational biology, bioinformatics, artificial intelligence, and big data science, medical and life science research has entered the era of big data. Globally, researchers have moved from the "reductionist theory" to a "system theory," from a single, isolated research mode to a multi-faceted and systematic one. An important facet of this approach is to analyze the association between disease occurrence and mechanism of drug action from the biomolecular network perspective, and to use the network to regain the "whole." This has lead to major changes and new challenges in medical research [1]. In this era, systematic medicine [2], network biology [3], and the theme of this book—network pharmacology [4] came into being, bringing unprecedented opportunities for systematic research of TCM.

Network pharmacology is an emerging discipline, integrating systems biology, multi-directional pharmacology, computational biology, network science, and other related disciplines. It analyzes the molecular association between drugs and diseases in a holistic manner, thus revealing the systematic pharmacological mechanism of drugs through scientific verification. This ultimately guides research and development of new drugs and clinical treatment. Globally, network pharmacology is regarded as the "Next Generation Medicine Research Mode." [5] Network pharmacology is characterized by calculation and experimentation and aims at systematic treatment. This coincides with the characteristics of holistic treatment with TCM, and also creates favorable conditions for exploring the characteristics of TCM.

Network pharmacology is not only a breakthrough in the interdisciplinary research of systems biology and network medicine, but also a breakthrough in the cross-functional research of artificial intelligence and medicine. For example, the concept of new drug research and development based on network pharmacology is exactly in line with the TCM prescriptions. This provides an opportunity to explain the mechanism of action and rationale for TCM prescriptions. The chemical components contained in TCM formulae are bound to the target protein in an instantaneous and low-affinity form, and the whole disease network is used as the target for systematic intervention. The desired therapeutic effect is achieved when each component interacts with the network, to increase efficacy and reduce toxicity. Also, based on the key technology in network pharmacology, it is possible to analyze the distribution of targets affected by the ingredients contained in the prescriptions, thus helping to explore the network characteristics of prescriptions, such as drug properties, TCM formulation, Qiqing Hehe, etc. Furthermore, network characteristics are used to predict clinical biomarkers of prescription drugs and the rationale for the prescription, and are being used to promote new technology groups in China and integrate with Western drug R&D groups studying network pharmacology. This would lay a foundation for industrial innovation and technological transformation for the entire pharmaceutical industry.

Network pharmacology and related research fields such as bioinformatics, systems biology, systems pharmacology, network medicine, artificial intelligence, and big data science are emerging and developing simultaneously. Systems biology understands organisms holistically rather than as an isolated part, and studies the overall relationship between macroscopic and microscopic behaviors of organisms through mathematical modeling, while exploring theories and methods for designing and controlling cellular or multicellular systems. Systems pharmacology [6] emphasizes that under a unified time–space multi-scale framework, the research of body function changes from the macro to the micro level and is caused by the treatment of diseases and syndromes with these drugs, and lays emphasis on the integration of multiple sets of scientific data from a holistic perspective, while correlating at all levels. The concept of network medicine [7] derives from complex networks in a broad sense, including social networks, etc. It is believed that diseases with similar phenotypes or coexisting ailments have common components in biological networks. The description and verification of compound intervention in multiple targets have laid the foundation for network pharmacology and several powerful analytical tools and research methodology. The above related fields collectively reflect the innovative and systematic thinking of researchers on drug and syndrome interactions, and have made great contributions to the development of network pharmacology in terms of research ideas, algorithms, and data. Compared to traditional drug research strategies, network pharmacology is an innovative new discipline, and has its own originality that analyzes the interaction between drugs and complex biological systems from the biological network perspective and emphasizes on the transformation from a single target to a network target.

Recently, a variety of high-throughput and multi-component experimental technologies have evolved. Rapid computing methods and technologies represented by big data and artificial intelligence have also effectively promoted the development and wider application of network pharmacology. Furthermore, network pharmacology provides new ideas and methods for analyzing massive amounts of biomedical data and has established the process transformation from data to knowledge. Network pharmacology has developed rapidly, and its influence has also expanded gradually. As shown in Fig. 1.1, subject retrieval and statistics in network pharmacology were conducted on Web of Science and in the CNKI database, and it was found that the number of articles published on network pharmacology both in China and overseas has been steadily and rapidly increasing. The term "network

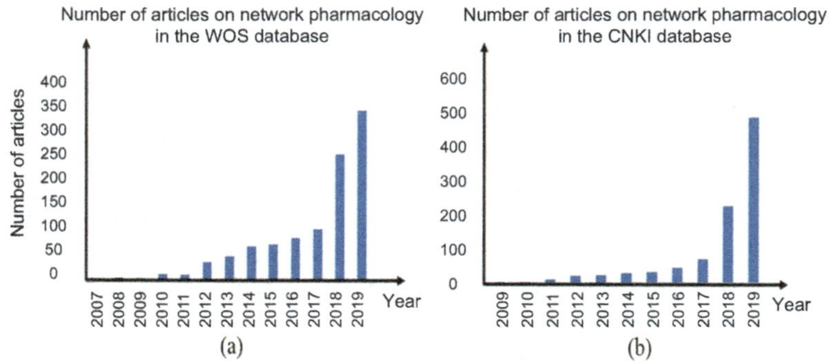

Fig. 1.1 Number of articles on "network pharmacology" listed on Web of Science and in the CNKI database based on annual statistics

pharmacology" was first proposed by British scholar Hopkins in October 2007 [4]. He believed that drug intervention in disease can be achieved through multi-target interactions in biological networks. In 2009, Chinese researchers published a Chinese paper titled "Network Pharmacology" in the *Chinese Journal of New Drugs and Clinical Remedies* [8].

However, as an emerging research area with a little more than a decade's development history, network pharmacology still faces several challenges in terms of theory, methods, and application. On the one hand, these challenges come from the limitations of basic biological, medical, and pharmaceutical knowledge, while, on the other hand, they come from insufficient data accumulation in network pharmacology, imperfect calculation methods, and unclear research systems. Public databases provide vital information on network pharmacology. However, there are still some shortcomings in existing public databases, such as the quality of the data and the quantum of data that needs to be expanded, and brings challenges for researchers in integrating the information from multiple data sources comprehensively and systematically to obtain reliable results. Network-based computational methods provide key technical support for objective scientific pharmacological research. For related algorithms, however, highlighting the holistic characteristics of network pharmacology based on methodology, building a quantitative and dynamic network model, and application of network pharmacology methods to solve burning issues such as complex diseases and drug research still need more in-depth thinking and exploration. In terms of research, we have noticed that high-level research on network pharmacology indicates an in-depth integration of calculations and experiments of multi-component data and an interdisciplinary integration of mathematics and biology. Further exploration of network pharmacology in the study of complex diseases, syndrome mechanisms, and drug action through in-depth analysis of various cross-functions is also a breakthrough worth exploring. The hypothesis of relationships between TCM and biological network was originally proposed by Shao Li [9], which was 8 years ahead of the proposing of the term "network pharmacology" by Hopkins [4] (see 1.2). Development of network pharmacology and progress of research in this field are expected to provide more reliable information to study the interaction between diseases, syndromes, and drugs, as also to provide key technical support for drug R&D, mechanism interpretation, efficacy evaluation, drug dosage, and the wider application of "Next Generation Medicine Research Mode."

1.2 Key Role of TCM in the Origin and Development of Network Pharmacology

TCM is a treasure of the Chinese nation and the essence of Chinese people's experience in fighting diseases for thousands of years. Medical research is important to the national economy and people's livelihood. It has long been an important driving force for promoting scientific and technological innovation and revolution. TCM has accumulated many treatments from long-term clinical practice. TCM prescriptions contain many natural chemical components, such as artemisinin and arsenic trioxide, which are also valuable sources of original drug research in China. It is worth noting that TCM is a traditional systematic medicine, and the holistic nature is a distinctive feature common in TCM diagnosis and treatment. Complex diseases need to develop from single-target treatment to holistic and systematic network regulation. However, research methods that accord with the holistic characteristics of TCM have not yet been established. The methods of reduction and trial-and-error analysis commonly used in modern science are quite different from the holistic treatment characteristics of TCM. Also, the current medical research mode of "single target, single disease and single drug" results in increasing costs and lower success rate, which makes it difficult to adapt to the treatment demands of complex diseases. Therefore, TCM and modern medicine both look forward to the innovation of research models and methods.

Holistic practices in TCM also highlight the limitations of reductionist medicine and research mode. To systematically reveal the biological basis of the overall diagnosis and treatment of TCM, Professor Shao Li of Tsinghua University took the lead in proposing a new concept of "network target." The hypotheses, methods, and case studies related to network target were prior to the introduction of network pharmacology and were proposed internationally, and several Chinese and US invention patents have been awarded in this field, as shown in Fig. 1.2. In 1999, Professor Li put forward a hypothesis of the association between biomolecular networks and TCM [9], and thus began a series of exploratory studies on the overall analysis of the complex system of TCM. In 2002, the functional gene network was used to depict the overall regulatory effect of TCM prescriptions on complex diseases and syndromes. It was observed that TCM prescriptions intervened in diseases and syndromes through network regulation of "multi-cause and micro-effect," and finally achieved an "emerging" effect [10]. In January 2007, Professor

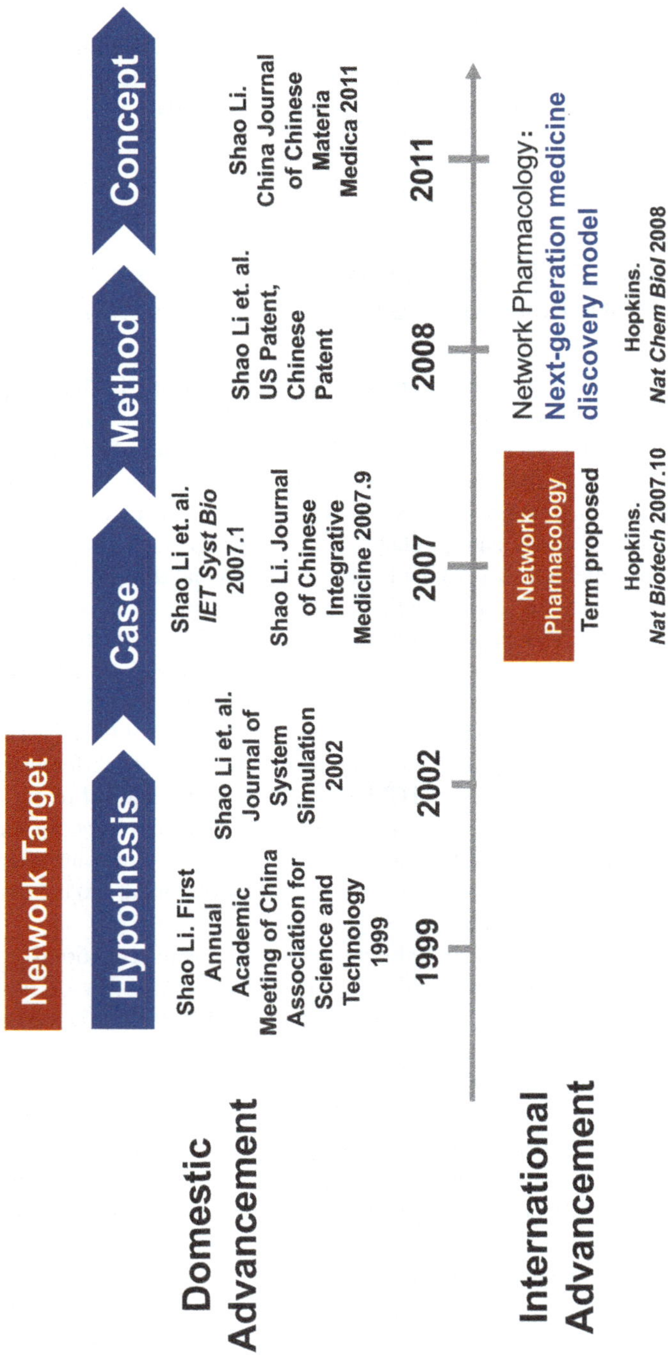

Fig. 1.2 Origin and development of network pharmacology

Li first published relevant research results in the international community, depicting the biological molecular network of cold and heat syndromes, and described the regulatory effects of cold–heat prescriptions on the network [11]. In September of the same year, a research framework of TCM prescriptions based on biological network was established [12], and a method for determining the synergistic effect of drug combinations based on network pharmacology was developed, and was awarded both Chinese and American invention patents. In April 2009, the internal network system of TCM syndromes and prescriptions was explained. In September 2009, the concept and research of TCM syndrome biomarkers was proposed. The concept of network target was then formally proposed in 2011 [13]. The hypotheses, cases, concepts, and methods related to network target originated from TCM research have played a key role in the origin and development of network pharmacology (as shown in Table 1.1).

Since 2007, the concept of network target has continuously explored new frontiers and applications, explained the original advantages of TCM, identified a series of innovative methods and applications, injected new impetus and vitality into the coordinated development of network pharmacology in Chinese and Western medicine. Based on the network target theory, a series of high-precision intelligent algorithms were established, as well as new experimental methods created for both the detection of intervention intensity of TCM network target and the synergistic effects of TCM (as shown in Table 1.2). Importantly, Shao Li's research group revealed the overall associated modular rules of the relationship between "Chinese and Western medicine phenotypes-biomolecules-Chinese and Western medicines," and thus took a lead in modeling and realizing genome-wide disease-causing genes and medicine target predictions, achieving the highest precision globally at that time. It also realized for the first time the whole genome de novo prediction of TCM syndrome-related gene profiles and TCM component target profiles, to establish a series of high-precision intelligent algorithms such as large-scale prediction of the synergistic effect of medicine (TCM components) based on biological networks. Further, Shao Li et al. introduced a variety of network-level high-throughput, parallel experimental methods and multinomial detection methods. Furthermore, a key technology platform (Using Network target for Intelligent and Quantitative analysis on drug actions, UNIQ) for network pharmacology with independent intellectual property rights was proposed based on the network target theory, which led to the construction of a disease/biological network of TCM syndromes, disease biomarker discovery, drug–drug combination discovery, network regulation mechanism of TCM prescriptions and new indication discovery, qualitative and quantitative analysis of drug–gene–disease coordination modules, etc., providing new support for the precise prevention and treatment of major diseases and innovative development of TCM (as shown in Fig. 1.3).

For example, as shown in Table 1.3, with reference to network pharmacology essentially being termed a reinforcer by Chinese and Western medicine for the precise prevention and control of major diseases such as the regulatory issues of gastric cancer with a long occurrence time, tedious monitoring, and difficulties in early warning, the research group of Shao Li employed the CIPHER algorithm along

Table 1.1 The key role of TCM in the origin and development of network pharmacology

Timeline	Research attribute	Author	Research content	Country	Journal/Conference
1999	Hypothesis	Shao Li	TCM Syndromes Are Related to Molecular Networks	China	First Annual Academic Meeting of China Association for Science and Technology [9]
2002	Hypothesis	Shao Li et al.	Network Regulating Effect of TCM Prescriptions	China	Journal of System Simulation, 2002, 14 (11):1429–1432 [10]
January 2007	Case	Shao Li et al.	Biological Network of Cold-Heat Syndrome Prescriptions	China	IET Systems Biology, 2007, 1(1):51–60 [12]
September 2007	Framework	Shao Li	Research Framework of Prescriptions Based on Biological Network	China	Journal of Chinese Integrative Medicine, 2007, 5(5):489–493 [11]
October 2007	Concept	Andrew L Hopkins	Network Pharmacology	UK	Nature Biotechnology, 2007, 25 (10):1110–1111 [4]
October 2008	Concept	Andrew L Hopkins	Network Pharmacology: First Generation Medicine Research Mode	UK	Nature Chemical Biology, 2008, 4 (11):682–690 [5]
November 2008 (application) December 2011 (authorized)	Method	Shao Li et al.	Determination Method for Synergy of Medicine Combination Based on Gene Network	China	Chinese Patent, US Patent
April, 2009	Concept	Shao Li	Internal Network System of TCM Syndromes and Prescriptions	U.S.A	Current Bioinformatics, 2009, 4 (3):188–196
December 2008 (application) February 2012 (authorized)	Method	Shao Li et al.	Method of Network-Based Identification of Multicomponent Synergy and Compositions for Use as Effective Component of Anti-Angiogenesis Medicines	U.S.A	US Patent
September 2009	Concept	Shao Li	Concept and Research on Biomolecular Network Markers of TCM Syndromes	China	Journal of Traditional Chinese Medicine, 2009, 50(9):773–776
2011	Concept	Shao Li	Network Targets: An Entry Point of Network Pharmacology Research on TCM Prescriptions	China	China Journal of Chinese Materia Medica, 2011, 36:2017–2020 [13]
2015	Model	Shao Li	On/Off Effect Model Based on Network Targets	U.S.A	Science (Supplement) 2015, 350(6262 Suppl):S72–S74

Table 1.2 Methods constructed based on network target and network pharmacology

Category	Timeline	Name	Introduction	Journal
Disease/TCM Syndrome Biological Network	2006	LMMA	Disease-specific Molecular Network Construction Algorithm Combining Articles and Omics Data	Bioinformatics, 2006, 22(17):2143–2150
	2008	CIPHER	Prediction Algorithm of Pathogenic Genes Based on "Phenotype Network-Molecular Network"	Molecular Systems Biology, 2008, 4:189
	2010	CSPN	Disease Signaling Pathway Network Construction Algorithm	BMC Bioinformatics, 2010, 11(Suppl 1):S32
	2010	ClustEx	Disease-specific Gene Module Identification Algorithm	BMC Systems Biology, 2010, 4:47
	2011	CIPHER-HIT	Disease Gene Prediction Based on Modularization	BMC Systems Biology, 2011, 5:79
	2013	sGSCA	Pathway Crosstalk Network Analysis Algorithm	Molecular BioSystems, 2013, 9(7):1822–1828
	2017	Multiscale modeling	Molecular-cell-system Multi-scale Network Computational Model for Inflammation-Cancer Transformation	Cancer Research, 2017, 77(22):6429–6441
Drug/TCM Target Network	2010	drugCIPHER	Target Prediction Algorithm Based on the Overall Association of "Drug Network-Molecular Network"	PLoS ONE, 2010, 5(7):e11764
	2010	DMIM	Network Construction Algorithm of Chinese Medicine Compatibility	BMC Bioinformatics, 2010, 11(Suppl 11):S6
	2010	NADA	Network-based Drug (Chinese Medicine Ingredient) Action Evaluation Algorithm	Chinese Science Bulletin, 2010, 55:2974–2980
	2010	SAF	Synergy Evaluation Factor of Drug Combination	BMC Systems Biology, 2010, 4:50
	2011	NIMS	Combined Prediction Algorithm of Network-based Synergistic Drugs (Chinese Medicine Ingredient)	BMC Systems Biology, 2011, 5(Suppl 1):S10
	2015	SidePro	Network-based Algorithm for Inferring the Relationship Between Protein and Drug Side Effects	Quantitative Biology, 2015, 3(3):124–134

(continued)

Table 1.2 (continued)

Category	Timeline	Name	Introduction	Journal
	2015	GIFT	Prediction Algorithm of Drug Substructure-Protein Domain Relationship	Bioinformatics, 2015, 31(15):2523–2529
	2019	UNIQ	Network Pharmacology Computing Platform Based on Network Targets	Chinese Patent CN201910902205.1
	2020	VISAR	Algorithm and Visualization Tool for Analyzing Drug-Protein Binding Patterns Based on Neural Networks	Bioinformatics, 2020, 36(11):3610–3612
Drug-Gene-Disease Synergy Module	2008	dbNEI	Construction Algorithm of Drug-NEI-disease Multi-level Networks	Bioinformatics, 2008, 24(20):2409–2411
	2012	comCIPHER	Drug-Gene-Disease Related Common Module Analysis Algorithm	Bioinformatics, 2012, 28(7):955–961
	2014	DGPsubNet	Drug-Gene-Disease Related Sub-Network Analysis Algorithm	CPT: Pharmacometrics and Systems Pharmacology, 2014, 3(11): e146

with other network pharmacology methods, in combination with experiments and clinical multi-omics detection to divulge the multi-level biological network associated with gastritis-cancer transformation, and established the biological molecular network of cold and heat syndrome in TCM; they further investigated the biological basis of the phenomena of stomach heat and cold, as well as tongue coating flora markers, in an attempt to augment the process of integration and innovation of Chinese and Western medicine in the biological network mechanism. Furthermore, based on the multi-level biological framework of gastritis-cancer transformation, the evolution law emerging from molecular to clinical phenotype of gastritis-cancer transformation was discovered, leading to the development of the first intelligent early warning system of traditional Chinese and Western medicine for gastric health. For the first time, a single-cell network of gastritis-cancer transformation was constructed in patients suffering from TCM's stomach heat-related manifestations, and this unprecedented step led to the breakthrough discovery of "extremely early" gastric cancer cells, facilitating a new staging and target method for the prevention and control of gastric cancer. Besides, the network pharmacology method was upgraded to predict the prognosis of the biological framework associated with pancreatic cancer, and after clinical verification through a multi-center large sample, it was ascertained that the pancreatic cancer precise chemotherapy markers,

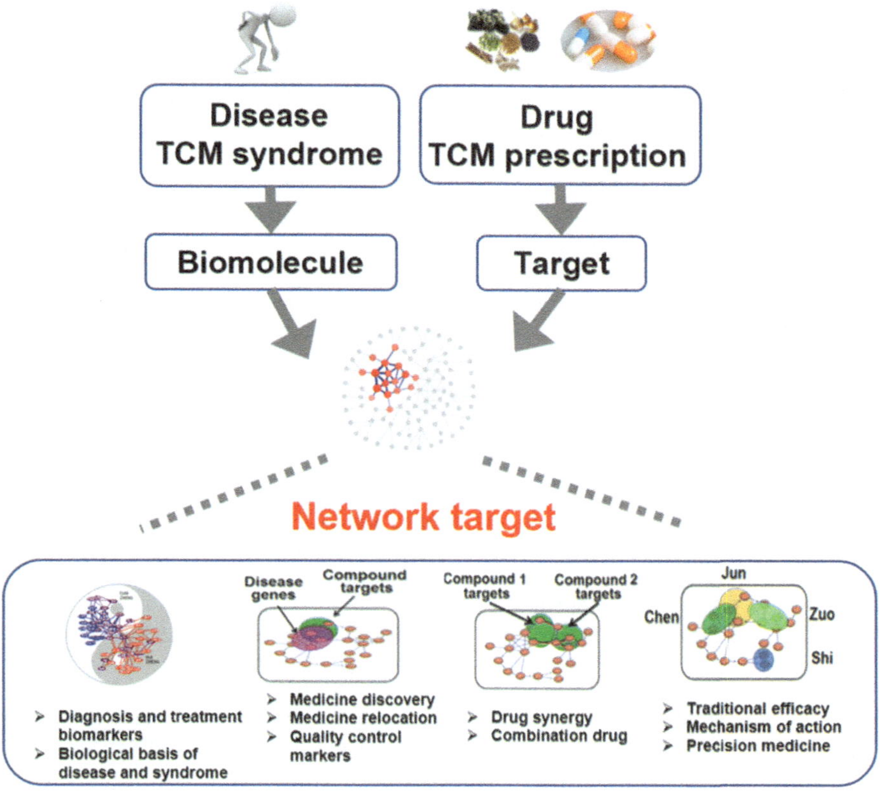

Fig. 1.3 Key technology platform of network pharmacology based on network target (UNIQ)

constituting of five network key node molecules, were significantly finer than the existing markers.

Considering the network pharmacology analysis of classic, famous, and proven prescriptions from credible doctors, pertaining to network target theory and method with disease-syndrome biological network as the intervention target, traditional efficacy, modern indications, effective substances, and action mechanism of Liuwei Dihuang prescription (nourishing Yin, enhancing body's disease resistance or immunity) and Gegen Qinlian Decoction (clearing heat and removing dampness) were elucidated. Additionally, several latest activities of Chinese medicine ingredients, for body heat and cold, were discovered (as shown in Table 1.3). Targeting the molecular network of cold–heat syndrome and related diseases and employing the "core prescription of Traditional Chinese Medicine-molecular network-indications" co-module analysis, Traditional Chinese Medicine prescriptions and constituents combination for angiogenesis regulation were discovered. Furthermore, a series of investigations were conducted on the clinical prescriptions of various eminent doctors. For example, the compatibility law of 871 Anti-rheumatism Clinical Prescriptions by Professor Li Jiren, the first Master of Traditional Chinese Medicine,

Table 1.3 Application of network target theory and methods in Chinese and Western medicine

Category	Timeline	Research object	Discovery of network target analysis	Journal
Diagnosis and Treatment BioMarkers	2006	Biological processes or diseases related to cold or heat	Angiogenic network	Bioinformatics, 2006, 22(17):2143-2150
	2010	Patients with cold syndrome	Characteristics of network biology	Molecular BioSystems, 2010, 6 (4):613-619
	2010	Biological processes or diseases related to cold or heat	Pathway networks related to inflammation, angiogenesis, and cancer	BMC Bioinformatics, 2010, 11(Suppl 1):S32
	2012	Tongue coating of atrophic gastritis patients with cold or heat syndrome	Cold and heat microbial network	Scientific Reports, 2012, 2:936
	2013	Different stages of gastritis patients with cold or heat syndrome	Metabolism-immune imbalance, network biomarkers	Scientific Reports, 2013, 3:1543
	2019	Inflammation induced tumorigenesis	Gene collaboration module based on biomolecular networks	ACS Synthetic Biology, 2019, 8(3):482-490
	2019	Tongue coating in patients with atrophic gastritis at different stages	Tongue coating flora network of atrophic gastritis	Protein & Cell, 2019, 10(7):496-509
	2019	Cell network of gastric cancer	Cell network of gastritis-cancer transformation	Cell Reports, 2019, 27(6):1934-1947
	2020	Patients with pancreatic cancer	Network markers of precise chemotherapy for pancreatic cancer	EBioMedicine, 2020, 55:102767
Drug/Drug Combination Discovery	2011	TCM Ingredients in Qingluo Decoction	Screening of anti-angiogenesis synergistic combination	BMC Systems Biology, 2011, 5(Suppl 1):S10
	2013	Vitexicarpin	New anti-tumor angiogenesis activity	Evidence-based Complementary and Alternative Medicine, 2013:278405
	2015	Ligustrazine	Alleviate oxidative organ damage caused by methotrexate	Journal of Ethnopharmacology, 2015, 175:638-647
	2016	Nuciferine	Anti-tumor activity and mechanism	Acta Pharmacologica Sinica, 2016, 37 (7):963-972
	2018	Matrine, the main ingredient of Qingluo Decoction	New activity that induces macropinocytosis	Frontiers in Pharmacology, 2018, 9 (10):1-11

(continued)

Table 1.3 (continued)

Category	Timeline	Research object	Discovery of network target analysis	Journal
	2018	Qingluo Decoction and methotrexate	Network regulation mechanism of anti-rheumatoid arthritis	Frontiers in Pharmacology, 2018, 9 (1472):1-17
	2019	Tanshinol borneol ester	New synthetic small molecules promote angiogenesis	British Journal of Pharmacology, 2019, 176(17):3143-3160
Prescription mechanism/ Precision prescription	2010	Liuwei Dihuang Pill	TCM network and collaboration modules for the treatment of different diseases	BMC Bioinformatics, 2010, 11(Suppl 11):S6
	2013	Qingluo Decoction	Network regulation mechanism of Traditional Chinese Medicine formulation	Evidence-based Complementary and Alternative Medicine, 2013:456747
	2014	Liuwei Dihuang Pill	Anti-tumor network regulation mechanism, potential new activity of active ingredients	Molecular BioSystems, 2014, 10(5):1014-1022
	2014	Gegen Qinlian Decoction	Network regulation mechanism of type 2 diabetes mellitus	Evidence-based Complementary and Alternative Medicine, 2014:138460
	2015	Discovering Qingluo Decoction from 871 proven prescriptions	Network regulation effect on rheumatoid arthritis	Evidence-based Complementary and Alternative Medicine, 2015:451319
	2018	Fuzheng Chinese Medicine	Network biology foundation of the anti-tumor Fuzheng Chinese Medicine	Cancers, 2018, 10 (11):461:1-23

was taken into consideration. Core prescriptions such as "Qingluo Decoction" were examined. The network regulatory mechanism of Traditional Chinese Medicine formulation of Qingluo Decoction was analyzed. The combination of matrine with other anti-cancer drugs exhibiting anti-angiogenesis effect was discovered. (as shown in Fig. 1.4). The following chapters of this book feature the research methods and representative cases in detail.

The original theory, method, and application of network target technique have promoted extensive international research on network pharmacology. The theory and methodology of network target being at the core of network pharmacology influences the field of modern and traditional medicine immensely. The representative paper was published in the English version of the Chinese Journal of Natural Medicines [14] (According to statistics by scholars in Taiwan, it was considered to

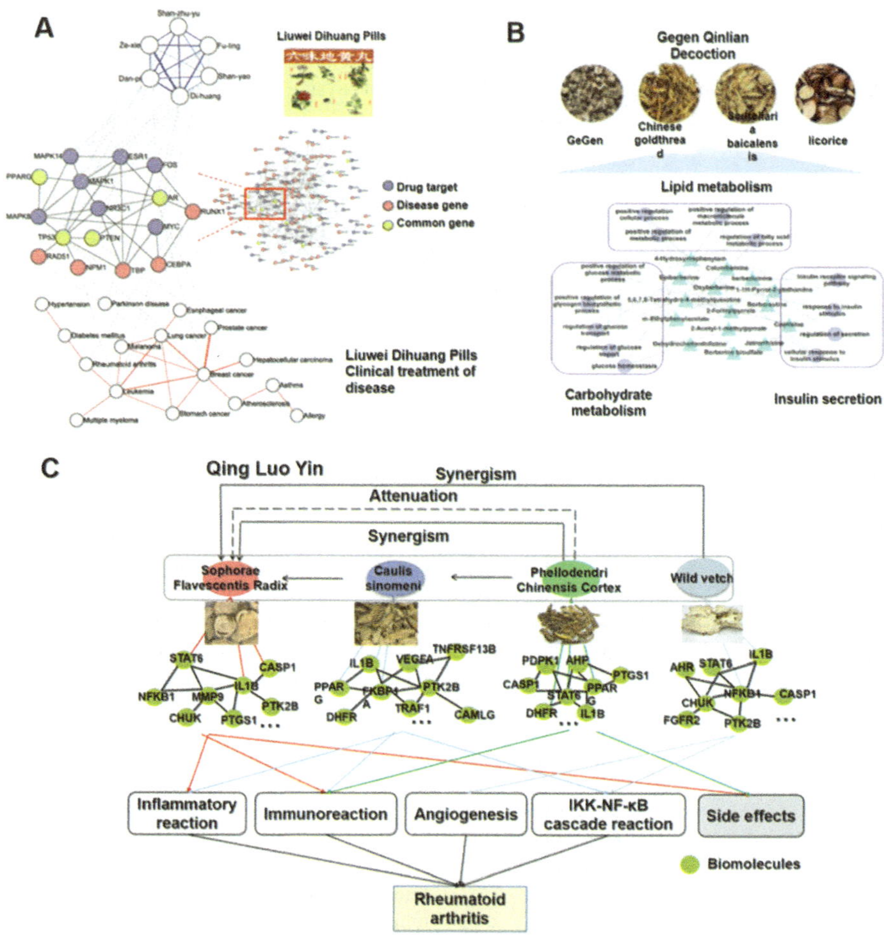

Fig. 1.4 Cases of network pharmacology analysis of Liuwei Dihuang Pill, Gegen Qinlian Decoction, and Qingluo Decoction

be the most cited paper in PubMed's "Traditional Chinese Medicine" themed articles from 2013 to 2017) [15] and remained highly acclaimed by peers in China and researchers abroad (see Appendix B). According to the statistical analysis conducted in 2019, the theory, methods and cases of network targets were cited by 609 syndrome studies and 728 prescription studies internationally, leading to the global acknowledgement of the Chinese medicine; simultaneously, it was cited by researchers from almost 73 countries and regions, demonstrating substantial support for the innovative development of the 16 kinds of traditional medicines and characteristic diagnosis and treatment worldwide, especially in countries situated along the "One Belt and One Road," making the network target theory and method with the original characteristics of Traditional Chinese Medicine a global phenomenon with a widespread international influence.

The original theory and methods of network target have made pioneering contributions to the evolving research of Traditional Chinese Medicine. In 2017, the three research results of network target model, cold–heat syndrome biomolecular network, and Liuwei Dihuang network pharmacology analysis were utilized as representative examples in the *White Paper on Cancer Complementary and Alternative Medicine Research Strategy* issued by the National Institute of Health (NIH)/National Cancer Institute (NCI), signifying that Network Pharmacology is a "crucial" paradigm for revealing complex mechanisms of Traditional Chinese Medicine and designing effective integrative clinical trials [16]. Academician Boli Zhang and others commented in the *Twenty Years of Modernization of Chinese Medicine*: "In 2007, Shao Li from Tsinghua University first proposed a research framework for TCM prescriptions based on biological networks. By constructing a key technological platform for network pharmacology, it has broken through key technologies such as network-based disease gene and Chinese medicine target prediction, Chinese medicine discovery and combination screening of Chinese medicine compatibility, as well as the construction and analysis of biological network of disease-syndrome-prescription." In recent years, Professor Shao Li has been appraised as the pioneer and forerunner of TCM network pharmacology time and again by domestic and overseas peers (see Appendix B). The above deduction illustrates that network pharmacology with the network target methodology at its core has not only emerged as an original scientific research technique of Chinese medicine and modern medicine research, but also as an academic progressive juncture capable of being a vanguard of international science setup in the context of contemporary science and technology.

1.2.1 Original Method of Network Target Analysis

It is essential to understand the "relationship" between the key elements to infer the micro pathogenic genes, drug targets, etc., from large-scale complex biological networks. The discovery of the law of "relationship," along with qualitative and quantitative description plays a significant role in studying the mechanism of complex diseases and the revealing of the scientific connotation of TCM. By learning from and exploring the TCM holism and based on the network target theory, Shao Li's research group skillfully expressed the disease phenotype, biomolecules, drugs, and their interactions as "relationships" with multilevel biological networks, and created "relationship inference" analysis methods for prediction of pathogenic genes and drug targets, e.g., CIPHER, drugCIPHER, comCIPHER, and CIPHER-SC [17–20], revealed the modular coding rule of "Phenotype of Traditional Chinese and Western Medicine-Biomolecules-Traditional Chinese and Western Medicine" on the network, realized the quantitative description of diseases and syndromes (diseases and syndromes) and the overall effect of TCM according to biomolecular network, and established a new model of TCM holistic view and biological basic research of syndrome differentiation and treatment as shown in

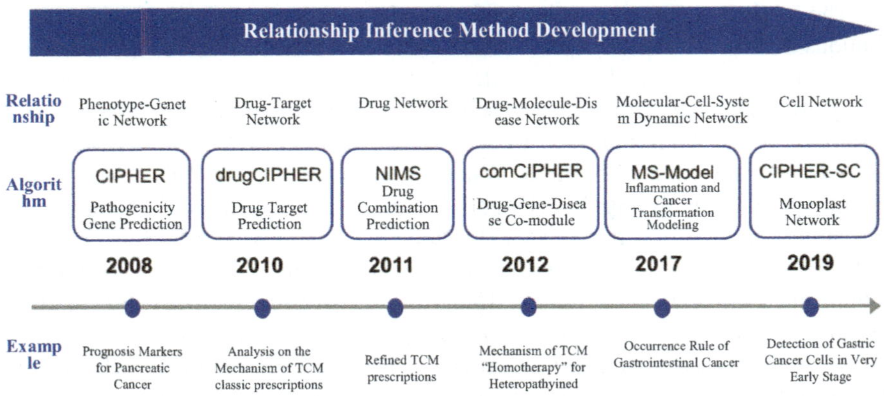

Fig. 1.5 Relationship inference method development of network target analysis

Fig. 1.5. Compared with the best international methods at that time, the series of "relational inference" methods have increased the prediction enrichment of pathogenic genes by 2 times and the drug target prediction enrichment by 6 times. The purpose of cipher algorithm, a typical method of "relationship inference," is looking for related intervention genes from a group of candidate genes based on a given phenotype. CIPHER algorithm has established a mathematical model of "relationship inference" on the basis of multilevel biological network and quantitative inference of pathogenic genes from an overall picture. It has realized the whole-genome prediction of disease pathogenic genes and the prediction of TCM syndrome concerned biomolecules for the first time, been successfully applied to the research of complex diseases, TCM syndromes and TCM prescriptions, and has made a series of original discoveries.

The "relationship inference" analysis method is divided into three main steps:

1. Relationship network construction, i.e., to obtain the relationship between complex biosystem elements from literature, experiment, or genomics data, including the relationship between macro level elements, micro level elements, and macro–micro level elements. Relational network is a common way to show the relationship of complex biosystem elements.
2. Relationship representation and modeling, i.e., to conduct mathematical modeling of macro micro elements of complex systems, including the definition of module local and the mathematical presentation of the correlation between modules. What is worthwhile to be paid attention to is that the established model needs to indicate the relationship between macro and micro element modules in the whole complex system, that is to say, it needs to reflect the overall nature of inference. This is the core of relation inference method which can reflect the integrity of complex system.
3. Inference of unknown relations, i.e., to present with the model established in (2), and take full advantage of the known relations of complex system elements to infer the pending key elements. Taking inferring phenotype related pathogenic

genes as an example, for a given phenotype, we initially start with the known pathogenic gene nodes close to the phenotype, and regard them as the seed node module of prior knowledge, and then determine the candidate node modules which are close to the phenotype as per the relationship obtained from big data. It is presumed that there is a certain "relationship" (model representation) between a given phenotype and a known close phenotype, as well as between the seed node and the node to be found. We can find the pathogenic gene of a given phenotype from the known phenotype and the seed node by making use of this relationship.

1.2.2 Common Methods of Network Target Analysis

As a common method in network target analysis, the enrichment of functional modules uses the enrichment of network nodes and known functional gene sets to study the correlation between the network and the known biological processes. (The following is the original content of the second section.)

1.3 Core Theory of Network Pharmacology: Network Target

1.3.1 Proposal and Development of Network Target Theory

Network pharmacology has not only triggered major alterations to drug research, but also created some major opportunities and challenges for Chinese and Western medicine research. The opportunities emerge with the anticipation of network pharmacology leading to innovative ideas in drug research and development, systematically comprehending and dealing with the complexity of chemical and biological systems, and accomplishing the transformation of modern drug research from description to prediction. However, the challenges lie in organic integration of the ideas and techniques of network pharmacology with the internal mechanisms and system interventions of complex diseases, as well as the complex system of TCM prescriptions with long-term clinical practices, in order to achieve a major breakthrough in the field of Chinese and Western medicine research on complex diseases. In response to the aforementioned requirements and challenges, the network target theory abolishes the limitations of the long-term "single target, partial confrontation" research mode. The research mode and method of "network target and system regulation" dispensed a novel approach of thinking and comprehensive methodology for interpreting the interactions between complex chemical and biological systems of the human body, which has transpired as the core theory originating from Traditional Chinese Medicine and unraveling new frontiers for network pharmacology.

1.3.2 The Concept of Network Target

The core theory of network pharmacology is network target, which was first proposed by Shao Li [13]. This section firstly introduces the concept of biological network in network pharmacology, and then the concept of network target. Further, adopting the perspective of concept definition and qualitative and quantitative analysis, it evaluates and compares the concept of network target with that of the single and multiple targets, with the aim of further accentuating the readers' understanding of the network target concept.

1. Biological Network
Biological network not only serves as the foundation for the establishment of complex biological systems of an organism, but also as a vital method that aids in describing the relationship between elements in biological systems. Being at the core of the essence for the construction of biological systems, biological networks present diverse manifestations in a narrow and a broad sense. In a narrow sense, there are gene regulatory networks, protein interaction networks, signal transduction networks, metabolic networks, etc.; whereas a broader sense encompasses systems like biological function networks, TCM ingredient networks, TCM compatibility networks, disease-disease networks, and TCM-disease networks. Being pivotal in describing the relationship between elements in biological systems, biological networks can be described and analyzed by employing complex network theory and methods with respect to the calculations. For example, taking cognizance of the topology of a biological network by examining properties such as node degree, degree distribution, intermediate number, and shortest path of biological network; identifying the key regulation links of network by studying the network phantom and network module of the biological network, and simulating the evolution in time and space by performing network dynamics analysis on biological networks via differential equations.

2. Network Target
Network target refers to key links in network which can associate drug and diseases from mechanism and quantitatively represent the holistic regulatory mechanism, including key molecules, key pathways or key modules, etc. [12]. Network target can be understood from a narrow and a broad sense. From a narrow sense, network target appears as a key link in the disease-syndrome biological network intervenable by drugs. In a broad sense, network target can be acknowledged as a research mode that make the association between drugs and disease-syndromes. In other words, qualitative and quantitative analysis of the network topology and dynamic characteristics of the local biological network modules related to the disease-syndrome phenotype in the disease-syndrome biological network, identifying its key mechanisms, and then designing the key link of drug intervention in the disease-syndrome biological network leads to the realization of the overall regulation of disease-syndrome phenotype. Noticeably, the network target concept appears essentially distinct from that of single target and multi-target. The single target concept refers to

the drug with high affinity and high selectivity for a single target, treating a disease by intervening with a target. Multi-target concept refers to a method that administers the drug onto two or more related targets in the disease-syndrome biological network at the same time, generating a synergistic effect on the action of each target, hence, the total effect is greater than the sum of all individual effects. The differences between network target, single target, and multi-target are as follows: Firstly, single target and multi-target concepts are defined from the perspective of the nature of drug action, while network target is defined from the perspective of drug interaction with the organism, taking into account the drug action mechanism and molecular mechanism of the disease and syndrome. In addition, the concepts of single target and multi-target are explanatory and descriptive, with a lack of clear quantification, while the hypothesis of network target emphasizes on the qualitative as well as quantitative analysis of the mechanism of action meant to comprehend the holistic effect of drugs.

The research theory of network pharmacology outlines the mapping of drug targets and disease-syndrome related molecules to biological molecular networks, establishing the association mechanism between drugs and disease-syndromes derived from the biological molecular networks, and analyzing the network target-system regulation mechanism of drugs administered. Considering the network pharmacology research on TCM intervention of a disease and syndrome as an example, the intervention effect of TCM on a disease and syndrome is characterized by the complex chemical composition of Traditional Chinese Medicine, diverse compound combination forms, relatively mild biological activity of each effective ingredient of Traditional Chinese Medicine, and the synergistic effect of "multi-cause and micro-effect" comprehensive regulation. The curative effect mechanism of Traditional Chinese Medicine is the novel emerging system based on "multi-cause and micro-effect." [10] The applications of computer simulation, system modeling, and experimental verification to the study of the nonlinear, open, and complex system of Traditional Chinese Medicine seem highly beneficial in elucidating the mechanism of network target-system regulation in TCM, comprehending the nature of complex biological network imbalance, and deciphering the mechanism of curative and toxic effect of Traditional Chinese Medicine. For example, the ingredients of Traditional Chinese Medicine can intervene onto a set of targets with specific associations on the network, and utilize the network connection of the target effect in time and space such as to generate the holistic effect in an "on and off" manner [17].

Ideally, the target effect of the optimized TCM prescription ingredient is bound to superimpose or synchronize with the disease and syndrome biological network, and spread through this network, exceeding the threshold of the desired effect, so that the holistic effect "turns on," which is manifested as a curative effect. Simultaneously, the target effect is dispersed or antagonized in the biological network related to toxicity and other side effects, which seem to be lower than the effect threshold, so that the overall holistic effect "turns off" without toxicity or with minimal toxicity. Specifically, on a time scale, differential equations and other methods are utilized in order to simulate the variation shown in the effects of drug targets on disease and syndrome biological networks over time. On a space scale, the key links of drug treatment are illustrated by measuring the topological properties of drug targets distributed on the disease-syndrome biological network and by obtaining other details. Finally, the effects of time and space scales are integrated to form a comprehensively holistic effect, and the relationship between the comprehensive effect and the threshold of the effect is investigated. If the threshold of the effect is exceeded, the holistic effect is "turned on" and manifested as "emerging." By means of this time–space multi-scale, biomolecule-biological function module-multilevel phenotype simulation, qualitative and quantitative analyses of the variations of biomolecules at the micro level affecting the dynamic process of drug treatment at the macro level [18] become feasible.

1.4 Overview of Network Pharmacology Research Methods and Characteristics

1.4.1 Characteristics of "Single Target-Partial Confrontation" Research Mode

The research mode in traditional pharmacology is determined from a single drug ingredient to the determined target of action, then to the downstream signaling pathway and finally to the disease-related phenotype. The disease-related phenotype here often manifests as an abnormal increase or decrease of certain macroscopic indicators. In actual research, it is characterized by substitute indicators in an animal, at the cellular or molecular level. This mode studies the process from the drug molecules to a determined molecular target then to the drug's actions.This is known as linear transmission process.

The "Single Target-Partial Confrontation" research mode is based on the theoretical hypothesis of "one gene, one drug, one disease." The main aim of traditional drug discovery is to find specific ligands. The theory of "one gene, one drug, one disease" contains two implicit hypotheses. One includes a single target that is connected with a phenotype through a mechanical process, and the activity of the target is strongly in line with the effects of the target phenotype. Secondly, the main drug action is only on a single target—stronger the drug selectivity, more specific the mechanism of action and higher the degree of correlation with the target phenotype. Based on these two hypotheses, specific ligands can selectively interfere with the target at very low concentrations to achieve effective control. Therefore, discovering specific ligands plays a vital role in drug design.

However, with advancing pharmacological research, these implicit hypotheses were found to have limitations, and use of specific traditional ligands as candidate drugs has also been questioned by researchers. Using drugs administered in schizophrenia, for example, the first generation of antipsychotic drugs was mostly dopamine receptor inhibitors that alleviated symptoms of schizophrenia by blocking dopamine binding with the respective receptors. However, these drugs have serious and even life-threatening side effects, including agranulocytosis, epilepsy, weight gain, diabetes, etc. The side effects are caused by four dopamine receptor involved pathways—midbrain-limbic system, midbrain-cortical system, nodule-infundibulum, and substantia-nigra striatum, in the central nervous system (CNS). Highly selective inhibition of dopamine receptors can affect many of the physiological functions related to these four pathways, therefore, although they can alleviate the symptoms of schizophrenia to a certain extent, they also cause severe side effects. Studies on a new generation of antipsychotics have shown that drugs with more complex target spectrum on the CNS may have better efficacy. Many updated research findings also highlight that specific target spectrum binding characteristics are better than strong selectivity for a single target [19].

Common diseases and TCM-defined syndromes belong to a category of complex diseases, which are collectively referred to as those occurring in organisms with complex interactions due to environmental exposure, genetic susceptibility, age, and other factors. The eight-cardinal syndrome differentiation, viscera differentiation, qi-blood differentiation, etc., summarized by TCM doctors based on long-term diagnosis and treatment practices still have significant application in current clinical practices. Complex diseases and TCM syndromes are difficult to describe and study using the "Single Target-Partial Confrontation" research mode. The problem of drug action calls for a new and more holistic research mode, and development of a suitable research mode is important in the innovation and development of modern Chinese medicine.

1.4.2 Characteristics of "Network Target-System Regulation" Research Mode

Compared to the "Single Target-Partial Confrontation" mode, in the "Network Target-System Regulation" mode, the drugs act on a certain phenotype-related network target, and then affect the static key structure or dynamic balance of the network target, thus regulating diseases in a systematic manner. The "Network Target-System Regulation" research mode comprehensively and systematically considers many phenotype-related molecules and their relationships. It also describes and establishes the network target model in a network format, and then analyzes the mechanism of action of drugs, while predicting the intervention results on the phenotype, based on the network target. The following describe key links and common methods involved in "Network Target-System Regulation" research mode.

1. Constructing a Biological Network

The construction of a biological network is the basis of network pharmacology. At the molecular level, traditional biological networks include gene regulatory networks, protein interaction networks, signal transduction networks, and metabolic networks. With the development of technology and enrichment of data, hierarchical network construction including the interaction networks between organisms and the environment is being constantly developed and updated. Biological networks are being constructed based on literature mining, omics technology, and global association analysis. The following are some representative construction methods.

Data sources for biological network construction based on literature mining include Medical Subject Headings (MeSH), biomedical literature database (PubMed), National Knowledge Infrastructure (CNKI), and Online Mendelian Inheritance in Man (OMIM) [20]. MeSH provides a standardized description of a disease phenotype, biomedical literature databases can be used to retrieve literature and information on molecules related to diseases and syndromes, and OMIM can provide related information on phenotypes and genotypes. Commonly used biomedical literature mining methods include co-occurrence, natural language processing, etc. The co-occurrence method checks biomedical entities based on whether they are in the same sentence, number of separated words, co-occurrences, etc. These are indicators to determine the strength of correlation between biomedical entities, and help to construct a disease-syndrome biological network. In addition to the co-occurrence method, natural language processing in artificial intelligence also helps in literature mining in biomedicine. Currently, there are several online resource platforms such as the STRING data platform that can realize biomedical data integration, and provide multi-faceted evidence for constructing various disease and syndrome biological networks through literature mining.

The data sources used in biological network construction methods based on omics technology include Gene Expression Omnibus (GEO) [21] and The Cancer Genome Atlas (TCGA). GEO mainly includes high-throughput gene expression data, while TCGA provides a large number of genomic data helpful for cancer research. Biological network of disease-syndrome can be constructed based on the literature and omics database, and supported by various interaction data (such as protein interaction data), thus fully integrating the relationship between disease-syndrome and currently existing biomolecular information.

Global association is based on literature and omics data, and is an emerging method to predict pathogenic genes and construct disease syndrome-related biological networks. Similar to TCM, global association analysis mainly considers the relationship between two phenotypes, phenotype and molecule, and between two molecules, based on all phenotypes and whole genomes. It uses a specific calculation model to score and evaluate the correlation between phenotypes and genes, and gene products at the genome-wide level. This helps in systematic prediction and sorting of disease-syndrome phenotype-related genes and gene products, thus building a disease-syndrome biological network. The commonly used indicators for evaluating prediction accuracy include fold enrichment, accuracy rate, and recall rate.

2. Network Target Analysis Method

2.1 Original Method of Network Target Analysis

It is essential to understand the "relationship" between the key elements to infer the micro pathogenic genes, drug targets, etc., from a large-scale complex biological network. The discovery of the law of "relationship," along with qualitative and quantitative description plays a significant role in studying the mechanism of

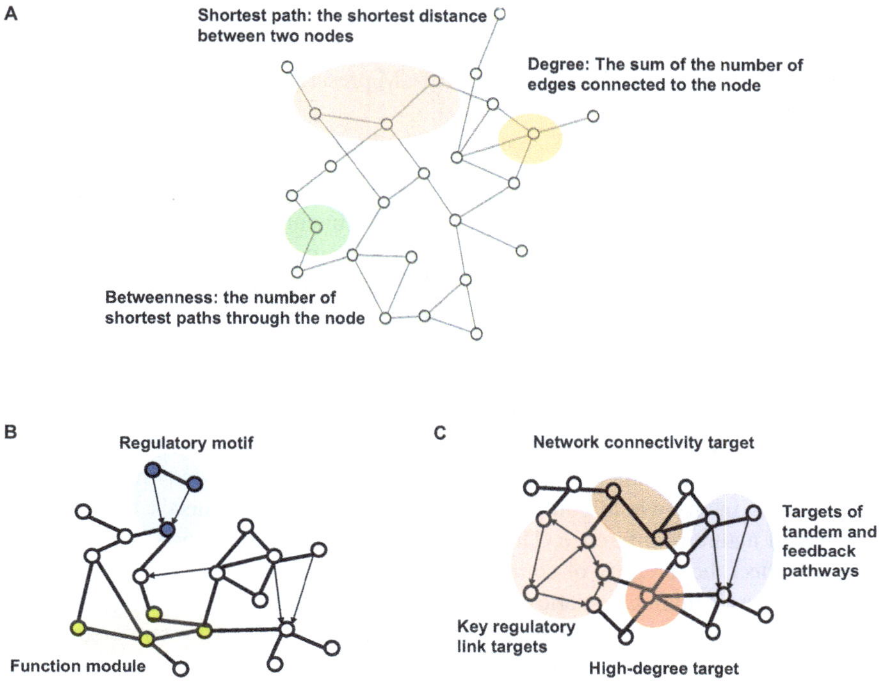

Fig. 1.6 Schematic diagram of related concepts of static network topology attribute analysis [34]

complex diseases and the revealing of the scientific connotation of TCM. By learning from and exploring the TCM holism and based on the network target theory, Shao Li's research group skillfully expressed the disease phenotype, biomolecules, drugs, and their interactions as "relationships" with multi-level biological networks, and created "relationship inference" analysis methods for prediction of pathogenic genes and drug targets, e.g., CIPHER, drugCIPHER, comCIPHER, and CIPHER-SC [22–25], revealed the modular coding rule of "Phenotype of Traditional Chinese and Western Medicine-Biomolecules-Traditional Chinese and Western Medicine" on the network, realized the quantitative description of diseases and syndromes (diseases and syndromes) and the overall effect of TCM according to biomolecular network, and established a new model of TCM holistic view and biological basic research of syndrome differentiation and treatment as shown in Fig. 1.6. Compared with the best international methods at that time, the series of "relational inference" methods have increased the prediction enrichment of pathogenic genes by 2 times and the drug target prediction enrichment by 6 times. The purpose of cipher algorithm, a typical method of "relationship inference," is looking for related intervention genes from a group of candidate genes based on a given phenotype. Cipher algorithm has established a mathematical model of "relationship inference" on the basis of multi-level biological network and quantitative inference of pathogenic genes from an overall picture. It has realized the whole genome prediction of disease pathogenic genes and the prediction of TCM syndrome concerned biomolecules for the first time, been successfully applied to the research of complex diseases, TCM syndromes and TCM prescriptions, and has made a series of original discoveries.

The "relationship inference" analysis method is divided into three main steps:

(1) Relationship network construction, i.e., to obtain the relationship between complex biosystem elements from literature, experiment, or genomics data, including the relationship between macro level elements, micro level elements, and macro-micro level elements. Relational network is a common way to show the relationship of complex biosystem elements.
(2) Relationship representation and modeling, i.e., to conduct mathematical modeling of macro-micro elements of a complex system, including the definition of module local and the mathematical presentation of the correlation between modules. What is worthwhile to be paid attention to is that the established model needs to indicate the relationship between macro and micro element modules in the whole complex system, that is to say, it needs to reflect the overall nature of inference. This is the core of relation inference method which can reflect the integrity of complex system.
(3) Inference of unknown relations, i.e., to present with the model established in (2), and take full advantage of the known relations of complex system elements to infer the pending key elements. Taking inferring phenotype-related pathogenic genes as an example, for a given phenotype, we initially start with the known pathogenic gene nodes close to the phenotype, and regard them as the seed node module of prior knowledge, and then determine the candidate node modules which are close to the phenotype as per the relationship obtained from big data. It is presumed that there is a certain "relationship" (model representation) between a given phenotype and a known close phenotype, as well as between the seed node and the node to be found. We can find the pathogenic gene of a given phenotype from the known phenotype and the seed node by making use of this relationship.

2.2 Common Methods of Network Target Analysis

As a common method in network target analysis, the enrichment of functional modules uses the enrichment of network nodes and known functional gene sets to study the correlation between the network and the known biological processes. Network target aims to analyze the biological processes involved in the disease syndrome-related biological network, and the key static and dynamic characteristics in the network. This is helpful in describing and predicting the mechanism of drug intervention. Table 1.4 shows a comparison between several representative network target analysis methods. The processes, hypothesis, advantages, and limitations of these analytical methods are described in detail below.

The enrichment of functional modules uses the enrichment of network nodes and known functional gene sets to study the correlation between the network and the known biological processes. If there is significant enrichment, there is a strong correlation between the network target and biological process. Commonly used

Table 1.4 Representative network target analysis methods

Analysis methods	Calculation methods involved	Analysis goals	Representative works
Relationship inference	Multi Level Network Correlation Analysis	Disease gene prediction, drug target prediction, biomarker discovery, TCM Mechanism Analysis, etc.	CIPHER [22] drugCIPHER [23] comCIPHER [24] CIPHER-SC [25] NIMS [26]
Enrichment analysis of functional modules	(1) Fisher's exact test, chi-square test, and binomial distribution test; (2) Non-parametric test	Analyze or verify the relationship between the constructed network targets and known biological processes	GSEA [27] DAVID [28] Enrichr [29] clusterProfiler [30]
Static topology attribute analysis	Complex network theory	Predict or verify which of the constructed network targets may be the key drug intervention action points	MCODE [31] Barabasi et al. [32] Li et al.
Effect signal switching analysis	Random walk on the network, network analysis theory	Predict or semi-quantitatively describe the effect switch changes of constructed network targets after drug intervention	Li et al. [21]
Dynamic balance analysis	Differential equation method; stochastic simulation method; rule-based method	Predict or quantitatively describe dynamic system changes of the constructed network targets after drug intervention	Zhang et al. [33] Guo et al. [18]

enrichment analysis tools include DAVID, GSEA, Enrichr, etc. DAVID [28] is a commonly used web application for enrichment analysis. The statistical method used is Fisher's exact test and p-value correction. The functional module gene set uses genes collected and labeled by authorities such as KEGG, BioCarta, Gene Ontology, and Reactome; GSEA [27] calculates the position of the maximum enrichment score of the functional gene set in Molecular Signatures Database (MSigDB). This shows the correlation of the gene set with the tested functional gene set. The Enrichr [29] method collects a large number of gene sets from different sources (not limited to diseases or biological processes, but also gene sets such as cell lines and changes after drug intervention). On the other hand, it introduces a fuzzy enrichment analysis method that considers the weight of each gene in the enrichment gene set in the calculation.

Static network topology attribute analysis involves statistical descriptors of network topology, including the following types of commonly used descriptors [34], as shown in Fig. 1.6.

(1) The distance between nodes is frequently measured by the shortest path.
(2) The clustering coefficient of a node represents the ratio of the actual number of edges to the total number of possible edges between the node sets connected

with the node. The clustering coefficient of the network is the mean value of the clustering coefficient of all nodes.

(3) Degree is an important description of the statistical characteristics of node interconnection and reflects important network evolution characteristics. The degree of a node represents the sum of edges connected to the node, while the distribution of the degree represents the probability of distribution of degrees in the network.
(4) Centrality analysis refers to adopting the quantitative method to depict the extent of each node in the center of the network so as to describe whether the core exists and which kind of core that exists in the whole network. "Degree centrality" analysis assumes that the node with the largest degree is the central point. "Closeness centrality" analysis considers the central point to be the least total distance of all other nodes to this point, and the "betweenness centrality" analysis assumes that the central point is the node with the heaviest load when information, substance, or energy are transferred on the network, which is the node with the largest number of shortest paths through this point. Centrality means that each node is arranged outward from the center according to the size of centrality to get a "centrality" network.
(5) "Network motif" refers to subnets with significantly higher occurrence in complex networks than in random networks. "Network module" refers to a collection of nodes that implement specific functions. The network module reflects the topology of the complex network, and the functional characteristics of the complex network.
(6) Biological networks also have some important topological properties, such as "scale-free network" and "small-world network". Scale-free network means that the degree of distribution of the network is a power law distribution, i.e., most of the nodes are low degree nodes, while only some are high degree nodes (central nodes). Small-world network refers to a network with large clustering coefficients. Each node in the network can reach other nodes through a small number of steps.

Static network topology attribute analysis focuses on the key links of biological networks related to drug intervention, such as the following three types of targets or sets: ① targets or sets with high degree and significant affect on network connectivity; ② targets or sets of key regulatory links; ③ targets or sets on series and feedback channels. The analysis of network phantoms and network modules can identify the key regulatory links of disease-related biological networks from structural and functional perspectives. This provides guidance for drug intervention. Researchers also continue to discover, design, and innovate better indicators to depict the topological characteristics of key nodes, to improve prediction accuracy, and explain the network intervention of drugs more clearly.

As a natural extension of static network topology analysis, the signal switching analysis can be performed on a more clearly defined network target (usually presented as a specific local network structure). The steps of such an analysis method include: ① Defining the rules of signal transmission at the network level, the measurement index of output, and the initial effects of network intervention; ② Use random walk and other computational methods to simulate the diffusion of signals within the network, and observe the ON/OFF effect, synergy, and superposition. This analysis method has gained importance in the intervention network target of TCM prescriptions [24]. In the biological molecular network of disease and syndrome, TCM ingredients exert synergistic or superimposed effects by acting on a group of interrelated target combinations on the disease and syndrome biological network, and this can spread through the network in time and space, to produce a curative effect. Finally, a collection of TCM ingredients with weak effects emerges, having significant curative effects. For biomolecular networks related to toxicity and side effects, TCM ingredients acting on network targets produce antagonistic effects, or the targets of TCM ingredients are relatively dispersed, which does not cause an effect.

Contrary to the above semi-quantitative analysis methods based on constraints in the network targets, dynamic balance analysis is quantitative and provides an accurate modeling analysis of network targets. The usual analysis steps are:

(1) Use differential equations or rules to describe the relationship between nodes in the network continuously or discretely.
(2) Set and adjust the initial state of each node in the network and the parameters of each differential equation/rule and conduct a computer simulation.
(3) Observe the network dynamics and the impact of interventions used.

Like the effect signal switching analysis, dynamic balance analysis also needs a defined local network structure as the network target. Also, due to quantitative calculation, several parameters are often introduced and a large number of time-series quantitative data are required for verification, which is difficult using an ordinary experimental system. These requirements limit the application of such analytical methods.

3. Network Target Analysis of Drug Action

Network target analysis of drug action mechanism is roughly divided into two links: the first link that determines or predicts drug action target, and the second link that analyzes drugs in the network target (as shown in Fig. 1.7). The first link relies on the identification of drug ingredients and the accumulation of drug–target data. The former is particularly important in the analysis of Chinese medicine ingredients, involving a series of processes such as extraction, separation, and identification of active ingredients. The latter can be mined from a large number of public databases, and can also be collected and accumulated through high-throughput experimental methods. There are also several published and newly developed drug–target prediction tools available based on reliable information on ingredients. Information about related databases and software tools are introduced in subsequent chapters.

Research methods for the second link are highly flexible and constitute active fields in network pharmacology research. In addition to the continued use of network target analysis methods described in the previous section, newer methods are also being developed. It is worth noting that the analysis of TCM syndromes and

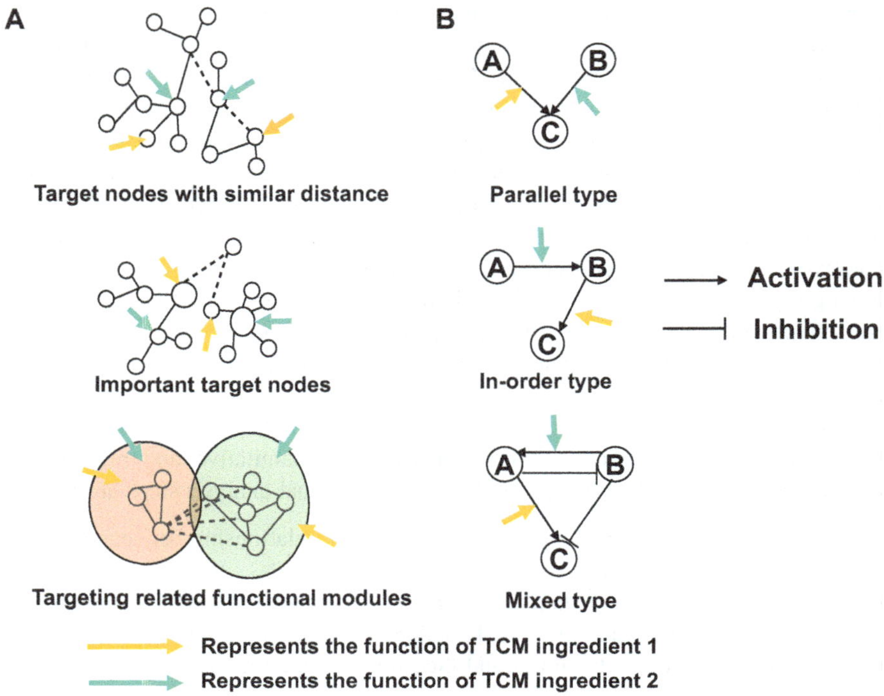

Fig. 1.7 Schematic diagram—drug mechanism analysis in network target

prescriptions and the design and prediction of optimal drug intervention constitute the network target analysis of the drug action mechanism by these network targets, specifically: ① Considering disease-syndrome biomolecular network links as the target, the relationship between the target spectrum of the prescription ingredients of medicinal substances can be measured and the action mechanism of TCM prescriptions can be understood; ② By analyzing the distribution pattern of targets in the ingredients on the biological network, characteristics such as medicinal properties, Traditional Chinese Medicine formulation, and Qiqing Hehe can be explored; ③ Prescription drugs can be rationally designed using the network to predict their clinical biomarkers. In the following chapters, several excellent studies on the mechanism of network pharmacology of drugs are analyzed in detail. The following only briefly introduces some representative analytical methods and tools.

(1) Network target-based multi-ingredient synergistic identification method (NIMS) mainly evaluates the synergistic effects of TCM ingredients, by measuring the interaction between the targets of different TCM ingredients on the biological network. A specific algorithm integrates the network topology between the targets and also maps similarities between target-related phenotypes. It further calculates and screens out ingredient combinations with potential synergistic effects from large-scale TCM ingredient combinations.

(2) Efficient screening methods of synergistic anti-cancer drug combinations (RACS) [35] are mainly based on the network effects of multi-ingredient and multi-target drugs, combined with the characteristics of cancer gene expression profiles. They then use machine learning algorithms to extract the network targeting characteristics of synergistic anti-cancer drug combinations and use it for sorting and screening potential synergistic drug combinations.
(3) The three-node enzymatic network was used to study the combined effects of the two drugs [36]. It also helped to determine and analyze the basic model of synergistic or antagonistic drug action and clarify the relationship between the topology of drug–target network and drug combination, which then helps in designing a new type of drug combination based on network topology;
(4) A network-based method for analyzing the compatibility of Traditional Chinese Medicine prescriptions [37] explores the network characteristics of the featured connotations such as "Traditional Chinese Medicine formulation," "Qiqing Hehe," and other prescriptions by analyzing the distribution pattern of the targets contained in these prescriptions and their effects on the disease-syndrome biomolecular network. This ultimately helps in designing holistic prescriptions.

4. Network Target Analysis and Verification

Researchers can obtain prediction results of key targets, key modules, key pharmacodynamic components, together with key biological pathways through the above network pharmacology analysis method. The next step is to verify the prediction results. It is urgent to establish a rigorous, standardized, scientific, and unified evaluation system in order to ensure the healthy development of the discipline due to the uneven quality of network pharmacology research, lack of standardized data, inadequate scientific testing, and other phenomena. In February 2021, the World Federation of Chinese Medicine Societies approved the first international Guideline on Evaluation Methods of Network Pharmacology (hereinafter referred to as the Guideline) compiled by Shao Li [38]. The Guideline specifies that the evaluation shall be conducted from three aspects: reliability, normalization, and rationality. Specifically, the main evaluation contents of reliability include whether the data are accurate, complete, and publicly available, the accuracy and stability of network analysis methods, the reliability and validity of experimental verification methods and repeatability of results; The normalization mainly covers the complete description of data information, whether the description of data collection and processing methods is clear, whether the algorithm design or network analysis process is clear, whether the algorithm development has rigorous methodology evaluation, whether the analysis methods and technical indicators can be traced, whether the adopted models and operation processes are vividly described, and whether the evaluation index and result description are clear and objective; The rationality mainly comes to whether the data extraction and screening conform to the research purpose and screening requirements, whether the selected network analysis method and indicator can meet the requirements, and whether the models and indicators adopted for verification are suitable for the research content.

1.4.3 Typical Scenarios of Network Pharmacology Analysis

A summary of typical application scenarios of network pharmacology analysis is shown in Table 1.5. Among them, the drug/single herbal medicine treatment of specific indications, the material basis and mechanism of TCM prescriptions are commonly used application scenarios of network pharmacology, embodying the advantages of network pharmacology in practice. The research on the material basis and mechanism of action of TCM prescriptions is mainly for the analysis of the

Table 1.5 Some typical scenarios of network pharmacology analysis

Category	Typical analysis objectives	Typical analysis modules
Drug–target prediction	Identify drug intervention targets	Based on ligand structure data analysis, interaction network analysis
Mechanism of action of single medicinal materials of medicine/single medicinal materials of TCM in the treatment of specific indications	Identify the key ingredients in medicinal materials, indications, related key targets, and biological mechanisms	Chemical composition identification, target prediction, enrichment analysis, network construction, topological structure analysis of network
Analysis of materials and action mechanism of TCM syndromes and prescriptions	Identify the key active ingredient groups in the prescriptions and identify syndrome-related network targets	Chemical composition identification, omics data analysis, target prediction, enrichment analysis, network construction, topological structure analysis of network
Analysis of TCM quality markers	Analyze the effective material basis of TCM and quality control marker ingredients	Chemical composition identification, target prediction, network construction, network analysis
Analysis of biological basis of disease and syndrome	Identify disease-related phenotypes or biomarkers related to TCM syndromes and Western medicine	Omics data analysis, network construction, network analysis
Study on the compatibility laws of TCM prescriptions	Identify the law of action of each active ingredient of the prescription "Traditional Chinese Medicine formulation" on network targets	Compatibility analysis, target prediction, network construction, network analysis
Drug relocation	Identify new uses of known drugs	Chemical structure analysis, omics data analysis, target prediction, network construction, network analysis
Combinatorial drug development	Identify drug combinations with synergistic effects	Target prediction, cluster analysis, network construction, network analysis
Analysis of indications for drugs	Identify diseases or clinical phenotypes that drugs can effectively treat	Omics data analysis, target prediction, network construction, network analysis

target and biological function of each component in the prescription, and to measure the relationship between the target and the key modules of disease and syndrome biomolecular network through the combination of calculation and experiment. The scientific connotation of the compatibility law of TCM prescriptions can be explored, the therapeutic mechanism of traditional Chinese medicine prescriptions can be explained, and new indications can be found with the analysis of the distribution of these targets in the biological molecular network. More and more research cases are in other types of application scenarios, while new methods are still being explored and developed. The determination of drug targets is a key step in drug discovery, and many drug–target interaction prediction algorithms have been developed for drug–target prediction. Drug–target interaction, combined with disease gene relationship, can be employed to find drug indications and provide guidance for drug relocation. More and more attention has been paid to the research of network pharmacology which combines experimental and clinical research to help people deepen their understanding of the occurrence and development of diseases and the mechanism of drug action.

1.4.4 Characteristics, Advantages, Challenges, and Developmental Direction of Network Pharmacology Research

Network pharmacology emphasizes on multi-channel regulation of biological systems based on a holistic concept. Network pharmacology can be used to understand and deal with the complexity of pharmaceutical and biological systems, to understand the mechanism of disease and syndrome development, and evaluate the overall drug intervention to restore the biological network balance.

Network pharmacology research is a systematic, relevant, and predictable approach. Biological molecular network and its relatedness to disease and syndrome is understood from this research. This approach indicates a shift from reductionism to a more holistic system. In terms of relevance, it maps drug targets and disease-syndrome phenotype-related molecules to biomolecular networks, and then analyzes the interactions and correlation between the two. Qualitative and quantitative analysis can be done by observing the combined effects of drugs, based on the biomolecular network of disease and syndrome, thus predicting the action mechanism of drugs.

The advantages of network pharmacology in understanding the biological mechanism of disease and syndrome, studying pharmacodynamic substances and their action mechanisms, and developing new drugs are as follows: ① Network pharmacology organically combines the macro phenotype and microbiological indicators, thus making research on the biological mechanism of complex diseases and syndrome more predictive than descriptive, and from entity research to relationship inference, to provide insights into biological mechanisms of complex diseases and syndromes. ② Network pharmacology adopts the "Network Target-System Regulation" mode, and breaks through the limitation of "Single Target-Partial Confrontation" mode, by conducting integrated research on the pharmacodynamics, biological effects, and action mechanism of drugs. This is done by predictive analysis calculations based on experiments and clinical practice. The research hypothesis is generated by analysis and calculations derived from experiments and uses this approach to overcome shortcomings of more traditional research methods, thus providing a new method in line with the holistic characteristics of TCM. This method can significantly shorten the R & D cycle and save costs.

One key challenge in network pharmacology is to integrate a massive amount of clinical and experimental data, to promote precision-oriented diagnosis and treatment, as well as promote innovation and development of Traditional Chinese Medicine. At the same time, uncontrollable data quality, heterogeneous processing, network-level system analysis, calculation and experimental methods pose some issues that need to be resolved urgently. Network pharmacology understands complex biological systems from a network perspective. Thoroughly understanding the network regulation mechanism of disease and syndrome, drug efficacy and its action mechanism, and to evaluate the overall effects of drugs is also challenging in theory, algorithm development, and practical application.

With its increasing influence, network pharmacology is being applied more frequently. However, the quality of research lacks standardization and there is an urgent need to establish unified norms and rigorous scientific standards to ensure appropriate development of this emerging discipline. In view of the above challenges and limitations, the World Federation of Chinese Medicine Societies has developed the first international standard of network pharmacology, *Network Pharmacology Evaluation Method Guidance* [33]. This guideline aims at the main stages of the research process: data collection, network analysis, and experimental verification, and standardizes the principles, procedures, and evaluation indexes to promote the healthy development of network pharmacology. Also, the core theory and method of network target needs to be explored and improved. For example, finding the efficacy indicators of drugs acting on specific diseases and syndromes based on "Network Target-System Regulation," discovering effective substances of Traditional Chinese Medicine based on network target system, discovering new drugs and their combinations. In order to establish a new evaluation and optimization method of drug effectiveness and safety based on network target, extensive efforts are required in network pharmacology to accelerate the pace of exploration and innovation, jointly promote the progress of this discipline and usher in a new generation Chinese and Western medicine research paradigm.

Network pharmacology related research is on the rise due to increasing use of big data and artificial intelligence in the biomedicine field. "Network Target-System Regulation" has received increasing attention and application and is of great significance to modern Chinese and Western medicine research. This chapter introduces the basic ideas and development network pharmacology, focuses on the theory of network targets, and introduces "Network Target-System Regulation." Network pharmacology and network target theory will continue to lead the development of new drug design and the modernization of Chinese medicine.

References

1. Greene JA, Loscalzo J. Putting the patient back together - social medicine, network medicine, and the limits of reductionism. N Engl J Med. 2017;377(25):2493–9.
2. Wang RS, Maron BA, Loscalzo J. Systems medicine: evolution of systems biology from bench to bedside. Wiley Interdiscip Rev Syst Biol Med. 2015;7(4):141–61.
3. Barabasi AL. Network medicine—from obesity to the "diseasome". N Engl J Med. 2007;357 (4):404–7.
4. Hopkins AL. Network pharmacology. Nat Biotechnol. 2007;25(10):1110–1.
5. Hopkins AL. Network pharmacology: the next paradigm in drug discovery. Nat Chem Biol. 2008;4(11):682–90.
6. Apsel B, Blair JA, Gonzalez B, et al. Targeted polypharmacology: discovery of dual inhibitors of tyrosine and phosphoinositide kinases. Nat Chem Biol. 2008;4(11):691–9.
7. Berger SI, Iyengar R. Network analyses in systems pharmacology. Bioinformatics. 2009;25 (19):2466–72.
8. Pan J. New paradigm for drug discovery based on network pharmacology. Chin J New Drugs Clin Rem. 2009;28(10):721–726 (in Chinese) [潘家祜. 基于网络药理学的药物研发新模式. 中国新药与临床杂志. 2009;28(10):721–726].
9. Li S. Possible relationship between TCM syndromes and molecular network regulation mechanism. Scientific and technological progress and social and economic development in the 21st century (volume I), Beijing, China Science and Technology Press. 1999. p. 442 (in Chinese) [李梢. 中医证候与分子网络调节机制的可能关联. 面向21世纪的科技进步与社会经济发展(上册), 北京, 中国科学技术出版社,1999:442].
10. Li S, Wang Y, Ji L, et al. A discussion and case study of complexities in traditional Chinese medicine. J Syst Simul. 2002;14(11):1429-1432 (in Chinese) [李梢,王永炎, 季梁, 等. 复杂系统意义下的中医药学及其案例研究. 系统仿真学报. 2002;14(11):1429-1432].
11. Li S. Framework and practice of network-based studies for Chinese herbal formula. J Chin Integr Med. 2007;5(5):489–493 (in Chinese) [李梢. 基于生物网络调控的方剂研究模式与实践. 中西医结合学报. 2007;5(5):489–493].
12. Li S, Zhang ZQ, Wu LJ, et al. Understanding ZHENG in traditional Chinese medicine in the context of neuro-endocrine-immune network. IET Syst Biol. 2007;1(1):51–60.
13. Li S. Network target: a starting point for traditional Chinese medicine network pharmacology. Chin J Chin Mater Med. 2011;36(15):2017-2020 (in Chinese) [李梢. 网络靶标:中药方剂网络药理学研究的一个切入点. 中国中药杂志. 2011;36(15):2017-2020].
14. Li S, Zhang B. Traditional Chinese medicine network pharmacology: theory, methodology and application. Chin J Nat Med. 2013;11(2):110–20.
15. Chien TW, Kan WC, Wang HY, et al. Using choropleth maps to show the most cited articles and authors on the topic of traditional Chinese medicine from 2013 to 2017 in Pubmed Central. Chin Tradit Med J. 2018;1(1):1–6.
16. Xi D, Bao T, Chen Q, et al. State of the science: cancer complementary and alternative medicine therapeutics research—NCI Strategic Workshop Highlights of Discussion Report. J Natl Cancer Inst Monogr. 2017;(52):lgx003.
17. Guo YC, Nie Q, Maclean AL, et al. Multiscale modeling of inflammation-induced tumorigenesis reveals competing oncogenic and oncoprotective roles for inflammation. Cancer Res. 2017;77(22):6429–41.
18. Li S. Mapping ancient remedies: applying a network approach to traditional Chinese medicine. Science. 2015;350(6262 Suppl):S72–4.

19. Roth BL, Sheffler DJ, Hroeze WK. Magic shotguns versus magic bullets: selectively non-selective drugs for mood disorders and schizophrenia. Nat Rev Drug Discov. 2004;3 (4):353–9.
20. Hamosh A, Scott AF, Amberger JS, et al. Online Mendelian Inheritance in Man (OMIM), a knowledgebase of human genes and genetic disorders. Nucleic Acids Res. 2005;33:D514–7.
21. Barrett T, Wilhite SE, Ledoux P, et al. NCBI GEO: archive for functional genomics data sets-update. Nucleic Acids Res. 2013;41(D1):D991–5.
22. Wu XB, Jiang R, Zhang MQ, et al. Network-based global inference of human disease genes. Mol Syst Biol. 2008;4:189.
23. Zhao SW, Li S. Network-based relating pharmacological and genomic spaces for drug target identification. PLoS One. 2010;5(7):e11764.
24. Zhao SW, Li S. A co-module approach for elucidating drug-disease associations and revealing their molecular basis. Bioinformatics. 2012;28(7):955–61.
25. Zhang YD, Chen LJ, Li S. CIPHER-SC: disease-gene association inference using graph convolution on a context-aware network with single-cell data. IEEE/ACM Trans Comput Biol Bioinform. https://doi.org/10.1109/TCBB.2020.3017547.
26. Li S, Zhang B, Zhang NB. Network target for screening synergistic drug combinations with application to traditional Chinese medicine [J]. BMC Syst Biol. 2011;5(Suppl 1):S10.
27. Subramanian A, Tamayo P, Mootha VK, et al. Gene set enrichment analysis: a knowledge-based approach for interpreting genome-wide expression profiles. Proc Natl Acad Sci U S A. 2005;102(43):15545–50.
28. Huang DW, Sherman BT, Lempicki RA. Systematic and integrative analysis of large gene lists using DAVID bioinformatics resources. Nat Protoc. 2009;4(1):44–57.
29. Kuleshov MV, Jones MR, Rouillard AD, et al. Enrichr: a comprehensive gene set enrichment analysis web server 2016 update. Nucleic Acids Res. 2016;44(W1):W90–7.
30. Yu G, Wang LG, Han Y, et al. clusterProfiler: an R package for comparing biological themes among gene clusters. Omics A J Integr Biol. 2012;16(5):284–7.
31. Bader GD, Hogue CW. An automated method for finding molecular complexes in large protein interaction networks. BMC Bioinformatics. 2003;4:2.
32. Barabasi AL, Gullbahce N, Loscalzo J. Network medicine: a network-based approach to human disease. Nat Rev Genet. 2011;12(1):56–68.
33. Zhang T, Brazhnik P, Tyson JJ. Exploring mechanisms of the DNA-damage response: p53 pulses and their possible relevance to apoptosis. Cell Cycle. 2007;6(1):85–94.
34. Bian YM, He XB, Jing YK, et al. Computational systems pharmacology analysis of cannabidiol: a combination of chemogenomics-knowledgebase network analysis and integrated in silico modeling and simulation. Acta Pharmacologica Sinica. 2019;40(3):374–86.
35. Sun Y, Sheng Z, Ma C, et al. Combining genomic and network characteristics for extended capability in predicting synergistic drugs for cancer. Nat Commun. 2015;6:8481.
36. Xu H, Zhang Y, Lei Y, et al. A systems biology-based approach to uncovering the molecular mechanisms underlying the effects of Dragon's Blood Tablet in Colitis, involving the integration of chemical analysis, ADME prediction, and network pharmacology. PLoS One. 2014;9 (7):e101432.
37. Li S, Zhang B, Jiang D, et al. Herb network construction and co-module analysis for uncovering the combination rule of traditional Chinese herbal formulae. BMC Bioinformatics. 2010;11 (Suppl 11):1–12.
38. Li S. Network pharmacology evaluation method guidance-draft. World J Tradit Chin Med 2021;7(1):146–154.

Chapter 2
Application of Network Pharmacology Based on Artificial Intelligence Algorithms in Drug Development

Wenxia Zhou, Xuejun Li, Lu Han, and Shengjun Fan

Guide to This Chapter

The continuous development and progress of biotechnology and information technology provides data for pharmaceutical research and application. It is difficult to fully utilize large-scale data with simple statistical analysis methods. In order to improve data utilization, pharmaceutical research must be promoted using advanced information analysis. Artificial intelligence has experienced half a century of development since its inception and has been successfully applied to many industrial and technological fields. Recently, breakthroughs in machine learning represented by deep learning have made artificial intelligence one of the most popular research directions. Artificial intelligence algorithms use different types of data based on various strategies to do multiple tasks such as search and discrimination, and are suitable for solving massive data analysis problems faced in network pharmacological research. This chapter briefly introduces artificial intelligence algorithms and their applications in network pharmacology research, and provides references for researchers to better understand and apply artificial intelligence.

W. Zhou (✉) · L. Han
Beijing Institute of Pharmacology and Toxicology, Beijing, China

X. Li · S. Fan
Peking University, Beijing, China
e-mail: xjli@bjmu.edu.cn

S. Li (ed.), *Network Pharmacology*, https://doi.org/10.1007/978-981-16-0753-0_2

2.1 Introduction to Artificial Intelligence Methods in Network Pharmacology

Network pharmacology [1] is a research method based on systems biology. The concept includes recognizing and discovering drugs based on the overall relationship between an organism and drugs. In recent years, the growth of high-throughput omics data and the accumulation of pharmacological knowledge have promoted the rapid development of network pharmacology. With the accumulation of different types of data resources and knowledge bases, mining effective information like drug targets, mechanism of action, and drug and organism interaction from massive, heterogeneous data has become increasingly important in network pharmacology research. Therefore, the demand for more accurate and efficient analysis algorithms has also increased [2].

There are three common problems that may be encountered in network pharmacology research: ① Optimal solution search; ② prediction and classification; ③ automatic construction of networks and pathways. Artificial intelligence can effectively perform feature extraction and potential relationship mining from complex big data, and is beneficial for solving common problems in network pharmacology. Combining artificial intelligence and network pharmacology has great potential to overcome the problems faced in the latter field.

Since the emergence of network pharmacology research, artificial intelligence has been closely integrated with it and widely applied. For example, when the drug–target interaction is evaluated using simulation, it is necessary to perform optimal solution search operation, such as genetic algorithm [3] or simulated annealing algorithm [4], as the core of molecular docking and molecular dynamics simulation technology to implement the conformation search strategy. During network analysis and prediction, classification and prediction are required, hence unsupervised learning clustering algorithms (Affinity propagation clustering algorithm, K-means clustering algorithm) and supervised learning are widely used. In mechanism research, it is necessary to construct the network and path automatically, hence various network construction-related artificial intelligence algorithms such as the Bayesian network algorithm are often applied.

This chapter briefly reviews the development history of artificial intelligence, and the classification and characteristics of the main algorithms applied in network pharmacology, in order to promote the better understanding of the applications and evaluation methods for researchers.

2.1.1 Introduction to Artificial Intelligence Algorithms

Artificial intelligence is an important branch of computer science. The definition of artificial intelligence has not yet been unified, but it can be summarized as studying the laws of human intelligence activities and constructing artificial systems with certain intelligent behavior [5]. Thanks to high-performance scale computing equipment, big data accumulation, and algorithm innovation, artificial intelligence has been widely applied in image recognition [6, 7], speech recognition [8, 9], medical diagnosis [10], drug R&D [11], and many other fields, and its achievements cover all aspects of human life. Artificial intelligence algorithms that widely used in network pharmacology can be divided into three types: heuristic algorithms, machine learning, and network construction algorithms according to their problem-solving scope and application characteristics.

1. Introduction to Heuristic Algorithms

Heuristic algorithms are based on intuitive or empirically constructed algorithms that give feasible solutions to problems in acceptable time and space. Its classic algorithms include: simulated annealing algorithm [4], genetic algorithm [3], etc. Heuristic algorithms perform optimal solution search with limited computational cost and time. The optimal solution search often be applicable to specific problems such as sub-network, optimal conformation, and specific sequence search.

Network pharmacology problems using heuristic algorithms usually have two basic characteristics. First, the search results can be measured by quantitative index; second, the search target can be constructed in a certain way. Taking optimal conformation as an example, the change in binding free energy is used as the quantitative index, and new binding conformations can be constructed through operations such as translation and rotation of chemical bonds and atoms in molecules.

2. Introduction to Machine Learning

Machine learning is currently the most rapidly developing artificial intelligence algorithm. For large and high-dimensional complex data, machine learning method can effectively perform data classification, data fitting, prediction model establishment, feature selection, and other tasks.

Supervised machine learning methods mainly include two categories: regression and classification [12], by which the mapping relationship could be established from input X_i to output Y_i from a large amount of input data, to construct a prediction model or analyze the weight of input features. The commonly used regression algorithms include: LASSO (Least Absolute Shrinkage and Selection Operator) regression, ridge regression, and elastic net. Classification algorithms include logistic regression, Bayesian classifier algorithm, support vector machine, K-nearest neighbor, random forest, and artificial neural network. Additionally, deep learning [13] is a rapidly developing supervised learning method in recent years, which is an improvement of the artificial neural network structure. It is characterized by more hidden layer structures between the input and output layers. Its classic structure includes: Convolutional neural networks (CNN) and recurrent neural network (RNN).

Unsupervised machine learning methods include clustering [14] and dimension reduction [15], which do not rely on input data labels to establish the feature-to-label mapping, but focus on the characteristics and interrelationships of a large amount of data. Based on various measurement relations, the input data is divided into different categories (clustering), or the dimension of input feature vector is reduced, to remove noise and reduce redundant features (dimension reduction). Commonly used clustering algorithms include K-means clustering algorithm, hierarchical clustering, and affinity propagation clustering algorithm. Commonly used dimension reduction algorithms include principal component analysis (PCA) and factor analysis.

3. Introduction to Network Generation Method

Network generation method can be divided into network construction and sub-net extraction methods based on new network connection relationships and their generation.

In network pharmacology research, the network nodes are composed of elements related to Drug property such as compounds, targets, genes, and diseases. Networks related to biological processes are usually the most complex. For example, gene expression regulation is a dynamic process involving time and space factors. Static networks often cannot effectively reflect the temporal and spatial specificity of biological processes [16]. However, to achieve a relatively accurate characterization of the dynamic regulation of biological networks, a large amount of data with temporal and spatial differences is required. Therefore, limited data volume, and uncertain knowledge expression and reasoning can be used to make predictions and generate new network connection relations. Network construction methods include association, Boolean model, dynamic Bayesian network, and differential equation.

The sub-net extraction method does not aim at discovering new network relationships, but can extract the most relevant sub-nets from the known background network, and is often used to explain the effects of drugs or disease mechanisms. Extracting key sub-networks and identifying overlapping networks from complex relationships are important components of network analysis. Identifying key sub-networks is often closely related to the discovery of drug targets, and identification of pathways and key regulatory factors. Heuristic algorithms such as simulated annealing algorithm, genetic algorithm, and Steiner's forest algorithm [17] are often used to find the sub-net with the highest score.

2.1.2 Performance Evaluation Method for Artificial Intelligence Algorithms

Although artificial intelligence algorithms solve specific problems in network pharmacology research through a reasonable computational model, blindly trusting the computational results of artificial intelligence algorithms is detrimental. The performance of artificial intelligence algorithms to solve problems needs to be systematically evaluated by scientific metric or measures in order to effectively reduce errors caused by various risks such as low data quality or overfittings.

Table 2.1 Evaluation indicators of typical artificial intelligence methods

Artificial intelligence methods	Introduction to the methods	Performance evaluation method and evaluation index
Heuristic algorithm	Based on the specific construction algorithm, artificial intelligence is used to search an optimal solution within a certain calculation consumption. The representative algorithms include annealing algorithm, genetic algorithm, etc.	Number of iterations, convergence time, etc.
Machine learning algorithm	A class of algorithms for knowledge learning and acquisition by simulating human learning behavior is usually used for prediction and classification in pharmacological research. Representative algorithms include deep learning algorithm and clustering algorithm.	Precision rate, recall rate, ROC curve, mutual information, contour coefficient, etc.
Network generation algorithm	The method of comprehensively generating the network using multidisciplinary analysis methods such as probability theory and graph theory is mostly used in molecular network construction and drug mechanism analysis. Representative algorithms include Bayesian network algorithm and shortest path method.	Precision rate, recall rate, etc.

To evaluate the performance and generalization ability of artificial intelligence algorithms, some performance evaluation methods are required. The most well-known "Turing test" [18] is the first evaluation method proposed to gauge whether a machine is intelligent. However, it has limitations and a smaller application scope. There are several different methods or metrics could be adopted according to the algorithm and data characteristics.

Different artificial intelligence methods need to use different performance evaluation metrics and approach to evaluate the performance of the methods. General evaluation indexes include loss value, accuracy, etc., and there are also commonly used evaluation indexes for different algorithms and data characteristics. Relevant evaluation indexes are briefly summarized in Table 2.1.

1. Heuristic Algorithm Evaluation

Multiple solutions may be obtained by heuristic algorithm due to its characteristics, hence evaluation metrics could be set according to different purposes. For example, in order to save time in large-scale calculations, genetic algorithm can involve relatively few iterations and use shorter convergence time as indexes while searching for feasible solutions, whereas higher global search ability can be used as the evaluation index to get better solutions.

2. Machine Learning Algorithms Evaluation

The evaluation metrics of machine learning are applied to different algorithms, purposes, and data characteristics. The essence is to evaluate the gap between predicted and actual values through biased functional loss, and later by optimizing the parameters. This part mainly introduces the evaluation metrics of supervised classification algorithm, regression algorithm, and clustering algorithm.

Supervised classification algorithm can divide a given object *X* into a predefined category *Y*. In supervised classification, all samples can be divided into a training set, validation set, and test set. The training and validation set data are used to train the prediction model. The trained model then uses the test set to test its accuracy and generalization ability. Additionally, *k*-fold cross-validation method can be used to divide the training data into two parts based on the ratio of $(k-1)/K$ and $1/K$. The former is used for model training, and the latter is used to evaluate model performance and generalization ability. The most common evaluation index in supervised classification algorithm is accuracy, to predict the proportion of accurate classification in all samples. However, due to "imbalanced data" [19] problems, evaluation indicators with characteristics such as precision and recall indicators are often used. The former is focused on the correct proportion of positive samples predicted by the classifier, while the latter is more concerned with whether it is possible to predict more positive samples. The two evaluation indexes are applicable to various scenarios. For example, when predicting effective drugs from large amount of unrelated molecules, less false positive predictions are better for researchers in order to avoid subsequent invalid biological experiments. Therefore, the accuracy rate is often used as the classification index. However, when constructing a global network regulation relationship, it is more important to cover all targets nodes, so it has greater tolerance for false positive results, and the recall rate can be used as a classification index. In addition, there are also evaluation metrics that consider both accuracy rate and recall rate, such as F1 score, receiver operating characteristic curve (ROC curve), precision-recall curve, and confusion matrix.

The regression algorithm is a statistical analysis method to determine the interdependent quantitative relationship between two or more variables. The commonly used evaluation indicators of regression algorithm include: Mean absolute deviation (MAE), root mean squared error (RMSE), mean-square error (MSE), Huber loss, log-cosh loss, etc. Using different evaluation indicators may have a greater impact on constructing prediction models. For example, "mean absolute deviation" (also known as L1 loss) is less sensitive to the output error and is relatively more stable when an abnormal point exists. At the same time, the regression model is not unique, and there may be multiple optimal solutions. Whereas, the mean-square error (also known as L2 loss) squares the output error, so the error can be optimized to a greater extent, and it is easier to obtain a stable regression model. Also, it may be more sensitive to the response of abnormal points with lower robustness.

Clustering is an important representative of unsupervised learning. They can divide samples into different categories according to similarity measures. When the sample data has a given label, a matching degree of the real label and clustering can be calculated. Mutual information, Rand index, and other indicators are commonly used. When the sample data does not have a given label, a silhouette coefficient can be used to evaluate the rationality of the clustering division.

3. Network Generation Algorithm Evaluation

In case the complete regulatory network is known, the constructed network can be compared with the complete network to calculate the precision rate, recall rate, and other indicators. The evaluation method is the same as that of the classification algorithm in machine learning.

Several network pharmacology studies using artificial intelligence use individual case verification, such as comparing model results with literature or conducting experimental verification, instead of the above evaluation indicators. This approach is usually feasible, and combined with systematic validation can be persuasive and the result can be more reliable.

2.1.3 Applications of Artificial Intelligence

Network pharmacology research involves several application requirements such as optimal solution search, target and drug prediction, and regulatory network construction. Artificial intelligence can play a key role in solving various application needs of network pharmacology. Different artificial intelligence methods can solve problems and satisfy different needs. Therefore, it is important to determine whether the algorithms suit for research problem. The following helps classify and introduce the applied fields of artificial intelligence methods.

1. Applications of Heuristic Algorithm

The main application of the commonly used heuristic algorithm is optimal solution search, which is widely used in biology and pharmacy. For example, the heuristic algorithm based tool Blast (Basic Local Alignment Search Tool) [20] is used for protein or gene sequence matching, and Open Babel [21] uses the genetic algorithm to generate small molecule conformations that are used for searching in molecular docking [22] and molecular dynamics simulation [23], heuristic algorithm is also the core algorithms in the sub-net extraction process. If the problems in network pharmacology research have the following characteristics, heuristic algorithm can be applied: ① Quantifiable scoring system: The generated results of the heuristic algorithm can judge whether calculations meet the requirements of certain scoring indicators. ② New scheme generation based on current optimal solutions: Based on the known optimal solution, a new feasible solution is generated by evaluating the distance between the calculation and the optimal solution. ③ There are corresponding convergence or termination conditions. Taking Open Babel as an example, when generating small molecule conformations, to determine whether the conformation is stable, it can either use a quantitative scoring system such as the energy of the generated conformation, or by evaluating the RMSD (Root Mean Square Deviation) coordinate deviation between the generated conformation and natural conformation.

2. Applications of Machine Learning

There are differences in the application scope and analysis between unsupervised and supervised learning methods. The purpose of unsupervised learning is to explore the relationship between input data, while supervised learning establishes mapping from input to output data from the training data, to achieve the learning purpose.

Unsupervised learning can be divided into clustering, dimension reduction, association, and other types, in which clustering and dimension reduction algorithms are widely used in network pharmacology research. Commonly used clustering algorithms include K-means clustering algorithm, AP clustering algorithm, and hierarchical clustering. Input data can be divided into various categories according to the measurement relationships. For example, Iorio et al. [24] evaluated the similarity of gene expression profiles between pairs of 1309 drugs, and used the AP clustering algorithm to construct a drug–drug similarity network for drug repurposing.

Commonly used linear dimension reduction algorithms include principal component analysis (PCA), factor analysis, etc. In the analysis of high-dimensional data, the problem of "dimension disaster" is often encountered, hence the dimension reduction algorithm is often needed to reduce the dimensionality of feature vectors, so as to reduce noise and redundant features. For example, Subramanian et al. [25] used PCA and clustering algorithm to reduce the dimension of the transcriptome data, and compressed the expression data of more than 12,000 genes to 978 landmark genes. Moreover, the 978 landmark genes can be used to infer 80% of the network regulatory relationship at the transcription level, thereby greatly reducing the cost of transcriptome data measurement.

Since linear dimension reduction algorithm often cannot meet the analytical needs when processing complex data, nonlinear dimension reduction algorithm is also widely used. For example, the t-SNE [26] algorithm, which is often used for data visualization, can retain the proximity characteristics of high-dimensional data and reduce it to two-dimensional or three-dimensional space, which plays an intuitive role in the systematic research of complex omics data [27, 28].

The supervised learning method commonly used in network pharmacology [29] includes two main types: regression and classification, both of which are used to establish the mapping relationship between input X_i and output Y_i. The output Y of regression is continuous quantitative data, such as blood pressure, blood drug concentration, while the output of classification is often qualitative data, such as negative/positive diagnosis results, tumor classification. This indicates that different types of functional losses need to be used in the calculations; however, regression and classification problems can often occur simultaneously. Supervised learning helps establish a reliable prediction model, and the model is used to predict new potential relationships.

Regression algorithms can quantitatively describe the mapping relationship between variables, so they are widely used in omics analysis and network pathway inference. For example, Gamazon et al. [30] used linear regression to infer gene expression from single nucleotide polymorphisms and predicted biological phenotypes. Xiong and Zhou [31] used linear regression to infer the regulatory network relationship of genes from the biological experimental data level. The classification algorithm is often used in the qualitative prediction of drug–target interactions. For example, Yamanishi et al. [32] integrated multiple types of biological data (such as chemical structures, drug side effects, amino acid sequences, and protein domains), and used machine learning to train user-submitted data and to predict unknown drug–target interaction network.

Deep learning [13], as an extension of artificial neural networks, is the most rapidly developing and applied artificial intelligence algorithm in recent years. It has similar functions to traditional machine learning methods, but also has new characteristics: ① Deep neural network structure is conducive to expressing complex mapping relationships: Traditional machine learning algorithms are mostly shallow structures, hence it is difficult to display highly complex functions, whereas deep learning introduces multiple hidden layers between the input and output ends to achieve a nonlinear network structure, thus, it has the ability to express complex functions. ② Multi-hidden layer structure is capable of autonomously extracting features: Traditional machine learning algorithms rely on humans to manually extract features, while deep learning can autonomously extract features. Due to the emergence of deep structures, the input features may be transformed into new feature space, whereas the hidden layers and irrelevant features are suppressed. The above two points ensure that deep learning has better performance in processing complex big data.

3. Applications of Network Generation

Network construction is the first step in the study of network pharmacology. The commonly used methods are association, Boolean model, Bayesian network, differential equation. Artificial intelligence algorithms in network construction lay more emphasis on logical reasoning and relationship discovery, which is different from deep learning and other predictive models.

High false positive rate often occurs in the process of network construction, the complex and huge networks are not conducive to further identification of key components in the network. Therefore, it is important to extract key sub-networks from complex relationships and identify overlapping networks [34]. For example, Steiner's forest algorithm can be used to extract protein and gene–gene interaction networks from complex networks and quickly identify key interaction pathways and factors.

2.1.4 Frontiers and Prospects of Artificial Intelligence

Artificial intelligence technology has penetrated all aspects of network pharmacology research. From molecular docking, function, and target prediction, to network construction and analysis, artificial intelligence is playing an increasingly important role. On the other hand, the molecular structure of drugs, therapeutic uses, clinical response, and multi-latitude omics data obtained from laboratory measurements constitute big data in the research field, which also brings opportunities for the application of new artificial intelligence technologies [34].

Among all types of artificial intelligence algorithms, the one with the most noticeable development in recent years is undoubtedly the deep learning algorithm [6]. Its outstanding performance in large-scale data analysis and in solving a variety of computing problems has rendered it the research frontier of artificial intelligence. In the performance evaluation and comparison of large-scale training of pharmaceutical data, deep learning surpasses traditional machine learning algorithms [35, 36]. The feature extraction ability of deep learning is convenient for analyzing complex high-dimensional data. Although it has become an emerging research direction in various industries, its application in many specific directions is still a question worth exploring.

However, the application of artificial intelligence in network pharmacology research also has corresponding technical and application problems. The most common one is over-fitting problems in the training process [37]; it is usually necessary to ensure sufficient sample amount of training data, and adopt appropriate training parameters and reliable performance evaluation methods to reduce the over-fitting problem. In addition, the deep learning algorithm also brings about the interpretability of predictive models and the computational efficiency of the big data fitting process. In order to solve these potential problems, possible future research directions include studying and understanding the function of each layer of the neural network in deep learning, optimizing deep neural network training methods to ensure efficiency and speed, introducing time and space information to achieve complex data as input, and carrying out application research.

2.2 Application of Artificial Intelligence in Network Pharmacology Research

Network pharmacology aims to promote research by using network tools. Artificial intelligence in network pharmacology plays an important role in solving drug target discovery, Drug property mechanism determination, discovery of new uses of compounds, and research on Traditional Chinese Medicine. Artificial intelligence technology is used in target discovery based on analysis methods such as structural docking, structural comparison, network simulation, and machine learning. Artificial intelligence is also used in mechanism research such as pathway and molecular function prediction and Drug property pattern analysis. In terms of discovery of new uses, artificial intelligence is used in the prediction of new uses based on multiple phenotypes and molecular data after drug perturbation. In terms of TCM research, artificial intelligence is used in the research of Chinese medicine targets, mechanisms, and syndrome theories. The following sections introduce the application status of artificial intelligence in these aspects.

2.2.1 Prediction and Discovery of Drug Targets

The discovery of drug targets is a long-standing topic in network pharmacology research. According to the strategy and data differences in the discovery of drug targets using artificial intelligence, the analysis can be divided based on ligand structure similarity and quantitative structure–activity relationship, reverse molecular docking, action network simulation, and machine learning.

1. Analysis Based on Ligand Structure Similarity and Quantitative Structure–Activity Relationship

Structural data of drugs/compounds is easily available and not only fully reflects the basic characteristics of molecules, but can also be easily counted and compared. It was used earlier in network pharmacology research. Many artificial intelligence algorithms such as intelligent search and classification are used in structural comparison analysis methods. According to the research characteristics, the analysis can be divided into structural similarity comparison method, quantitative structure–activity relationship analysis method, and docking method. They are as follows:

The importance of structural similarity mainly comes from the similar property principle [38]: molecules with similar structures may bind to the same target and have similar biological functions. By comparing the chemical similarity of ligands, it can be inferred that they may have similar targets and pharmacological effects. New pharmacological effects can be found through this method. Also, biomacromolecules (targets) with different functions may have similar drug binding domains. Therefore, the similarity between the chemical characteristics of a drug that binds to a target and the structure of the target molecule can be used to predict the unknown target of drugs [39]. Similarity measurement includes three parts: structural characterization, weight calculation, and similarity coefficient [40]. Vilart et al. [41] proposed a method to identify new DDI (Drug–Drug Interactions) based on the similarity of molecular structures of drugs involved in the established DDI. The basic assumption is that if drug A and drug B interact to produce a specific biological effect, a drug similar to drug A (or drug B) may interact with drug B (or drug A) to produce the same effect. This study collected 9454 pairs of known DDI resources, and identified DDI candidates [41] by calculating the structural similarity of all drug pairs in DrugBank. Yan et al. [42] proposed a SDTRLS (substructure-drug-target Kronecker product kernel regularized least squares) method based on sub-structure similarity, Gaussian interaction profile (GIP), similarity network fusion (SNF), RLS-Kron classifier, and other technologies. In the independent verification of G protein-coupled receptors (GPCRs), the predictions are better than in the SDTNBI algorithm (substructure-drug-target network-based inference) [42]. Keiser et al. [43] compared 3665 drugs approved by the US FDA (Food and Drug Administration) and drugs that still in the research stage, with hundreds of drug targets. By comparing the chemical similarity between the drug and the ligand set, they predicted thousands of new associations. Thirty of these associations were experimentally verified, and 23 new drug–target associations were confirmed, of which 5 have higher binding strength with the predicted target. In addition, there is a compound N, and the physiological significance of the interaction between n-dimethyltryptamine and 5-hydroxytryptamine receptor has been verified in gene knockout mice [43].

In addition to structural similarities, quantitative structure–activity relationship (QSAR) is another commonly used research method based on structural data. It refers to a quantitative relationship that links the structural parameters of a compound with its biological activity data through a corresponding algorithm. The basic idea is that similar molecules usually bind to similar proteins. The interaction is predicted by comparing new ligands with known protein ligands [40, 44]. The predictive ability of the QSAR model depends largely on the structural similarity between the training set and the test set molecules [45]. Zhang et al. [46] used a data set of 3133 compounds to build a QSAR model. The model was built using dragon descriptors (0D, 1D, and 2D), ISIDA-2D fragment descriptors, and support vector machine (SVM) method. In the QSAR modeling and verification process, the data set is randomly divided into modeling and external evaluation sets; and the sphere exclusion algorithm is used in the training set and the test set to divide the modeling set multiple times. Then, using the consensus approach, the QSAR model is applied to the VS (virtual screening) of the ChemBridge database. The 42 inactive compounds predicted by the model have been experimentally verified [46]. Melo-Filho et al. [47] developed a continuous combi-QSAR model for the oxadiazole inhibitor data set of smTGR, and further evaluated the top 10 compounds in vitro on *Schistosoma japonicum* and adult worms, and found that two compounds containing new chemical scaffolds had high activity in various life stages of parasites at low molecular concentrations [47]. Marcelo et al. [48] combined QSAR to develop SAR rules and a binary QSAR model of antituberculosis compounds based on chalcone. Then, these models were used to conduct synthesis and biological evaluation of 33 compounds, and candidate drugs [48] with low activity to symbiotic bacteria, good selectivity to mycobacterium tuberculosis, and low cytotoxicity to Vero cells were found.

Comparison of structural similarity and QSAR is based on the hypothesis that similar structures correspond to similar activities, and molecular docking is the most intuitive application of receptor–ligand hypothesis. Molecular docking is a traditional method for evaluating the chemical complementarity of small molecules and target molecules based on the three-dimensional (3D) structure of the target. DTIs (drug target interactions) were evaluated by using a scoring function to provide a quantitative docking score associated with binding affinity [49]. Molecular docking has a wide range of applications in DTI prediction. Starting from known target proteins, screening ligands with the best affinity from many known three-dimensional structure molecules are suitable for large-scale screening of candidate ligand compounds after obtaining disease targets. Ordinarily, for one or several given targets, such as estrogen receptor [50], HIV-1 integrase [51], potential active compounds can be prioritized by molecular docking. Web applications based on molecular docking, such as TarFisDock [52], DRAR-CPI [53], rDock [54], are all built for target search based on docking. Although molecular docking is widely used, it still has its limitations, such as not being suitable for situations where the number of proteins is large and the three-dimensional structure is not available, it cannot be applied to membrane proteins with complex structures, such as ion channels and G protein-coupled receptors (GPCRs), and the extremely low efficiency of docking computing due to the huge consumption of computing resources [45].

The key assumption of drug target analysis based on calculation of similarities is that similar drugs tend to share similar targets [29]. Thus, internationally, Yamanishi et al. [30, 31] proposed a method to predict drug target relationship by combining chemical drug similarity and genetic similarity; Keiser et al. [32] compared the chemical structure of the drug with ligands known to regulate the function of protein receptors, and obtained indirect connections between the drug and the target through these ligands. In addition, there are methods to predict drug targets based on chemical similarity [33, 34] and side effect similarity [35].

Another type of method focuses on indirect drug–gene relationships and uses additional similarity measures to obtain drug-related genes. For example, Hansen et al. [36] used the similarity of protein–protein interaction networks to predict the drug–gene genetic association, and combined the gene expression data with the drug response data provided by Kutalik et al. [37] to infer the common module relationship between genes and drugs.

In China, Cheng et al. [38] developed three supervised inference models to predict the interactions between drugs and targets, namely drug similarity inference, target-based similarity inference, and network-based inference. Li et al. [39] developed the target prediction algorithm drugCIPHER based on the overall association of "drug network–molecular network." In this method, the authors developed a computational framework called drugCIPHER, based on the interrelationships observed in the fields of pharmacology and genomics, to infer drug target interactions on a genome-wide scale. Based on the protein–protein interaction network, three linear regression models are proposed, which connect the drug treatment similarity, chemical similarity, and the correlation between the combination of the two and the target, respectively. Experiments have shown that the model (drugCIPHER-MS) that combines drug treatment similarity and chemical similarity has achieved good results on the training set and test set. The model process is shown in Fig. 2.1.

2. Reverse Molecular Docking

In recent years, with the development of computer-aided drug design, a reverse molecular docking based on the "lock-key theory" has become a new means of drug target discovery in network pharmacology [55]. For a drug or new chemical entity, reverse molecular docking works opposite to molecular docking. Small molecular compounds are used as probes to search for biomacromolecules that may be combined with them in the database of candidate targets with known structures. Possible molecular complexes can be identified using space and energy matching and potential drug targets can then be predicted [56–58].

The concept of reverse molecular docking was proposed by researcher Chen Yuzong from the National University of Singapore. Chen connected a single small molecule with multiple biological targets by means of molecular docking and by downloading the protein structure of a biomolecule in the PDB database and the

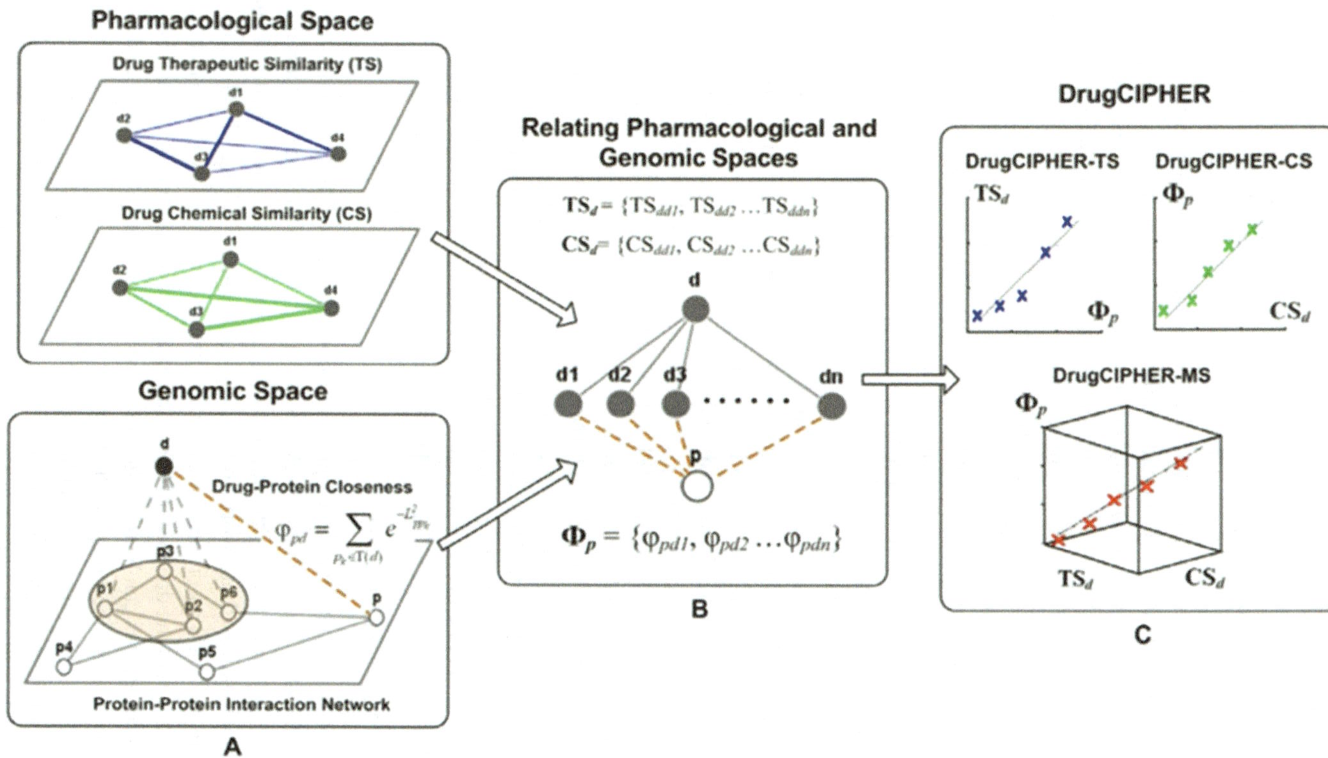

Fig. 2.1 Schematic diagram of target prediction algorithm drugCIPHER based on the overall association of "Drug Network–Molecular Network" [39]

INVDOCK platform. He then evaluated the binding energy of the ligand-compound, and preliminarily evaluated potential biological targets [59] of smaller active molecules. Subsequently, more convenient and rapidly reversing molecular docking network platforms have been developed, such as TarFisDock [60], PharmMapper [61], Reverse Screen 3D [62], and idTarget [63].

Guo et al. demonstrated that ganoderic acid D exerts an anti-cervical cancer effect [64] through the direct binding of 14-3-3 protein using bidirectional gel electrophoresis technology and INVDOCK. Subsequently, they used a similar method to clarify that the cardioprotective action of salvianolic acid B is through direct binding with human epidermal growth factor receptor (EGFR) [65]. Park et al. investigated potential biological targets of ginsenoside based on reverse molecular docking with their own protein target database, and found that dozens of biological targets such as MEK1 and EGFR could be directly regulated by ginsenoside [66].

3. Analysis Based on Action Network Simulation

The analysis based on interaction network simulation is different from the one based on structural comparison. It relies on an interaction database presented in the form of a network. Therefore, the advantage of this analysis is that it makes more extensive use of the observed interaction network to find targets. These network-based methods are usually based on algorithms in recommendation systems and relational algorithms in complex networks, which cover a larger target space and can predict potential DTIs by executing simple physical processes such as "resource diffusion," "collaborative filtering," and "random walk" on the network [67]. Topological similarity reasoning of drug target bipartite network and in vitro experiments have also been conducted. Cheng et al. [68] confirmed that five kinds of old drugs had multi-directional pharmacological properties on human estrogen receptor or dipeptidyl protease IV, and found that simvastatin and ketoconazole showed strong antiproliferative activity on human MDA-MB-231 breast cancer cell line [68]. The MD-Miner (Mechanism and Drug Miner) method proposed by Wu et al. [69] has found potentially effective drug candidates by constructing a patient-specific signal transduction network that integrates known disease-related genes with patient-derived gene expression profiles. This is based on the number of common genes between the patient-specific dysfunction signal transduction and the Drug property network, and also by a drug mechanism of action network, which integrates drug target and drug-induced expression profile data. This method has been evaluated on PC-3 prostate cancer cell line, which shows that compared to random selection, the success rate of finding effective drugs is significantly improved, and can provide in-depth understanding of potential mechanisms of action [69]. Isik et al. [70] studied whether biological responses and protein interaction networks of drug interference with cancer cells could reveal drug targets and key pathways. Through systematic analysis of more than 500 drugs in cMAP (connectivity map, gene expression profile database), it has been proven that drug interference usually has no significant effects on the expression of drug target genes, hence the changes in expression after drug treatment are insufficient to identify drug targets. However, network topology measurement and local radiance measurement that combine perturbed gene and functional interaction network information are conducive to discovering cancer-specific pathways [70].

Link prediction in the network refers to predicting the possibility of a connection between two nodes in the network that have not yet been connected through information, such as known network nodes and structures [40]. This prediction includes both the prediction of unknown connections and the possibility of possible new connections.

Chen et al. [41] developed a rebooted random walk model—NRWRH, based on heterogeneous networks, to predict potential drug–target interactions by implementing random walks on heterogeneous networks. This work assumes that similar drugs often interact with similar targets and integrate the drug–drug similarity network, protein–protein similarity network, and known drug–target interaction network, into a heterogeneous network. In this work, NRWRH was used to predict potential drug–target interaction by integrating drug-related information. The originality of this method lies in the integration of three different networks (drug similarity network, target similarity network, and known drug–target interaction network) into a heterogeneous network. NRWRH is applied to four target proteins, including enzymes, ion channels, GPCR, and nuclear receptors, using cross-validation to predict potential drug–target interactions, and demonstrated superior performance of NRWRH over previous methods.

Abhik et al. [42] extended the experimental data set on the basis of NRWRH. This method also integrates the three networks of drug–drug similarity network, protein–protein similarity network, and known drug–target interaction network into a heterogeneous network, and expands relevant drug–target network data and uses external data sets for verification.

This section follows a brief demonstration of the link prediction analysis steps in the Python language.

(1) Description of Question

Let G (V, E) be an undirected graph network, where V is a set of nodes and E is a set of edges. Given the link prediction method, assign a score value "S" to each pair of unconnected node pairs, and then sort all pairs according to the score value from the largest to smallest, with the first node pair having the highest probability of connecting edges [40].

(2) Link Prediction Method

Common link prediction methods are based on similarity, maximum likelihood estimation, and probability model [43, 44]. The similarity-based link prediction methods are divided into three main categories [45]—similarity based on nodes, pathways, and random walks. The concept of the method based on node similarity is: the greater the similarity between two nodes, greater the possibility of links between them. Therefore, there are many definitions of node similarity, including common neighbor index [46], Salton index [47], Jaccard index [48], HDI [49], etc. Based on the similarity index of pathways, there are mainly local path index [50], Katz index [51], and LHN-II index [56]. Similarity indexes based on random walk include

Table 2.2 Code implementation

Core codes	
import networkx as nx	# Import networkx toolkit
data = open("ppi.txt")	# Load PPI data
G = nx.Graph()	# Create empty graph, G network undirected graph
for i, line in enumerate(data):	
line = line.split("\t")	
G.add_edge(line[0], line[1])	# Add data to undirected graph
preds = nx.jaccard_coefficient (G,[(0,1),(2,3)])	# Calculate the Jaccard coefficients of all the unconnected nodes
for u, v, p in preds:	# Triple iterator in the form of (u,v,p), wherein print (% D,% d) -> %.8f' % (u, v, p)
P(u,v) = preds(u,v)	# (u, v) is a pair of nodes and P is their Jaccard coefficient.
>>>	# Program running results
(ATP6V1B1, ATP6V1A) -> 0.75000000	
(17, 1546) -> 0.75000000	

average commute time [56], restarted random walk [57], Cos+ index [58], and SimRank index [52].

(3) Algorithm Implementation Case

In this paper, the Jaccard coefficient in network topology similarity [48] and PPI network data have been used as inputs for predicting links to unconnected nodes in the PPI network.

Jaccard coefficient definition: Given two sets *A* and *B*, Jaccard coefficient is the ratio of the size of the intersection of *A* and *B* to the size of the union of *A* and *B*, which is defined as follows:

$$J(A,B) = \frac{|A \cap B|}{|A \cup B|} = \frac{|A \cap B|}{|A| + |B| - |A \cap B|}$$

The implementation of Python core code is shown in Table 2.2. The program input is PPI network data (the node number represents the number corresponding to the protein), and the results are shown in Fig. 2.2.

The number of nodes in the above figure represents the number of nodes in the PPI network in this program. We retained the mapping relationship between the numbers and protein molecules. As observed, using Jaccard coefficient, we calculated the relationship index between ATP6V1B1 (node 17) and ATP6V1A (node 1546) as 0.75.

(4) Application of Link Prediction in Network Pharmacology

Link prediction is not limited to social networks, but also has great application value in the biomedical field. With the development of network medicine, researchers have begun to analyze and predict the interaction between proteins,

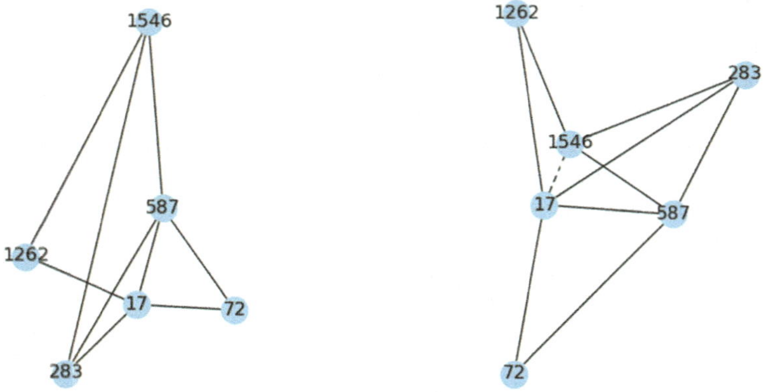

Fig. 2.2 Effect diagrams before and after operation of link prediction program

drugs, and targets at the molecular level [53]. There are links between nodes of protein interaction and the metabolic network [54, 71], which indicates that there is an interaction between them. The prediction of missing drug–target network and suspicious link is helpful to explore the mechanism of action of different drugs and to predict and evaluate drug efficacy. However, revealing the hidden interaction in such networks increases the cost of biological experiments, while the results of link prediction guide these experiments, improving the success rate of experiments, and thus reducing experimental costs. In addition, link prediction can also be used to find similar drugs in the drug network, as well as to find new drug targets, opening up a new path for the research and development of new drugs [72].

4. Analysis Based on Machine Learning

This analysis is different from analytical strategies based on structural comparison or action network simulation. Machine learning-based analytical methods have a more flexible database. It can be a structure, a network, or any other detection index that can be quantified. Many machine learning-based methods have been used to identify relationships between drugs and targets. Machine learning is an analysis method that generates prediction models based on some underlying algorithms and given data sets. It can be divided into unsupervised learning methods (clustering, dimension reduction, association, etc.), supervised learning methods (regression, classification, etc.), and semi-supervised learning methods. In most machine learning-based approaches, biological data sets from multiple sources are integrated, such as chemical structures of drugs, target protein sequences, and known drug–target interactions.

In terms of supervised learning, Yamanishi et al. [31] proposed a nuclear-regression-based method to infer drug target interaction by integrating chemical structure information of compounds, sequence information of target proteins, and topology of known drug target interaction network, to study the interaction of four kinds of drug targets in humans. Bleakley and Yamanishi [30] developed a supervised learning approach based on a two-part local model (BLM) to predict unknown drug–target interactions, by transforming the edge prediction problem into a binary classification problem. Further, Yamanishi et al. [67] believed that pharmacological action similarity was related more to drug–target interaction than chemical structure similarity, so they further proposed a correlation-based model to infer the unknown drug–target relationship based on chemical structure information, genome sequence information, and large-scale pharmacological action information.

In terms of semi-supervised learning, Xia et al. [73] developed NetLapRLS, a semi-supervised learning method that combines chemical space, genomic space, and known drug–protein interaction network information into a heterogeneous biosphere to predict potential drug–target interactions.

In terms of deep learning, Wang and Zeng [74] proposed a method based on restricted Boltzmann machine (RBM). This framework of multidimensional drug target network not only predicts the binary interaction between drugs and targets, but also predicts the interactions between different types of drugs (i.e., how drugs interact). Ramsundar et al. integrated millions of data points, representing both positive and negative examples of DTI with more than 200 specific goals [34]. They used a multi-tasking framework in which each target prediction is considered a separate task that requires its own (linear) classifier. The AUC (area under the receiver operation curve) of the maximum cross-validation achieved by the deep learning method is 0.87, and it is proven that the multi-tasking aspects of their method always provide slight improvement (AUC increases about 0.01) with the same amount of data compared with the same single task analysis. Wen et al. [59] proposed Deep DTIs, a drug target prediction algorithm framework based on Deep Learning. This method first uses unsupervised pre-training to extract the characterization from the original input descriptor, and then uses the known drug target relationship tags to construct a classification model. Compared to other methods, DeepDTIs perform better and can be further used to predict whether a new drug target is associated with other existing targets or whether a new target interacts with some existing drugs. In addition to improving the prediction performance of deep learning models, the analysis of key chemical characteristics learned by machine learning models for predicting drug activity is also important for understanding the performance of the model, screening models with better generalization ability, and for further protein-compound binding modes. Ding et al. proposed a method to analyze the chemical characteristics learned from the QSAR model based on the neural network hidden layer functions and backtracking gradients. They then developed an interactive tool to identify the molecular characteristics of the GPCR family protein targets binding to compounds, which can be verified by eutectic structural analysis.

In DTI prediction, the general machine learning process is divided into three steps. Firstly, the input data of drugs and targets are preprocessed. The underlying model is then trained based on a set of learning rules. Finally, the test data set is predicted by using the prediction model [45]. Kumari et al. [95] developed a sequence-based prediction method to identify and distinguish human non-drug and drug target proteins. Training features include amino acid sequence characteristics, composition, and dipeptide compositions used to produce prediction models.

Through 10-fold cross-validation and leave-one-out validation tests, the sensitivity, specificity, and accuracy of the model (above 80%), and the Matthews correlation coefficient (above 0.7), can help in evaluating the composition pattern of human drug targets [75]. Zhang et al. [76] proposed a clustering-based multi-view DTI prediction method to achieve more accurate DTI predictions by integrating drug and target data from different views and maximizing clustering consistency in each view, to predict 54 kinds of potential DTI [76]. Jamali et al. [77] used machine learning method to analyze 443 sequence-derived protein features to predict whether proteins had drug properties, and compared the properties of different machine learning methods and conducted feature selection. New drug targets have been identified in cell signaling pathways, gene expression, and signal transduction [77].

In addition, this section provides a description of HTINet [78], a TCM target prediction method based on representation learning. In recent years, with the continuous development of network medicine and pharmacology, multi-source biological network data and databases have been widely accumulated, providing adequate data support for researchers. Meanwhile, representation learning [79] is developing rapidly in the field of deep learning. It is a method that learns the feature representation of each node in the network through the network structure and makes the node feature representation fit the original network structure. This method has been applied in many fields (image, video, and natural language understanding) and achieved good results. The HTINet model integrates TCM and Western medicine data (including Traditional Chinese Medicine, disease, symptoms, Western medicine, and targets) based on symptoms, and integrates a multi-source heterogeneous data network. It also obtains feature representations of Chinese medicine and genes based on the network representation method and finally builds a supervised classification model obtained from previous learning to predict the interaction relationship between Chinese medicine targets. The method flow is shown in Fig. 2.3.

The HTINet model has achieved a maximum of 95% AUC and 94% AUPR on the test set, and its performance has been greatly improved compared with the baseline model, indicating its potential in the prediction of TCM targets. In addition, this work also carried out external validation on some experimental results, randomly selected three Traditional Chinese Medicines (Polygonum bistorta, flos farfarae, and *Rhododendron dauricum*), and predicted its targets through the HTINet model and effectively verified the predicted targets in external databases and literature.

2.2.2 Study on the Drug Property Mechanism

One of the central research objectives of network pharmacology is to completely characterize the biological process under Drug property, i.e. to clarify the mechanism of Drug property. The clarification of intracellular chemical reactions and pathways is the most challenging issue in this field. Common biological pathways are related to metabolism, gene expression regulation, and molecular signaling.

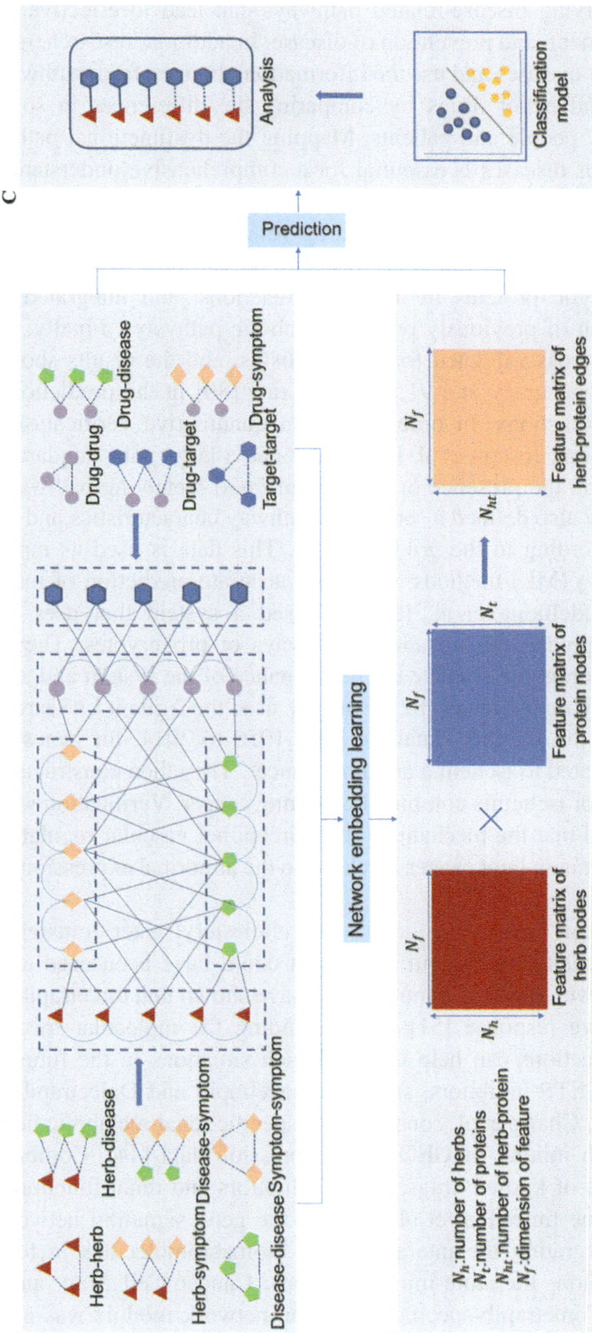

Fig. 2.3 HTINet model construction [78]

Pathways play a key role in the advanced research of functional genomics. For example, identifying disease-related pathways can lead to effective strategies for diagnosis, treatment, and prevention of disease. In addition, researchers can discover the root cause of diseases and use the information obtained from pathway analysis to develop new and better drugs by comparing the differences in some pathways between healthy people and patients. Mapping the dysfunctional pathways associated with various diseases is essential for a comprehensive understanding of these diseases.

One of the common problems in drug research is the accurate prediction of pathways and molecular functions. Pireddu et al. [80] proposed a model for predicting catalytic proteins in important reactions, and integrated these into a prototype system of previously proven metabolic pathways. Finally, 10 metabolic pathways were cross-validated for 13 organisms, and the results showed a 71.5% cross-validation accuracy and 91.5% recall rate [80] in the prediction of catalytic proteins of all reactions. In order to find a quantitative verification method for pathway prediction, Joseph et al. [81] developed a large gold standard data set that contained data on the presence or absence of 5610 metabolic pathways in various organisms. They also defined a set of 123 pathway characteristics and evaluated the information according to the gold standard. This data is used as input in various machine learning (ML) methods to achieve accurate prediction of metabolic pathways [81]. Boudellioua et al. [82] proposed a system that uses "rule mining techniques" to predict the metabolic pathways of prokaryotes. They used cross-validation technology to evaluate the performance of the system and achieved good results in identifying pathways [82]. Fan et al. used the Agilent LitSearch tool [67] to dig deeper into the Pubmed database from 1950 to 2014, for genes that regulate angiogenesis related to ischemia and lung cancer. They then constructed the disease target network for ischemia combined with lung cancer. Verification with molecular biology revealed that the mechanism of bidirectional vascular regulation in animal models of ischemia in lung cancer is related to the abnormal expression of elastase in centrioles [73].

Torcetrapib can inhibit the activity of cholesteryl ester transfer protein and increase high density lipoprotein in vivo. It could have been used as a new anti-lipid drug; however, phase III clinical trials have shown that torcetrapib can induce a fatal hypertensive response [51]. Understanding the molecular mechanisms that induce lethal reactions can help to avoid such situations in the future and clarify whether other CETP inhibitors, such as Anacetrapib and Dalcetrapib should continue to be used. Chang et al. constructed a specific renal metabolic network model through in-depth mining of GEO gene expression data [44]. Combined with the off-target effects of known drugs, CETP inhibitors and renal function were evaluated. At the same time, Fan et al. mapped the gene signaling network of human diseases by integrating the interactions of biomacromolecules in four databases including BioCarta, literature-mined network, Cancer Cell Map, and the HPRD database [45]. Torcetrapib-specific regulation network module was mined by analyzing the GEO database, and the abnormal gene set regulation of torcetrapib was drawn. The possible explanation of torcetrapib-induced hypertension was thus clarified from a systematic view point.

Drug property model is the key to drug development. It usually involves a target through which a drug can induce pharmacological effects, including understanding the drug influence pathway and biological processes. This information can be used to support treatment hypotheses in animal models, clinical indications, and patient selection. It is also important to distinguish new drugs from current standards, treatments, and competing molecules. Although the mode of action of drugs is not necessary for FDA approval, most researchers hope to understand the function of drugs at the molecular level. There are already some examples of artificial intelligence usage to solve the discovery of Drug property patterns. Pang et al. [83] used "random forests" to analyze gene expression data and established a path based classification and regression method. This approach allows researchers to sequence important pathways from externally available databases, and identify important genes to take advantage of a continuous outcome variable in regression settings [83]. Hancock et al. [84] proposed a new classification model, HME3M. This probabilistic model is a combination of a mixed Markov model, which is used to identify frequently observed path clusters in a specific network structure, and proves that the HME3M algorithm is superior to the comparison method in the case of increasing network complexity and path noise. It is an accurate and reliable classification of metabolic pathways [84].

Carfilzomib is a conventional drug for treating multiple myeloma. However, clinical studies have found that long-term use of Carfilzomib can induce drug resistance in multiple myeloma. Zheng et al. analyzed KMS-11 cell lines that are resistant and sensitive to Carfilzomib in the GEO database, through a string biological macromolecule interaction platform [52]. This helped to model a gene regulatory network related to Carfilzomib resistance. The enrichment analysis results showed that abnormal changes in cytokine and receptor, autophagy, ErbB signaling, microRNA, and fatty acid metabolism pathways may be related to drug resistance exhibited in patients treated with Carfilzomib for multiple myeloma [53].

2.2.3 Discovery of New Drug Uses

Network pharmacology is not only used for drug target discovery and mechanism interpretation, but also for the discovery of new drug uses. Phenotypic and omics data generated in drug experiments and clinical applications provide important clues for the discovery of new drug uses. Artificial intelligence plays an important role in the use of this data.

1. Analysis of Drug-Phenotype Data

Drug phenotypic analysis is a method for analyzing the phenotypic changes in an organism after Drug property. It identifies the effects of a drug by analyzing cell and animal models in a disease state. Although drug discovery based on drug targets once dominated the scene, several new disease targets determined by genomics and systems biology methods are categorized as non-usable [85]. Moreover, the function of these new targets is unclear. These issues have prompted researchers to refocus on the discovery of drug phenotypes as a complement to target-based drug discovery [86]. The phenotype of the drug includes characteristics of the drug's indications, side effects, etc., which are reflected at the individual level. Drug phenotypes can be attributed to many molecular interactions, including on-target or off-target binding, drug–drug interactions, dose-dependent pharmacokinetics, metabolic activity, downstream pathway interference, aggregation effects, and irreversible target binding. Although certain drug phenotypes such as side effects are unexpected results of drug intervention, they help in understanding the physiological changes caused by drugs. Phenotype-based methods for discovering new uses of drugs are being valued increasingly by researchers.

PubChem's bioassay function contains more than 740 million data points from biochemistry and phenotypic screening, covering more than 1 million biologically active molecules. Several compounds have hundreds or even thousands of analysis results [21, 22]. ChEMBL contains biometric data with more than 12 million data points. NPCPD29 contains a drug-phenotype matrix of nearly 35 clinically approved compounds, covering cardiovascular disease, diabetes, and cancer. In addition, the Center for Chemical Genomics of the National Institutes of Health has compiled a data set of approximately 2500 approved compounds that are screened in approximately 200 phenotypic and target-based tests, focusing on various cancers, malaria, nuclear receptors, and signal pathways [23].

Research on the sensitivity of cancer cell lines is the most important task in network pharmacology based on cell phenotype screening. The Cancer Therapeutic Response Portal assessed the sensitivity of 242 cancer cell lines with genetic characteristics to 354 types of small molecule probes and drugs [16]. The GDSC (Genomics of Drug Sensitivity in Cancer) database measured 138 anticancer drugs in 700 cell lines [18]. The Cancer Cell Line encyclopedia provides detailed genetic characterization of 1000 cancer cell lines and can be used to assess cell line similarity and predict drug perturbation growth rates in other cell lines [24].

SIDER (Side Effects Resources) is a public side effect database that contains compiled information from FDA package specifications, linking 888 drugs with 1450 side effects [27]. The OFFSIDES database analyzed more than 400,000 adverse reactions not listed on the official FDA drug labels, and determined that each drug had an average of 329 off-label ADEs [28]. Finally, the FDA Adverse Event Reporting System (FAERS) is the database of information on adverse event and drug error reports submitted to the FDA by manufacturers, health-care professionals, and the public [29, 30].

Relationships between drugs and phenotypes can be used to identify shared target proteins among chemically different drugs and to infer new indications using their phenotypic similarities [87]. One of the underlying principles behind this theory and related approaches is that drugs that share a large number of similar phenotypes may be associated with common mechanisms of action associated with the treatment of a disease, and may serve as phenotypic biomarkers for specific diseases

[88]. Currently, several new indications and targets have been found by using drug phenotypes using artificial intelligence methods. For example, Dimitri et al. developed DrugClust [89], a machine learning algorithm for drug side effects prediction. According to the Bayesian score, the first batch of drugs was clustered based on their characteristics, and then the side effects were predicted. Biological validation of the clustering can be completed using enrichment analysis. The process of drug discovery is realized by verifying obtained clusters and possible new interactions between some side effects and non-targeted pathways. Luo et al. [90] constructed a drug side effect network based on SIDER2 (Side Effect Resource 2) database, and introduced the link prediction method into the network to develop and evaluate the framework of drug side effect prediction. Ferrero et al. [91] developed the drug re-positioning hypothesis on the basis of disease genetics by mining the public repository and transcriptome profiles of GWAS (Genome-Wide Association Studies) data [91]. Yin et al. [92] used the drug indications in the Medicine Indications Resource (MEDI) as the gold standard to evaluate whether the drug indications found from GWAS and Phewa (Phenome-Wide Association Studies) have clinical indications [92]. Yang et al. [88] extracted the relationship between 3175 diseases and SEs (Side Effects). A naive Bayesian model was then established based on SEs' features to predict the indications of 145 diseases. In addition, the QSAR model of SEs was used to predict the indications of 4200 clinical molecules [88]. Ye et al. [93] constructed a drug–drug network based on the similarity of clinical side effects. The indication of a drug can be inferred by enriching the function of its neighboring FDA-approved drug in the network. It has high accuracy in drug prediction for diabetes, obesity, laxatives, and mycobacteria infection. A large number of predicted results were approved by the FDA or supported by preclinical/clinical studies [93]. Previous studies have shown that chemical structure, target protein, and side effects can provide rich information for drug similarity evaluation. However, each individual data source plays an important role on its own, and data integration is expected to reposition drugs more accurately. Wang et al. [94] established a new drug re-positioning method (predicted drug re-positioning) by integrating the molecular structure, molecular activity, and phenotypic data, and by characterizing drugs by analyzing their chemical structure, target proteins, and side effect data, and defining their disease-related core functions. Then, an SVM was trained to calculate and predict new drug–disease interactions, which has advantages over other methods in terms of accuracy and coverage rate [94].

Scheiber et al. used the known drug–ADE (adverse drug event) association, and the extension of NaïveBayes modeling to connect specific chemical characteristics of drugs with 4210 ADE terms [56]. Liu et al. used the causal relationship analysis based on Bayesian network structure to connect the chemical and biological characteristics of drugs with ADE, which can be interpreted as causality [57]. Vilar et al. used the GBA method in large insurance claims databases to estimate drug associations with four different ADE: acute kidney failure, acute liver failure, acute myocardial infarction, and upper gastrointestinal ulcer [58].

2. Transcriptome Data Analysis

The omics data generated from drug trials undoubtedly provides valuable information for the discovery of new uses of drugs. Compared with other omics data such as proteomics and metabolomics, transcriptome data have many advantages such as high throughput, low cost, precise quantification, and sufficient complexity. Therefore, the large-scale use of transcriptome data for drug discovery is the most rapidly developed and mature method.

(1) Integrated Library Project Based on Network Cellular Response Imprinting (LINCS) [95]

The CMap project [96] and LINCS (The Library of Integrated Network-Based Cellular Signatures) project [97] promoted the development of a comprehensive and large-scale transcriptome database with drug research as an important goal. Drugs and target perturbation data collected and recorded have been used to determine the connections, similarities, or differences between diseases, drugs, genes, and pathways, which provide great opportunities for computational pharmacogenomics and drug design. Unlike classic pharmacology that only focuses on one target at a time, the transcriptomics data provided by CMap and LINCS opens the door for systems biology methods at the pathway and network level [98]. The LINCS project highlights the potential of gene transcription analysis as a universal language for linking chemistry, biology, and clinical practice by inferring genome-wide similarities or differences [99]. In recent years, several studies have used various machine learning methods to analyze Cmap data and LINCS data for target discovery and drug re-positioning. For example, Xie et al. [100] systematically explored and predicted the re-positioning of 480 marketed drugs with other therapeutic attributes using LINCS drug-induced transcript level data, which was based on the machine learning algorithm Softmax for multiple classification problems. Young et al. [101] used the gene silencing perturbation data in LINCS, adopted the linear regression model, and combined the prior and posterior probability to infer the regulatory relationship in genes, thus verifying the relationship identified in the TRANSFAC (TRANScription FACtor database) and JASPAR. Lee et al. [102] used LINCS data to evaluate the ability to predict novel re-positioning of drugs based on several perturbations in four cancer types [102]. Sawada et al. [103] proposed a new computational method for predicting inhibition and activation targets of drug candidate compounds. Integrating chemical induction and gene interference with the gene expression profile of human cell lines helps avoid excessive dependence on the chemical structure of compounds or proteins. Based on the transcriptomic changes of the overall gene expression profile after chemical treatment, as well as the transcriptomic changes after gene knockout and overexpression, the combined learning algorithm was used to build a prediction model of a single target protein. This method can distinguish inhibition targets from activation targets, and can accurately identify therapeutic effects [103]. Liu et al. analyzed the CMap transcription profile and revealed its hidden factors by weighted gene co-expression network analysis (WGCNA). Simultaneously, seven common modules associated with protein binding, extracellular matrix tissue, and translation were identified. Finally, the drugs were clustered by module expression, and the mechanism of action (MoA) was inferred according to their common activity profiles. Sirota et al. systematically compared the gene expression profiles of 164 small molecule compounds from CMAP with a set of expression profiles derived from the GEO database for 100 different diseases. Based on this model, more than 1000 drug repurposing predictions were generated, linking at least one of 164 compounds to each of the 53 diseases [48].

(2) Gene Expression Omnibus (GEO) [104, 105]

The Gene Expression Omnibus (GEO) is a public information storage platform managed and maintained by the National Center for Biotechnology Information (NCBI) of the United States. The database mainly provides gene expression data retrieval, browsing, query, and download services, and is an important source for obtaining high-throughput chip expression profiles data. GEO includes two sub-databases: Datasets and Profiles database. The Datasets database stores the data of gene chip centered on experiments. The Profiles database stores gene-centric chip data. Currently, GEO has more than 900 drug perturbation experiments and can be another direct source of drug–target perturbations in network pharmacology research.

(3) ArrayExpress Database [106]

The ArrayExpress database is a microarray common repository of gene expression data developed and operated by the European Bioinformatics Institute (EMBI). Its main purpose is to store and record annotated high-throughput data sets and original image sets from all over the world. The ArrayExpress interface is simple and supports multiple retrieval methods. So far, the database includes more than 6000 sets of high-throughput experimental data, including expression data such as RNA-seq, ChIP-seq, GRO-seq, epigenetic profiles, and FAIRE-seq.

3. Docking Profiles Data Analysis

The combination of listed drug targets that are not thoroughly studied with different targets leads to a wide range of side effects. Hence, the cost of screening all potential molecular targets in biological experiments is high. The "molecular docking profiles" using virtual large-scale molecular docking is helpful to study the drug–target relationship, and plays an important role in the development of new clinical indications of drugs. Yang et al. [107] used molecular docking and logistic regression to construct a real-time prediction server DPDR-CPI based on small molecular structures. When a user submits a molecule, the server docks it with 611 human proteins to generate predictive CPI (chemical–protein interactome) characteristic profiles. It shows the correlation between the input molecules and about 1000 human diseases, and gives the highest prediction results [107]. Chen et al. [108] proposed a new ligand-based pipeline: given a set of experimental data, first, use principal component analysis (PCA) and genetic algorithm (GA) to establish a segment descriptor with the signature of the SVM model, and then the pipeline develops QSARs in the form of the SVM prediction model, and applies the model in virtually screen compound databases [108].

Chavali et al. used the metabolic model to generate lists of 15 genes and 8 dual-gene combinations that were predicted to be relevant targets for neglected tropical diseases (mainly Leishmaniasis) [70]. By associating these genes with 254 FDA-approved compounds based on drug–target interactions, it was found that 14% (10 of 71) of these compounds were validated in overlapping with high content screening data for leishmaniasis. In addition, Chen et al. integrated information such as drug–target interaction, disease–gene association, and protein–protein interaction networks into heterogeneous networks (DrugNet, linking drugs, targets, and diseases) [35]. Using the ProphNet network propagation algorithm, we can define the input query node, drug, or disease, and rank the remaining nodes of other types, that is, the drug for the disease query, and vice versa.

4. Web-Based Drug Indication Analysis

With advancement in the interaction group detection methods and the accumulation of data resources, the discovery of drug indications based on network analysis is widely used in network pharmacology. Relevant studies have shown that drug–target network, drug–drug, drug–disease, protein–protein interaction, transcriptional, and signal transduction networks can be used to identify the efficacy characteristics of drugs, thus providing new opportunities for drug discovery or indication discovery.

Li et al. [109] developed a binary drug–target network approach to identify potential new indications for existing drugs through their relationship with similar drugs. In the bipartite network model, drug pair similarity integrates chemical structure similarity, common drug targets, and protein interactions. The author established a causal network (CauseNet) [110] based on the previous work, which is based on a multi-layered approach to genes, diseases, and drug targets to determine new therapeutic uses of existing drugs. In the causal network, the transition probability of each chain is estimated based on the known drug–disease treatment association.

Wu et al. [111] used the known relationship between disease genes and drug targets in the KEGG database to construct a heterogeneous drug network. Nodes represent drugs or diseases, and edges represent shared genes, biological processes, pathways, phenotypes, or combinations of these characteristics. The network is then clustered to identify modules that can be used to extract potential drug–disease pairs for drug re-positioning. This method not only considers genes, but also other features of constructing disease drug networks.

Chen et al. [68] developed a method based on functional linkage network (FLN) to find modules negatively related to drugs. FLN is a network in which nodes (proteins or genes) are connected by weighted edges to measure the probability of sharing a common biological function. The network is constructed by using different biological information sources (such as mutation and transcription level). These information sources act as the features of a Bayesian classifier, and calculate the possibility of each edge. FLN's filtering method is to remove all genes that are not within the user-specified genetic distance from the disease mutation and display differential expression below a certain threshold. Such networks are processed to determine the extent to which drugs and disease-related genes are associated with possible re-positioning of candidate genes.

Ali et al. [69] used centrality measurement commonly used in social network analysis to identify drugs with better positioning in the side effect and drug indication networks. The basic assumption of this work was that drugs with similar phenotype profiles (e.g., side effects) can share similar therapeutic properties based on relevant mechanisms of action and vice versa. The development of side effect resources includes unique drugs with side effects and indications. Drugs are ranked according to their centrality scores, thus identifying 18 major drugs from the drug side effect network and 15 major drugs from the drug indication network. Indications and side effects of prominent drugs were inferred from profiles of their network neighbors and compared with existing clinical studies, while seeking optimal similarity threshold values between drugs. Threshold values can then be used to predict indications and side effects for all drugs. The similarities are measured by the extent to which they share a phenotypic profiles and neighbors.

Campillos proposed in 2008 that drug–target interaction networks using the principle of side-effect similarity might be overlooked in new drug discovery. By analyzing the side effects of 746 drugs already in the market, his team constructed a drug-side-target network with 1018 nodes, and found some new activities and new indications of some drugs through biological verification [87].

5. Analysis of Drug Indication Based on Machine Learning

The prediction of drug indication is also a typical machine learning problem [70]. Specifically, the interaction between drugs and the human body can be gauged and predicted through a series of clinical and biological characteristics. In this section, we summarize the general principles and types of drug indication analysis algorithms based on machine learning.

An important advantage of machine learning algorithm is its richness and rapid development. Any existing or new algorithm can be applied to drug indication analysis with some modification. In this section, the drug expression profile data combined with the machine learning algorithm is taken as an example to predict its indications, i.e. drug expression profile is used as a predictor (i.e., feature) for the therapeutic potential of drugs. The resulting variable can be a drug, for example, cardiovascular or anticancer drug or a drug targeted at a specific disease like diabetes. In the former case, consideration may be given to the classification of a drug in a category other than its own indications, for re-positioning. In the latter case, a drug with a high predictive probability but not shown as a disease, may be a candidate for re-positioning. Existing indications for drugs are readily available from public web resources such as the Anatomical Therapeutic Chemistry (ATC) classification system. The following is a detailed introduction of different types of drug indication prediction methods:

In terms of the prediction of drug indications, a linear model has advantages of rapid calculation speed, intuitiveness, and can be easily realized by a variety of programming languages and statistical software. For example, the glmnet package in R language supports rapid implementation of normalized linear models and has detailed documentation available online [112]. Linear models are also easy to explain, as the importance of features can be gauged from the size of the regression coefficient, and methods have recently been developed to assess statistical significance [113]. However, linear models capture only linear relationships between input characteristics and output variables, which may not be the case in many real-world scenarios, including biomedical applications. A recent study [114] identified transcriptional response as a multi-label classification problem, identified novel therapeutic properties of drugs, and pointed out that multi-label logistic regression is superior to other methods such as random forest and convolutional neural networks.

In terms of drug indication prediction methods based on classification and regression models, Napolitano et al. [115] integrated a variety of drug characteristics, including chemical structure and proximity of targets in the interaction network and expression profiles, and used support vector machine (SVM) to predict the treatment category. Menden et al. [116] developed a machine learning model to predict the response of cancer cell lines to drug treatment, which was quantified by a semi-inhibitory concentration (IC50) value. In this model, the feed-forward perceptron neural network model and random forest regression model were established using the oncogenome characteristics and chemical properties (such as structural fingerprints) of the cell line. The predicted IC50 value was further cross-validated and independent blind tests were done. Gottlieb et al. [117] integrated various disease-related characteristics (such as phenotype and genetic characteristics), calculated the similarity of drugs and diseases, constructed classification features and further used logistic regression classifiers to predict new drug indications.

In terms of predicting drug indications based on collaborative filtering technology, Zhang et al. [118] proposed a unified calculation framework for integrating the multidimensional features of drug similarity and disease similarity. Simply put, drug similarity matrix and disease similarity matrix are extracted by integrating genome (e.g., drug target protein, disease gene), phenotype (e.g., disease phenotype, drug side effect), and chemical structure (e.g., drug chemical structure). Based on this information, this author turns the drug–disease network analysis into an optimization problem. This computational framework shows the effectiveness of exploring new indications for drugs. Yang et al. [119] used causal inference probability matrix factorization to infer drug–disease correlation. In this model, they integrate multi-level relationships, construct causal networks linking drug–target–pathway–gene–disease and learn PMF patterns based on known interactions. This approach can predict new drug–disease associations and thus be of value for drug indication analysis.

2.2.4 Traditional Chinese Medicine and Its Therapeutic Theory

The composition of TCM prescriptions is complex, and research on its ingredients and treatment is more complex than that of chemical drugs. Network pharmacology plays an important role in revealing the material basis of TCM and the theoretical research of treatment with TCM. Researchers are increasingly using artificial intelligence to solve important problems such as prediction of Chinese medicine target in theoretical research of TCM, molecular mechanism of Chinese medicine prescriptions, and molecular mechanism of syndrome theory.

1. TCM Target Prediction

The determination of drug targets is the key to drug R & D. TCM usually needs to have a synergistic effect between different ingredients due to its complex compound composition, resulting in the complex TCM mechanism of action. In terms of actual target prediction, Zhang et al. [120] proposed a systematic pharmacology method to predict the complexity of compound components and related multiple targets. This was done by identifying bioactive compounds of TCM, to clarify its molecular mechanism of action. System pharmacology method also helps to understand the complex interactions between biological systems, drugs, and diseases from a network perspective. Modern technologies such as drug screening (high-throughput screening, high content screening, and virtual screening) and omics methods (proteomics, genomics, metabolomics) have also been widely used in the identification of bioactive ingredients and drug targets in TCM. Wang et al. [121] introduced high content screening technology and used the HCS instrument to screen TCM-derived compounds and promoted technology development. In order to promote research on the function and mechanism of TCM, ETCM [122] provides the predicted target genes of Chinese medicine ingredients, TCM, and prescriptions according to the similarity of chemical fingerprints between TCM ingredients and known drugs. In the ETCM system, researchers also explored the relationship between TCM, formula, ingredients, gene target, and related pathways or diseases, to finally establish a network structure.

With the development of artificial intelligence, especially the progress made in natural language processing, drug target prediction and discovery have been combined to greatly improve research efficiency. Biomedical literature information can be obtained from the network. Sometimes the abstracts of these literatures contain important frontier research information of drugs and targets. If we can capture the latest research trends of drug targets on time, it will help to advance the process of target prediction. Extracting valuable information from massive amount of literature is the main aim of natural language processing. Real-time literature is collected through web crawler technology, and then large-scale distributed storage is carried out, which can be cleaned by data extraction, exchange, and loading, to preprocess structured data. Then, by using methods such as part-of-speech analysis, grammatical analysis, and semantic analysis in natural language processing technology, combined with the similarity analysis, cluster analysis, topic mining, and relationship extraction in machine learning, the relationship between drugs and targets is established. Combined with the database of known drug targets, the knowledge mining system is conversely applied to improve the accuracy of drug target knowledge, thus further improving the efficiency of drug target prediction and reducing costs.

2. Study on the Molecular Mechanism of TCM Prescriptions

TCM and its formulations contain many active molecules with complex ingredients, resulting in complex interactions and mechanisms of action. Only by further understanding the mechanism of action and clinical efficacy can we help users. The basic form of TCM for disease prevention and treatment is TCM compound prescription, which is a quantitative mixture of several specific Chinese herbal medicinal plants. There are a lot of chemical substances in TCM compound prescriptions, which may interact with multiple disease-related targets. Therefore, at the molecular level, the TCM compound mechanism used for disease treatment is like that of multi-directional pharmacology or network pharmacology. TCM has existed since ancient times in China. Molecular biology originated in modern times, and its effective combination with TCM is a topic that needs to be explored. If we can prove the rationality of TCM prescriptions and formulas at the molecular level, it will help to integrate modern science and technology with ancient Chinese medicine prescriptions, which will not only provide a more reasonable scientific basis for further optimization of TCM prescriptions, but also provide a solid backing for TCM's growth in the international market. At present, many pharmacological studies have been used to reveal the mechanism of action of TCM and its molecular mechanism. For example, research in the field of aging shows that hemopoietic stem cell autophagy has anti-aging effects, and there are many new discoveries in the field of plant extracts and Chinese herbal medicine [123]. Among them, Chinese herbal medicine extracts represented by curcumin and resveratrol, some single Chinese medicine extracts, and classical Chinese medicine prescriptions have partial anti-aging effects by regulating the molecular mechanism of aging in vivo and in vitro. Research on the molecular mechanism of TCM prescriptions can be carried out with the help of the TCM information database TCM-ID [124], which provides comprehensive information on TCM, including prescription ingredients, molecular structure, and functional characteristics of TCM ingredients and active ingredients, TCM formula, clinical indications, and application of each Chinese herbal medicine. Zhu et al. designed the framework of the TCM prescription analysis system based on existing TCM prescription data resources and TCM prescription analysis systems, using artificial intelligence and data mining technology. This system assists in various applications, such as knowledge extraction and knowledgebase construction, establishment and improvement of prescription database, medication experience sorting and mining, and new drug development [125].

3. Study on Biomolecular Network Mechanism of TCM Syndromes

The biological basis of syndromes is the key to modernizing TCM. Currently, research is being conducted on blood stasis, cold syndrome, heat syndrome, etc. Research on syndromes includes several aspects such as the nature and essence of the syndrome and micro-syndrome differentiation [126]. The syndrome usually refers to the overall physiological and pathological state of the human body and diagnosis based on it. The TCM theory of disease treatment has gradually developed on the basis of syndrome differentiation. Syndrome theory has accompanied the development of TCM and has been guiding clinical work as well. However, syndromes and their classification have not been effectively developed in recent years. The main reason lies in the lack of appropriate supportive scientific data, and what information exists, is often obtained through subjective inquiry from TCM doctors. In recent years, the basic research of syndrome biology has shifted from inquiry to theoretical research and has made a lot of progress. Some studies have tried to correlate the phenotype of the syndrome with the microbiological molecules, and then studied the syndrome. They have further combined it with modern scientific means to prove some of the already existing syndrome theories. Domestically, some scholars have studied the theory of syndrome biology from the perspective of biomolecular network [126], and have established a multi-layer architecture from phenotypic network, biomolecular network to drug network. Based on this network framework, some typical syndromes such as cold and heat syndromes were studied, which laid a good foundation for the scientific theoretical research of syndromes. At the same time, the characteristics of diseases and syndromes on the biological molecular network were studied, thus providing additional means of finding methods and drugs for systematic intervention of these disease syndromes. Therefore, the old topic of TCM syndrome differentiation and treatment has been extended to the modern field of molecules.

2.3 Application of Artificial Intelligence

This chapter briefly introduces the application of artificial intelligence technology in network pharmacology. With the rapid accumulation of effective data in the life science and pharmaceutical research fields, it has led to unique perspectives on the application of machine learning in new drug development or drug re-positioning. Information on the structure of small drug molecules is available on the PubChem [127] and drug bank [128] databases. These databases contain information of listed drugs, and QSAR is often used to study drugs with annotated information, to find potential new drugs [44]. The PDB (Protein Data Bank archive) [129] database reveals drug–target interaction relationship, based on ligand–target structure related data, information on side effects from Sider [130], and vector data for drug–target interaction relationships. These can be used to predict potential new targets for drugs [45]. In terms of omics data, there is a GEO (Gene Expression Omnibus) database that stores high-throughput chip data [131], TCGA (The Cancer Genome Atlas) [132], etc. There are databases on expression profile based on cell response to drugs under different conditions, used to predict drug interactions/indications [100, 133] and side effects [134]. In summary, these expansive, high-dimensional databases provide relevant information on artificial intelligence, which plays an important role in drug research. The use of artificial intelligence to guide drug screening and discovery in future drug development may become the norm and bring revolutionary changes to the pharmaceutical industry.

References

1. Hopkins AL. Network pharmacology: the next paradigm in drug discovery. Nat Chem Biol. 2008;4(11):682–90.
2. Zhang Y. Progress in network pharmacology and modern research of traditional Chinese medicine. Chin J Pharmacol Toxicol. 2015;29(06):883–92 (in Chinese).
3. Maulik U, Bandyopadhyay S. Genetic algorithm-based clustering technique. 2000;33.
4. Selim S, Alsultan K. A simulated annealing algorithm for the clustering problem. 1991;24.
5. Zou L. Artificial intelligence and its development and application. Inf Network Secur. 2012 (02):11–3 (in Chinese).
6. Krizhevsky A, Sutskever I, Hinton GE. ImageNet classification with deep convolutional neural networks. Commun ACM. 2017;60(6):84–90.
7. Lecun Y, Boser B, Denker J, et al. Handwritten digit recognition with a back-propagation network. 1997;2.
8. Mikolov T, Deoras A, Povey D, et al. Strategies for training large scale neural network language models. 2011.
9. Mohamed A, Dahl GE, Hinton G. Acoustic modeling using deep belief networks. IEEE Trans Audio Speech Lang Process. 2012;20(1):14–22.
10. Kalinin AA, Higgins GA, Reamaroon N, et al. Deep learning in pharmacogenomics: from gene regulation to patient stratification. Pharmacogenomics. 2018;19(7):629–50.
11. Gawehn E, Hiss JA, Schneider G. Deep learning in drug discovery. Mol Inf. 2016;35(1):3–14.
12. Kotsiantis S. Supervised machine learning: a review of classification techniques. 2007;31.
13. Lecun Y, Bengio Y, Hinton G. Deep learning. Nature. 2015;521(7553):436–44.
14. Jain AK, Murty MN, Flynn PJ. Data clustering: a review. ACM Comput Surv. 1999;31 (3):264–323.
15. Van Der Maaten L, Postma E, Herik H. Dimensionality reduction: a comparative review. 2007;10.
16. Zhou W. Network construction technology in network pharmacology research. Int J Pharm Res. 2016;43(05):797–812 (in Chinese).
17. Akhmedov M, Kedaigle A, Chong RE, et al. PCSF: an R-package for network-based interpretation of high-throughput data. PLoS Comput Biol. 2017;13(7):e1005694.
18. Turing AM. Computing machinery and intelligence// computers and thought. American Association for Artificial Intelligence; 1950.
19. He H, Garcia EA. Learning from imbalanced data. 2009;21.
20. Altschul S, Gish W, Miller W, et al. Basic local alignment search tool. 1990;215.
21. O'Boyle NM, Banck M, James CA, et al. Open Babel: an open chemical toolbox. J Cheminformatics. 2011;3(1):33.
22. Trott O, Olson AJ. AutoDock Vina: improving the speed and accuracy of docking with a new scoring function, efficient optimization, and multithreading. J Comput Chem. 2009:455–61.

23. Case DA, Cheatham TE, Darden T, et al. The Amber biomolecular simulation programs. J Comput Chem. 2005;26(16):1668–88.
24. Iorio F, Tagliaferri R, Bernardo DD. Identifying network of drug mode of action by gene expression profiling. J Comput Biol. 2009;16(2):241–51.
25. Subramanian A, Narayan R, Corsello SM, et al. A next generation connectivity map: L1000 platform and the first 1,000,000 profiles. Cell. 2017;171(6):1437–52.e17.
26. Van Der Maaten L, Hinton G. Visualizing data using t-SNE. J Mach Learn Res. 2008;9:2579–605.
27. Shekhar K, Lapan SW, Whitney IE, et al. Comprehensive classification of retinal bipolar neurons by single-cell transcriptomics. Cell. 2016;166(5):1308–23.e30.
28. Grimes M, Hall B, Foltz L, et al. Integration of protein phosphorylation, acetylation, and methylation data sets to outline lung cancer signaling networks. Sci Signal. 2018;11(531): eaaq1087.
29. Vidyasagar M. Identifying predictive features in drug response using machine learning: opportunities and challenges. Annu Rev Pharmacol Toxicol. 2015;55(1):15–34.
30. Gamazon E, Wheeler H, Shah K. A gene-based association method for mapping traits using reference transcriptome data. 2015;47.
31. Xiong J, Zhou T. Gene regulatory network inference from multifactorial perturbation data. 2012.
32. Yamanishi Y, Kotera M, Moriya Y, et al. DINIES: drug-target interaction network inference engine based on supervised analysis. Nucleic Acids Res. 2014;42(W1):W39–45.
33. Gopalan PK, Blei DM. Efficient discovery of overlapping communities in massive networks. Proc Natl Acad Sci. 2013;110(36):14534–9.
34. Chen H, Engkvist O, Wang Y, et al. The rise of deep learning in drug discovery. Drug Discov Today. 2018;23(6):1241–50.
35. Mayr A, Klambauer G, Unterthiner T, et al. Large-scale comparison of machine learning methods for drug target prediction on ChEMBL. Chem Sci. 2018;9(24):5441–51.
36. Korotcov A, Tkachenko V, Russo DP, et al. Comparison of deep learning with multiple machine learning methods and metrics using diverse drug discovery data sets. Mol Pharm. 2017;14(12):4462–75.
37. Teschendorff AE. Avoiding common pitfalls in machine learning omic data science. Nat Mater. 2019;18(5):422–7.
38. Bero SA, Muda AK, Choo YH, et al. Similarity measure for molecular structure: a brief review. J Phys: Conf Ser. 2017;892:012015.
39. Zhang Y, Cheng X, Zhou W. Drug reorientation: an important application field of network pharmacology. Chin J Pharmacol Toxicol. 2012;26(6):779–85 (in Chinese).
40. Willett P. The calculation of molecular structural similarity: principles and practice. Mol Inf. 2014;33(6–7):403–13.
41. Vilar S, Harpaz R, Uriarte E, et al. Drug—drug interaction through molecular structure similarity analysis. J Am Med Inform Assoc. 2012;19(6):1066–74.
42. Yan C, Wang J, Lan W, et al. SDTRLS: predicting drug-target interactions for complex diseases based on chemical substructures. Complexity. 2017;2017:1–10.
43. Keiser MJ, Setola V, Irwin JJ, et al. Predicting new molecular targets for known drugs. Nature. 2009;462(7270):175–81.
44. Neves BJ, Braga RC, Melo Filho CC, et al. QSAR-based virtual screening: advances and applications in drug discovery. Front Pharmacol. 2018;9:1275.
45. Chen R, Liu X, Jin S, et al. Machine learning for drug-target interaction prediction. Molecules. 2018;23(9):2208.
46. Mitchell JBO. ChemInform abstract: the relationship between the sequence identities of helical proteins in the PDB and the molecular similarities of their ligands. ChemInform. 2002;33(10): no-no.
47. Bleakley K, Yamanishi Y. Supervised prediction of drug–target interactions using bipartite local models. Bioinformatics. 2009;25(18):2397–403.

48. Yamanishi Y, Araki M, Gutteridge A, et al. Prediction of drug–target interaction networks from the integration of chemical and genomic spaces. Bioinformatics. 2008;24(13):i232–40.
49. Michael J, et al. Predicting new molecular targets for known drugs. Nature. 2009;462 (7270):175–81.
50. Martin YC, Kofron JL, Traphagen LM. Do structurally similar molecules have similar biological activity? J Med Chem. 2002;45(19):4350–8.
51. Schuffenhauer A, Floersheim P, Acklin P, et al. Similarity metrics for ligands reflecting the similarity of the target proteins. J Chem Inf Comput Sci. 2003;43(2):391–405.
52. Cheng F, et al. Prediction of drug-target interactions and drug repositioning via network-based inference. PLoS Comput Biol. 2012;8(5):e1002503.
53. Zhao SW, Li S. Network-based relating pharmacological and genomic spaces for drug target identification. PLoS ONE. 2010;5:e11764.
54. Zhang L, Fourches D, Sedykh A, et al. Discovery of novel antimalarial compounds enabled by QSAR-based virtual screening. J Chem Inf Model. 2013;53(2):475–92.
55. Fan S, Li X. Reverse molecular docking: a new approach to discovery and identification of drug targets. Adv Physiol Sci. 2012;043(005):367–70 (in Chinese).
56. Kuhn M, Campillos M, González P, et al. Large-scale prediction of drug-target relationships. FEBS Lett. 2008;582(8):1283–90.
57. Hansen NT, Brunak S, Altman RB. Generating genome-scale candidate gene lists for pharmacogenomics. Clin Pharmacol Ther. 2009;86(2):183–9.
58. Kutalik Z, Beckmann JS, Bergmann S, et al. A modular approach for integrative analysis of large-scale gene-expression and drug-response data. Nat Biotechnol. 2008;26(5):531–9.
59. Chen YZ, Zhi DG. Ligand–protein inverse docking and its potential use in the computer search of protein targets of a small molecule. Proteins. 2001;43(2):217–26.
60. Li H, Gao Z, Kang L, et al. TarFisDock: a web server for identifying drug targets with docking approach. Nucleic Acids Res. 2006;34(Web Server):W219–W224.
61. Liu X, Ouyang S, Yu B, et al. PharmMapper server: a web server for potential drug target identification using pharmacophore mapping approach. Nucleic Acids Res. 2010;38(Web Server):W609–W614.
62. Kinnings SL, Jackson RM. ReverseScreen3D: a structure-based ligand matching method to identify protein targets. J Chem Inf Model. 2011;51(3):624–34.
63. Wang JC, Chu PY, Chen CM, et al. idTarget: a web server for identifying protein targets of small chemical molecules with robust scoring functions and a divide-and-conquer docking approach. Nucleic Acids Res. 2012;40(W1):W393–9.
64. Yue QX, Cao ZW, Guan SH, et al. Proteomics characterization of the cytotoxicity mechanism of ganoderic acid D and computer-automated estimation of the possible drug target network. Mol Cell Proteomics. 2008;7(5):949–61.
65. Feng LX, Jing CJ, Tang KL, et al. Clarifying the signal network of salvianolic acid B using proteomic assay and bioinformatic analysis†. PROTEOMICS. 2011;11(8):1473–85.
66. Gormley GJ, Stoner E, Bruskewitz RC, et al. The effect of finasteride in men with benign prostatic hyperplasia. J Urol. 2002;167(2, Part 2):1102–7.
67. Wu Z, Li W, Liu G, et al. Network-based methods for prediction of drug-target interactions. Front Pharmacol. 2018;9:1134.
68. Feixiong C, Chuang L, Jing J, et al. Prediction of drug-target interactions and drug repositioning via network-based inference. PLoS Comput Biol. 2012;8(5):e1002503.
69. Wu H, Miller E, Wijegunawardana D, et al. MD-Miner: a network-based approach for personalized drug repositioning. BMC Syst Biol. 2017;11(S5):86.
70. Isik Z, Baldow C, Cannistraci CV, et al. Drug target prioritization by perturbed gene expression and network information. Sci Rep. 2015;5(1):17417.
71. Melo Filho CC, Dantas RF, Braga RC, et al. QSAR-driven discovery of novel chemical scaffolds active against Schistosoma mansoni. J Chem Inf Model. 2016;56(7):1357–72.
72. Gomes MN, Braga RC, Grzelak EM, et al. QSAR-driven design, synthesis and discovery of potent chalcone derivatives with antitubercular activity. Eur J Med Chem. 2017;137:126–38.

73. Shen J, Tan C, Zhang Y, et al. Discovery of potent ligands for estrogen receptor β by structure-based virtual screening. J Med Chem. 2010;53(14):5361–5.
74. Hu G, Li X, Zhang X, et al. Discovery of inhibitors to block interactions of HIV-1 integrase with human LEDGF/p75 via structure-based virtual screening and bioassays. J Med Chem. 2012;55(22):10108–17.
75. Kumari P, Nath A, Chaube R. Identification of human drug targets using machine-learning algorithms. Comput Biol Med. 2015;56:175–81.
76. Zhang X, Li L, Ng MK, et al. Drug-target interaction prediction by integrating multiview network data. Comput Biol Chem. 2017;69:185–93.
77. Jamali AA, Ferdousi R, Razzaghi S, et al. DrugMiner: comparative analysis of machine learning algorithms for prediction of potential druggable proteins. Drug Discov Today. 2016;21(5):718–24.
78. Tang Y, Zhu W, Chen K, et al. New technologies in computer-aided drug design: toward target identification and new chemical entity discovery. Drug Discov Today: Technologies. 2006;3 (3):307–13.
79. Rognan D. Structure-based approaches to target fishing and ligand profiling. Mol Inf. 2010;29 (3):176–87.
80. Pireddu L, Poulin B, Szafron D, et al. Pathway analyst automated metabolic pathway prediction// IEEE Symposium on Computational Intelligence in Bioinformatics & Computational Biology. IEEE, 2005.
81. Dale JM, Popescu L, Karp PD. Machine learning methods for metabolic pathway prediction. BMC Bioinformatics. 2010;11(1):15.
82. Boudellioua I, Saidi R, Hoehndorf R, et al. Prediction of metabolic pathway involvement in prokaryotic UniProtKB data by association rule mining. PLoS ONE. 2016;11(7):e0158896.
83. Pang H, Lin A, Holford M, et al. Pathway analysis using random forests classification and regression. Bioinformatics. 2006;22(16):2028–36.
84. Hancock T, Mamitsuka H. A Markov classification model for metabolic pathways. Algorithms Mol Biol. 2010;5(1):10.
85. Pammolli F, Magazzini L, Riccaboni M. The productivity crisis in pharmaceutical R&D. Nat Rev Drug Discov. 2011;10(6):428–38.
86. Swinney DC, Anthony J. How were new medicines discovered? Nat Rev Drug Discov. 2011;10(7):507–19.
87. Campillos M, Kuhn M, Gavin AC, et al. Drug target identification using side-effect similarity. Science. 2008;321(5886):263–6.
88. Yang L, Agarwal P. Systematic drug repositioning based on clinical side-effects. P. Csermely. PLoS ONE. 2011;6(12):e28025.
89. Dimitri GM, Lió P. DrugClust: a machine learning approach for drugs side effects prediction. Comput Biol Chem. 2017;68:204–10.
90. Luo Y, Liu Q, Wu W, et al. Predicting drug side effects based on link prediction in bipartite network. Proceedings - 2014 7th International Conference on BioMedical Engineering and Informatics, BMEI 2014; 2015. p. 729–33.
91. Ferrero E, Agarwal P. Connecting genetics and gene expression data for target prioritisation and drug repositioning. BioData Mining. 2018;11(1):7.
92. Yin W, Gao C, Xu Y, et al. Learning opportunities for drug repositioning via GWAS and PheWAS findings. 2018.
93. Ye H, Liu Q, Wei J. Construction of drug network based on side effects and its application for drug repositioning. PLoS ONE. 2014;9(2):e87864.
94. Wang Y, Chen S, Deng N, et al. Drug repositioning by Kernel-based integration of molecular structure, molecular activity, and phenotype data. PLoS ONE. 2013;8(11):e78518.
95. Duan Q, Flynn C, Niepel M, et al. LINCS Canvas Browser: interactive web app to query, browse and interrogate LINCS L1000 gene expression signatures. Nucleic Acids Res. 2014;42 (W1):W449–60.

96. Lamb J. The connectivity map: using gene-expression signatures to connect small molecules, genes, and disease. Science. 2006;313(5795):1929–35.
97. Keenan AB, Jenkins SL, Jagodnik KM, et al. The library of integrated network-based cellular signatures NIH program: system-level cataloging of human cells response to perturbations. Cell Syst. 2018;6(1):13–24.
98. Musa A, Ghoraie LS, Zhang SD, et al. A review of connectivity map and computational approaches in pharmacogenomics. Brief Bioinformatics. 2017:bbw112.
99. Iorio F, Rittman T, Ge H, et al. Transcriptional data: a new gateway to drug repositioning? Drug Discov Today. 2013;18(7–8):350–7.
100. Xie L, He S, Wen Y, et al. Discovery of novel therapeutic properties of drugs from transcriptional responses based on multi-label classification. Sci Rep. 2017;7(1)
101. Young WC, Raftery AE, Yeung KY. A posterior probability approach for gene regulatory network inference in genetic perturbation data. Math Biosci Eng. 2016;13:1241–51.
102. Lee H, Kang S, Kim W. Drug repositioning for cancer therapy based on large-scale drug-induced transcriptional signatures. E. PLoS ONE. 2016;11(3):e0150460.
103. Sawada R, Iwata M, Tabei Y, et al. Predicting inhibitory and activatory drug targets by chemically and genetically perturbed transcriptome signatures. Sci Rep. 2018;8(1):156.
104. Edgar R, lash A. 6. The Gene Expression Omnibus (GEO): a gene expression and hybridization repository. 2002.
105. Barrett T, Wilhite SE, Ledoux P, et al. NCBI GEO: archive for functional genomics data sets--update. Nucleic Acids Res. 2013;41(Database issue):D991.
106. Parkinson H, Kapushesky M, Shojatalab M, et al. ArrayExpress--a public database of microarray experiments and gene expression profiles. Nucleic Acids Res. 2007;35(Database issue): D747–50.
107. Luo H, Zhang P, Cao XH, et al. DPDR-CPI, a server that predicts drug positioning and drug repositioning via chemical-protein interactome. Sci Rep. 2016;6(1):35996.
108. Chen JJF, Visco DP. Developing an in silico pipeline for faster drug candidate discovery: virtual high throughput screening with the signature molecular descriptor using support vector machine models. Chem Eng Sci. 2016:S0009250916300914.
109. Li H, Gao Z, Kang L, et al. TarFisDock: a web server for identifying drug targets with docking approach. Nucleic Acids Res. 2006;34(Web Server):W219–W224.
110. Luo H, Chen J, Shi L, et al. DRAR-CPI: a server for identifying drug repositioning potential and adverse drug reactions via the chemical-protein interactome. Nucleic Acids Res. 2011;39 (suppl_2):W492–W498.
111. Ruiz Carmona S, Alvarez-Garcia D, Foloppe N, et al. rDock: a fast, versatile and open source program for docking ligands to proteins and nucleic acids. PLoS Comput Biol. 2014;10: e1003571.
112. Lu L. Link prediction of complex networks. J UESTC. 2010;39(5):651–61 (in Chinese).
113. Chen X, Liu MX, Yan GY. Drug-target interaction prediction by random walk on the heterogeneous network. Mol Biosyst. 2012;8(7):1970.
114. Seal A, Ahn YY, Wild DJ. Optimizing drug-target interaction prediction based on random walk on heterogeneous networks. J Cheminform. 2015;7:40.
115. Zhang Y, Feng Y. Methods and development of link prediction. Measure Control Technol. 2019; 38(2):8–12 (in Chinese).
116. Liu W, Lü LY. Link prediction based on local random walk. EPL (Europhys Lett). 2010;89 (5):58007.
117. Chen B. Link prediction of complex networks and its application in recommendation. Nanjing University of Aeronautics and Astronautics, 2016;126 (in Chinese).
118. Lorrain F, White HC. Structural equivalence of individuals in social networks. Soc Networks. 1977;1(1):67–98.
119. Chowdhury G. Introduction to modern information retrieval. McGraw Hill; 1983.
120. Zhang W, Huai Y, Miao Z, et al. Systems pharmacology for investigation of the mechanisms of action of traditional chinese medicine in drug discovery. Front Pharmacol. 2019;10

121. Wang J, Wu MY, Tan JQ, et al. High content screening for drug discovery from traditional Chinese medicine. Chin Med. 2019;14(1):5.
122. Xu HY, Zhang YQ, Liu ZM, et al. ETCM: an encyclopaedia of traditional Chinese medicine. Nucleic Acids Res. 2019;47(Database issue):D976.
123. Liu BH, Gu YH, Tu Y, et al. Molecular regulative mechanisms of aging and interventional effects of Chinese herbal medicine. Zhongguo Zhong Yao Za Zhi. 2017;42(16):3065–71.
124. Chen X, Zhou H, Liu YB, et al. Database of traditional Chinese medicine and its application to studies of mechanism and to prescription validation. 2006.
125. Zhu Y, Gao B, Cui M. Design and implementation of TCM prescription analysis system framework. Chin J Tradit Chin Med. 2014;29(5):1543–46 (in Chinese).
126. Li S. conception and Research on biomarkers of TCM syndromes. J Tradit Chin Med. 2009 (9):7–10 (in Chinese).
127. Li Q, Cheng T, Wang Y, et al. PubChem as a public resource for drug discovery. Drug Discov Today. 2010;15(23–24):1052–7.
128. Wishart DS, Feunang YD, Guo AC, et al. DrugBank 5.0: a major update to the DrugBank database for 2018. Nucleic Acids Res. 2018;46(D1):D1074–82.
129. Burley SK, Berman HM, Bhikadiya C, et al. RCSB Protein Data Bank: biological macromolecular structures enabling research and education in fundamental biology, biomedicine, biotechnology and energy. Nucleic Acids Res. 2019;47(D1):D464–74.
130. Kuhn M, Letunic I, Jensen LJ, et al. The SIDER database of drugs and side effects. Nucleic Acids Res. 2016;44(D1):D1075–9.
131. Edgar R, lash A. 6. The Gene Expression Omnibus (GEO): a gene expression and hybridization repository. 2002.
132. Tomczak K, Czerwińska P, Wiznerowicz M. Review the Cancer Genome Atlas (TCGA): an immeasurable source of knowledge. Współczesna Onkologia. 2015;1A:68–77.
133. Aliper A, Plis S, Artemov A, et al. Deep learning applications for predicting pharmacological properties of drugs and drug repurposing using transcriptomic data. Mol Pharm. 2016;13 (7):2524–30.
134. Wang Z, Clark NR, Ma'ayan A. Drug-induced adverse events prediction with the LINCS L1000 data. Bioinformatics. 2016;32(15):2338–45.

Chapter 3
Common Network Pharmacology Databases

Haiyu Xu, Yanqiong Zhang, and Feifei Guo

Guide to This Chapter
Network pharmacology research is set against the background of vast biological databases and artificial intelligence. Traditional Chinese Medicine (TCM) involves ancient manuscripts, documents, and innumerable prescriptions belonging to various dynasties. Modern research implements many prescriptions or Chinese medicinal resources for ingredient separation method and analysis, especially in contemporary molecular pharmacological research. This implementation has taken place due to the fact that TCM in itself serves as a huge holistic database and currently aids in systematically sorting out a number of authoritative databases. Majority of these databases are predicated on the ingredients suggested by TCM compound prescriptions or medicinal resources; the association between TCM and the diseases or syndromes is established by employing network pharmacology to potential drug targets. These databases provide valuable input and resources, which are not only instrumental for the comprehension of the TCM treatment mechanism for diseases but also strengthen the understanding of TCM theories.

In addition to TCM databases, network pharmacology research is highly dependent on various prominent international public databases. For example, the drug and chemical databases equip us with valuable data to recognize the physical and chemical properties, biological activities, targets of action, and druggability of natural products such as TCM ingredients. Additionally, the statistics of FDA-approved drugs listed in these databases furnishes the gold standard for pharmaceutical informatics research. Furthermore, various disease databases like OMIM, HPO, DisGeNet, etc., endow researchers with ample and reliable annotation details meant for exploring disease-related genes and disease pathogenesis. The protein–protein interaction database, including STRING, provides a bridge for

H. Xu (✉) · Y. Zhang · F. Guo
Institute of Chinese Materia Medica; China Academy of Chinese Medical Sciences, Beijing, China
e-mail: yqzhang@icmm.ac.cn; ffguo@icmm.ac.cn

S. Li (ed.), *Network Pharmacology*, https://doi.org/10.1007/978-981-16-0753-0_3

establishing the correlation between drugs and diseases, as well as for the construction of a drug intervention disease network.

Therefore, this chapter meticulously explains the databases commonly used in network pharmacology from three major aspects: Chinese medicine database, chemical and drug database, and disease and protein interaction database.

3.1 TCM Databases Commonly Used in Network Pharmacology

A typical TCM compound prescription comprises various Chinese herbal medicines, each of which further contains multiple active ingredients, leading to an extensive target range of TCM. However, this "multi-ingredient, multi-target and multi-pathway" approach is precisely the reason for superior efficacy of TCM in treating some complex diseases such as cancer and diabetes. Based on the above characteristics of Chinese medicine, the idea of network pharmacology framework proves to be efficacious in studying the mechanism of action of Chinese medicine. The research of network pharmacology is an amalgamation of many entities such as Chinese medicine ingredients, targets, pathways, phenotypes, syndromes, and diseases. ETCM [1], TCMID [2, 3], and several other databases concentrate on the collection of data about various chemical ingredients and targets of TCM, whereas SymMap [4] and TCMGeneDIT [5] focus on the relationship between TCM entities. Among them, SymMap collects and evaluates the correlation between TCM syndromes, western medicine symptoms, and TCM ingredients and targets. TCMGeneDIT creates and investigates the relationship between Chinese medicine, genes, and diseases via literature mining. TCMSP [6] and BATMAN-TCM [7] aim at the ingredient-based target prediction and network analysis. Hence, these databases serve as the major reservoir of vital data and resources for the mechanism research of TCM. This chapter briefly introduces the network pharmacology related databases and analysis platforms set up in recent years, with the aim to get familiar with the Traditional Chinese Medicine database analogous to network pharmacology, so as to efficiently comprehend the TCM data resources and data platforms crucial to network pharmacology research. This chapter introduces each of the TCM databases from the aspects of database introduction, database structure, main functions, database characteristics, etc.

3.1.1 ETCM: Encyclopedia of Traditional Chinese Medicine

ETCM [1] is an all-inclusive resource database of TCM designed and developed in 2018 by Xu Haiyu's team, Institute of Chinese Materia Medica, China Academy of Chinese Medical Sciences and Professor Liu's team from the State Key Laboratory of Natural and Biomimetic Drugs, and Peking University School of Pharmaceutical Sciences. The main purpose of ETCM includes: I. Providing comprehensive and standardized information about commonly used Chinese herbal medicines, Chinese herbal compound prescriptions and their ingredients, and making available convenient resources to cater to the users' need of acquiring inclusive information about various Chinese medicines and prescriptions; II. Considering the resemblance of chemical fingerprints between TCM ingredients and several known drugs, carry out target prediction of TCM ingredients; III. System analysis function—enables the users to establish a network within the website in order to explore the relationship between TCM, compound prescriptions, distinct ingredients, gene targets, and related pathways or diseases. According to the network pharmacology strategies, ETCM seeks to clarify the potential relationship between TCM, targets, and modern diseases, as well as reveal the action mechanism of this traditional system of health and well-being. ETCM has become instrumental in promoting basic research, clinical application, and drug development of TCM.

3.1.1.1 Data Structure

ETCM exhibits 402 Traditional Chinese Medicines (origin, flavor and meridian tropism, indications, ingredients, quality control standards, etc.), 3959 TCM compound prescriptions (name, dosage form, composition, indications, ingredients, etc.), 7284 chemical ingredients of TCM, 2266 effective or predicted drug targets, and 3027 related diseases (as shown in Fig. 3.1 [1]). Besides, the Traditional Chinese Medicines are further classified according to their taste (acid, bitter, sweet, pungent, and salty), medicinal properties (chilly, hot, warm, cold, and steady), and meridian tropism (lung meridian, liver meridian, etc.). By analyzing the pie chart of each category above, users can obtain a complete list of Chinese herbal medicines belonging to each category. The details of each listed Chinese herbal medicine can be retrieved by clicking on its Chinese or Pinyin name, including origin, best harvest time, flavor, meridian tropism, indications and chemical ingredients, images of each herb, its distribution in China, and quality control standards. The TCM information page also dispenses the names of all compound prescriptions containing the medicine. Click on each name of the compound prescription to directly access the link to the information page of a particular compound prescription. *Gene Ontology (GO)* or pathways enriched by specific ingredients, Traditional Chinese Medicines, and compound prescriptions or genes related to certain distinctive diseases remain incorporated in ETCM.

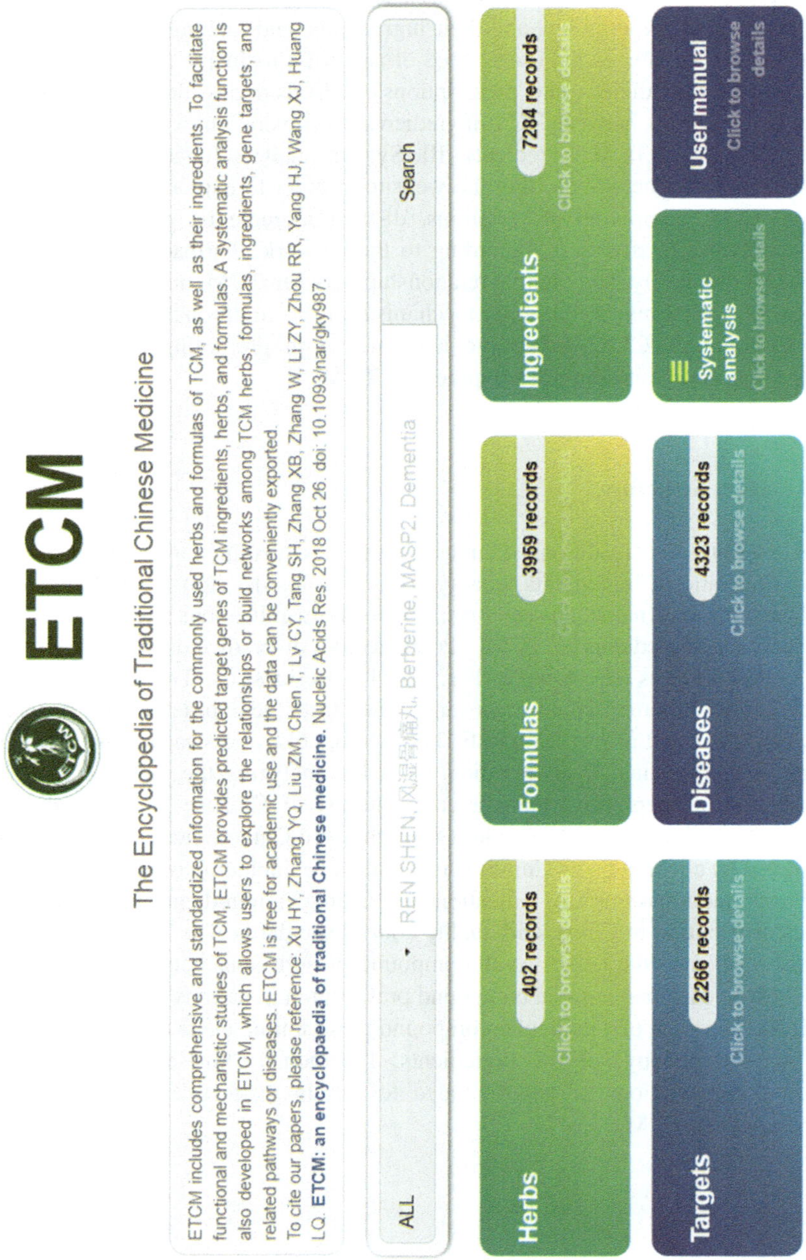

Fig. 3.1 Main functions of ETCM [1]

3.1.1.2 Function Introduction

(1) Target Prediction of Traditional Chinese Medicine Ingredients

This database employs the MedChem Studio (version 3.0) to predict the potential targets of TCM ingredients. MedChem Studio—a drug similarity search tool, is utilized to find known drugs that possess high structural similarity (Tanimoto > 0.8) with TCM ingredients, facilitating target prediction. The value range of Tanimoto or Jaccard coefficient is set within the scope of [0,1], where "0" indicates that the structure of the ingredient is completely different from that of the known drug, and "1" indicates that the two ingredients possess the same structure. Based on the TCM ingredients inserted by users, MedChem Studio generates a list of target candidates of Tanimoto > 0.8 after screening. Physiological functions and participation pathways of drug target candidates are retrieved from Gene Ontology and KEGG databases.

(2) Network Analysis

In a bid to competently decipher the relationship among ingredients, Traditional Chinese Medicines, compound prescriptions, targets, pathways involved in targets and diseases, ETCM provides a system analysis function, enabling users to establish networks linking two or more of the items mentioned above. By inputting query items and selecting one or more categories, users can construct TCM–ingredient–target, compound prescription–TCM–pathway, compound prescription–TCM–target–disease, and other networks in the system, as shown in Fig. 3.2 [1]. The nodes and edges of a network can also be marked or modified to facilitate supplemental research.

(3) Prediction and Evaluation of Drug-like Properties of Ingredients Based on Compound ADMET

To conduct the investigation of drug-like properties of each concerned ingredient, the pharmacokinetic parameters calculated by the ADMET module based on the Pipeline Pilot platform are also provided in ETCM, including water solubility, permeability of blood–brain barrier, CYP450 2D6 inhibition rate, hepatotoxicity, human intestinal absorption, and plasma protein binding rate. The QED (Quantitative Estimate of Drug-Likeness) was used to quantitatively analyze the drug-like properties of the ingredient. The value range of QED is set to (0,1), where a 0 QED value indicates that all the properties of the compound are not conducive to the preparation of a medicine; and a 1 QED value indicates that the compound has excellent druggability. Various investigations have shown that the average QED value of attractive ingredients in drug development is 0.67, and that of unattractive ingredients is 0.49. According to the QED values (i.e., druggability), all 7274 TCM ingredients assembled by ETCM were divided into three groups ranging by their attractiveness: good (QED > 0.67), medium (0.49 ≤ QED ≤ 0.67), and weak (QED < 0.49), providing a certain basis for the follow-up study of the ingredients.

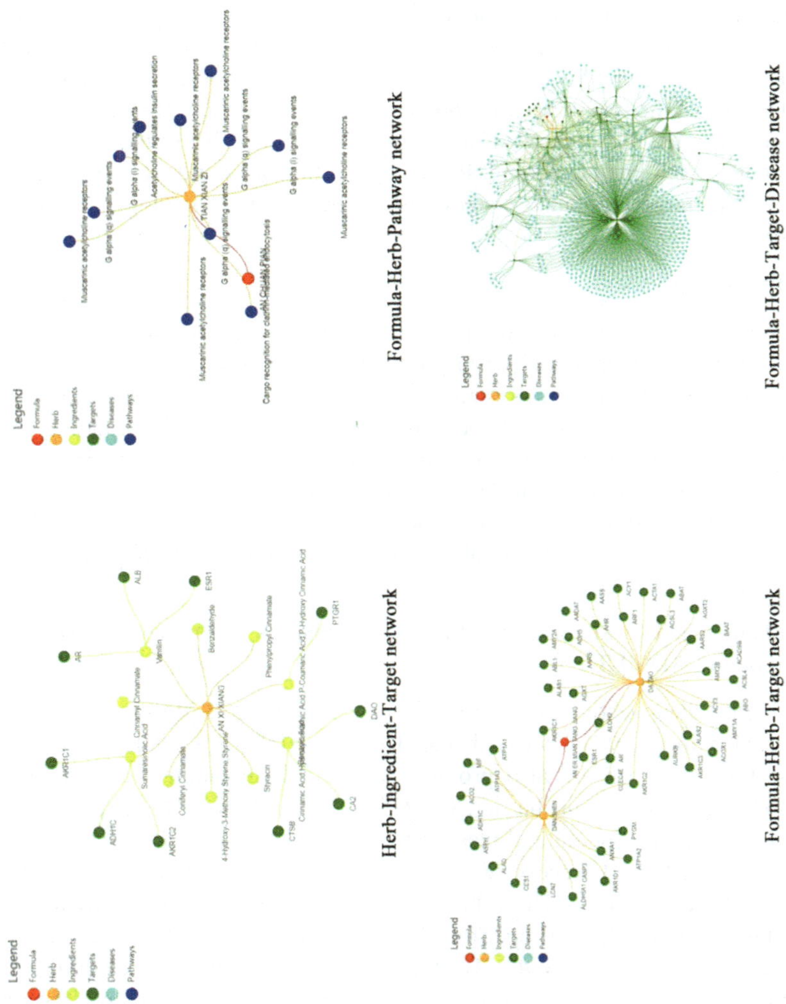

Fig. 3.2 Various network examples constructed by ETCM system analysis function [1]

3.1.1.3 Characteristics

(1) The signs and symptoms provided in the 2015 edition of *Chinese Pharmacopoeia* appear different from modern diseases. Therefore, ETCM strives to exploit the genetic relationship between TCM ingredients and modern diseases so as to establish the relationship between TCM indications and modern diseases.
(2) Network analysis: For a proficient understanding of the correlation between ingredients, TCM, compound prescriptions, targets, gene-related channels, and diseases, ETCM employs the dynamic browser-based visualization library vis.js (4.21.0) network module, which allows users to create a multi-level interaction network between Traditional Chinese Medicine, compound prescriptions, targets, and diseases.
(3) Compared to other TCM-related databases, ETCM has upgraded itself with several innovative modules and functions, including: origin distribution maps of TCM, images of Chinese herbal medicines, quality control standards of TCM and compound prescriptions, quantitative information of index ingredients, ADME parameters of ingredients, drug similarity evaluation, link to ChEMBL and PubChem databases, network construction and analysis, etc.

3.1.2 SymMap: Integrated TCM Database Focusing on the Association of Syndromes

SymMap [4] is an integrated TCM database that focuses on the association of syndromes. The database includes TCM syndromes, Chinese herbal medicines, Western medicine symptoms, syndrome-associated diseases, Chinese herbal medicine ingredients, and drug targets. The association between these six entities generates a heterogeneous network. In this way, SymMap associates TCM with modern medicine at both the phenotypic and molecular level. SymMap analyzes and grades the associations between the six types of entities based on statistical tests, aiding pharmacists in screening the entities based on their importance and thus regulating drug discovery.

3.1.2.1 Data Structure

The six types of entity libraries of SymMap include 1717 types of TCM syndromes, 961 types of western medical symptoms, 499 types of Chinese herbs, 19,595 types of drug ingredients, 4302 types of drug targets, and 5235 types of diseases. The direct association among the six types of entities in SymMap includes 6638 types of Chinese herbal medicines–TCM syndrome association, 2978 types of TCM syndromes–Western medicine symptom association, 48,372 types of Chinese herbal medicines–medicine ingredient association, 12,107 types of Western medicine symptoms–disease association, 29,370 types of medicine ingredients–drug target association, and 7256 types of genes–disease association (as shown in Fig. 3.3 [4]). For example, under the TCM symptom–Chinese herbal medicine association, each Chinese herbal medicine appears associated with an average of 13.30 types of TCM syndromes, and each TCM symptom appears associated with an average of 3.87 types of Chinese herbal medicines. Under the association set of TCM syndromes–Western medicine symptoms provided by SymMap, each TCM syndrome appears associated with 1.74 types of Western medicine symptoms, and each Western medicine symptom appears associated with 3.13 types of TCM syndromes.

In the middle of the picture are the six entity sets included in SymMap. The blue associations between the six categories of entities represent the six direct entity associations, whose names and numbers are listed on the left. Nine indirect entity associations between six types of entities are listed on the right.

3.1.2.2 Function Introduction

(1) Retrieval Methods

Users can browse, search, and download SymMap's six sections and interrelationships through the SymMap webpage. One can click the search button on the home page and enter a search item to complete the search. Each part of the SymMap is capable of providing a multi-type search box with different keywords. For example, on searching for specific western medicine symptoms, three different keywords are allowed, including the name of the symptom, the symptom ID included in other public databases, and the synonyms of the symptom. Users are also allowed to download the search results of SymMap. Additionally, after entering the search item, SymMap's automatic search function provides related entries for users to choose from, and then complete the SymMap search.

(2) SymMap Retrieval Results

After completing a SymMap search, the items that meet the criteria are displayed in a summary table at the bottom of the search interface; the first column is the SymMap ID. Users can click on the SymMap ID hyperlink in order to get detailed information about that item. In the detail interface, SymMap consists of detailed description information and searches the network visualization images and tables associated with the other five parts, by retrieving entries. Furthermore, the list of all items in the six sections can be viewed in the browsing interface, and all the lists can be downloaded from the webpage.

After browsing or searching SymMap, users can click on the SymMap ID of each specific entry to enter the details interface. The interface provides a summary of the entry, a web panel that visualizes the relationship between the six parts, and a list displaying the association between the searched item and the other five entities.

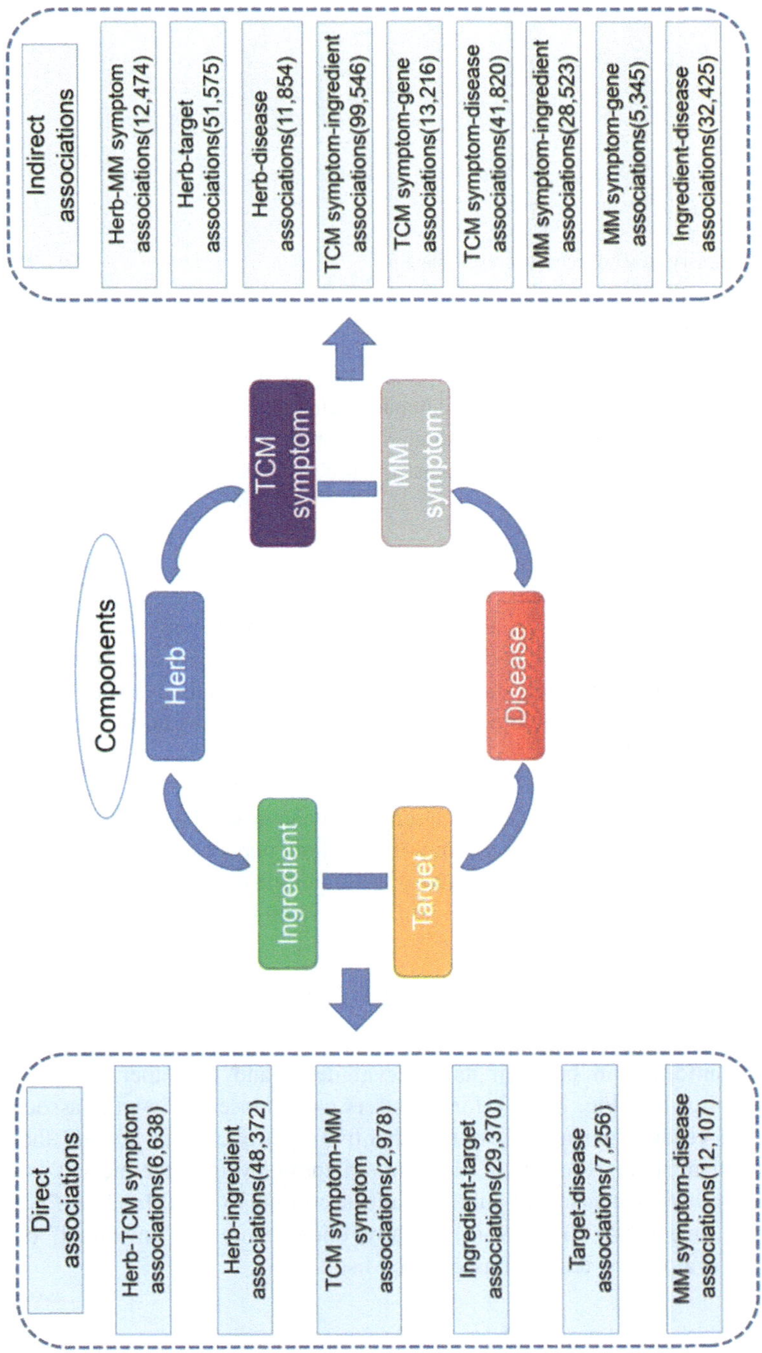

Fig. 3.3 SymMap data architecture diagram [4]

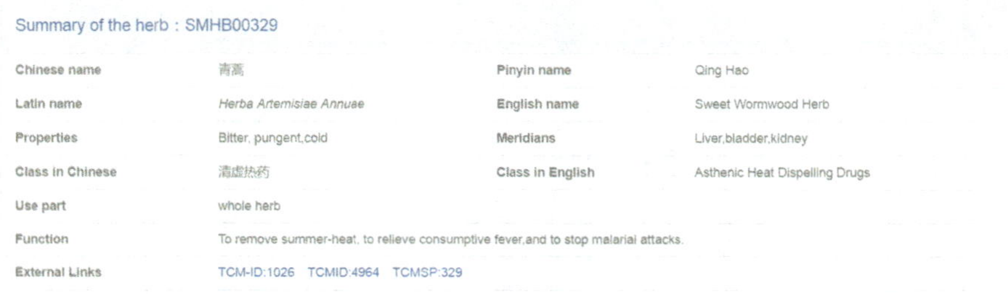

Fig. 3.4 Summary panel of retrieval result page [4]

(3) Summary Panel

The summary panel displays the summary information of the retrieved items, as shown in Fig. 3.4 [4]. The SymMap database generates three kinds of information: (1) name and gene symbol; (2) explanation information (definition and classification); (3) external links for other databases, which are directly accessible.

(4) Network Panel

The network panel provides a visual interface of the network associated with the retrieval items and other entities, as shown in Fig. 3.5 [4]. Nodes in the network are marked with different colors in accordance with their types and assigned different positions. The size of a node is determined by the range of its connectivity in the network. When the user hovers the mouse over a node, the node is expanded and its related associations are highlighted. In addition, the name of the node is displayed in a balloon textbox next to it.

Each node in the image is linked to the detailed information interface of its corresponding entity via hyperlinks. Users can change the layout of the network using the control panel, zoom in and out of the whole network, as well as download network images. To avoid having plenty of nodes in the network, SymMap tends to show only the indirect association between entities with FDR (BH) < 0.05 [8], in the network panel.

(5) Association List

The association list provides information on network visualization, including the association information between its retrieval items and the other five types of entities, as shown in Fig. 3.6 [4]. Firstly, users can choose to view the association between the retrieval item and one of the other five types of entities. Second, they can select statistical analysis results of different strictness levels to the present association. Thirdly, users can also sort out the results according to SymMap IDs, *P*-values, FDRs (BH), and FDRs (Bonferroni). Finally, clicking on the "download" button, users can download the adjusted association list.

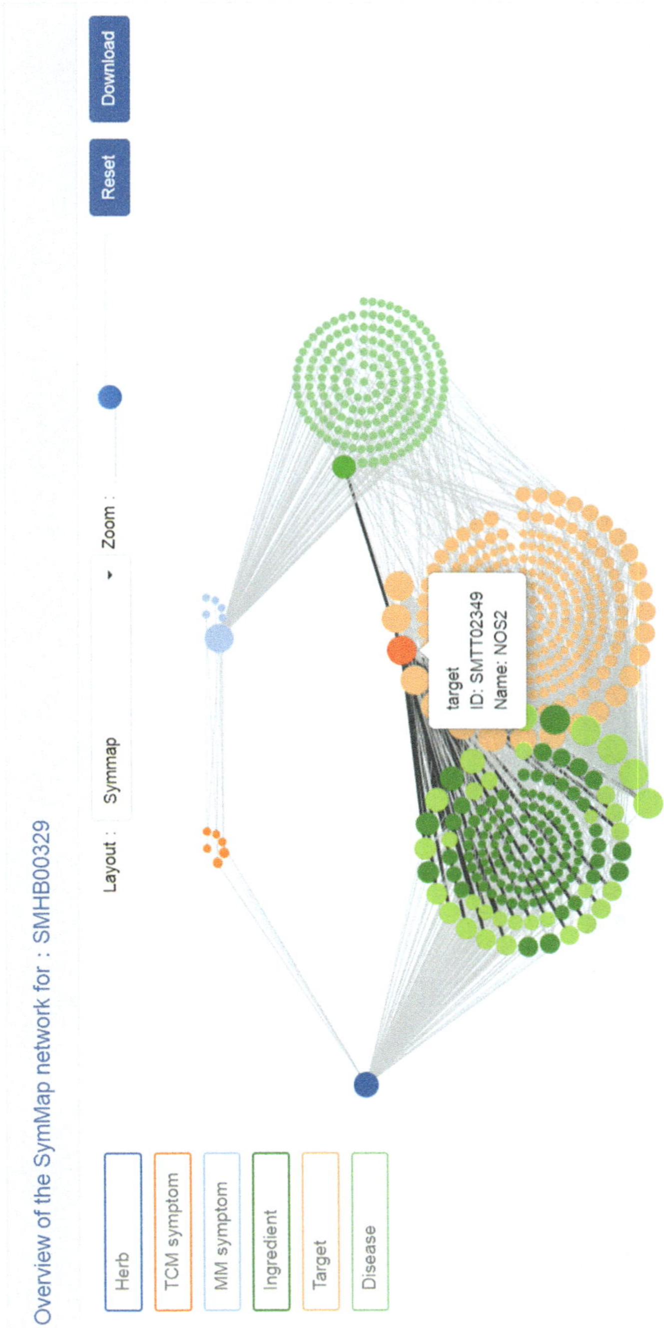

Fig. 3.5 Network panel of retrieval result page [4]

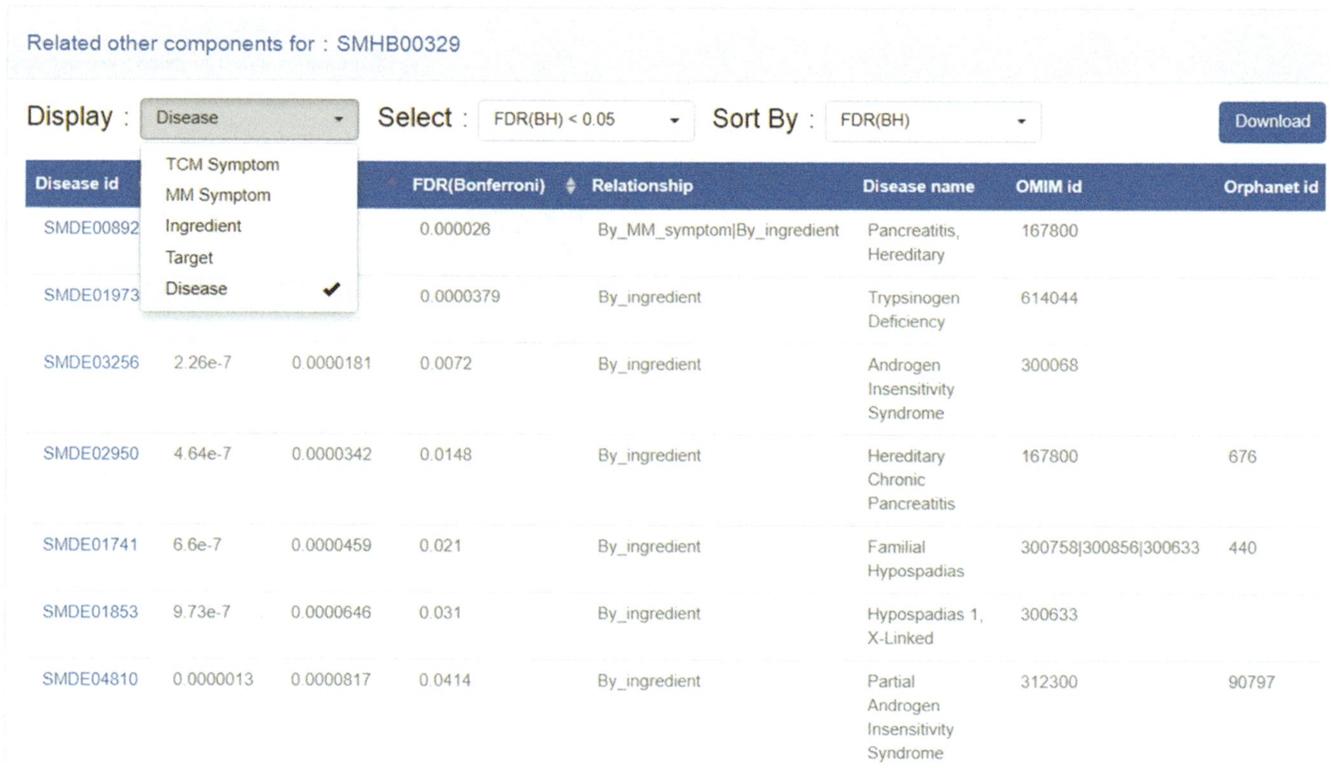

Fig. 3.6 Association list of retrieval result page [4]. The association relationship in the Association List corresponds to the content of network visualization in Fig. 3.5

3.1.2.3 Characteristics

SymMap centers around the association between syndromes and Chinese medicine data. Establishment of the relationship between TCM syndromes and Western medicine symptoms and Western medicine diseases gives rise to the bridge between TCM and modern medicine. Furthermore, SymMap also quantitatively illustrates the relationship between entity data, and offers quantitative association data for the association study amid the entity data of Chinese medicine.

3.1.3 BATMAN-TCM: Bioinformatics Analysis Platform for the Molecular Mechanism of Traditional Chinese Medicine

BATMAN-TCM [7] is an online bioinformatics analysis platform for evaluating the action mechanism of TCM, and is used to reveal the complex interaction between the material basis of TCM and the physiological process of the human body. The main functions of BATMAN-TCM include: 1. Target prediction of TCM ingredients; 2. Target functional analysis; 3. Visualization of the interaction network of ingredient–target–pathway/disease; 4. Comparative analysis of multiple Traditional Chinese Medicines. The BATMAN-TCM tool was successfully applied to predict the possible effect of Qishen Yiqi Droplet on the renin–angiotensin system. Subsequent experimental verification revealed that Qishen Yiqi Droplet provided myocardial protective function by regulating the renin–angiotensin system. The BATMAN-TCM platform is committed to revealing the action mechanism of TCM by engaging the integrated strategy of "multi-component, multi-target, and multi-pathway." The prediction of this platform is anticipated to provide valuable clues for subsequent experimental verification, thereby endorsing the research endeavors on the action mechanism of TCM.

3.1.3.1 Data Structure

BATMAN-TCM supports three kinds of input: 1. Pinyin names of Chinese herbal compound prescription, for example, Huo Xiang Zheng Qi San; 2. A list of Chinese herbal medicine with various Pinyin, English, or Latin names (Ren Shen, Ginseng, or Panax Ginseng); 3. List of compound prescriptions that requires the input of the compound structures in the PubChem_CID or InChI format. For the above three input types, including compound prescription, Chinese herbal medicine, and compound structure, BATMAN-TCM further retrieves their constituent compounds from the background database, for subsequent analysis.

Parameter setting: Score cut-off: Default value is considered to be 20. For each compound, the predicted candidate targets are assigned a target predicted score with a score range of [0,1000]. Only potential targets (including known targets) with a score greater than 20 are included in the subsequent functional analysis.

Adjusted *P*-Value: Default value is considered to be 0.05. Functional items with statistically significant enrichment are determined based on this parameter. The enrichment of a feature entry is considered statistically significant only if the adjusted *P*-value is less than the value set by the user. Adjusted *P*-value refers to the *P*-value obtained after correction, employing various Benjamini–Hochberg tests [8].

3.1.3.2 Function Introduction

(1) Function 1: Target Prediction of TCM Ingredients

For the Chinese medicinal compounds entered by the users, a list of targets with a score greater than the score cut-off is obtained after BATMAN-TCM predicts the ingredients through the target. These targets are considered as potential targets that satisfy the screening requirements (as shown in Fig. 3.7 [7]). All subsequent analyses depend on the potential target results of this step. Score cut-off can be fixed by the user while submitting the analysis, or can be adjusted on the results page.

(2) Function 2: Functional Analysis of Potential Targets

This function undertakes the enrichment analysis of KEGG pathway, GO function entries, and OMIM/TTD disease phenotypes for potential targets (as shown in Fig. 3.8 [7]). Adjusted *P*-value parameter set by the user is used to decide whether an item is enriched or not. The result table of functional enrichment analysis enlists details on the adjusted *P*-value corresponding to the enriched item and the number and list of potential targets contained in a particular item. In response to the enrichment results of the KEGG pathway, an additional coverage map of potential targets in this pathway is also provided.

(3) Function 3: Visualization of Ingredient–target–pathway/disease Interaction Network

In the ingredient–target–pathway/disease interaction network view, three types of associations are displayed, namely, the association between the user's input of TCM ingredients and their potential targets, the association between the potential targets and biological pathways, and the association between the potential targets and the enriched disease entries (as shown in Fig. 3.9 [7]). The visualization network can also be adjusted by modifying the number of associated compounds of potential targets, in order to focus on the association between crucial targets and their related functions.

(4) Function 4: Comparative Analysis

Users can submit multiple tasks for analysis simultaneously, and the Batman-TCM tool compares the calculation results from target, function, network, and other

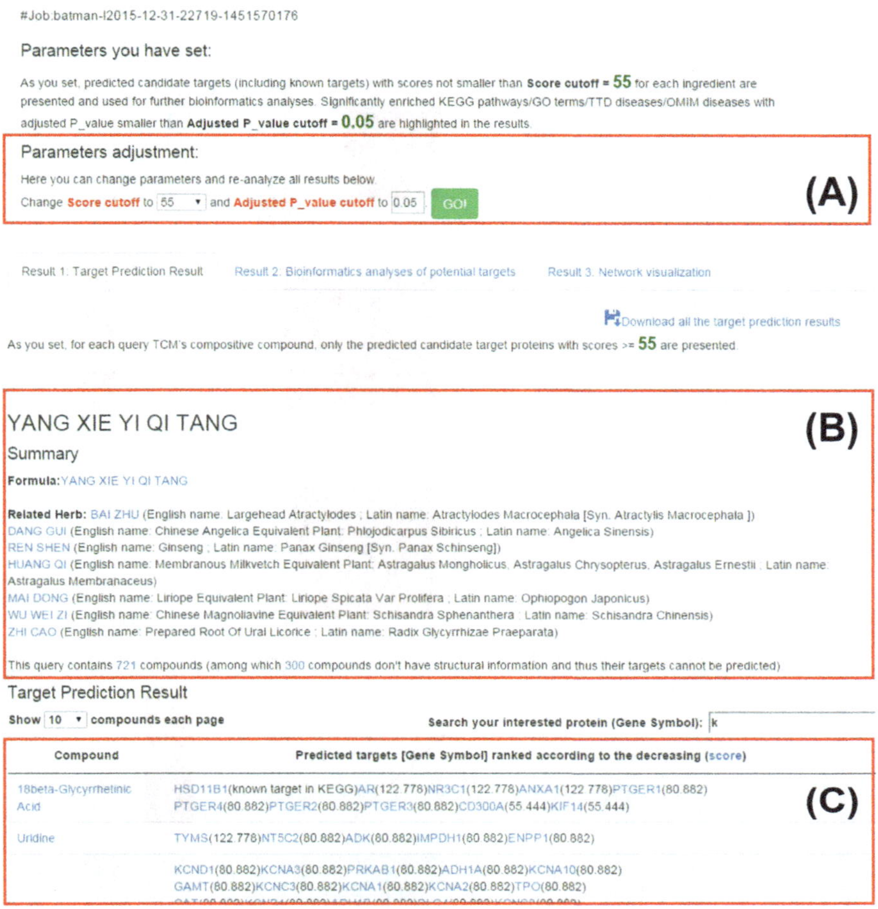

Fig. 3.7 TCM target prediction results page [7]. (**a**) Both the parameters, Score cut-off and Adjusted *P*-value cut-off, can be reset on this page. Once the above two parameters are adjusted, the analysis results of all the tests are updated accordingly. (**b**) User inputs overview, including user input of compound prescription name, composition of Chinese herbal medicine, and retrieval of compound list (**c**) Target prediction table: In this table, each ingredient lists its potential target and predicted score. In addition, potential targets listed in DrugBank, KEGG, or TTD databases are marked as known targets

aspects. In BATMAN-TCM, each submitted task is defined as a cluster. The Venn diagram of target comparison between different clusters can be viewed on the target prediction results page. The enrichment and coverage of different clusters on the same functional item are displayed on the function enrichment analysis result page.

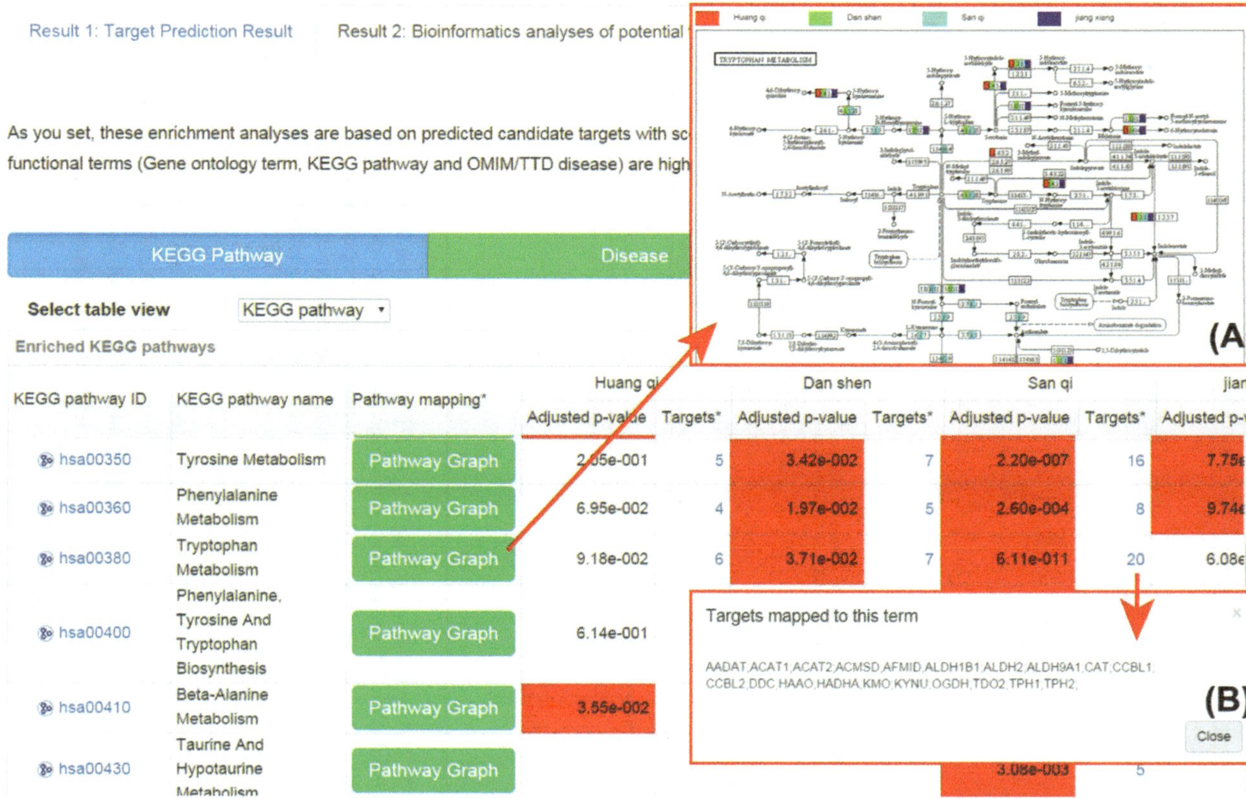

Fig. 3.8 Target enrichment analysis results page [7]. This page presents KEGG pathways, GO functional entries, and disease entries with significant enrichment of potential targets. A feature item whose Adjusted *P*-value is less than the card value is marked in red. (**a**) Click on the "Pathway Graph" button on the result page of KEGG Pathway to display the coverage of potential targets on the KEGG Pathway Graph. (**b**) Click the number under the "Target" field to display a detailed list of potential targets included in the feature entry

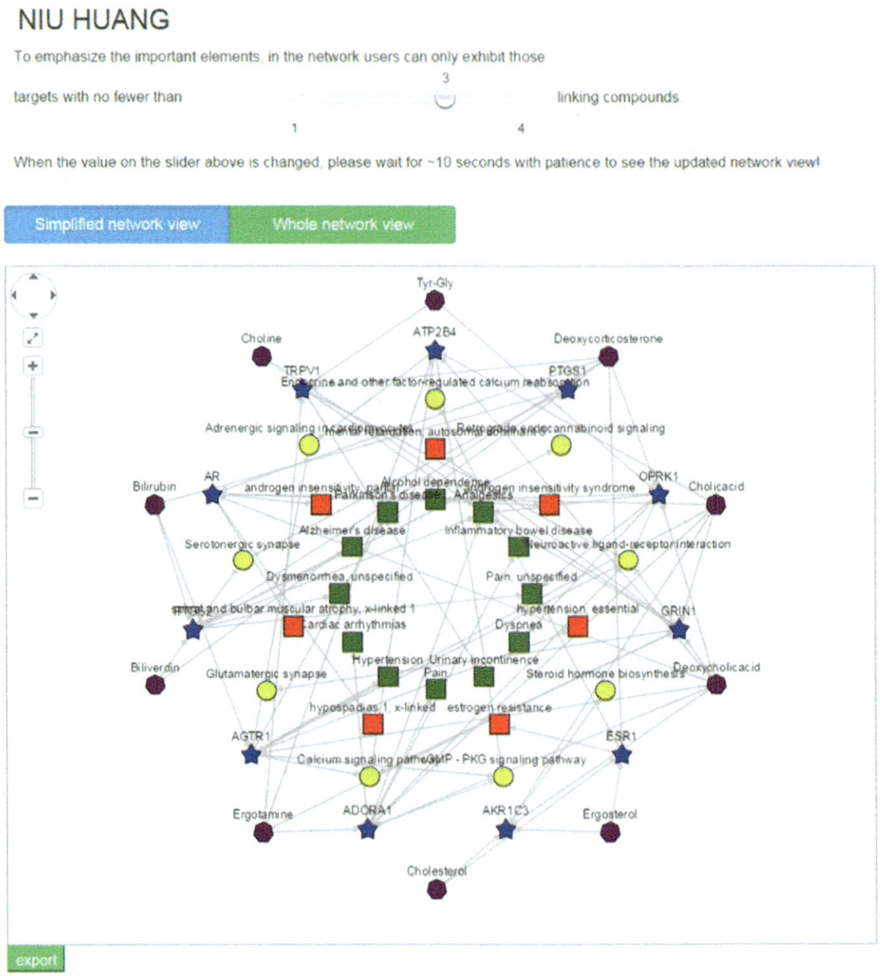

Fig. 3.9 Ingredient–target–pathway–disease association network [7]. In this network, TCM ingredients, potential targets, pathways, and diseases are classified into four different types of nodes, which are distinguished by different colors and shapes. In addition, there are three types of associations, namely, the association between the user input of TCM ingredients and their potential targets, the association between the potential targets and biological pathways, and the association between the potential targets and the enriched disease entries

(5) Function 5: Retrieving TCM Through Function

By clicking the Function2TCM button on the home page, users can view a list of TCM compound prescriptions and Chinese herbal medicines associated with a particular pathway, disease, or GO entry.

3.1.3.3 Characteristics

BATMAN-TCM is an online bioinformatics analysis tool used to evaluate the action mechanism of TCM. It is developed by a team led by distinguished Academician He Fuchu of the Academy of Military Medical Sciences. It is a highly proficient data analysis tool that is capable of completing target prediction and functional analysis of TCM with just one click. Moreover, the system provides a comparative analysis between different drugs, which facilitates the comparison of drugs with different roles in TCM formulation, as well as a retrieval function of TCM through pathways.

3.1.4 TCMID: TCM Integrated Database for Molecular Mechanism Analysis of TCM

TCMID [2, 3] records TCM-related information derived from different resources via text mining. TCMID consists of six data fields: prescription, medicinal material, ingredient, target, drug, and disease. The main goal is to establish a relationship between Chinese herbal medicinal ingredients and diseases through disease genes/proteins, which may also serve as potential drug targets. The platform's web-based software represents an integrated relationships network portraying the association between Chinese herbal medicines and the diseases they treat, and the active ingredients and their targets, which greatly assists in the research of combination therapies and provides a comprehensive approach to study the underlying mechanisms of TCM at the molecular level. The main networks TCMID has built are: 1. Chinese herbal medicine–disease network; 2. Ingredients of Chinese herbal medicine–target interaction network; 3. Chinese herbal medicine–target–disease–medicine network.

3.1.4.1 Data Structure

The internal relationship of the six data fields in the database system is shown in Fig. 3.10 [3]. The prescription is mainly composed of herbs and the herbal drugs are known to contain various ingredients (compounds). Any ingredient (or drug) can interact with its target (protein), and the disease may be caused by gene/protein function.

Database structure: A–E: six data fields for prescriptions, medicinal materials, ingredients, diseases, targets, and drugs.

1–5: 1. The prescription is composed of Chinese herbal medicine. 2. Chinese herbal medicine contains ingredients. 3. Interaction between ingredients and targets. 4. Target determination of drugs. 5. Target causes disease.

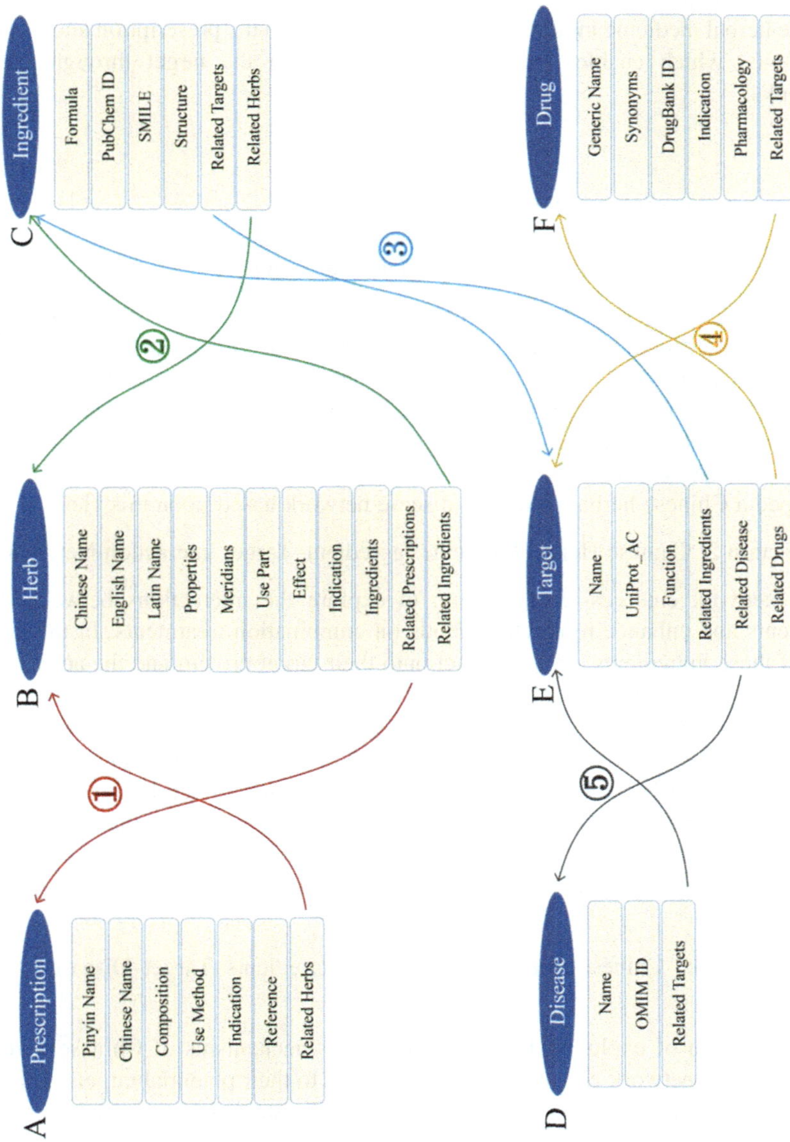

Fig. 3.10 Six data fields in the database system and their internal relations [3]

Since the information and data derived from six different fields is connected, users can utilize any of the data fields to generate an inquiry into the database and follow the link to retrieve relevant information.

For example, the user can select herb as the entry point and use the English name of the herb to make an inquiry; the result page displays the information of the Chinese herbal medicine inquired, and display its links to the prescription and herbal ingredients, which enables the user to interact with the target through these hyperlinks.

3.1.4.2 Function Introduction

(1) Function 1: Chinese Herbal Medicine–Disease Network

In the TCM framework, Chinese herbal medicines or prescriptions are formulated under a specific "mode" (called "syndrome" in Chinese), which is a description of a specific functional state, while modern medicinal drugs are designed to treat only certain diseases. Therefore, it proves to be highly beneficial to associate Chinese herbal medicines or prescriptions with the diseases they treat. Since a certain disease-causing gene/protein may be the target of a certain herb component, TCMID developed a Chinese herbal medicine–disease network based upon this view.

(2) Function 2: Chinese Herbal Medicine Ingredient–Target Interaction Network

The network emerges as a medium to explore the interactions between the ingredients and enhance research methods on combination treatments. In this network, if these ingredients are able to act onto their target protein and the activity is supported by experimental data or calculation methods, then the protein and the ingredient are said to be related to each other. Therefore, based on the network, if both the ingredients can interact with the same protein or different proteins interact with each other, users can infer the potential synergy/antagonism between the two ingredients. However, TCMID exhibits a shortcoming concerning the association between ingredients and targets, that is, the corresponding ingredients can only be identified by inputting the target, but the targets of TCM or the ingredient cannot be identified.

(3) Function 3: Chinese Herbal Medicine Ingredients–Target–Disease–Drug Network

With the aim of exploring the potential action mechanisms of Chinese herbal ingredients, the network connects these ingredients to their potential targets, related diseases, and related medicines. In addition, a tool is established to reveal relationships in a network. This tool provides the users with an intuitive perspective in order to conclude the mechanism of disease treatment and identify potential component targets through their connections. If an ingredient of a Chinese herbal medicine is able to interact with protein targets associated with a disease, it indicates that the ingredient exhibits a potential mechanism for treating the disease. Besides, if a

Chinese herbal ingredient has the same target as a medicine, it implies that the ingredient has a potential pharmacological effect.

3.1.4.3 Characteristics

TCMID proves immensely valuable as it contains a relatively comprehensive variety of Traditional Chinese Medicines and ingredients; it contains 8159 Traditional Chinese Medicines and 43,413 chemical components. Although the current version of the TCMID database displays the “target” option, it can only be used to inquire about compounds by means of targets. It can neither be used to inquire through Chinese herbal medicine or compounds, nor can it display the Chinese herbal medicine–target–disease network. The TCMID system gives rise to novel research ideas for studying the molecular level mechanism of Chinese medicine modernization. As the TCM treatment of diseases tends to become more comprehensive, adopting a systematic approach to explore the potential mechanisms and therapeutic effects of TCM becomes even more essential. Therefore, this system strives to merge the knowledge accumulated over 2000 years of clinical practices with the modern experiences or calculation methods, by uniting the common features of modern Western medicine and TCM—Chinese herbal medicine ingredients/compounds with their goals. This comprehensive information is not only conducive to the moderate development of TCM, but also facilitates the development of network pharmacology. Moreover, with the progress of system biology, several new omics methods, such as proteomics and metabolomics, have been gradually embraced in TCM research. As a result, the amalgamation of such information proves immensely beneficial in promoting the systematic research of TCM.

3.1.5 Other TCM Databases

TCMID [9] serves as an information platform, it provides information on all aspects of TCM, including prescriptions, Chinese herbal medicine that constitutes each prescription, Chinese herbal medicine ingredients, molecular structure and functional properties of active compounds, clinical indications and applications of each prescription, efficacy and toxic effects of Chinese herbal medicine ingredients, and related literature. Currently, TCMID contains information on 1588 prescriptions, 1313 Chinese herbal medicines, 5669 Chinese herbal ingredients, and 3725 3D structures of drug ingredients. The value of the data in TCMID lies in that it can help solve problems such as active constituents identification and the molecular mechanism research of TCM to a certain extent [10]. To solve this problem, two separate studies used some data from TCMID. Firstly, the three-dimensional structures of specific herbal ingredients were used to predict their molecular targets through computer simulation. The identified targets were further tested to determine whether the known therapeutic effects of these ingredients could be explained by interfering with the intended effects of these targets. Secondly, we developed an artificial intelligence (AI) system to verify the new TCM compound preparations using known TCM prescriptions. The AI system used some newly published TCM prescriptions that have not been included in TCMID, for testing.

In TCMSP [6], the systematic pharmacology of TCM is used as the framework to establish a systematic TCM pharmacology database and analysis platform. It contains the drug target and disease action of each active compound, and can automatically establish the compound target and target disease network, allowing users to view and analyze the drug action mechanism. TCMSP aims to promote the development of Chinese herbal medicines, the integration of modern and traditional medicine, and the discovery and development of medicines. TCMSP contains a large number of Chinese herbal ingredients and can be used to identify drug target networks and drug disease networks, which is helpful in revealing the mechanism of action of TCM and its formulation, and to discover drugs and drug combinations.

TCMGeneDIT [5] is a database that provides association relationships among TCM, genes, diseases, TCM functions, and TCM ingredients, which have been mined from a large number of biomedical documents by researchers from Taiwan University. The relationship between TCM, genes, and diseases can be examined by transmission of intermediate objects. Information on the interaction between integrins and proteins and biological pathways is also used to investigate gene regulation relationships related to the effects of Chinese medicine. TCMGeneDIT helps people understand the possible mechanism of action of TCM through gene regulation relationships and the contribution of synergistic and antagonistic effects.

3.2 Biological Databases Commonly Used in Network Pharmacology

In recent years, the establishment of various biological databases has provided reliable and powerful data support for network pharmacology research. Biological databases commonly used in network pharmacology include disease phenotype and genotype association databases (OMIM, HPO, DisGeNET), drug target information databases (TTD, PDB, KEGG), and biological molecular interaction databases (BioGRID, DIP, IntAct, MINT, STRING). Based on these biological databases containing clinical and basic research results, network pharmacology research can be used to construct the "disease phenotype–gene–target–drug" interaction network, and investigate the characteristics and mechanism of drug intervention on the disease network.

3.2.1 *Online Mendelian Inheritance in Man-OMIM*

3.2.1.1 Database Content and Its Application in Network Pharmacology Research

The OMIM database is a comprehensive and authoritative database on human genes and hereditary traits. This database focuses on the relationship between disease phenotypes and genotypes [11, 12], and contains information on all Mendelian genetic diseases and more than 15,000 human genes, including all known genetic diseases, genetically determined traits, and their genes. In addition to briefly describing the clinical characteristics, diagnosis, differential diagnosis, treatment, and prevention of various diseases, the linkage relationship of known pathogenic genes, chromosomal location, composition structure and function, animal model, and other information are also provided, with reference to related literature that have been manually checked and verified [11]. The genetic diseases, traits, and genes established in OMIM (data classification and entries are detailed, as shown in Table 3.1) are classified with OMIM numbers. Reports about diseases must be prefixed with the appropriate OMIM numbers to clarify which genetic disease is being discussed [12]. The OMIM database provides detailed, updated, real-time, and freely downloadable data on disease-related genes for network pharmacology research, and provides reliable data support for constructing and mining the interaction between disease-related genes and drug-target genes.

3.2.1.2 Data Structure

OMIM not only contains the related data of all single-gene diseases that follow the Mendelian inheritance pattern, but also contains the data of chromosomal diseases,

Table 3.1 Overall OMIM data status

MIM identifier	Autosomal inheritance	X-linked inheritance	Y-linked inheritance	Mitochondrial inheritance	Total
Well-defined locus	15,281	733	49	37	16,100
Locus of known phenotypes	44	0	0	0	44
Descriptions that usually have phenotypes	5195	336	5	33	5569
Mendelian genetic traits with unknown molecular mechanism	1438	119	4	0	1561
Whether the main phenotype is Mendelian phenotype has not been determined	1644	105	3	0	1752
Total	23,602	1293	61	70	25,026

polygenetic diseases, and mitochondrial diseases, covering an unusually wide range of diseases. OMIM provides information on everything from the basics to the clinical aspects of every item, that is, every disease. The specific information includes Description (basic description), Mapping (genetic positioning), Molecular Genetics, Inheritance (mode of Inheritance), Mapping (genetic positioning), Molecular Genetics, and Population Genetics. Each aspect of the description provides links to the corresponding reference literature.

3.2.1.3 Function Introduction

There are many types of genetic diseases, but they are relatively rare, and it is difficult for clinicians and geneticists to know every genetic disease. OMIM provides a large amount of information on clinical features, diagnosis, clinical management, and gene therapy of Mendelian genetic diseases. It also provides a concise and pragmatic clinical synopsis, and more relevant information can be obtained through the references links connected to other databases such as GeneTests, which can provide diagnostic test information on a variety of genetic diseases. OMIM is a powerful tool for clinical and genetic counseling professionals. At the same time, OMIM can provide information on clinical phenotypes and pathogenic genes of specific diseases (such as polygenic diseases), including gene positioning, molecular mechanism, pathology, animal model, mode of inheritance, etc. The description of each aspect includes a link to the corresponding literature, so that researchers can quickly and comprehensively grasp the main information and the latest developments in the disease.

3.2.1.4 Characteristics

OMIM is a comprehensive database of human genes and genetic diseases; it contains information on all Mendelian inherited diseases and human genetics, in addition to a brief description of the clinical features, diagnosis, treatment, and preventive measures of various diseases. It also provides information on the linkage relationship, chromosome positioning, function, and animal model of known disease-causing genes, and provides reference to relevant carefully curated literature. OMIM provides real-time, authoritative, comprehensive, and practical information. However, the OMIM database schema and data model are not open, hence, SQL query statements cannot be used to write your own query statements to query information in the database. For complex diseases such as asthma, due to the extremely complex types of data that need to be analyzed, the solutions currently provided by OMIM are unable to meet the growing research needs. Moreover, OMIM does not contain as much information as the Locus-Specific Database: mutation data is not comprehensive, and the database lacks primer design information, gene expression profiles, etc. Furthermore, data annotation is limited to genetics.

3.2.2 *Human Phenotypic Ontology Database-HPO*

3.2.2.1 Database Content and Its Application in Network Pharmacology Research

The HPO database was established in 2007 by Peter N Robinson and Sebastian Köhler of the Charité University Hospital in Berlin. It provides information on medical-related phenotypes, disease phenotype annotations, and ontology information based on phenotypes. HPO covers more than 13,000 terms and more than 156,000 genetic disease annotations in several fields such as anatomy, cell types, biological functions, embryology, and pathology. Most of the ontological information is in the form of Directed Acyclic Graphs (DAG), for example, the term metatarsal hypoplasia/dysplasia refers to the hypoplasia/dysplasia and abnormal metatarsal morphology that involve children's foot bones. Encoding multiple parent terms in DAG increases the flexibility and descriptiveness of the ontology information. The term "parent–child relationship" is transitive, which means that annotations inherit all paths to the root, for example, abnormal left ventricular morphology—abnormal ventricular morphology. At present, HPO is widely used in computing deep phenotype and precision medicine, integrating clinical data into translational research, and has been used as the criteria for determining phenotypic abnormalities by multiple international organizations for rare diseases, registration authorities, clinical laboratories, biomedical resources, clinical software tools, and other groups [13–15]. In network pharmacology research, HPO can provide specific phenotype description of disease symptoms and related gene sets, which can help users to collect relevant gene information based on the pathological link of the target disease, so as to explore the network regulation mechanism of drugs to a certain pathological link in the progression of the target disease. The phenotypic classifications covered by HPO are listed in Table 3.2 [13–15].

Table 3.2 Phenotypic classifications covered by HPO

Phenotypic type	Examples of entries
Morphological Abnormality	Arachnodactyly (HP:0001166)
Abnormal Process (organ)	Epistaxis (HP:0000421)
Abnormal Process (cellular)	Abnormality of Krebs Cycle
	Metabolism (HP:0000816)
Abnormal Laboratory Finding	Glycosuria (HP:0003076)
Electrophysiological Abnormality	Hypsarrhythmia (HP:0002521)
Abnormality by Medical Imaging	Choroid Plexus Cyst (HP:0002190)
Behavioral Abnormality	Self-Mutilation (HP:0000742)

3.2.2.2 Data Structure

Each term in HPO describes a clinical phenotype. These terms may be general terms, such as abnormal ear morphology, or specialized terms, such as chorioretinal atrophy. Each term is also assigned to five sub-ontology information, namely phenotypic abnormality, mode of inheritance, clinical modifier, clinical course, and frequency of phenotype. Each of these terms has a unique identity, namely an HPO label, for example "HP:0001140" for "globular ectoderm." The database has specific definitions and descriptions for most phenotypes and provides sources of evidence. For example, bulbar epithelioma is a benign tumor usually found at the junction of the cornea and the sclera (limbal epithelioma of the cornea).

3.2.2.3 Function Introduction

HPO is often used in clinical diagnosis, phenotypic genomic diagnosis, bioinformatics data mining, and other tools and algorithms [16]. Commonly used tools include: ① Clinical diagnostic tools: HPO provides a calculation basis for fuzzy and specific weighted phenotype matching algorithms to support differential diagnosis. Users can click on the representative phenotypic abnormalities (signs, symptoms, laboratory measurements, etc.) in the HPO term list to query. ② Exome/genome diagnosis and research tools: HPO includes a series of algorithm-based Java tools to achieve phenotype-driven optimization of Mendelian disease variants. These tools can be used to export VCF files and HPO term lists extracted from exomes or genomes related to phenotypic abnormalities. ③ Copy number variation diagnostic tools: Microarray comparative genomic hybridization and related tests are often used as screening tests for indications such as developmental retardation and congenital malformations. These tests can detect copy number variation (deletion and replication). Several copy number variations are found in all individuals, so it is difficult to determine whether copy number variations are associated with disease. Based on HPO, it is possible to analyze whether the gene copy number variation is related to the phenotypic abnormalities observed in patients, and then determine the correlation between copy number variation and disease. ④ Clinical phenotype tools: HPO focuses on accurate clinical phenotyping to facilitate disease classification and the discovery of candidate marker genes.

3.2.2.4 Characteristics and Deficiencies

HPO provides researchers and clinicians with well-defined, comprehensive, and interoperable resources for computational analysis of human disease phenotypes. It is used as a basic tool for disease phenotype analysis in clinical and research environments, and integrates complex phenotype information from different disciplines and databases. At first, HPO terms focused on rare diseases, mainly

Mendelian genetic diseases. Although HPO terms can now also be used for common diseases, its resources also cover precision medicine, cancer, and non-Mendelian genetic diseases; however, the coverage needs to be further extended.

3.2.3 Disease Gene Association Database-DisGeNET

The DisGeNET database is an open source database that integrates disease and gene-related information and related drug information, and links to other source databases and literature. The current version of DisGeNET (V6.0) contains 17,549 genes associated with 24,166 diseases, abnormalities, traits, and clinical or abnormal human phenotypes, totaling 628,685 gene–disease associations (GDAs). There are also 210,498 mutation–disease associations (VDAs) consisting of 117,337 variants and 10,358 diseases, traits, and phenotypes. The information sources of GDAs are mainly composed of the following 4 parts: ① CURATED: GDA information provided by UniProt, PsyGeNET, Orphanet, CGI, CTD (Human Data), ClinGen, and Genomics England PanelApp professional databases; ② ANIMAL MODELS: RGD, MGD, and CTD (mouse and rat data). These data include GDAs provided by disease information resources of animal models (currently rats and mice), and homology analysis is used to map the association with human genes. The data includes GDAs provided by animal model (currently for rats and mice) disease information resources, and use homology analysis to map the association with human genes; ③ INFERRED: This part of the data refers to GDAs inferred from Human Phenotype Ontology (HPO) and VDAs. Its database sources include HPO, CLINVAR, GWAS Catalog, and GWAS DB; ④ LITERATURE: Including LHGDN and BeFree databases. Information sources of VDAs mainly include: ① CURATED: Including UniProt, ClinVar, GWAS Catalog, and GWAS db databases; ② INFERRED: SETH tool. As a multifunctional information platform, the DisGeNET database is being widely used in basic molecular research of human diseases and their complications, the mining of disease gene characteristics, the biological basic research on drug therapy effect and adverse drug reactions, as well as for the validation of calculated predicted disease genes and the evaluation of the performance of text mining methods [17, 18].

3.2.3.1 Data Structure

To integrate gene–disease association data, the DisGeNET database has developed association type ontology. If there is a relationship between gene/protein and disease, then all association types found in the original source database are formally constructed by the parent gene–disease association class and expressed as ontology classes. It is an OWL Ontology that has been integrated into the Sematic Science Integrated Ontology (SIO), and provides necessary types and relationships for the description of abundant objects, processes, and their properties.

3.2.3.2 Function Introduction

In the DisGeNET database, most GDAs are identified through BeFree text mining literature and are integrated with human genetics databases from various authoritative sources. Each GDA is clearly annotated with its supporting evidence sources, which makes DisGeNET a reference resource for evidence-based knowledge discovery [19, 20]. DisGeNET contains a compilation of disease-related genes from different open source databases. DiGeNet can be used to obtain disease information related to gene mutations, information related to diseases and genes, types of associations between specific genes and disease, and newly discovered information on related genes and mutations for a particular disease.

3.2.3.3 Characteristics

The major feature of the DisGeNET database is data integration, standardization, and tracking and querying of evidence sources. The integration is performed through gene and disease vocabulary mapping and the use of the DisGeNET associated type ontology. In addition, GDAs are organized according to their types and levels of evidence, such as CURATED, PREDICTED, and LITERATURE, and are also graded according to supporting evidence, to prioritize and simplify their exploration. The goal of DisGeNET is to integrate the basic genetic information of all diseases for reference in a knowledgebase, to fill in genotype and phenotype differences. Currently, the DisGeNET platform is used to study biomedical problems.

3.2.4 Disease Information Data—MalaCards

The MalaCards Human Disease Database is a comprehensive searchable database integrating human diseases and their annotations from major database websites [21]. It has been jointly developed by Weizmann Institute of Science, the world's leading interdisciplinary basic research institution for natural and precision sciences in Israel, and Utah Valley University. The database is a comprehensive disease summary mined from 68 data sources and contains 20,000 disease entries in 6 categories worldwide. Each disease contains 15 small notes, including a summary, symptoms, anatomical background, drugs, genetic testing, mutation information, and some literature related to the disease. The database integrates information from complementary sources, and through its sophisticated search capabilities, relational database structure, and convenient data transfer capabilities, enables the processing of a large number of disease annotation resources. It also facilitates functions such as system analysis and genome sequence interpretation.

3.2.4.1 Introduction and Usage of the Database

(1) Disease Query

The database integrates the information of 68 databases, and users only need to input the disease name to search the corresponding diseases. The search interface is shown in Fig. 3.11 [21].

Take any disease as an example. MalaCards divides the search results about the disease into 14 sections (as shown in Fig. 3.12 [21]). Click "Jump to Section" to navigate to that section. At the same time, you can use the Summaries section to view the summary of the disease in multiple databases (as shown in Fig. 3.13 [21]).

(2) Network Analysis

MalaCards is a phenotypic disease network. We can see the relationship between interconnected diseases in Fig. 3.14 [21].

(3) Expansion of Disease-related Knowledge

(1) Some drugs and treatment methods currently being studied to treat diseases are shown in Fig. 3.15 [21].

(2) Articles related to heart failure are shown in Fig. 3.16 [21].

(3) MalaCards provides information on key genes related to the disease, as shown in Fig. 3.17 [21].

(4) Disease-related website entries are shown in Fig. 3.18 [21].

3.2.4.2 Characteristics

(1) Abundant database resources—72 databases.
(2) Extensive information on disease-related expansions, and provides further information on the disease from multiple aspects, including literature.

3.3 Related Databases of Commonly Used Gene Targets in Network Pharmacology

3.3.1 Therapeutic Target Database—TTD

The TTD was established by the Bioinformatics & Drug Design (BIDD) research group of the Faculty of Science, National University of Singapore. The database was last updated on September 15th, 2017. According to the 2018 TTD update statistics, the database covers a total of 3101 drug targets, among which 445 have been successfully verified, 1121 have been used for clinical treatment, and 1535 are in the research stage. There are a total of 34,019 drugs in the database, including 8103 drugs approved for clinical use, 18,923 drugs under study, 26,459 kinds of

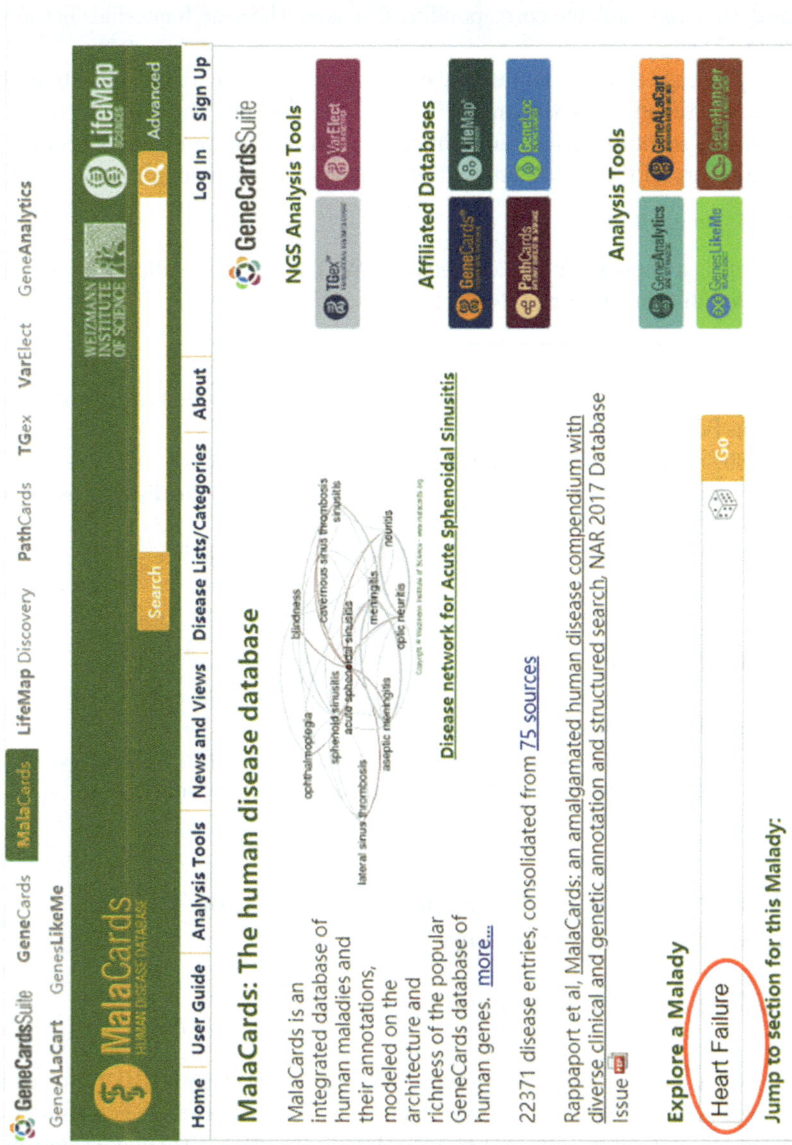

Fig. 3.11 Disease search interface [21]

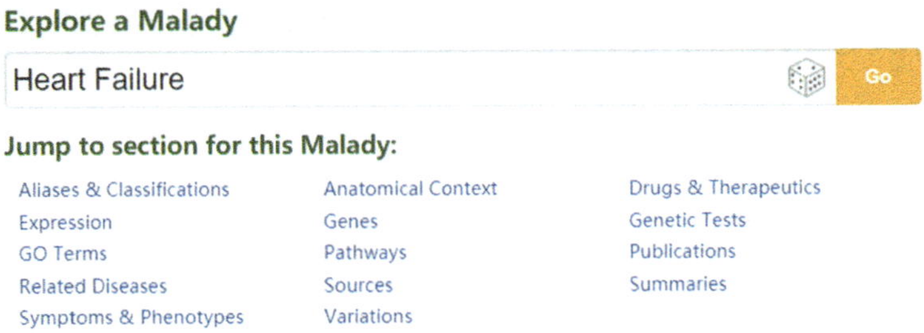

Fig. 3.12 14 sections for the disease [21]

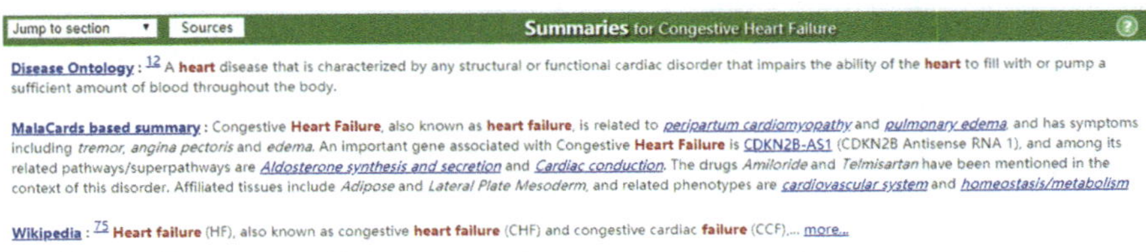

Fig. 3.13 Disease summary [21]

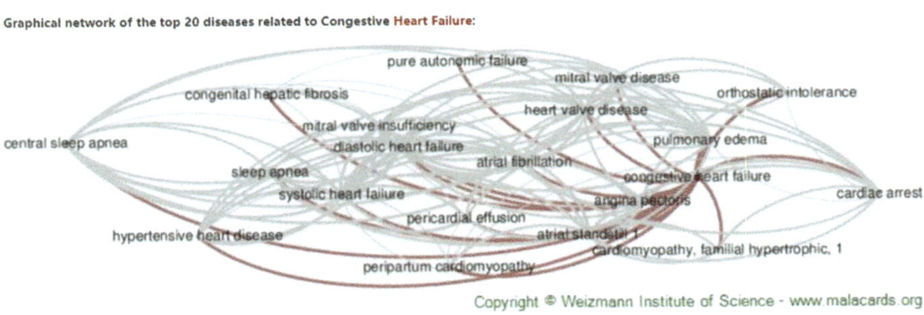

Fig. 3.14 Phenotypic disease network [21]

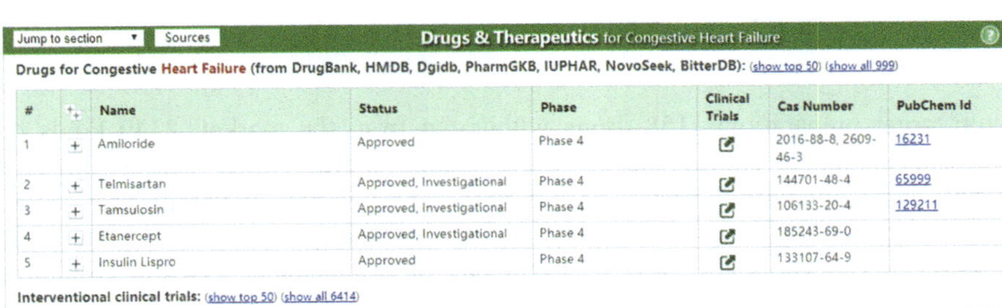
Jump to section | Sources | **Drugs & Therapeutics** for Congestive Heart Failure

Drugs for Congestive Heart Failure (from DrugBank, HMDB, Dgidb, PharmGKB, IUPHAR, NovoSeek, BitterDB): (show top 50) (show all 999)

#		Name	Status	Phase	Clinical Trials	Cas Number	PubChem Id
1	+	Amiloride	Approved	Phase 4		2016-88-8, 2609-46-3	16231
2	+	Telmisartan	Approved, Investigational	Phase 4		144701-48-4	65999
3	+	Tamsulosin	Approved, Investigational	Phase 4		106133-20-4	129211
4	+	Etanercept	Approved, Investigational	Phase 4		185243-69-0	
5	+	Insulin Lispro	Approved	Phase 4		133107-64-9	

Interventional clinical trials: (show top 50) (show all 6414)

Fig. 3.15 Known disease treatment methods and drugs [21]

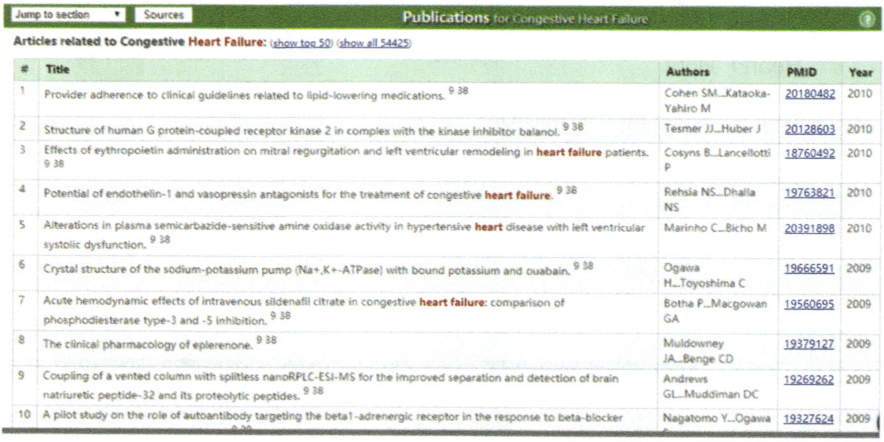

Jump to section ▼ Sources **Publications** for Congestive Heart Failure

Articles related to Congestive Heart Failure: (show top 50) (show all 54425)

#	Title	Authors	PMID	Year
1	Provider adherence to clinical guidelines related to lipid-lowering medications. [9] [38]	Cohen SM...Kataoka-Yahiro M	20180482	2010
2	Structure of human G protein-coupled receptor kinase 2 in complex with the kinase inhibitor balanol. [9] [38]	Tesmer JJ...Huber J	20128603	2010
3	Effects of eythropoietin administration on mitral regurgitation and left ventricular remodeling in **heart failure** patients. [9] [38]	Cosyns B...Lancellotti P	18760492	2010
4	Potential of endothelin-1 and vasopressin antagonists for the treatment of congestive **heart failure**. [9] [38]	Rehsia NS...Dhalla NS	19763821	2010
5	Alterations in plasma semicarbazide-sensitive amine oxidase activity in hypertensive **heart** disease with left ventricular systolic dysfunction. [9] [38]	Marinho C...Bicho M	20391898	2010
6	Crystal structure of the sodium-potassium pump (Na+,K+-ATPase) with bound potassium and ouabain. [9] [38]	Ogawa H...Toyoshima C	19666591	2009
7	Acute hemodynamic effects of intravenous sildenafil citrate in congestive **heart failure**: comparison of phosphodiesterase type-3 and -5 inhibition. [9] [38]	Botha P...Macgowan GA	19560695	2009
8	The clinical pharmacology of eplerenone. [9] [38]	Muldowney JA...Benge CD	19379127	2009
9	Coupling of a vented column with splitless nanoRPLC-ESI-MS for the improved separation and detection of brain natriuretic peptide-32 and its proteolytic peptides. [9] [38]	Andrews GL...Muddiman DC	19269262	2009
10	A pilot study on the role of autoantibody targeting the beta1-adrenergic receptor in the response to beta-blocker	Nagatomo Y...Ogawa	19327624	2009

Fig. 3.16 Articles related to the disease [21]

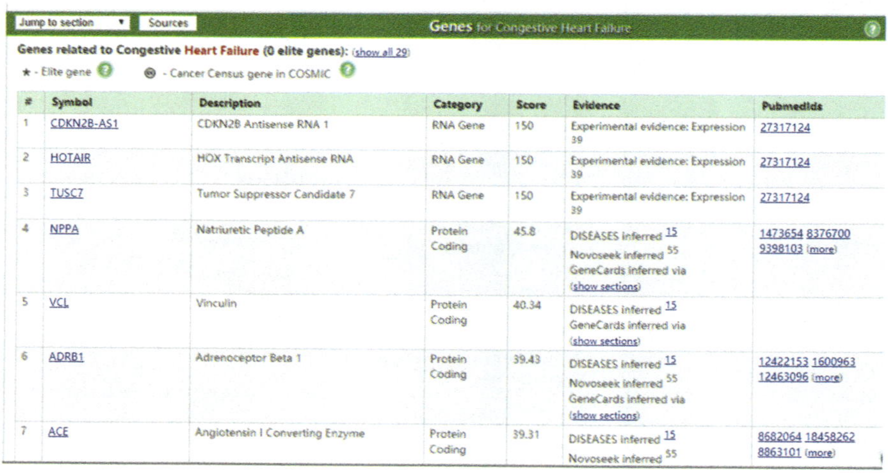

Jump to section ▼ Sources **Genes** for Congestive Heart Failure

Genes related to Congestive Heart Failure (0 elite genes): (show all 29)

★ - Elite gene ⊗ - Cancer Census gene in COSMIC

#	Symbol	Description	Category	Score	Evidence	PubmedIds
1	CDKN2B-AS1	CDKN2B Antisense RNA 1	RNA Gene	150	Experimental evidence: Expression [39]	27317124
2	HOTAIR	HOX Transcript Antisense RNA	RNA Gene	150	Experimental evidence: Expression [39]	27317124
3	TUSC7	Tumor Suppressor Candidate 7	RNA Gene	150	Experimental evidence: Expression [39]	27317124
4	NPPA	Natriuretic Peptide A	Protein Coding	45.8	DISEASES inferred [15] Novoseek inferred [55] GeneCards inferred via (show sections)	1473654 8376700 9398103 (more)
5	VCL	Vinculin	Protein Coding	40.34	DISEASES inferred [15] GeneCards inferred via (show sections)	
6	ADRB1	Adrenoceptor Beta 1	Protein Coding	39.43	DISEASES inferred [15] Novoseek inferred [55] GeneCards inferred via (show sections)	12422153 1600963 12463096 (more)
7	ACE	Angiotensin I Converting Enzyme	Protein Coding	39.31	DISEASES inferred [15] Novoseek inferred [55]	8682064 18458262 8863101 (more)

Fig. 3.17 Key genes of the disease [21]

multi-target preparations, 158 drugs withdrawn from the market, 2349 kinds of drugs suspended for clinical use, 417 pre-clinical trial drugs, 1929 drugs terminated during unspecified study phase, 21,936 kinds of effective small molecule drugs, 2326 approved drugs with effective structures, 4258 kinds of drugs that can be used in clinical trial structures, and 15,352 kinds of drugs under existing structural research. In addition, 21 bispecific antibodies and 10 stem cell drugs are included in the updated database. The database provides information about known or under exploration therapeutic protein targets and nucleic acid targets, the diseases targeted by such targets, pathway information, and corresponding drug ligand molecules. TTD also provides links to related databases, including target function, sequence,

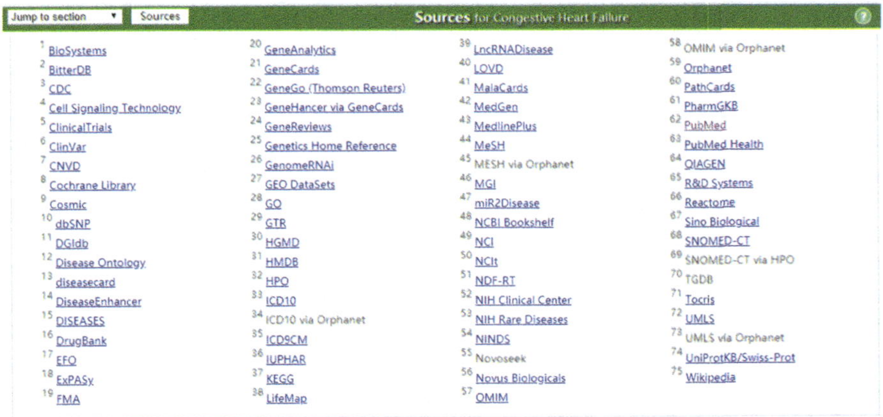

Fig. 3.18 Disease-related website entries [21]

three-dimensional structure, ligand binding characteristics, enzyme naming and drug structure, treatment category, clinical development status, etc. [22]. In network pharmacology research, the known drug structure and target information contained in TTD can be used as a positive control data set for predicting unknown drug targets. The candidate target spectrum of unknown drugs can be obtained through the comparison of compound structure and function similarity.

3.3.1.1 Data Structure

QSAR models developed to understand different molecular scaffolds for different targets are incredibly useful in facilitating drug development and optimization. Currently, TTD has 841 ligand based QSAR models for 228 chemically active compounds against 121 targets; the specific architecture of the models can be accessed on the related page.

3.3.1.2 Function Introduction

With the rapid development of bioinformatics, database technology plays an important role in bioinformatics. The difficulty of drug research lies in the discovery and determination of targets. TTD collects three types of validation data: Efficacy of drugs on their main targets through experiments, efficacy or effect of drugs on disease models (cell lines, in vitro, and in vivo models) related to their main targets, and observed effects of in vivo models of target knockout, RNA interference, and transgenic therapy.

3.3.1.3 Characteristics

The architecture and interface design of TTD are user friendly, and provide easy access to updated data and previous version data. TTD has been developed using the Drupal content management system (CMS) and provides easy and convenient data access. In the new TTD interface, the newly added resistance mutation and target expression data can be accessed through the patient data column, and the target combination information can be accessed through the target drug column. The Drugs Group column also includes search options for multi-target preparations and naturally derived drugs. The advanced search bar includes custom search, target similarity search, drug similarity search, and path search options. In addition, a JSME molecular editor has been added to facilitate users to draw molecules and then search for TTD drug entries with a similar structure to the input molecules. At present, the database is constantly updated and improved. There is an increasing amount of target information, which has great significance for the discovery of new drug targets, drug screening, disease treatment, and pharmacological mechanism research.

3.3.2 Protein Data Bank—PDB

The PDB is a biological macromolecular structure database initially established by Dr. Walter Hamilton of Brookhaven National Laboratory in the United States in 1971, and was officially made accessible to relevant laboratories around the world in 1973 [23]. In October 1998, PDB was transferred to the Research Collaboratory for Structural Bioinformatics (RCSB) and the transfer was completed in June 1999. RCSB is responsible for maintaining PDB. RCSB's main server and mirror servers all over the world provide database retrieval and download services. PDB collects three-dimensional structure data of 153,085 biomacromolecules determined by experiments (X-ray crystal diffraction, nuclear magnetic resonance, electron microscopy, etc.), proteins, including nucleic acids, polysaccharides, protein and nucleic acid compounds, and various compounds determined by X-ray crystal diffraction and nuclear magnetic resonance analysis methods. Irrespective of the way the structural data is obtained, it is stored in a spatial structure database in the same format in PDB, and is referred to as an entry. Each entry has its own unique PDB-ID, which is composed of four characters (capital letters A–Z and four digits 0–9), for example, 6A21. Users can query relevant information in PDB by entering the PDB-ID, including molecular name, date of inclusion of the molecule, source of sample, name of author, ID number, sequence, primary structure, secondary structure (α-helix, β-fold, and β-turn), heterogeneity (description of non-standard amino acid residues), connecting part (disulfide bond and some other chemical conditions), spatial coordinates and terminal composition of atoms, experimental methods used to determine the structure, resolution of diffraction data, relevant literature, and other information, as shown in Fig. 3.19 [24, 25]. All the data in the PDB can be accessed

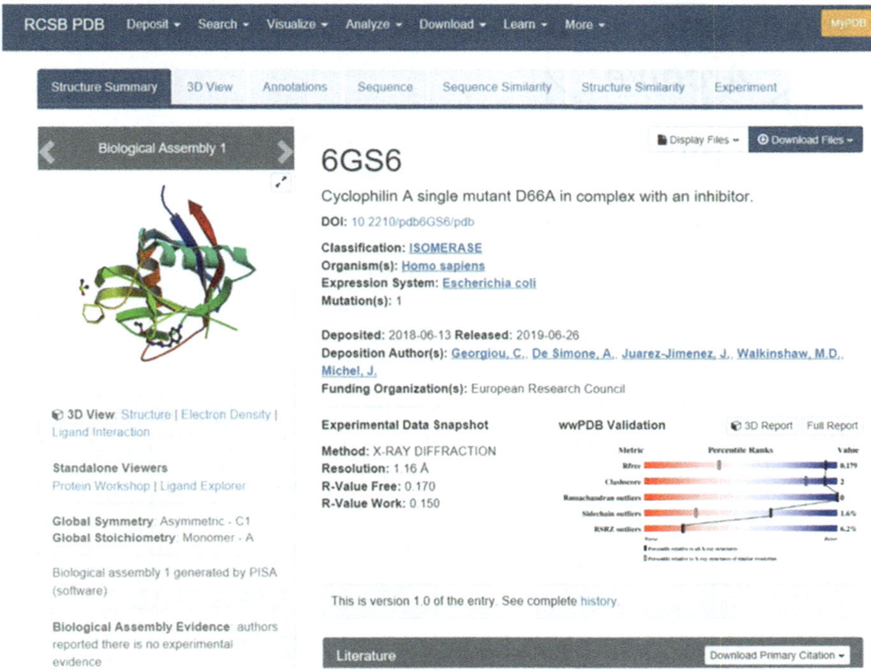

Fig. 3.19 6GS6 query result in PDB [24, 25]

online for free, and can also be accessed from CDs that are available. Data support is provided in the form of structure analysis and function mining of the network target.

3.3.2.1 Data Structure

The structure of biomolecules in PDB is expressed in terms of atomic space coordinate values and descriptions of their connection forms, connection orders, etc., in a specific format. Through specific software, such as PyMol, RasMol, Chimera, VMD, Swiss-PdbViewer, etc., the three-dimensional structure of the biological macromolecules can be visualized based on the PDB file, and the structure can be viewed and edited in detail, to apply for further research.

Users submit data to the PDB in mmCIF or PDB format via PDB's online AutoDep facility (see Fig. 3.20 [24]). AutoDep then calls a set of validators and returns the output diagnostic file online to the user within minutes of the data being sent to the PDB. The entries that pass the validation are published as LAYER-1. The PDB staff then evaluate the entries and output files that need to be validated, complete the annotations and return them to the user for comment and approval. After user approval and corrections, the final entry is published as Layer-2.

The three-dimensional structure records in PDB can be divided into two types: dominant sequence information and recessive sequence information. Both can be

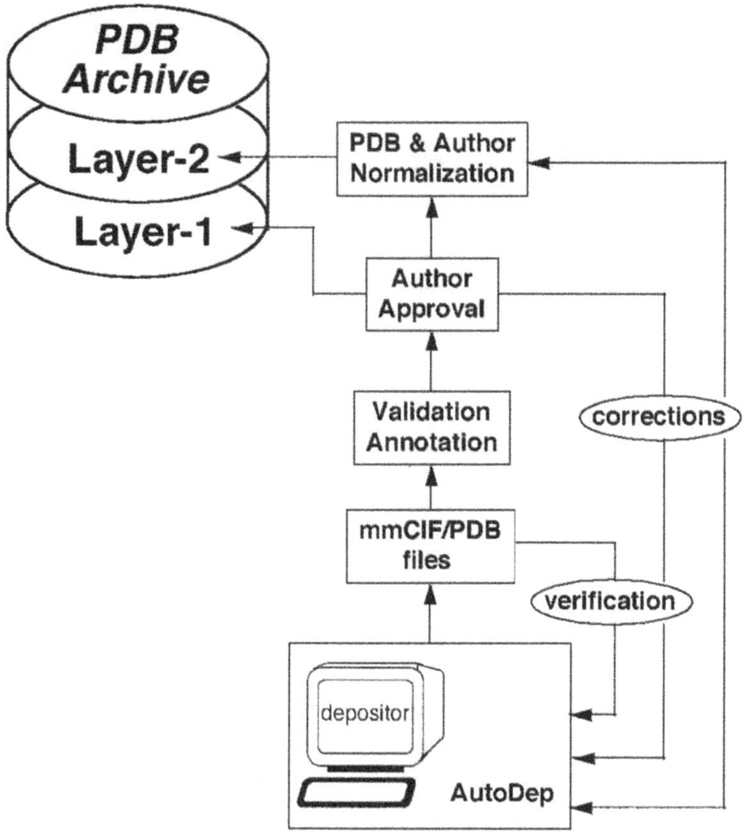

Fig. 3.20 Hierarchical submission method based on online AutoDep [24]

used to reconstruct chemical images of biopolymers. The dominant sequence is stored line by line in the PDB file starting with the keyword SEQRES. Unlike other sequential databases, PDB records use three-letter amino acid codes (as shown in Fig. 3.21 [24, 25]). The recessive sequence in the PDB record is the stereochemical information, which is contained in the ATOM record in the PDB file and the corresponding (*X*, *Y*, *Z*) three-dimensional coordinate structure. The ATOM record lists the atom name, residue name, residue sequence number, *X*, *Y*, and *Z* coordinates of each atom, occupancy rate, and temperature factor (as shown in Fig. 3.22 [24, 25]), which roughly account for more than 90% of the total number of records in each data file [26].

```
SEQRES   1 A  273  MET ARG GLN ILE ALA ILE TYR GLY LYS GLY GLY ILE GLY
SEQRES   2 A  273  LYS SER THR THR THR GLN ASN LEU THR ALA ALA LEU SER
SEQRES   3 A  273  THR MET GLY ASN ASN ILE LEU LEU VAL GLY CYS ASP PRO
SEQRES   4 A  273  LYS ALA ASP SER THR ARG MET LEU LEU GLY GLY LEU ASN
SEQRES   5 A  273  GLN LYS THR VAL LEU ASP THR LEU ARG SER GLU GLY ASP
SEQRES   6 A  273  GLU GLY ILE ASP LEU ASP THR VAL LEU GLN PRO GLY PHE
SEQRES   7 A  273  GLY GLY ILE LYS CYS VAL GLU SER GLY GLY PRO GLU PRO
SEQRES   8 A  273  GLY VAL GLY CYS ALA GLY ARG GLY ILE ILE THR SER ILE
SEQRES   9 A  273  GLY LEU LEU GLU ASN LEU GLY ALA TYR THR ASP ASP LEU
SEQRES  10 A  273  ASP TYR VAL PHE TYR ASP VAL LEU GLY ASP VAL VAL CYS
SEQRES  11 A  273  GLY GLY PHE ALA MET PRO ILE ARG GLU GLY LYS ALA LYS
SEQRES  12 A  273  GLU ILE TYR ILE VAL ALA SER GLY GLU LEU MET ALA ILE
SEQRES  13 A  273  TYR ALA ALA ASN ASN ILE CYS LYS GLY LEU ALA LYS PHE
SEQRES  14 A  273  ALA LYS GLY GLY ALA ARG LEU GLY GLY ILE ILE CYS ASN
SEQRES  15 A  273  SER ARG LYS VAL ASP GLY GLU ARG GLU LEU LEU GLU ALA
SEQRES  16 A  273  PHE ALA LYS LYS LEU GLY SER HIS LEU ILE HIS PHE VAL
SEQRES  17 A  273  PRO ARG ASP ASN ILE VAL GLN ARG ALA GLU ILE ASN ARG
SEQRES  18 A  273  LYS THR VAL ILE ASP PHE ASP ARG GLU SER ASP GLN ALA
SEQRES  19 A  273  LYS GLU TYR LEU THR LEU ALA ASP ASN VAL GLN ASN ASN
SEQRES  20 A  273  ASN LYS LEU VAL VAL PRO THR PRO LEU PRO MET GLU GLU
SEQRES  21 A  273  LEU GLU ALA MET MET VAL GLU PHE GLY ILE VAL GLU LEU
SEQRES   1 B  273  MET ARG GLN ILE ALA ILE TYR GLY LYS GLY GLY ILE GLY
SEQRES   2 B  273  LYS SER THR THR THR GLN ASN LEU THR ALA ALA LEU SER
SEQRES   3 B  273  THR MET GLY ASN ASN ILE LEU LEU VAL GLY CYS ASP PRO
SEQRES   4 B  273  LYS ALA ASP SER THR ARG MET LEU LEU GLY GLY LEU ASN
```

Fig. 3.21 Partial image of dominant sequence of 6QA8 PDB file [24, 25]

```
ATOM      1  N   MET A   1     -27.296  10.466  -9.085  1.00 60.81           N
ATOM      2  CA  MET A   1     -27.129  11.862  -8.690  1.00 58.02           C
ATOM      3  C   MET A   1     -28.472  12.594  -8.599  1.00 51.30           C
ATOM      4  O   MET A   1     -29.247  12.587  -9.549  1.00 54.67           O
ATOM      5  CB  MET A   1     -26.209  12.589  -9.676  1.00 45.14           C
ATOM      6  CG  MET A   1     -25.956  14.046  -9.312  1.00 50.94           C
ATOM      7  SD  MET A   1     -25.155  15.037 -10.600  1.00 60.91           S
ATOM      8  CE  MET A   1     -26.378  14.949 -11.908  1.00 57.37           C
ATOM      9  N   ARG A   2     -28.747  13.225  -7.459  1.00 48.49           N
ATOM     10  CA  ARG A   2     -29.942  14.053  -7.342  1.00 50.60           C
ATOM     11  C   ARG A   2     -29.745  15.367  -8.092  1.00 51.85           C
ATOM     12  O   ARG A   2     -28.657  15.957  -8.073  1.00 48.99           O
ATOM     13  CB  ARG A   2     -30.268  14.335  -5.873  1.00 48.21           C
ATOM     14  CG  ARG A   2     -30.578  13.104  -5.033  1.00 47.54           C
ATOM     15  CD  ARG A   2     -32.058  12.706  -5.111  1.00 49.73           C
ATOM     16  NE  ARG A   2     -32.934  13.548  -4.293  1.00 47.36           N
ATOM     17  CZ  ARG A   2     -33.068  13.440  -2.972  1.00 49.01           C
ATOM     18  NH1 ARG A   2     -32.372  12.531  -2.303  1.00 48.83           N
ATOM     19  NH2 ARG A   2     -33.902  14.242  -2.313  1.00 50.05           N
ATOM     20  N   GLN A   3     -30.808  15.830  -8.749  1.00 45.05           N
ATOM     21  CA  GLN A   3     -30.766  17.026  -9.590  1.00 44.03           C
ATOM     22  C   GLN A   3     -31.820  18.016  -9.095  1.00 45.48           C
ATOM     23  O   GLN A   3     -32.992  17.957  -9.479  1.00 40.95           O
ATOM     24  CB  GLN A   3     -30.975  16.651 -11.040  1.00 46.05           C
ATOM     25  CG  GLN A   3     -30.129  15.472 -11.466  1.00 45.26           C
ATOM     26  CD  GLN A   3     -30.345  15.109 -12.911  1.00 51.08           C
```

Fig. 3.22 Partial image of hidden sequence of 6QA8 PDB file [24, 25]

3.3.2.2 Function Introduction

(1) Prediction of secondary structure of proteins

Some researchers have used the protein secondary structure information available in the PDB to try to generalize more reliable secondary structure prediction methods, and many results have been published. With technological advances and emergence of new technologies, there may be a breakthrough in the near future in prediction.

(2) Research on protein evolution

In the past, the similarities and differences of sequences were mainly analyzed from the perspective of the primary structure. With the massive increase in protein stereostructure information in the PDB, some researchers are currently trying to study protein evolution based on the structural correlation of the stereostructure.

(3) Simulation of protein curing process

Researchers have proposed various possible curling paths and theoretically simulated the curling process, but the correctness of these hypotheses must be determined by comparison with an already clearly defined protein spatial structure. The PDB provides such a comparison standard, allowing researchers to modify the hypothesis based on the comparison results, to make it more in line with the actual situation.

3.3.2.3 Characteristics and Deficiencies

Unlike other databases on molecular stereostructure, most of the data available in PDB have not been published, but are directly provided by laboratories to PDB; whereas the data in other databases are mainly from information available in the public domain.

Although PDB's processing program has been greatly improved, there are still many errors that cannot be found by the system, and all entries need to be checked manually. Some types of problems still need manual intervention and processing, such as: dealing with heterogeneous (small molecules with complex structure) structures and solving the problem of crystal accumulation, and conflicts between the submitted amino acid sequences and the amino acid sequences found in the database. Sometimes it is necessary to refer to other publications and materials to clarify information such as crystal data, biological details, etc. It is necessary to further extend and improve the input and verification program components of AutoDep to meet the needs of some conflicts between information providers and users, and ensure the accuracy of information.

3.3.3 Gene Information Database—GeneCards

The GeneCards database covers the analysis data of human genes in various professional databases [27]; it is a relatively comprehensive and easy-to-use human genome annotation database. The GeneCards database was established in 1997 by the Crown Human Genome Center of the Weizmann Institute of Science in Israel. The initial goal of the database was to reasonably and systematically integrate the fragmented information in various databases. Through more than 20 years of research and development and maintenance, the GeneCards database has overcome the limitations of different database formats. It can automatically mine and integrate tens of thousands of human gene expressions, functions, positions, pathways, mutations, homologous genes, diseases, and related references from more than 190 databases. and integrate them into gene network cards for researchers to use for reference and application. As of November 2019, the GeneCards database has data on 268,549 human genes. This database is not only up to date, but also free to view.

The GeneCards database is a human genome compendium, containing genome, transcriptome, proteome, heredity, clinical, functional, and other gene-centric information [28]. To make the database website more compact, the detailed information, diagrams, tables, and references of some entries in GeneCards database can be viewed by clicking on the hyperlink, to see all available information of related genes.

3.3.3.1 Data Structure

Each gene entry in the GeneCards database is divided into 17 main chapters in the form of electronic web cards. Each gene card in the GeneCards database automatically integrates and annotates the genetic information of the original database to the corresponding section of the GeneCards database by compiling the genetic information of various databases. The GeneCards database has been updated to version 4.0, and while retaining the original information and functions, it provides a better user experience by improving the integration of data and information.

3.3.3.2 Applications/Functions in the Field of Molecular Biology

Each gene is described in detail in GeneCards database. In terms of genetic functions: ① Molecular function: The molecular function in the GeneCards database comes from other databases. The molecular function table of gene ontology has GO IDs, GO terms, evidence, and PubMed IDs. In addition, hyperlinks allow users to view other genes sharing the gene ontology. ② Phenotypes and animal models: This section lists the related phenotypes of human and mouse genes. Hyperlinks not only allow users to view other genes sharing this gene phenotype, but also enable users to navigate to animal models, such as mouse models with knockout genes. ③ Function-related products: This section provides product links to animal models, clones, and cell lines related to the gene. Pathways and interactions: ① Super metabolic pathways: The table of super metabolic pathways shows the pathways and dynamic links that may be involved in this gene, where G is KEGG pathway information and R is REACTOME pathway information. ② Pathway source: This part of the content is classified according to the pathway information source database. Only five related pathways are displayed in each database unit. Information of all pathways can be viewed by clicking the link. ③ Interacting proteins: The protein interaction network is shown in the form of pictures. Click the link to view the network pictures with more complex and interaction information. In addition, the interaction protein information is listed in table form, including the link to the gene name and gene card of each interacting protein, the link to the ID of interaction proteins and external databases, and the link to the interaction information in the protein interaction network. ④ Signaling Network Open Resource (SIGNOR): Displays the open resource link to the interaction signaling network, and the link to the interaction gene list and gene card. ⑤ Gene ontology biological process: This part shows the gene ontology biological process, including the gene GO ID, GO terms, evidence, and PubMed ID [29].

3.3.3.3 Characteristics and Deficiencies

Over the course of 20 years of development and dozens of revisions, the GeneCards database currently contains 268,549 human gene expressions, functions, positions, pathways, mutations, homologous genes, diseases, and related references, from more than 190 databases, which are integrated into gene network cards for researchers to use for reference. It is a comprehensive database of human genes that integrates a variety of professional database functions.

Although the gene information in the GeneCards database is rich and diverse, to make website more compact, the detailed information, diagrams, tables, and references of entries can be viewed by clicking on the appropriate hyperlink, to see all available information of related genes. This means that users need to frequently click hyperlinks or navigate to other databases to obtain comprehensive information of genes, which indirectly wastes the user's research time.

3.3.4 Kyoto Encyclopedia of Genes and Genomes—KEGG

One of the major challenges in the post-genomic era is how to fully display the biological information contained in cells and organisms with the help of computers. Scientists need to be able to calculate or predict complex cellular pathways or biological responses based on information in the genome. To this end, the Kyoto Encyclopedia of Genes and Genomes (KEGG Database) was established by Kanehisa Laboratory of Bioinformatics Center of Kyoto University in 1995. The database was last updated on May 1st, 2019, and the latest version is 90.1. KEGG is an integrated database divided into system information, genomic information, chemical information, and health information. KEGG combines genes, genomic information, and higher-level functional information to systematically analyze gene functions through the computerization of known biological processes in cells and standardization of the interpretation of existing gene function information [30]. It has many functions, such as describing of metabolic pathway, predicting gene function, accessing genomic information, identifying homology, and analyzing the interaction between proteins and other macromolecules. Researchers can not only obtain the data from the database for free, but also access the genome map and compare the genome map and transcriptome expression map using Java-based graphical tools.

3.3.4.1 Data Structure

So far, the KEGG database has 18 sub-databases, among which the 4 main databases are PATHWAY, GENES, LIGAND, and BRITE; the other sub-databases are derived from these 4 databases. The PATHWAY database provides artificial pathway maps of various reactions occurring in cells, presented in the form of a network. The GENES database stores the sequenced genome information registered in KEGG. The LIGAND database can be used to query information about compounds, polysaccharides, and enzymatic reactions. BRITE is a database that classifies and summarizes biological information according to hierarchy, and the KEGG ORTHOLOGY (KO) contained in it, is a system for gene homology identification [31].

3.3.4.2 Function Introduction

As a reference knowledgebase, KEGG is widely used for integrating and interpreting large-scale data sets obtained by genome sequencing and other high-throughput experimental techniques [32]. Its applications in bioinformatics include: ① Analysis of metabolic network: KEGG pathway map, BRITE hierarchical entries, and KEGG modules constituting KEGG reference information. By using the KEGG mapper to label the pathway, we can color the compounds or enzymes needed in the metabolic pathway, which is beneficial for the analysis of the metabolic pathway. In addition, the gene chip data can also be analyzed. For example, when analyzing the gene chip data in the KEGG Expression database, KegArray can be used to represent the expression changes of each gene in the pathway with different colors, with red indicating up-regulation and green indicating down-regulation. ② Application of disease and drug metabolism network analysis: The disease and drug information integrated using KEGG Mapping are widely used in related research. All known disease genes collected in KEGG DISEASE and all drug targets collected in KEGG DRUG are merged into KEGG PATHWAY and BRITE databases. KEGG mapping can be used to mark corresponding genes in different colors in the metabolic map. In the disease/drug map in the metabolic pathway map of diseases, the disease-related genes are shown in a pink box, and drug targets are shown in a bright blue box. ③ Genome comparison and merging: On the KEGG GENOME page, users can not only use Mapping to compare the metabolic capacity of different species, but also check the complementarity of human-pathogen and human-microform metabolism, and check the common characteristics between species. ④ Reconstruction of metabolic network and construction of enzyme database of target species: A list of all genes-enzymes and enzymes-reactions in the metabolic network of the reconstructed target species can be obtained from the ligand database. Among them, enzymes play a key role in connecting genes and corresponding metabolic reactions. Since the EC number of enzymes is unique, a list containing all metabolic components involved in cell metabolism and their metabolic reactions can be established accordingly. Then, through the information-assisted reference optimization of other databases, a database of all enzymes and reactions of the target species can be constructed. After obtaining a high-quality database, the metabolic network can be reconstructed by relevant software [33]. Therefore, the KEGG database can be widely used in constructing a metabolic network.

3.3.4.3 Characteristics and Deficiencies

The KEGG database is a large-scale comprehensive database that connects genes, enzymes, and reactions to construct the metabolic network. Its graphical interface for analysis and interpretation provides a good platform for the study of genes, enzymes, and their metabolic networks. In terms of biosynthesis, the output of the target product can be increased by controlling the metabolic flow. Not only that, the disease metabolism network developed by KEGG can help in studying the pathogenesis of diseases and the target of drug action.

KECG is a comprehensive database that includes data on metabolic pathways, genetic information, and compound reactions, but there are also some omissions. For example, the colored input boxes are case sensitive, incorrect data when starting KegArray, some enzymatic reactions have been recorded in the LIGAND database but do not occur in the specified species, so the reconstructed network contains false edges, etc. In the case of reconstructing multiple metabolic networks, in order to read data, we must visit KEGG's remote server frequently, which is very time-consuming.

3.4 Protein Interaction Databases Commonly Used in Network Pharmacology

3.4.1 Biological Universal Interaction Database—BioGRID

BioGRID is a free and open interactive repository dedicated to the management and storage of protein information, genetic material, and chemical interactions of all biological species and humans. BioGRID was initially established in 2003 as a general interactive dataset repository and later renamed as BioGRID [34]. The current version of BioGRID is 3.5.173. In this version, 1,690,901 protein–gene interaction information, 28,093 chemical associations, and 726,378 protein post-transcriptional modification information are sorted out from 69,644 literature sources, covering animals (including: human, zebrafish, mouse, fruit bat fly,

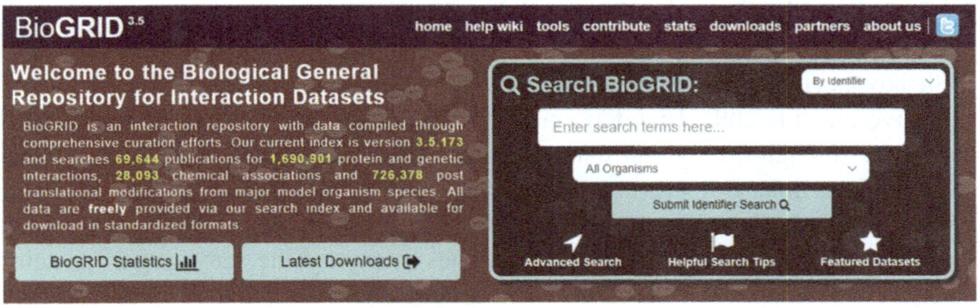

Fig. 3.23 Homepage of the BioGRID website [34]

Anopheles gambiae, European bee, cattle, dog, guinea pig, monkey, horse, chicken, rabbit, sheep, orangutan, pig, *Xenopus laevis*, sea urchin, etc.), plants (including *Arabidopsis thaliana*, honeysuckle, soybean, rice, tomato, potato, grape, corn, castor, etc.), bacterial viruses (including: *Bacillus subtilis*, *Candida albicans*, *Escherichia coli*, hepatitis virus, herpes virus, HIV virus, human papillomavirus, *Mycobacterium tuberculosis*, *Neurospora crassa*, tobacco mosaic virus, corn smut, *Vaccinia virus*), and others including *Caenorhabditis elegans*, amoeba, lice, Plasmodium, yeast, lichen, etc. All information can be viewed and downloaded free of charge through the search engine provided by the website. The database also provides several online analysis and visualization tools.

The homepage of the BioGRID website is shown in Fig. 3.23 [34]. It is relatively easy to use. You only need to enter a gene ID, keyword, or gene name, select the species, and click Search to get the gene interaction result. The search results mainly consist of 3 parts: ① Description of basic information: including retrieved protein names, aliases, post-transcriptional modifications, GO annotation information, and links to other databases; ② Information statistics: Statistics of each interaction type and proportion; ③ Detailed results display: Protein interaction information, interaction network of the protein, etc.

3.4.1.1 Data Structure

BioGRID is also developing related projects in areas related to biomedical science, such as ubiquitin–proteasome systems and interaction networks associated with various human diseases. The BioGRID strategy is coordinated through the Interactive Management System (IMS), which facilitates the compilation of interactive records through structured evidence codes, phenotypic ontologies, and gene annotations. The BioGRID structure has been improved to support a wider range of interactions and post-translational modification types, allowing for more complex representations of polygene/protein interactions.

3.4.1.2 Function Introduction

With advancements in the post-genomic era, protein research has become more extensive and in-depth. BioGRID currently has more than 1,670,000 interactions composed of high-throughput data sets and independent research, and more than 68,000 interactions from various literature sources. There are comprehensive literature reports on budding yeast (*S. cerevisiae*), fission yeast (*S. pombe*), and Arabidopsis (*A. thaliana*). BioGRID continues to expand the screening of proteins and genetic interactions from biomedical literature, as well as related attributes, such as protein variations, phenotypes, and chemical or drug interactions. The integration of these network datasets with other data types (including expression data, quantitative phenotypic data, and high-resolution sequence data) can help predict medicine and future drug discovery work.

3.4.1.3 Characteristics

The current focus is on specific areas of biology, and efforts are being made to expand the management of a variety of metazoans in order to gain insight into conservative networks and pathways related to human health. The BioGRID 3.5 web interface includes new search and display functions for quick queries across multiple data types and sources. BioGRID provides interactive data for several model biological databases, such as Entrez-gene, SGD, TAIR, FlyBase, and other interactive metadatabases. The entire BioGRID 3.2 dataset can be downloaded in a variety of file formats, including IMEx-compatible PSI-MI XML. For developers, BioGRID interaction is also available through REST-based web services and the Cytoscape plug-in. All BioGRID documents are available online in the BioGRID Wiki.

3.4.2 Database of Interacting Proteins—DIP

The Database of Interacting Proteins (DIP) was founded in August 1999 by the Laboratory of Structural Biology and Molecular Medicine of the Institute of Molecular Biology, UCLA. It aims to integrate various experimental evidence of protein–protein interaction (PPI) into an easily accessible online database to establish a simple and easy-to-use PPI public database. In addition, the DIP database is one of the member databases of the International Molecular Exchange Consortium (IMEx).

3.4.2.1 Data Structure

The DIP database contains experimentally confirmed PPI information and protein complexes from the PDB (Protein Data Bank) database, and contains the most

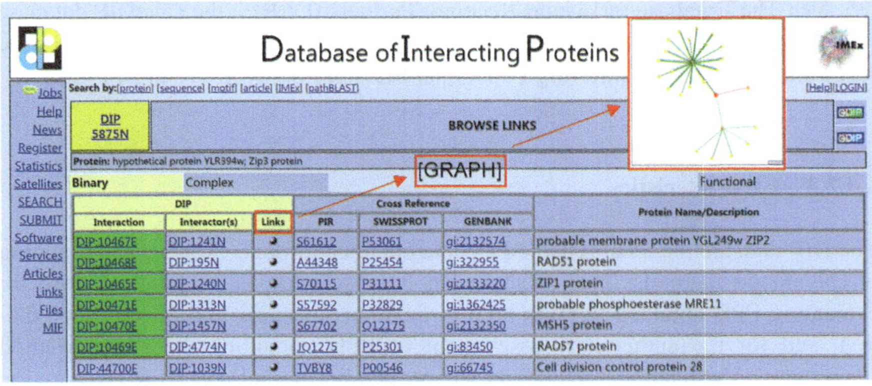

Fig. 3.24 Example of DIP database query results [38]

reliable PPI data obtained by manual mining or calculation by experts [35–37]. As of the latest update on February 13th, 2017, DIP has collected and classified 81,923 PPIs involving 28,850 proteins from 834 species, and 82,143 experiments from 8234 data sources.

The DIP database provides a variety of query methods. Users can directly query PPI based on protein, biological species, protein superfamily, keywords, experimental techniques, or cited literature, and can also query PPI based on sequence similarity using BLAST search, pattern search, and motif search. The query result is listed as two items: Node and Link. Nodes are used to describe the characteristics of the queried protein, including the functional domain and fingerprint of the protein, and some also include annotations of the enzyme code or the position in the cell. Link refers to the interaction relationship between two nodes. For each PPI, DIP provides evidence (experimental method) and literature, and records the number of experiments supporting the PPI in addition to providing big data analysis. An example of the query results is shown in Fig. 3.24 [38]. The DIP database provides standard data sets, including HiTHR high-throughput (genome scale) dataset, FULL (complete DIP dataset), SPECIES (specific species set), FASTA (DIP sequence), and DIP-IMEX dataset [38, 39].

3.4.2.2 Function Introduction

MiSink is a plug-in for the DIP database which can be used in Cytoscape (an open source platform used for visualization and integration of biological interactive data) and can be converted into an interactive graphical DIP interface. JDIP is a Java language-based visualization application tool provided by the DIP database that can display PPI data more intuitively in the form of a network, and allows users to integrate their experimental information such as mRNA expression data, function of functional domains, and post-translational modifications of proteins into the network of interactions between proteins. In addition, the DIP database has 3 sub-databases

[35, 39]: The Database of Ligand-Receptor Partners (DLRP), the LiveDIP database (LiveDIP), and the PPI database predicted by gene fusion method, Phylogenetic spectrum method, etc. (Inferring Functional Linkages between Proteins, Prolink).

3.4.2.3 Characteristics

The DIP data are the most reliable PPI data obtained through expert manual mining or calculation methods. This database has been selected as the gold standard for evaluating PPIs obtained through high-throughput screening and computer prediction, and for the authenticity assessment of PPIs, including the PVM Method (Paralogous Verification Method) based on parallel homology, EPR (Expression Profile Reliability) Method based on expression spectrum analysis, and DPV (Domain Pair Verification) Method based on structural domain interaction. However, due to the human intervention and processing, updates to the database are relatively slow.

3.4.3 Molecular Interaction Database—IntAct

The IntAct database was founded by the European Bioinformatics Institute (EBI) in 2003 [40, 41]. The main goal of this database is to help researchers access public PPI data, reduce redundancy, and provide a unified query tool to maximize the efficiency of data storage and retrieval. The IntAct database is one of the member databases of the IMEx Consortium. At present, this database also integrates all IMEx data. The IntAct database provides a free and open source database analysis tool for molecular interactions. All data comes from published literature reports and is manually annotated by biological experts to ensure high accuracy, and includes experimental methods, experimental conditions, and functional domains of interactions [41]. The IntAct database is updated monthly, the latest version is 4.2.12, which was updated on May 4th, 2019; the species covered include human, yeast, fruit fly, *Escherichia coli*, Arabidopsis (*A. thaliana*), and *Caenorhabditis elegans*. The database contains evidence of 585,731 interactions and 889,774 binary interactions of 110,643 proteins or molecules, covering 20,585 publications and 67,624 experiments. A total of 3829 controlled words are used to consistently describe the experimental details used to generate the data.

There are basic query and advanced query tools in the IntAct database. The basic query tool can be used to query based on gene name, protein name, PubMed ID, and biological function; the advanced query tool can be used to query according to experimental method and controlled vocabularies customized by IntAct; the result display tool displays the PPI network in a graphical format.

3.4.3.1 Data Structure

The IntAct database supports multiple formats including PSI-MI XML, PSI-MITAB, RDF/XML, RDF/ XML-ABBREV, N3, N-Triples, and Turtle. The IntAct research group suggests that biologists submit PPI information directly to the database prior to publication (in any format, IMEx format recommended) to facilitate the improvement and management of data, in the same manner as the nucleotide sequence is directly submitted to the GenBank database. The IntAct data can be retrieved through PSICQUIC service as well as many other data types, including through predictive interaction and genome and text-based mining for inferring molecular interactions.

3.4.3.2 Function Introduction

The IntAct database provides online visualization analysis of the PPI network and supports third-party network construction software such as Cytoscape and Proviz. In addition to storing and querying the interaction protein information, the IntAct database also provides the best bait protein information to predict pull-down based on the pay-as-you-go algorithm.

3.4.4 Database of Gene/Protein Interactions—STRING

The STRING database was established by the European Molecular Biology Laboratory in 2009 to collect and integrate known and predicted protein–protein related data information of numerous organisms [42–45]. It is a free and open source PPI search and prediction information database that integrates PPI from high-throughput experiments, text mining, biological information prediction, and interaction databases (such as BioGRID and IntAct). It uses a scoring system to assign different weights to the interactions obtained by different methods, and provides a reliability score of each PPI pair [35, 36]. Version 11.0, released on January 19th, 2019, is the latest version and covers about 24,600,000 proteins and over 2,000,000,000 interactions in 5090 organisms.

3.4.4.1 Data Structure

The associations in STRING database include direct (physical) and indirect (functional) interactions with specific and biological significance. At the same time, a scoring system is used to assign different weights to the interactions obtained by different methods, to provide the reliability score of each PPI pair. In addition to collecting and reassessing existing PPI data (sources: KEGG, EcoCyc, BIioCyc,

GO, Reactome, Biocarta, NCI-Nature Pathway Interaction Database, MINT, HPRD, BIND, DIP, PID, BioGRID), as well as introducing known pathways and protein complexes into the dataset, interaction predictions are derived from the following sources: ① System co-expression analysis, ② shared selective detection of cross genome signals, ③ automatic text mining of scientific literature (source: SGD, OMIM, FlyBase, PubMed), and ④ computational transfer of knowledge about interaction between organisms based on genealogy (Neighborhood, Co-Occurrence, Co-Expression, Gene Fusion).

Users can query by protein name (multiple concurrent input supported), sequence name (multiple concurrent input supported), organism, or protein family, and the results are presented in a clickable interactive network diagram of nodes and edges. Nodes represent proteins, and the connection between nodes represents the interaction between two proteins. Data from specific sources or the extended network graph can be selected for redrawing according to the user's requirements. The navigation options of the results include Viewers, Legend, Settings, Analysis, Exports, Clusters, and More/Less used to adjust the number of presented nodes in the interactive network diagram. When a protein is selected at a node, users can view the image of its crystalline protein (from PDB) and the image of the protein model (from SwissModel) in a pop-up window. The database supports the following operations: ① Find all proteins in STRING that interact with window proteins; ② Add the protein that interacts with the window protein to the network; ③ Display the protein sequence; ④ The homologue in STRING; ⑤ Redirect to the corresponding entry in the GeneCards database (only for human proteins); and ⑥ Redirect to the corresponding entry in the SMART database. In the Viewers page, users can get relevant information such as Network, Neighborhood, Co-occurrence, Co-expression, Fusion, Experiments, Databases, and Text mining. In the Legend page, the color of each protein and the score value corresponding to the queried PPI are displayed. In the Settings page, the user can set the PPI type and display type for the results. In the Analysis page, the GO and KEGG enrichment analysis results are provided for genes in the PPI network. In the Clusters page, users can perform cluster analysis of the genes using kmeans and MCL clustering, and results are available in a TSV format. An example of the query results is shown in Fig. 3.25 [46].

3.4.4.2 Function Introduction

The main purpose of the STRING database is to build the PPI network. It can be used to filter and evaluate functional genomics data and provide an intuitive platform for annotating the structure, function, and evolution of proteins. It is used to explore predictive PPI networks, targets new directions for experimental research, and provides cross-species prediction for interactive mapping. All PPI data are weighted, integrated, and have a calculated reliable value.

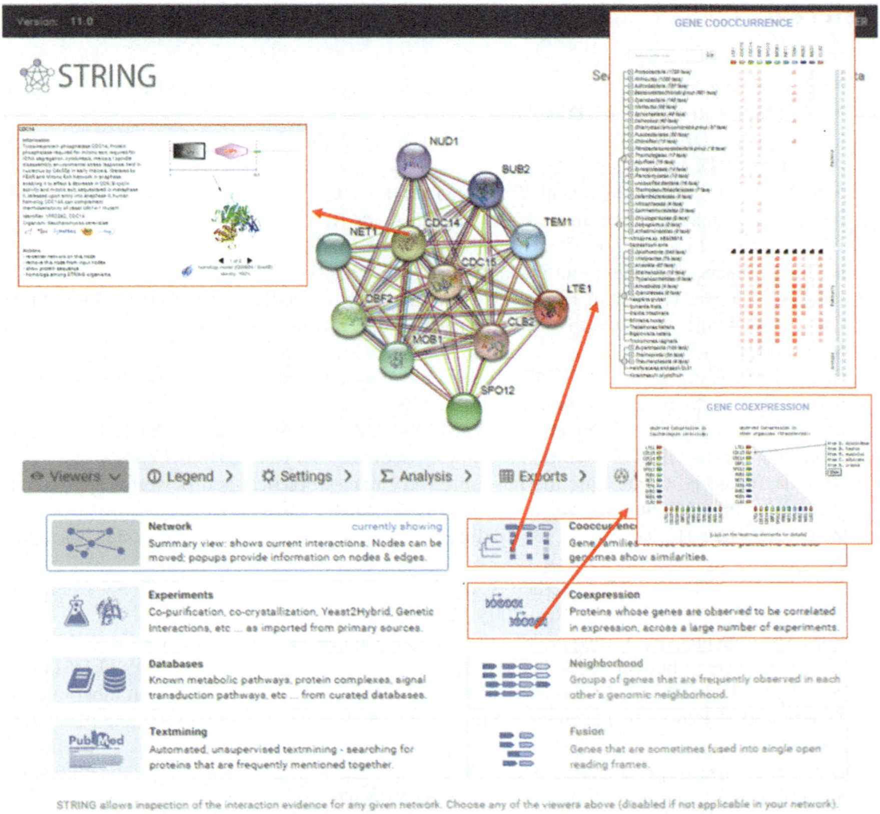

Fig. 3.25 Example of STRING database query results [46]

3.4.4.3 Characteristics

The STRING database is completely pre-calculated, so that all the information in the network at higher level or in a single PPI interface can be quickly obtained. It supports individual selection of various evidence types and can perform customized searches at runtime. At the same time, it includes a dedicated viewer to view all associated evidence. The STRING database is an exploratory resource that contains more related data than the basic PPI database. This database is recommended to quickly obtain preliminary PPI information of the queried protein, especially for proteins that are not well characterized.

References

1. Xu HY, Zhang YQ, Liu ZM, et al. ETCM: an encyclopaedia of traditional Chinese medicine. Nucleic Acids Res. 2019;47(D1):976–82.
2. Huang L, Xie DL, Yu YR, et al. TCMID 2.0: a comprehensive resource for TCM. Nucleic Acids Res. 2018;46(D1):1117–20.
3. Xue RC, Fang Z, Zhang MX, et al. TCMID: Traditional Chinese Medicine integrative database for herb molecular mechanism analysis. Nucleic Acids Res. 2013;41(D1):1089–95.
4. Wu Y, Zhang FL, Yang K, et al. SymMap: an integrative database of traditional Chinese medicine enhanced by symptom mapping. Nucleic Acids Res. 2019;47(D1):1110–7.
5. Fang YC, Huang HC, Chen HH, et al. TCMGeneDIT: a data-base for associated traditional Chinese medicine, gene and disease information using text mining. BMC Complement Altern Med. 2008;8(1):58.
6. Ru JL, Li P, Wang JN, et al. TCMSP: a database of systems pharmacology for drug discovery from herbal medicines. J Cheminf. 2014;6(1):1–6.
7. Liu ZY, Guo FF, Wang Y, et al. BATMAN-TCM: a Bioinformatics Analysis Tool for Molecular mechANism of Traditional Chinese Medicine. Sci Rep. 2016;6(1):82–3.
8. Yoav B, Yosef H. Controlling the false discovery rate: a practical and powerful approach to multiple testing. J R Stat Soc Ser B (Methodol). 1995;57(1):289–300.
9. Wang JF, Zhou H, Han LY, et al. Traditional Chinese medicine information database. Clin Pharmacol Ther. 2005;103(3):501.
10. Wheeler DL, Church DM, Federhen S, et al. Database resources of the National Center for Biotechnology. Nucleic Acids Res. 2003;31(1):28–33.
11. Hamosh A, Scott AF, Amberger JS, et al. Online Mendelian Inheritance in Man (OMIM), a knowledgebase of human genes and genetic disorders. Nucleic Acids Res. 2005;33:D514–7.
12. Amberger JS, Bocchini CA, Schiettecatte F, et al. OMIM.org: Online Mendelian Inheritance in Man (OMIM®), an online catalog of human genes and genetic disorders. Nucleic Acids Res. 2015;43:D789–98.
13. Groza T, Kohler S, Moldenhauer D, et al. The human phenotype ontology: semantic unification of common and rare disease. Am J Hum Genet. 2015;97(1):111–24.
14. Kohler S, Vasilevsky NA, Engelstad M, et al. The human phenotype ontology in 2017. Nucleic Acids Res. 2016;45(D1):D865–76.
15. Kohler S, Doelken SC, Mungall CJ, et al. The Human Phenotype Ontology project: linking molecular biology and disease through phenotype data. Nucleic Acids Res. 2014;42:D966–74.
16. Robinson PN, Mundlos S. The human phenotype ontology. Clin Genet. 2010;77(6):525–34.
17. Janet P, Àlex B, Nuria QR, et al. DisGeNET: a comprehensive platform integrating information on human disease-associated genes and variants. Nucleic Acids Res. 2017;45(D1):D833–9.
18. Pinero J, Queralt RN, Bravo À, et al. DisGeNET: a discovery platform for the dynamical exploration of human diseases and their genes. Database. 2015;2015:bav028.
19. Queralt RN, Pinero J, Bravo À, et al. DisGeNET-RDF: harnessing the innovative power of the Semantic Web to explore the genetic basis of diseases. Bioinformatics. 2016;32(14):2236–8.
20. Bravo À, Pinero J, Queralt RN, et al. Extraction of relations between genes and diseases from text and large-scale data analysis: implications for translational research. BMC Bioinformatics. 2015;16(1):55.
21. Rappaport N, Twik M, Plaschkes I, et al. MalaCards: an amalgamated human disease compendium with diverse clinical and genetic annotation and structured search. Nucleic Acids Res. 2017;45(D1):D877–87.
22. Li YH, Yu CY, Li XX, et al. Therapeutic target database update 2018: enriched resource for facilitating bench-to-clinic research of targeted therapeutics. Nucleic Acids Res. 2017;46(D1): D1121–7.
23. Bernstein FC, Koetzle TF, Williams GJ, et al. The Protein Data Bank. A computer-based archival file for macromolecular structures. Eur J Biochem. 1977;185(2):584–91.

24. Sussman JL, Lin D, Jiang J, et al. Protein Data Bank(PDB): database of three-dimensional structural information of biological macromolecules. Acta Crystallogr Sect D Biol Crystallogr. 1998;54(Pt 6 Pt 1):1078–84.
25. Drew HR, Wing RM, Takano T, Broka C, Tanaka S, Itakura K, Dickerson RE. Structure of a B-DNA dodecamer: conformation and dynamics. Proc Natl Acad Sci U S A. 1981;78 (4):2179–83.
26. Wang S. A brief introduction to spatial structure database of biomacromolecules (PDB). Chem Life (Bull Chin Biochem Soc). 1991(2):13–5 (in Chinese) [王三山. 生物大分子空间结构数据库(PDB)简介. 生命的化学(中国生物化学会通讯). 1991(2):13–5].
27. Safran M, Solomon I, Shmueli O, et al. GeneCards™ 2002: towards a complete, object-oriented, human gene compendium. Bioinformatics. 2002;18(11):1542–3.
28. Safran M, Dalah I, Alexander J, et al. GeneCards Version 3: the human gene integrator. Database. 2010;2010:baq020-baq020.
29. Stelzer G, Rosen N, Plaschkes I, et al. The GeneCards suite: from gene data mining to disease genome sequence analyses. Curr Protoc Bioinformatics. 2016;54(1):1.30.1–1.30.33.
30. Kanehisa M, Furumichi M, Tanabe M, et al. KEGG: new perspectives on genomes, pathways, diseases and drugs. Nucleic Acids Res. 2016;45(D1):D353–61.
31. Han Z, Tian P. Application of KEGG database in biosynthesis research. Biotechnol Bull. 2011 (01):76–82 (in Chinese) [韩增叶, 田平芳. KEGG数据库在生物合成研究中的应用.生物技术通报. 2011(01):76–82].
32. Kanehisa M, Sato Y, Furumichi M, et al. New approach for understanding genome variations in KEGG. Nucleic Acids Res. 2018;47(D1):D590–5.
33. Li X, Liu Z, Li J, et al. Progress of KEGG database and its application in bioinformatics. Pharmacobiotechnology. 2012;19(06):535–39 (in Chinese) [李向真, 刘子朋, 李娟, 等.KEGG数据库的进展及其在生物信息学中的应用.药物生物技术. 2012;19(06):535–39].
34. Stark C, Breitkreutz BJ, Reguly T, et al. BioGRID: a general repository for interaction datasets. Nucleic Acids Res. 2006;34:D535–9.
35. Wang J. Protein interaction database. Chin J Biochem Mol Biol. 2017;33(08):760–67 (in Chinese) [王建.蛋白质相互作用数据库.中国生物化学与分子生物学报. 2017;33 (08):760–67].
36. Yu X, Xu Z. Protein interaction database and its application. J Biochem Mol Biol. 2008 (03):189–96 (in Chinese) [余鑫煜, 许正平. 蛋白质相互作用数据库及其应用.中国生物化学与分子生物学报. 2008(03):189–96].
37. Salwinski L, Eisenberg D. Computational methods of analysis of protein-protein interactions. Curr Opin Struct Biol. 2003;13(3):377–82.
38. Xenarios I, Rice DW, Salwinski L, et al. DIP: the database of interacting proteins. Nucleic Acids Res. 2000;28(1):289–91.
39. Salwinski L, Miller CS, Smith AJ, et al. The database of interacting proteins: 2004 update. Nucleic Acids Res. 2004;32(suppl_1):D449–51.
40. Kerrien S, Aranda B, Breuza L, et al. The IntAct molecular interaction database in 2012. Nucleic Acids Res. 2011;40(D1):D841–6.
41. Hermjakob H, Montecchi PL, Lewington C, et al. IntAct: an open source molecular interaction database. Nucleic Acids Res. 2004;32(suppl_1):D452–5.
42. Von MC, Jensen LJ, Snel B, et al. STRING: known and predicted protein–protein associations, integrated and transferred across organisms. Nucleic Acids Res. 2005;33(suppl_1):D433–7.
43. Von MC, Jensen LJ, Kuhn M, et al. STRING 7—recent developments in the integration and prediction of protein interactions. Nucleic Acids Res. 2006;35(suppl_1):D358–62.
44. Szklarczyk D, Morris JH, Cook H, et al. The STRING database in 2017: quality-controlled protein-protein association networks, made broadly accessible. Nucleic Acids Res. 2017;45 (D1):D362–8.
45. Ensen LJ, Kuhn M, Stark M, et al. STRING 8-a global view on proteins and their functional interactions in 630 organisms. Nucleic Acids Res. 2008;37(suppl_1):D412–6.

46. Szklarczyk D, Gable AL, Lyon D, Junge A, Wyder S, Huerta-Cepas J, Simonovic M, Doncheva NT, Morris JH, Bork P, Jensen LJ, Mering CV. STRING v11: protein-protein association networks with increased coverage, supporting functional discovery in genome-wide experimental datasets. Nucleic Acids Res. 2019;47(D1):D607–13.

Chapter 4
Common Network Pharmacology Software

Xuezhong Zhou, Ning Wang, and Xing Zhai

Abstract As a growing trend in current pharmacology research and an important medical application in network science research, network pharmacology has become an indispensable complement to traditional pharmacology research with the immense accumulation and integration of large-scale pharmacology and disease molecular network data. In addition to emerging new methods and technologies, a large number of analytical techniques and methods, such as network analysis and molecular functional analysis have matured into related software or programs and are available for researchers to use for free or available as open source, which is an important factor and condition that has helped network pharmacology's robust and rapid development. From the perspective of information processing and computer systems, this chapter classifies and introduces commonly used network pharmacology software by refining the overall functional flow of network pharmacology-related software or programs and illustrates demonstrative application examples by combining actual data processing, analysis, and visualization operations. The practical steps and contents in this chapter, combined with the theoretical analysis, analysis methods, and research cases of network pharmacology in other chapters, can provide researchers or students with relevant software tools and practical operation methods that can be used for reference, as well as provide rapid and convenient software tool selection and practical guidance for actual research on network pharmacology.

X. Zhou (✉) · N. Wang
School of Computer and Information Technology, Beijing Jiaotong University, Beijing, China
e-mail: xzzhou@bjtu.edu.cn; wang_ning@bjtu.edu.cn

X. Zhai
Beijing University of Chinese Medicine, Beijing, China
e-mail: zhaix@bucm.edu.cn

S. Li (ed.), *Network Pharmacology*, https://doi.org/10.1007/978-981-16-0753-0_4

4.1 Software Functional Framework and Classification of Network Pharmacology

4.1.1 Overall Software Functional Requirements

Network pharmacology [1] uses network relationship data such as drug-target relationships, interaction group networks, and phenotype–genotype associations, with the goal of analyzing the regulatory role of drug intervention in molecular networks and using corresponding data analysis models and methods such as complex network, machine learning, and molecular functional analysis, to determine the research direction for the interpretation and discovery of drug molecular mechanisms. The focus of pharmacological research is to find the target of drugs and how to regulate the corresponding targets to achieve the effect of disease treatment. Network pharmacology research focuses on discovering and confirming the multi-target effect of drugs and their network pharmacodynamic mechanisms and analyzing and discovering the systemic therapeutic effect of drugs and their combination on diseases, by analyzing the overall effect of network regulation.

In general, classic network pharmacology research cases involve main links such as network data collection and integration, network structure analysis and prediction, molecular and network function analysis, drug-target (target) relationship analysis, drug interaction or combination analysis, and drug indication analysis. The first three links are the common steps and methods in classic network pharmacology research, while the last three links are typical tasks for specific applications. The core data involved in relevant links are described in detail in other chapters of this book, including the clinical efficacy information of drugs, drug composition structure and its interaction, drug-target relationship, interaction group network, phenotypic genotype association, drug side effects, and drug indications.

Network data collection and integration: Targeting research problems of specific drugs' action mechanism, the lack or limitation of main target relationship data, such as drug-target relationship, is relatively common. In addition to generating the corresponding target data through wet tests, network pharmacology research often uses automatic data extraction or generation methods to collect the target relationship data. At the same time, the integration of network data from different sources (medical literature, structured database, etc.) and different types (drug-target relationship, drug side effect relationship, disease gene relationship, etc.) is often used to integrate network data resources for specific research objectives. For example, as the core research task of network pharmacology, the prediction of drug-target relationship usually adopts relatively single data types in the initial stage, such as drug chemical structure information, drug-target relationship information, etc. However, due to the incompleteness and complementary characteristics of various types of information, in recent years, use of multi-source network data integration to construct the basic network pharmacology data resources has become a guiding research direction. In the following foreseeable future, network data integration will become the basic research method and foundation. Therefore, network data integration is one of the basic functional requirements of network pharmacology methods or software.

Network structure analysis and prediction: From the perspective of network science or complex network [2, 3], network pharmacology is a classic application of complex network in the pharmacology field, and its wider medical applications can be considered as network medicine [4]. Therefore, analysis methods and models based on complex networks such as node or edge centrality measure, shortest path, link prediction, and community analysis [5, 6] (community detection), and various statistical graph generation models (such as random graph [7], small world network [8], and scale-free network [9]) are the main supporting analysis methods in network pharmacology. For example, the problem of edge prediction using the adjacent structure of the network, the path connection mode of the network, or the attribute information of the node is called link prediction. Its most direct application is drug-target prediction (to determine whether the relationship between a specific drug node and a target node exists). The direct application of community analysis with relatively dense internal connections and relatively sparse external sub-network structures obtained from the overall network is the discovery and confirmation of the disease module [10] or drug-target module. Therefore, the above two methods naturally become the core complex network analysis methods in network pharmacology. In addition, due to the above two kinds of network analysis problems, we can also directly model typical machine learning problems [11], such as the drug-target relationship problem can be regarded as an information recommendation problem [12], a binary classification problem of edge judgment, or a corresponding sorting learning problem [13], and the analysis of disease module can be regarded as a clustering problem of network data. Therefore, supervised learning methods [11] such as regression analysis, support vector machine, Bayesian network, and deep neural network in machine learning can be used in drug-target prediction. However, unsupervised learning methods, such as k-means, spectral clustering, and hierarchical clustering, can be applied to the discovery of disease modules. Moreover, all kinds of community analysis methods, such as graph partition-based method and modularity evaluation-based optimization method, can be considered as clustering methods based on network data. Common complex network analysis and even some machine learning software based on network data are tools and methods that can be used in network pharmacology research.

Molecular and network function analysis: Determining the specific biological functions of drug-targets and their molecular networks is an important task for analyzing drug molecular mechanisms and their pharmacodynamic effects. Therefore, systematic molecular function analysis methods have become an important technical means in network pharmacology to further explain the drug effects and pharmacokinetic mechanisms from the multi-tiered levels of molecules, cells, tissues, organs, and systems, as well as adverse drug reactions and side effects. Among them, gene ontology (GO) analysis is the main functional analysis at the gene or protein level, while molecular pathway analysis can be combined with corresponding pathway databases such as KEGG and Reactome for molecular function analysis of metabolic pathways, signal transduction pathways, and protein complexes.

Analysis and prediction of drug-target relationship: Drug-target analysis is network pharmacology's core analysis task and goal. Judging from the types of drugs involved and the scope of research, it can be divided into two main research approaches. The first category focuses on drug-target discovery of specific drugs (or TCM compound prescriptions) or diseases. The purpose of this task is to identify novel binding relationship between drugs (corresponding small-molecule chemical components) and targets by means of virtual screening, manual compilation, and review of literature and information extraction or wet tests, using clinical efficacy or phenotype information of specific drugs, to form relatively reliable research results through the interaction information between the target in the molecular network and disease-related genes or biomarkers. The second category focuses on the R&D of large-scale drug-target relationship prediction methods using integrated network pharmacology data or drug association attributes. The first type of research is actually a case-based drug-target relationship study based on network pharmacology, which aims to analyze the mechanism of clinically effective drugs and prescriptions, provide an understanding and interpretation of pharmacological mechanisms, and provide a new record for drug-target relationship data resources. This kind of research is extensively practiced and has varied applications in the field of TCM network pharmacology. Especially in the research of the target of Chinese medicine compound prescriptions and their molecular network, this research type has generated practical results and research value. The second type of research aims at the development of new analytical methods and models, which is one of the core research tasks of network pharmacology. This method mainly includes two kinds of models: complex network analysis and machine learning. So far, researchers have implemented a variety of related drug-target prediction algorithms and models that promote the progress of network pharmacology research. Various algorithms and models for related drug-target prediction implemented by researchers have also promoted network pharmacology research development. In view of the significant performance advantages of deep representation learning and deep neural network models where there is sufficient data volume, the current algorithm and its software research and development has formed a tide and trend that is focused on the deep learning model.

Analysis of drug interactions and combinations: Drug interactions (drug–drug interaction) refer to the mutual influence and action between ingredients caused by simultaneous use of food, beverages, food supplements, and other drugs in the process of drug use. These interactions often lead to side effects and adverse reactions, but may also lead to beneficial medicinal effects [14]. Drug combination analysis refers to the analysis and study of the clinical situation of complex diseases such as co-diseases and concomitant diseases, as well as complex chronic diseases such as cancer and complex infectious diseases such as HIV. It is necessary to analyze and study the simultaneous listing and administration of multiple drugs for the same patient (especially the elderly), so as to find the best combination of drugs and identify the combination of drugs that cause serious side effects. Therefore, given the widespread use of combination drugs (or even compound drugs), drug interaction analysis has become an important research direction, and drug interaction analysis is also an important cross-sectional research area in the R&D of combination drugs within the network pharmacology framework. The above two research tasks complement each other. As network pharmacology focuses on the multi-target and molecular network effects of drugs, drug interaction and combinatorial analysis have become important applications of network pharmacology methods, as they can help discover and confirm more systematic drug interactions and effective combination drugs. At the same time, network pharmacology research of TCM itself is a compound-oriented pharmacological research. The diversity of compound medicine ingredients makes the systematic research of drug interactions and combined drug mechanisms a research task and scientific problem that is both important and promising for breakthroughs. The discovery and conformation network effect index of optimal combination drugs [15] and even a compound network drug efficacy index that reflects the compatibility of TCM formulation is an important basic research task in TCM network pharmacology.

Analysis and prediction of drug indications: Drug indication analysis is the final goal of network pharmacology research, that is, determining the disease or clinical phenotype that can eventually be effectively treated by drugs. From the perspective of analysis methods, the analysis and prediction of drug indications and the very important drug repositioning (or drug repurposing) [16] issue in the context of new drug research and development are the same issue. For a given drug, to predict its total pharmacophore spectrum (disease or phenotype treated or acted upon), the novel pharmacodynamic phenotype is the target of drug redirection analysis [16]. In addition, in this sense, the side effects and adverse reactions of a drug can also be considered as an effector phenotype in the broad sense of the drug, but the side effects and adverse reactions of the drug are only an unexpected effector phenotype. In view of the concept of drug action based on extensive systematic data integration and network regulation, network pharmacology has natural advantages and characteristics in the overall analysis of drug indications. Therefore, drug redirection research based on network method and network pharmacology has become a widely recognized new idea and method in the research and development of new drugs.

4.1.2 *Software Functional Framework and Classification of Network Pharmacology*

In the previous section, the data processing and analysis requirements of network pharmacology research were briefly summarized. Network pharmacology research involves data resource collection and integration, network construction and analysis, drug-target relationship prediction, and other diverse methods and software functional requirements. From its functional framework and classification, it basically includes the data processing and analysis function module, as shown in Fig. 4.1. In

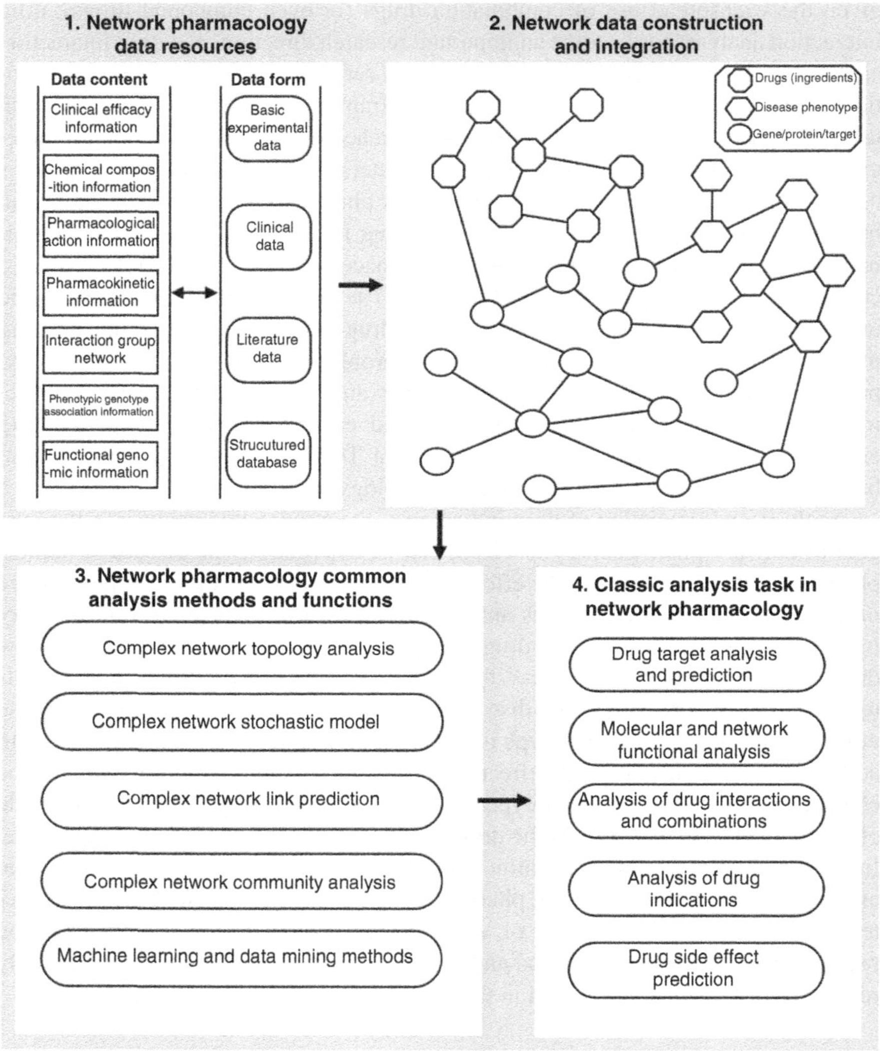

Fig. 4.1 Software functional module framework of network pharmacology

fact, the current research and development of network pharmacology methods and software research and development mainly focus on the following four aspects of functional requirements. For example, in terms of the formation and integration of network pharmacology data resources, a large number of network pharmacology databases have been constructed, such as DrugBank [17], STITCH [18], SIDER [19], PubChem, etc., as well as a large number of high-quality databases of functional genomics and interaction groups. Specifically, in the field of TCM network pharmacology, a database resource platform, including the relationship of TCM-chemical ingredients-targets has also been constructed, which is of immense help in the research and development of TCM network pharmacology. In addition, drug-target prediction methods and online software for specific diseases such as rare diseases, psychiatric diseases, and cancer, drug interaction prediction, drug combination analysis, drug redirection, and drug side effect analysis software are seeing rapid growth and development. At the same time, as complex networks, machine learning software, and programming language for big data analysis (such as Python) mature further, the applications in the biological field can provide strong technical support for network pharmacology research. The subsequent chapters illustrate and introduce typical methods, software, and practical programming operations related to the above aspects.

4.2 Online Software Commonly Used in Network Pharmacology

Based on the requirements of network pharmacology analysis introduced in the previous section, it can be seen that drug-target and drug indications are important applications. The research and development of convenient and fast online software is an important means to promote drug-target analysis, indication analysis, and other pharmacology research, especially for researchers who are new to network pharmacology technologies and methods. At present, several excellent online analysis tools have been developed for researchers. This section introduces the analysis tools from the perspective of established online software.

4.2.1 Online Software for Drug-Target Prediction

The design and development of new drugs has always been a complex, expensive, and time-consuming process. Moreover, the success rate of new drug research and development is quite low. Usually, only a few drugs can finally pass the FDA evaluation every year and be commercially available for treatment. Therefore, drug research faces problems of low drug development efficiency, rising demand for treatment, and serious shortage of existing therapeutic drugs. The determination of drug-target relationship is an important link in the development of new drugs; however, the screening method based on wet tests is still extremely challenging and difficult, therefore, drug-target prediction analysis is a hot research topic. Teams from research institutions and scientific research institutes around the world have made extensive research and contributions in this respect and have developed various computational models to predict potential drug-target relationships on a large scale. The prediction analysis methods introduced in previous chapters are mainly based on algorithms. In addition, there are also convenient and practical web-based service tools that can provide online drug-target prediction services, such as DINIES [20], SuperPred [21], and SwissTargetPrediction [22].

DINIES (Drug–Target Interaction Network Inference Engine based on Supervised Analysis) is an online platform that is used to infer potential drug–target interaction networks. DINIES can accept a variety of input data, such as chemical structures, side effects, amino acids, or protein domains. In addition, each dataset is converted into a nuclear similarity, and multiple state-of-the-art machine learning methods are used to predict the drug–target interactions.

SuperPred is an online platform used to predict the structure of small molecular targets. In SuperPred, drug-target prediction is based on similarity distribution through four input options (including the name of the compound searched in the PubChem database, the structure of the compound created through Simplified Molecular Input Line Entry Specification (SMILES), the structure diagram drawn with ChemDoodle, and the uploaded molecular file) to estimate individual threshold value and probability of a specific target.

SwissTargetPrediction is an online platform that is used to infer bioactive small molecular targets based on the two-dimensional and three-dimensional similarity values of known ligands. In addition, it can provide prediction results for five different biological tissues (human, house mouse, rat, cattle, and horse).

We use SwissTargetPrediction as an example to demonstrate the specific operation. First, the user can customize the species to be analyzed (in the case of humans, select homo sapiens) (as shown in Fig. 4.2); then, the user can enter the molecular structure of the compound and search for the specific SMILES string of the compound as the input on the ChEMBL website. Here, we take GINSENOSIDE RG1 as an example (as shown in Fig. 4.3); finally, the user can click the "Predict targets" button; the platform runs the calculations and finally the corresponding target prediction analysis results are displayed on the prediction interface (as shown in Fig. 4.4).

4.2.2 Online Software for Drug Indication Analysis

Indication is the phenotypic spectrum of the disease treated by drugs. The main goal of drug indication prediction is to establish the relationship between drugs and the indication spectrum, that is, to determine what is the complete spectrum of disease phenotypes that a specific drug can treat. In view of the different granularity of disease classification, there are two problems in the analysis of drug indications: Optimization of the classification of diseases that have been treated and prediction of new diseases. The view that predicted disease phenotype spectrum contains new major diseases is a widely studied drug repurposing or drug repositioning problem. The drug repositioning method has been successfully applied to the R&D of a variety of disease treatment drugs [23], which can shorten the time of drug R&D and reduce the cost and risk of drug R&D. Drug repositioning can not only expand the application scope of drugs and extend their service life, but also enable the reuse

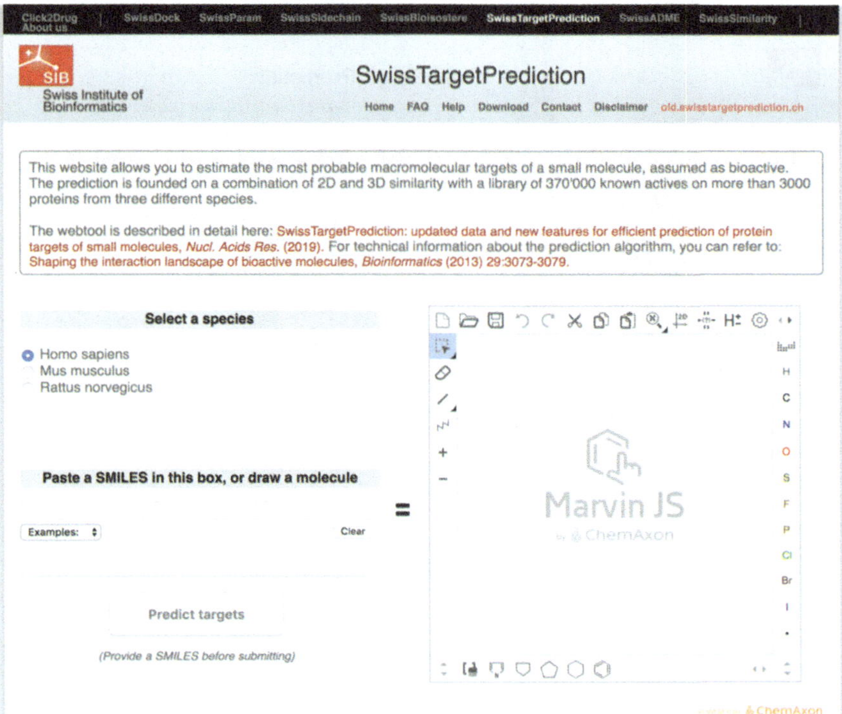

Fig. 4.2 SwissTargetPrediction front-page interface

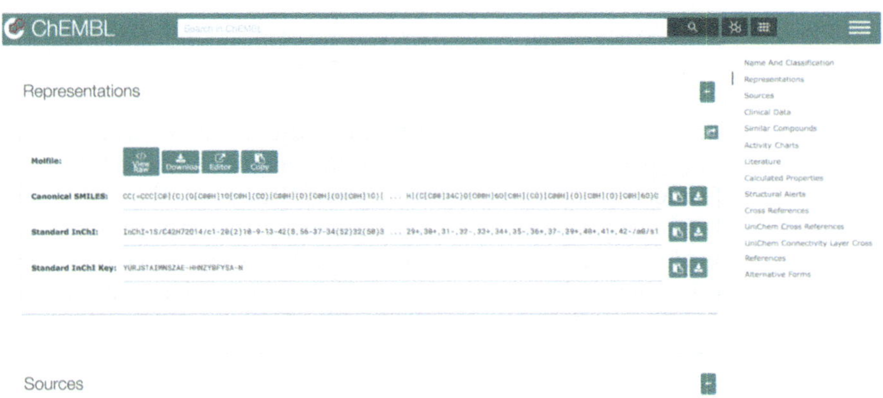

Fig. 4.3 ChEMBL search page

of withdrawn drugs. For example, the original intention of developing sildenafil was to treat cardiovascular diseases such as angina pectoris and hypertension, but it was unexpectedly found in clinical tests that it can be used to treat male erectile dysfunction [24]. Subsequent studies have shown that low doses of sildenafil can

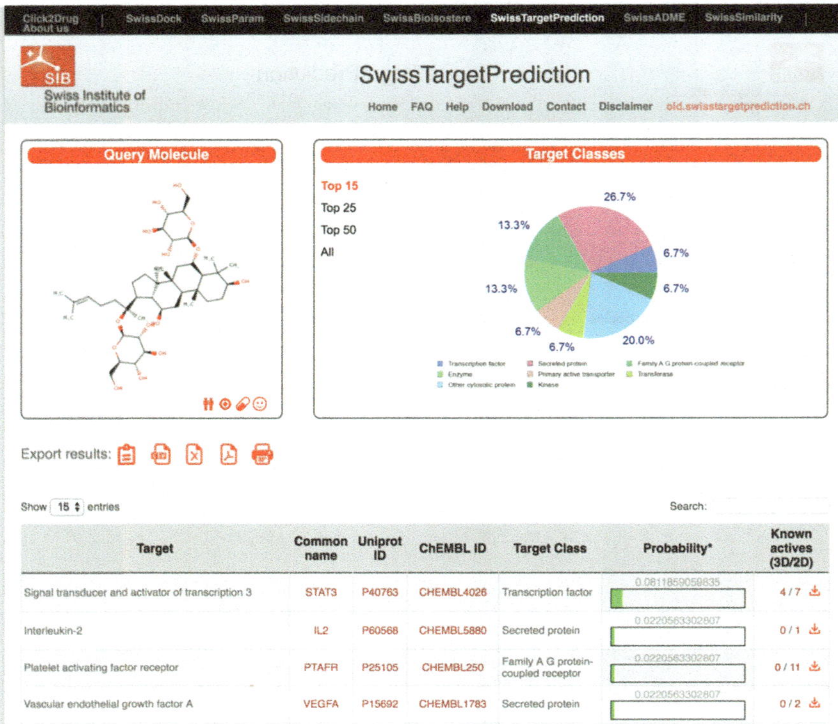

Fig. 4.4 Prediction result page

also be used for the treatment of pulmonary hypertension in rare cases [24]. The discovery of new uses for the above mentioned known drugs is mostly accidental, and not the result of rational design. Due to the large number of types of diseases and the number of known drugs, the cost of screening new uses of known drugs through experiments is still quite high. With the accumulation of omics data and the rapid development of various drug-related databases, such as DrugBank [17] and SIDER [19], drug repositioning prediction by computational methods has become a hot topic in computational biology and systems biology research in recent years [23]. The rational design of the clinical research scheme of drug repositioning assisted by computational methods can provide clues for large-scale experimental screening, further reduce the cost, and make drug repositioning enter the stage of combining rational design and experimental screening.

In recent years, there has been a growing trend in software R&D related to drug indication analysis, such as MeSHDD [25] and RE: fine Drugs [26]. Using the above software, researchers can analyze the properties of existing drugs through online methods to determine whether related drugs can be safely and effectively applied to specific diseases. The next section introduces a typical online tool: MeSHDD [25].

MeSHDD clusters drugs based on the drug–drug similarity of the Medical Subject Heading (MeSH) and then predicts new indications of the drug. Specifically,

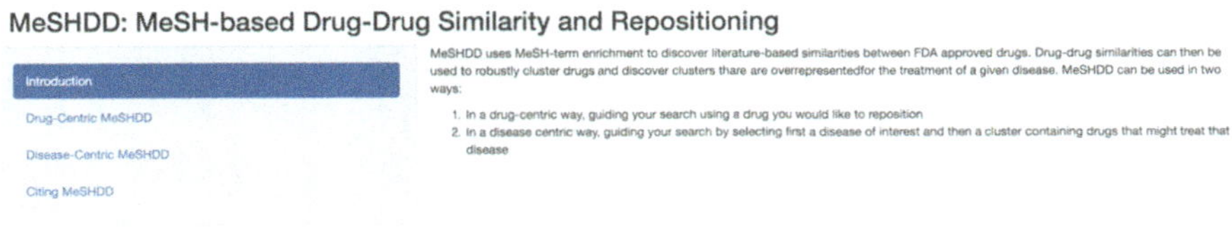

Fig. 4.5 Homepage of MeSHDD's official website

MeSHDD uses hypergeometric distribution to calculate the degree of co-occurrence of drug terms in MeSH and performs Bonferroni correction. Then, the drug–drug similarity is calculated by converting the above calculation result (represented by the P value) to the bit-by-bit distance obtained by the binary representation. Finally, pairing distance and clustering method are used to cluster the drugs, and the enrichment of disease indications is evaluated across multiple categories by comparing with data from TTD. In the verification experiment conducted by the author, it can be seen that MeSHDD can infer the indications for cystic fibrosis of antidiabetic drugs. The specific operation is as follows. First, navigate to the homepage of the official website (as shown in Fig. 4.5) and select the drug to be redirected from the drop-down list on the drug-centered page. Take quinine as an example, the indications corresponding to the drug can be obtained (as shown in Fig. 4.6), and related similar drugs can also be obtained (as shown in Fig. 4.7).

4.2.3 Online Software for Gene Function Enrichment Analysis

Several related gene expressions and interaction group data generated by high-throughput sequencing can provide abundant functional data resources for phenotypic genotype association research, however, they also put forward new requirements for efficient molecular function analysis. Enrichment analysis [27] is the main method to determine the common biological mechanism and medical phenotype association of batch differences or related genes by leveraging existing databases of gene function attributes, phenotypic genotype association data, and interaction group databases (such as molecular pathway database). According to the different related molecular function data used, enrichment analysis is mainly divided into GO enrichment analysis, pathway analysis, and differential gene enrichment analysis. Through gene function enrichment analysis, it is possible to discover the key biological pathways in the biological process in which gene sets are involved, which is an important analysis link in exploring the common rules from the complex omics data.

In short, gene enrichment analysis involves finding gene sets with certain gene functional characteristics and biological processes in a group of genes, which are often used in the follow-up analysis of differentially expressed genes and screened

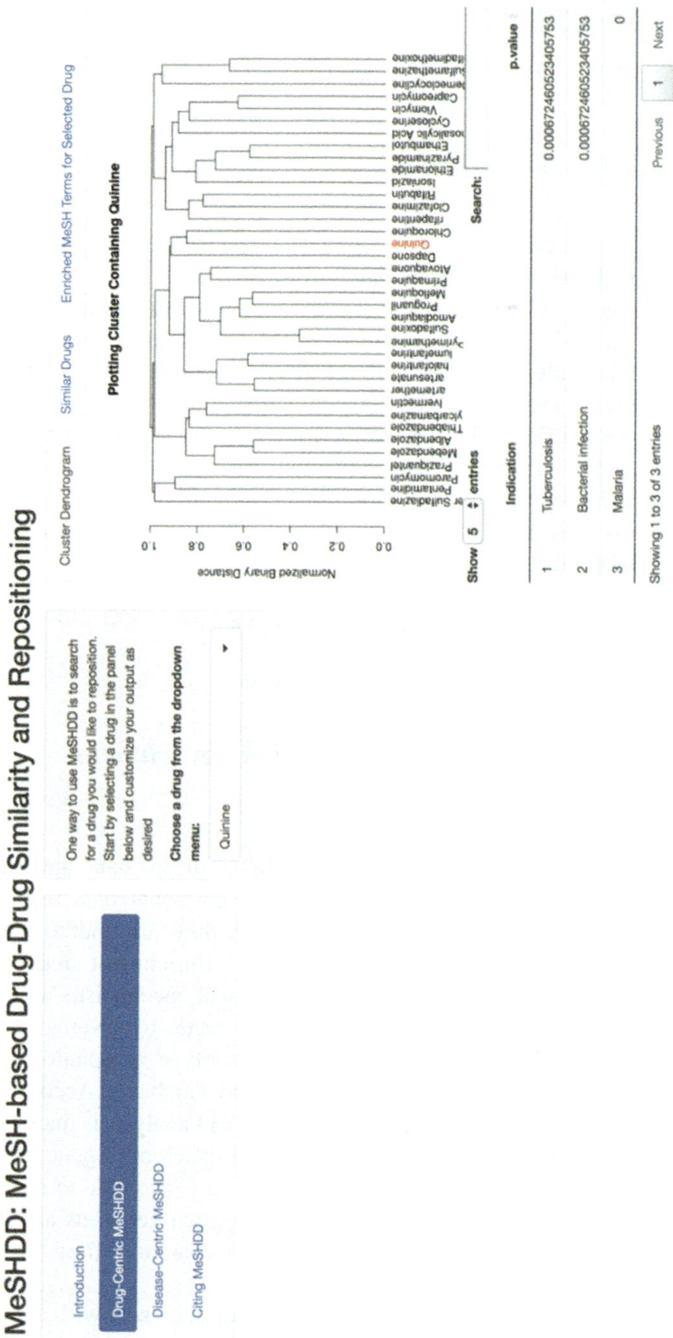

Fig. 4.6 MeSHDD prediction drug indications page

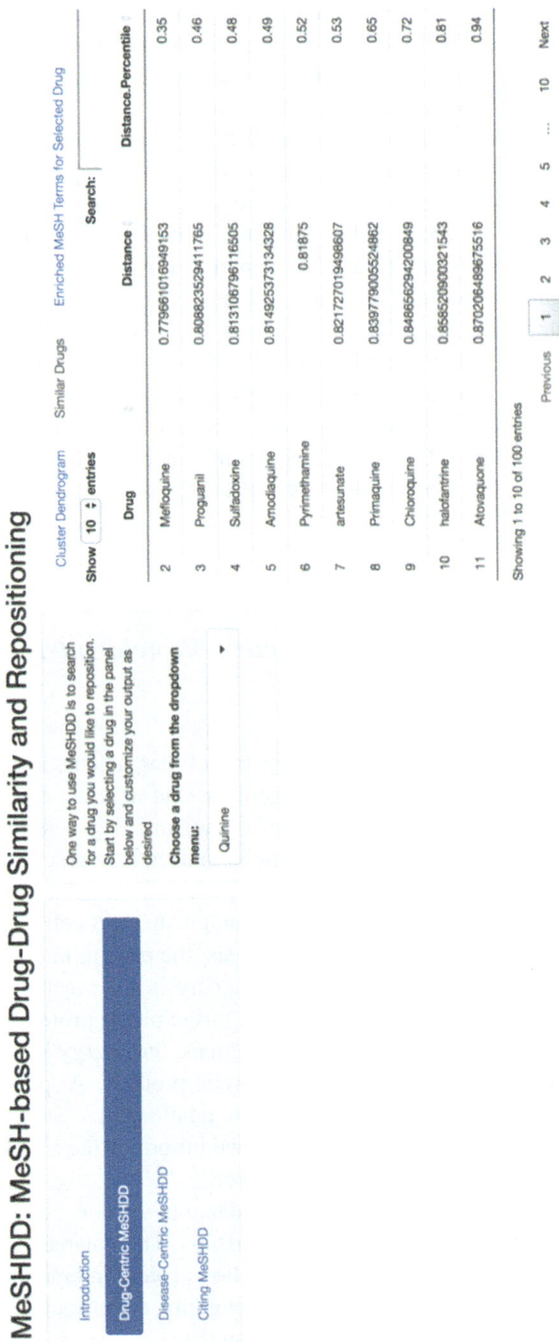

Fig. 4.7 MeSHDD prediction-related drug page

genes. At present, there are nearly 100 kinds of enrichment analysis tools developed by different research institutes. At present, many open source websites have integrated GO enrichment and KEGG pathway analysis functions, such as DAVID [28], KOBAS [29], and STRING [30]. In this section, we introduce DAVID, a well-known and commonly used enrichment analysis tool.

DAVID is taken as an example to conduct GO enrichment and pathway analysis for a given gene set. The homepage of the website is shown in Fig. 4.8. Step 1: Navigate to the Start Analysis page and input the gene set to be analyzed under Enter Gene List. Select Affy_ID under Select Identifier, then select the Gene List in List Type, and click the Submit List button, as shown in Fig. 4.9. Step 2: Select homo sapiens corresponding to the gene set under Select Species, then press the Use button under Select List and then click Functional Annotation Chart to initiate the analysis, as shown in Fig. 4.10; Step 3: Select the content to be analyzed, as shown in Fig. 4.11; select Gene_Ontology and Pathways, and click Functional Annotation Chart to display the analysis result, as shown in Fig. 4.12. The corresponding GO enrichment analysis and KEGG path analysis results can be obtained at the bottom of the analysis page, and the above analysis results can be downloaded by clicking the appropriate button.

4.2.4 Online Software for Constructing Protein Interaction Network

Proteins and their interactions are the pillars of cellular mechanism. Proteins are important macromolecules that constitute organisms and regulate a large number of basic life activities and biological behavior of organisms [31]. The protein interaction network is composed of individual proteins and their interactions, which can participate in all aspects of life processes such as biological signal transmission, gene expression regulation, energy and substance metabolism, and cell cycle regulation [32]. In network pharmacology correlation analysis, the protein interaction network is often used in drug-target and gene enrichment analysis and other studies and is of great significance for understanding the working principle of proteins in biological systems, the reaction mechanism of biological signals, the energy substance metabolism, as well as the functional connection between proteins. At present, there are many databases that provide protein interaction relationships, such as STRING, MINT [33], and BioGRID [34]. In this section, we introduce the STRING database that is well known and commonly used in research.

Currently, the STRING database has been updated to version 11, which includes known and predicted protein interaction relationships. The database contains 5090 species, 24.58 million proteins, and 3123.05 million protein interactions. The interaction relationships are derived from high-throughput experiments, text mining, other database data, and bioinformatics prediction data.

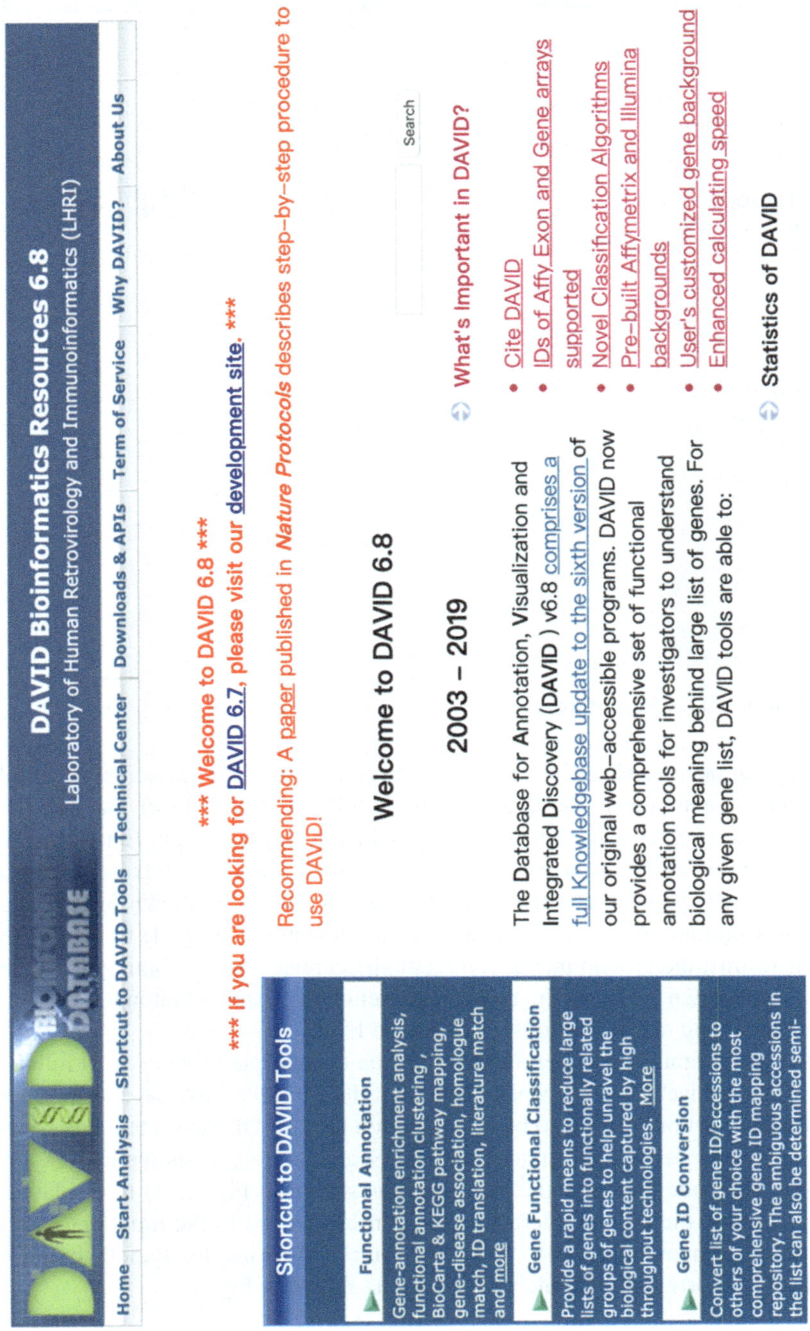

Fig. 4.8 Homepage of DAVID

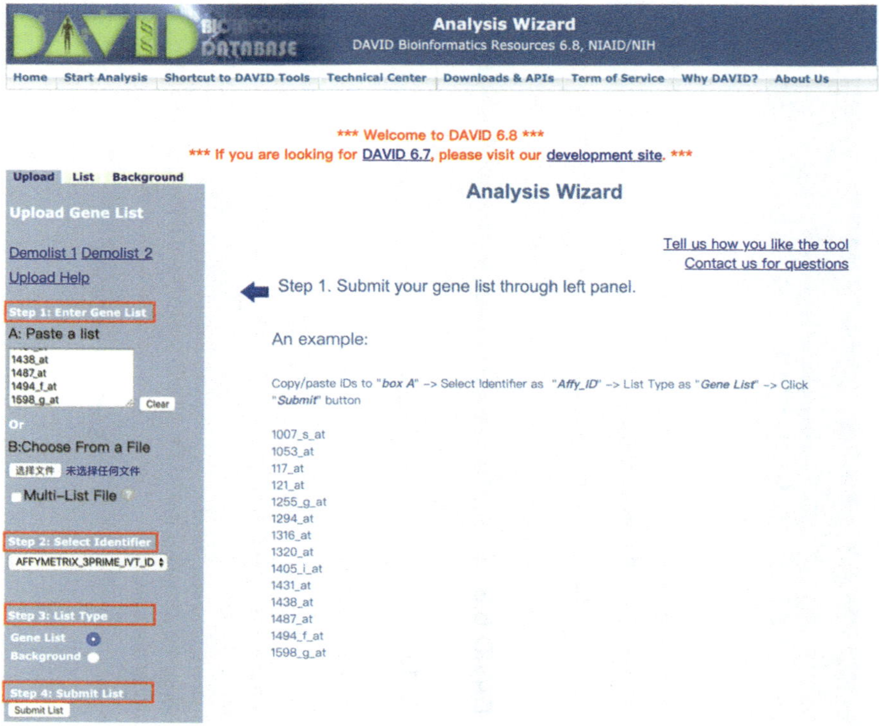

Fig. 4.9 Input data interface display

Users can query a single protein or a collection of multiple proteins. A sample operation for querying a single protein is as follows: Navigate to the website's homepage; the default page has the query tool for a single protein. Enter the gene to be analyzed (CASP3 as an example) into the Protein Name text box, select Homo sapiens under Organism, and then click the Search button, as shown in Fig. 4.13. Click the Continue button in the next page (as shown in Fig. 4.14) to display the analysis results; the protein interaction relationship related to the input gene can be obtained, as shown in Fig. 4.15. You can also click the Exports button to download the corresponding analysis results, as shown in Fig. 4.16.

A sample operation for querying a collection of multiple proteins is as follows: Navigate to the website's homepage and click the Multiple Proteins button. Then, enter the gene set or gene list to be analyzed into the List Of Names text box, select Homo sapiens under Organism, and click the Search button, as shown in Fig. 4.17. Click the Continue button in the next page (as shown in Fig. 4.18) to display the analysis results; the protein interaction relationship related to the input gene set is displayed, as shown in Fig. 4.19. Similarly, you can also click the Exports button to download the corresponding analysis results, as shown in Fig. 4.20.

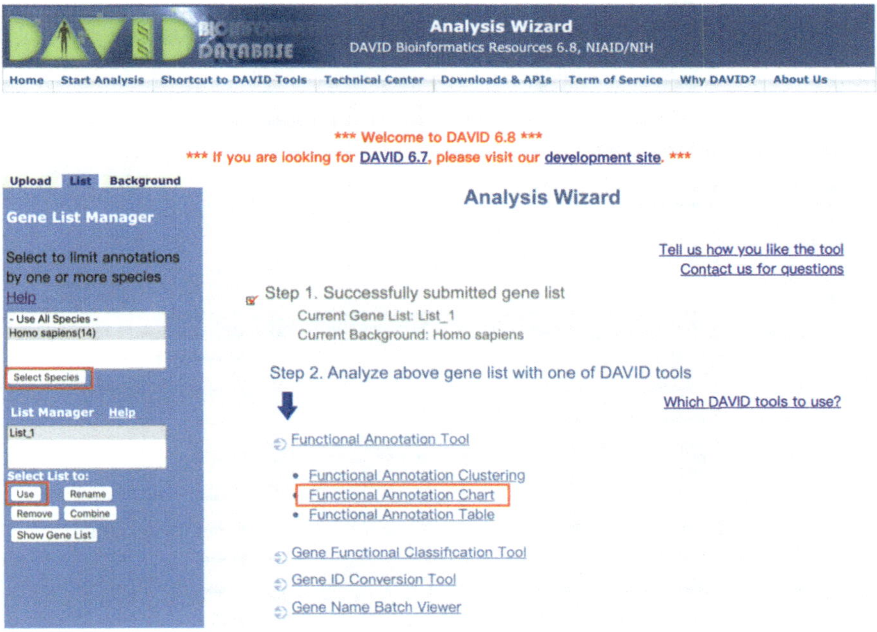

Fig. 4.10 Interface display for selecting and analyzing species

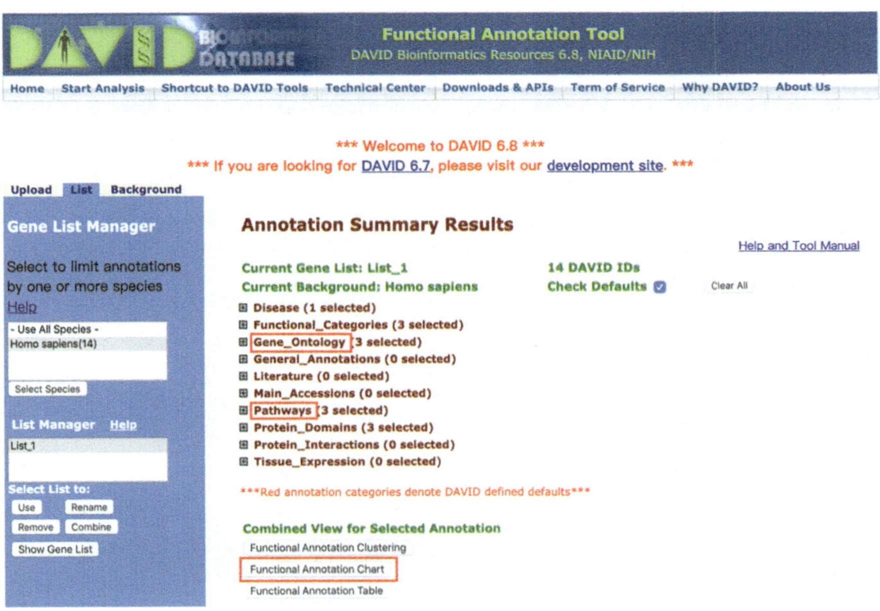

Fig. 4.11 Interface display for selecting and analyzing contents

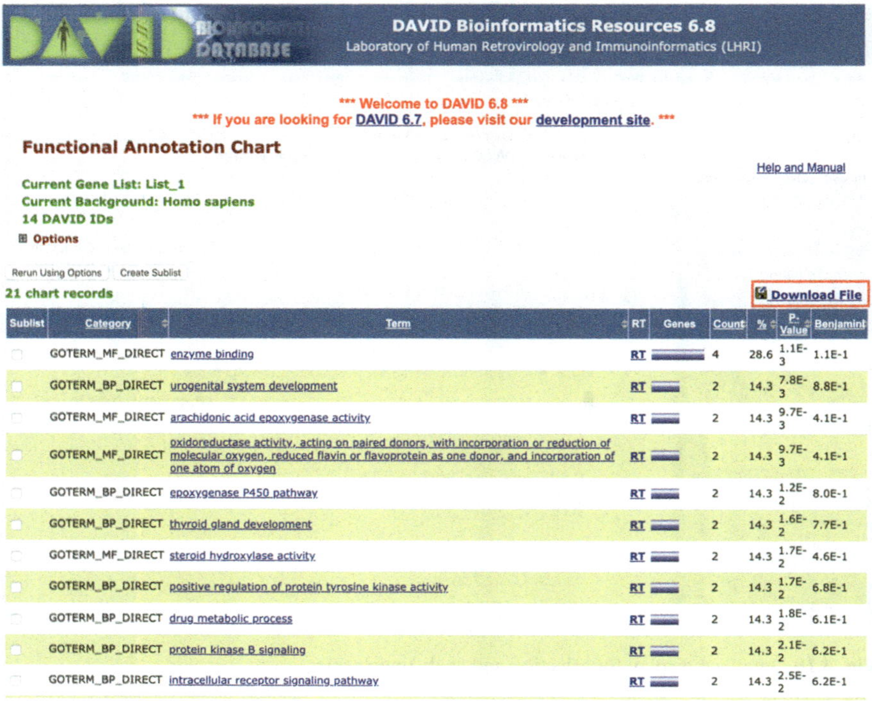

Fig. 4.12 Analysis results interface display

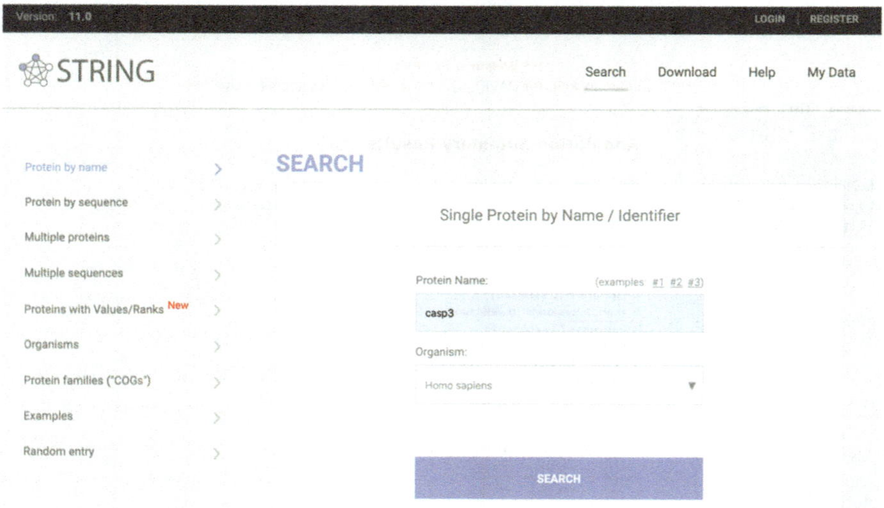

Fig. 4.13 Single gene query homepage

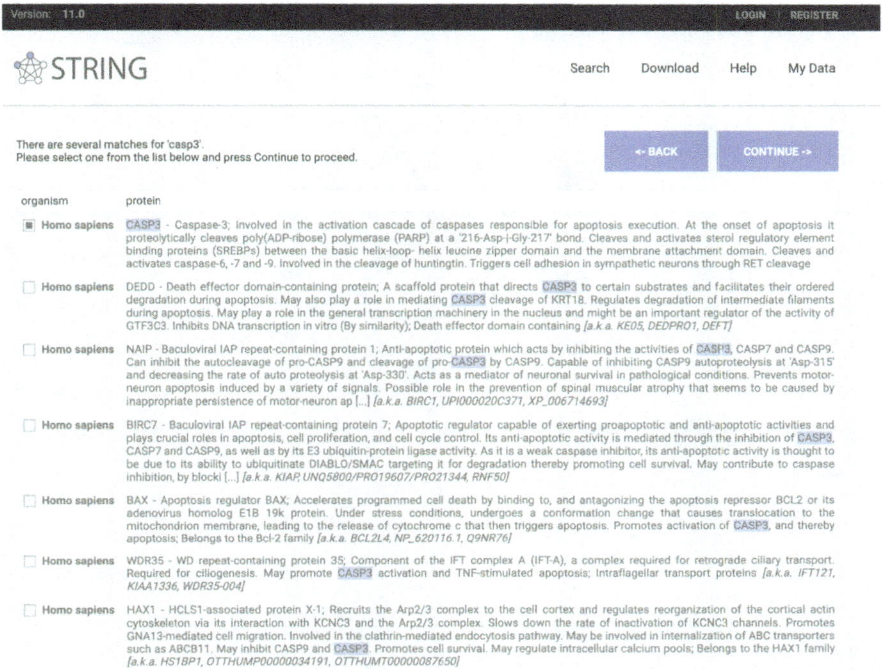

Fig. 4.14 Single gene query information confirmation page

4.3 Software Based on Graphical Interface Operation

Based on the network pharmacology analysis requirements introduced in the first section, we know that a complex network is one of the important methods. A complex network is not only a formal tool but also a scientific research method. Due to its universality for solving problems in various fields, it has been widely used in the fields of medicine, sociology, physics, information science, and ecology. At present, the accumulation of network data in various fields, such as protein interaction network [35], disease relation network [36], social network [37], power network, aviation network, and transportation network, has further promoted research on complex network methods. For example, in social network research, we study the law of group behavior [38] and the law of information dissemination [39] by constructing a social network, whereas in the biomedical field, we study drug interaction [40] and drug-target relationship [41] by using complex network methods. At present, a large amount of network data has a large scale and many network nodes and edges. Therefore, it is necessary to rely on visual network analysis methods to obtain effective results. In view of this, researchers have developed several excellent visual network analysis tools, including visual software based on graphical interfaces and software that can be programmed to call the package (For example: Python package, R language package, Java package, etc.),

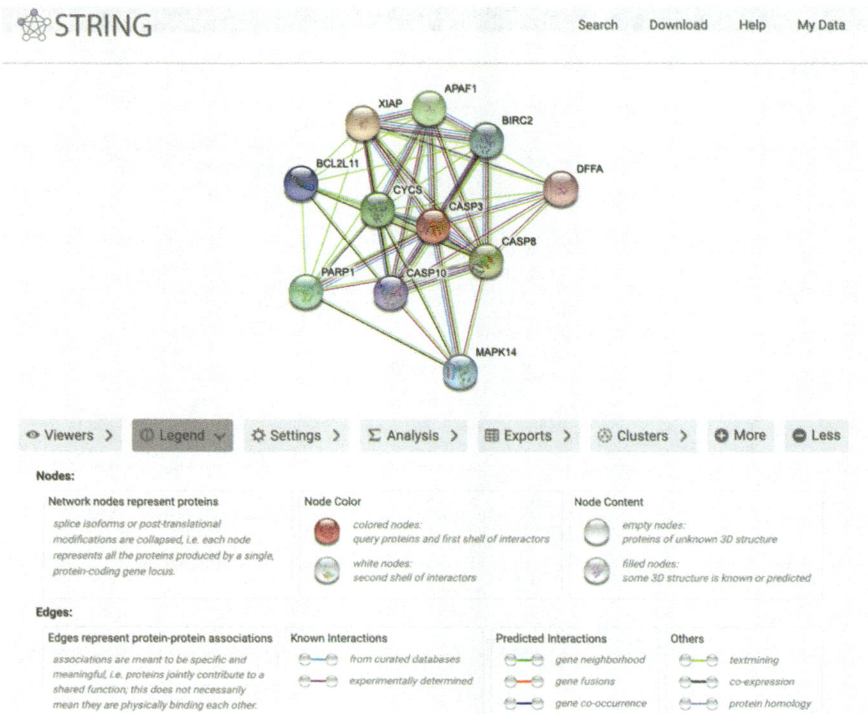

Fig. 4.15 Single gene query result page

among them, a visualization tool based on a graphical interface is easy to install and operate and is more intuitive to operate than a programming language package. Next, this section briefly introduces and demonstrates an independent system software from two aspects: differential gene enrichment analysis and network analysis.

4.3.1 Differential Gene Enrichment Analysis Software

The GO function and KEGG pathway enrichment analysis introduced in the previous section aims to discover the characteristic molecular function and pathway information of the identified gene set. In addition, another type of enrichment analysis is mainly used to identify differential genes for specific conditions such as phenotypes. For example: Gene Set Enrichment Analysis (GSEA) [42] is a widely used method that can be used to assess the distribution trend of genes in a gene set in phenotypic correlation ranking and determine their association with a specific phenotype. Different from KEGG pathway analysis, GSEA considers the influence of genes with little expression difference but important functions, on the pathway, and compared with KEGG pathway analysis, it can retain more relevant information.

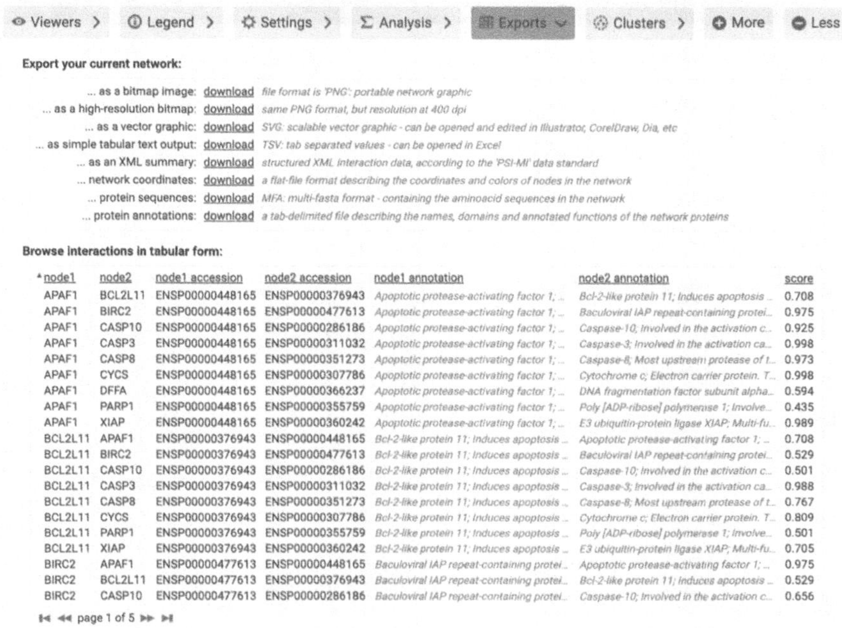

Fig. 4.16 Single gene query download page

The GSEA algorithm and software were developed by the Broad Institute in the USA. The installation and analysis process of GSEA software is introduced below.

4.3.1.1 Software Installation

Two methods are officially recommended. The first is the Java-based GSEA desktop application. Navigate to the GSEA official download page and click the Launch icon on the right to download (as shown in Fig. 4.21), however, the installation requires an internet connection. The second type is the Java-based GSEA application package. Click download on the right to download. The installation does not require an internet connection and starts quickly. The software startup interface is shown in Fig. 4.22. We use the second method as an example in the following analysis and introduction.

4.3.1.2 Data Preparation and Import

GSEA provides the sample dataset on its official website, as shown in Fig. 4.23. Users can download a selected gene expression matrix file and sample grouping information file for analysis.

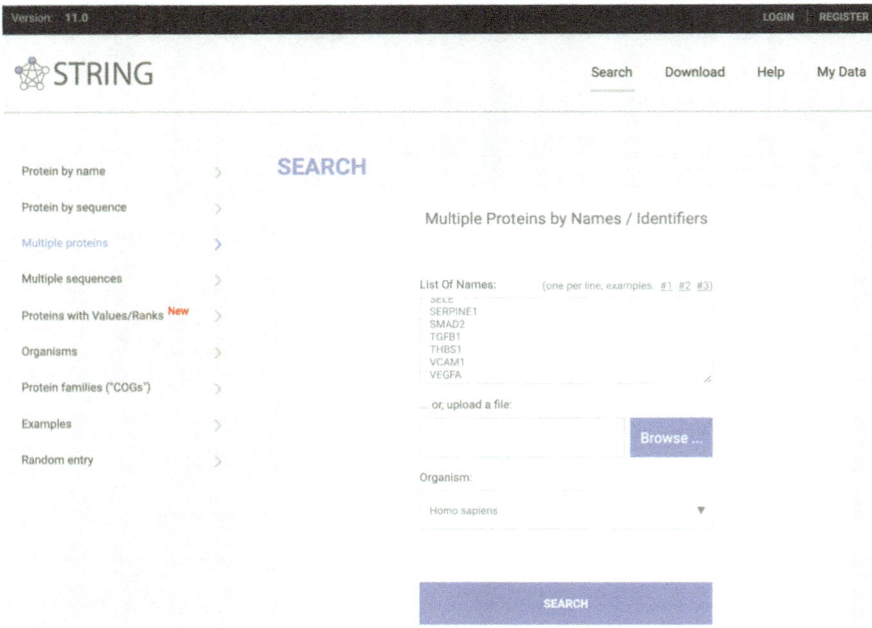

Fig. 4.17 Multiple gene query homepage

The gene expression matrix Diabetes_collapsed_symbols.gct, sample grouping information Diabetes.cls, and gene function classification data c5.all.v6.2.symbols.gmt provided by the GSEA website are selected here as an example. According to the steps shown in Fig. 4.24, click Load data— > Browse for File— > find the file to be imported in the pop-up box, select and click open to import data.

4.3.1.3 Setting Parameters and Running the Software

Click Run GSEA on the left panel of the interface; the parameter selection bar pops up. Parameter settings are divided into three parts: Mandatory parameter settings, basic parameter settings, and advanced parameter setting. Generally, the latter two parameters do not need to be modified, and the default value can be used. The following is a brief description of the fields in the mandatory parameter settings (as shown in Fig. 4.25).

Select the expression dataset file Diabetes_collapsed_symbols.gct in the Expression dataset field. Select the gene function set database c5.all.v6.2.symbols.gmt in the Gene sets database field. Number of permutations indicates the number of permutation tests, and the default value is 1000. Select the comparison method in the Phenotype labels field. GSEA automatically extracts the corresponding data from the expression dataset file for comparison based on the group information during the

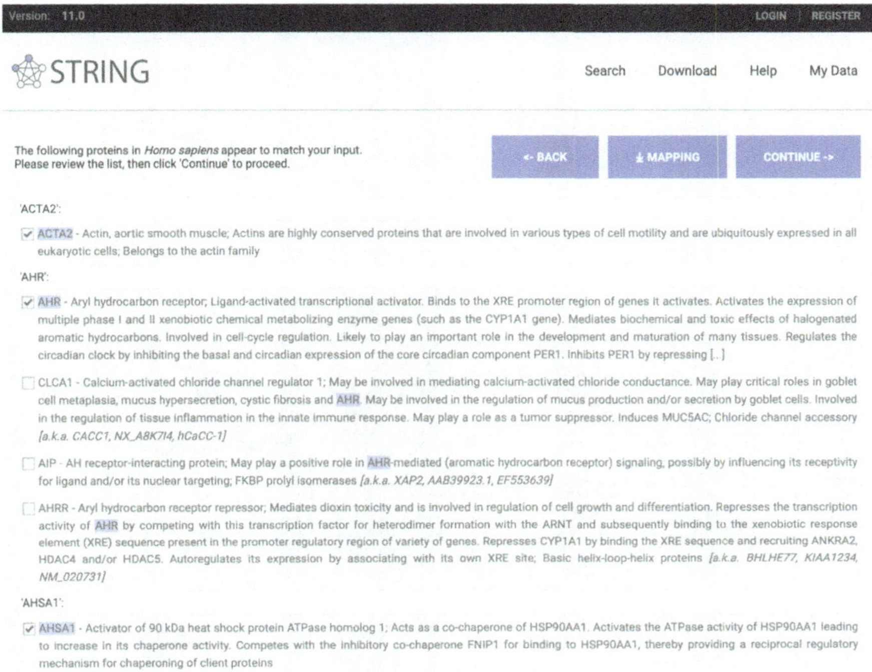

Fig. 4.18 Multiple gene query information confirmation page

analysis process. Select true in the Collapse dataset to gene symbols field. As the number of samples in each group is greater than 7, select phenotype in the Permutation type field. The Chip platform option is for the annotation conversion of the ID, which is not required in this example.

After the above parameters are set, click the Run button under the parameter settings column; the running status is displayed in the GSEA reports at the bottom left of the interface. If it displays Running, it means the operation is successful, and if it displays Error, it means the operation failed, as shown in Fig. 4.26. In case of an error, click Error to view the Error report.

4.3.1.4 View Results

The results of data analysis are saved to the set path. Click index.html to view the web version of the analysis report, as shown in Fig. 4.27.

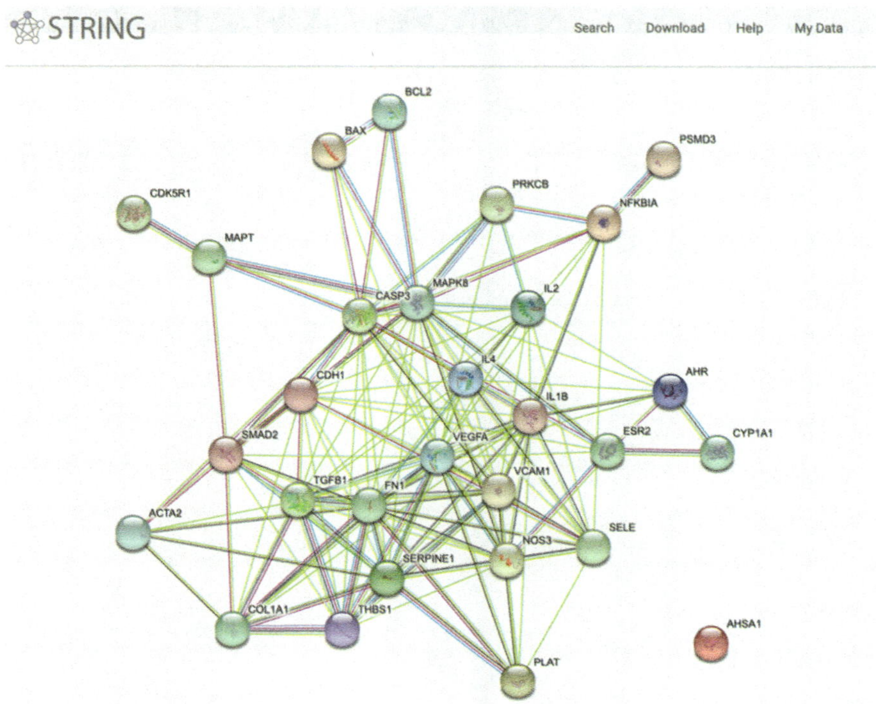

Fig. 4.19 Multiple gene query result page

4.3.2 Network Analysis Software

At present, there are many open source and commercial-use complex network construction and network analysis software. For example, Gephi [43] and Cytoscape [44] are open source and free, as shown in Table 4.1. These powerful software not only provide network graph creation, visualization, and abundant network graph layout methods, but also provide large-scale network analysis algorithms, such as community division algorithm, centrality measurement algorithm, and shortest path calculation method. Cytoscape currently has 14,650 citations and Gephi has 4704. Ruth et al. used Cytoscape to analyze the evolutionary network of mammals and their gut microbes [45], Zhong et al. used Cytoscape to analyze the overall distribution of Saccharomyces cerevisiae protein complex [46], Barberán et al. used Gephi to use network analysis to explore the symbiosis mode of soil microbial communities [47]. In this section, we imitate and introduce two common complex network visualization analysis software: Cytoscape and Gephi. To more intuitively and pragmatically explain the basic functions of software data processing and analysis, we use a small amount of Protein–Protein Interaction (PPI) network dataset (as shown in Table 4.2) to carry out a practical operation and demonstration in

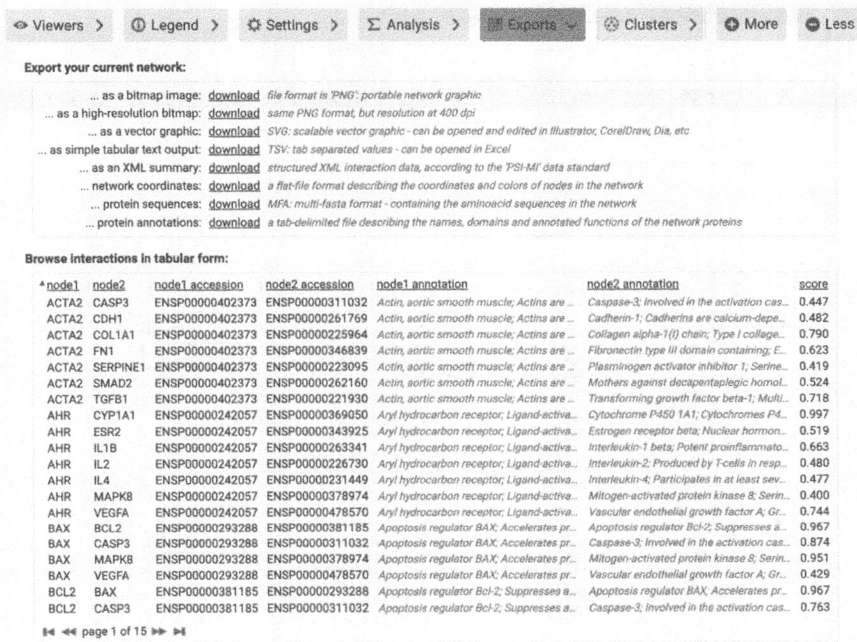

Fig. 4.20 Multiple gene query download page

combination with the functions of the corresponding software and generate relatively intuitive analysis results.

4.3.2.1 Cytoscape

Cytoscape is an open source software platform (latest version is 3.7.1) for visualizing molecular interaction networks and biological pathways, and integrating these networks with annotations, gene expression profiles, and other status data. Although Cytoscape was originally designed for biological research, it has become a universal platform for complex network analysis and visualization. Its dominant function is to analyze the relationships among large-scale protein interactions, protein–DNA, and genetic interactions. Cytoscape's core functions provide the basic components for data integration, analysis, and visualization. Additional extended functions are provided in the form of small programs (apps, formerly called plug-ins). Various apps can be used for molecular network analysis, new layouts, additional file format support, script writing, and connection with databases. The system also supports the development of open APIs based on Java, which can be published to the Cytoscape application store for free download or installation by users. As the software is developed and run on Java, the corresponding Java runtime library needs to be

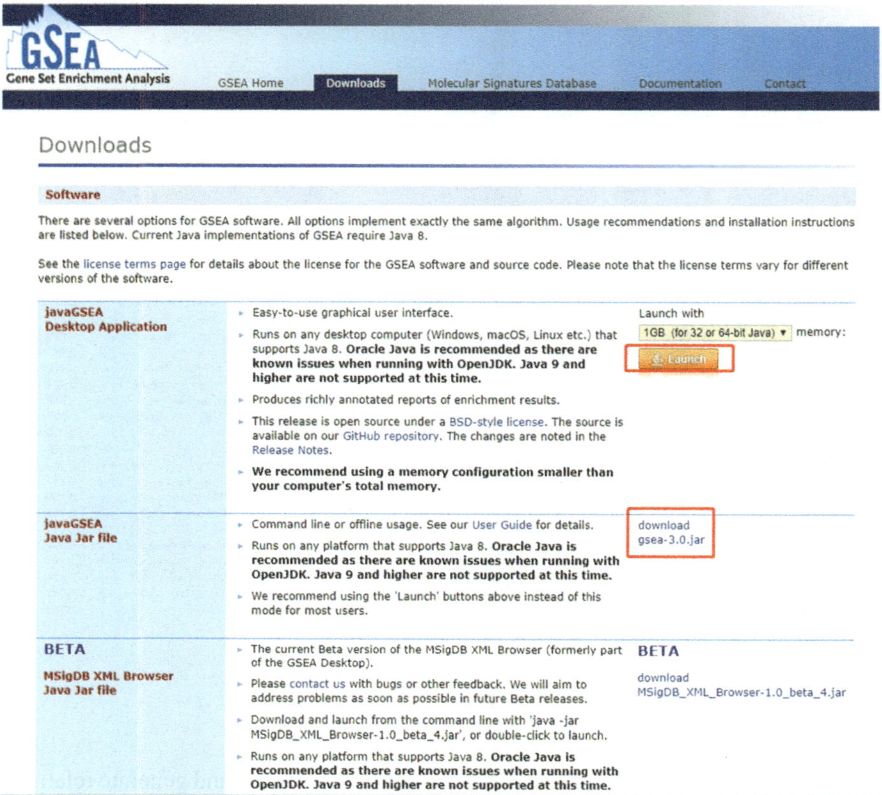

Fig. 4.21 GSEA official download page

installed beforehand. Cytoscape's main interface after an operation is shown in Fig. 4.28.

Basic Use

Launch the software, you can see the upper menu bar, select import under File to import the network; the imported data format for Cytoscape is as shown in Table 4.3. Interaction represents the relationship between nodes; this option can be defined according to actual data. Network layout can be selected as the Layout and includes grid layout, hierarchical layout, and circular layout. In addition to some basic software functions you can also search and install corresponding app plug-ins based on your needs. Cytoscape's core functions are also provided in the form of plug-ins. After importing the network diagram, you can select the layout mode and set the color, size, and shape of the nodes. The operation process is shown in Fig. 4.29.

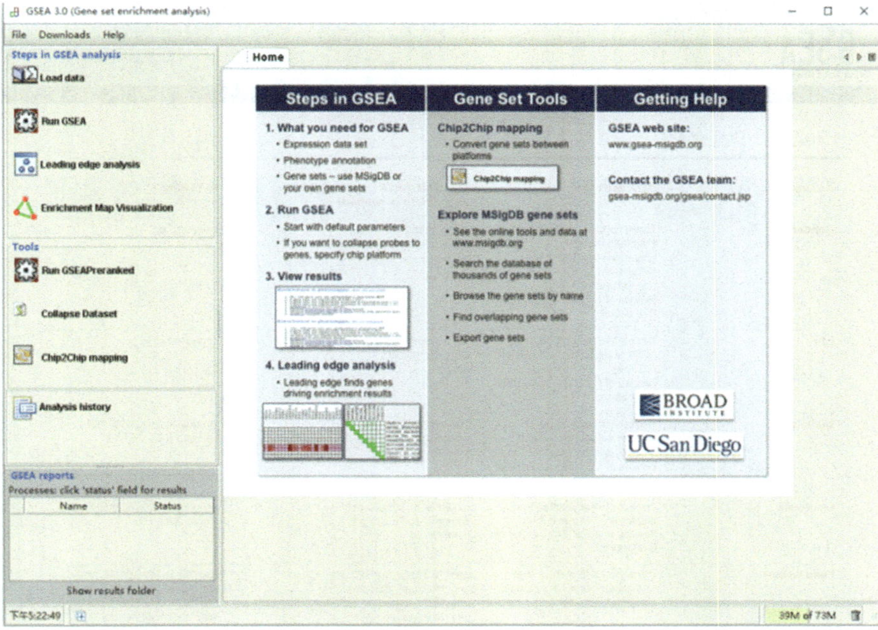

Fig. 4.22 GSEA software startup interface

Exemplary Functional Components

Common requirements in biological network analysis are analysis of network topology characteristics, community analysis, etc. To introduce the functions of Cytoscape more clearly, this chapter demonstrates the practical operation of apps such as CentiScaPe [49] and MCODE [50]. The data used in this section is the PPI network data, as shown in Table 4.3. The following is the actual operation of the above two components combined with PPI data:

Analysis of centrality measurement using CentiScaPe:

CentiScaPe is an app for network centrality measurement calculation, which can be used for analyzing undirected and directed networks. The supported centrality metrics can be divided into three aspects: network, node, and edge and include Network Diameter, Degree, Strength, Betweenness, Closeness, Eccentricity, etc. A simple operation demonstration of CentiScaPe is shown in Fig. 4.30.

Launch the Cytoscape software, select CentiScaPe from the Apps menu bar, the CentiScaPe menu is displayed. In this menu, select the network characteristics that need to be calculated, such as network diameter, node degree, etc. Then select undirected graph or directed graph and press the start button to start the calculation. Each indicator has a corresponding meaning and function. Click the button to the right of the indicator to view the details of that indicator.

Using MCODE for community analysis:

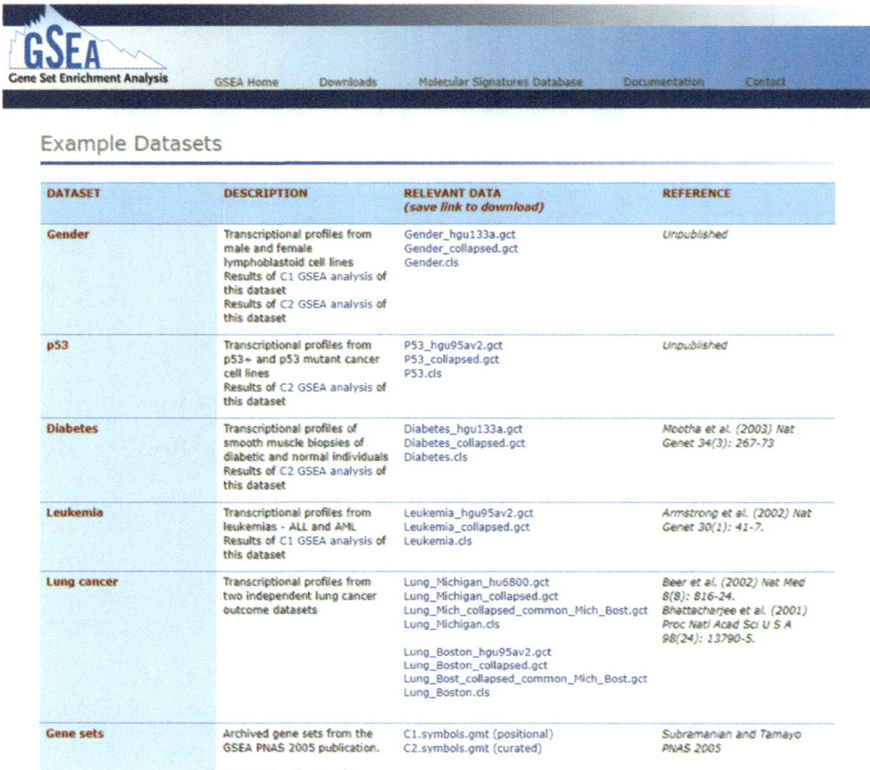

DATASET	DESCRIPTION	RELEVANT DATA (save link to download)	REFERENCE
Gender	Transcriptional profiles from male and female lymphoblastoid cell lines Results of C1 GSEA analysis of this dataset Results of C2 GSEA analysis of this dataset	Gender_hgu133a.gct Gender_collapsed.gct Gender.cls	Unpublished
p53	Transcriptional profiles from p53+ and p53 mutant cancer cell lines Results of C2 GSEA analysis of this dataset	P53_hgu95av2.gct P53_collapsed.gct P53.cls	Unpublished
Diabetes	Transcriptional profiles of smooth muscle biopsies of diabetic and normal individuals Results of C2 GSEA analysis of this dataset	Diabetes_hgu133a.gct Diabetes_collapsed.gct Diabetes.cls	Mootha et al. (2003) Nat Genet 34(3): 267-73
Leukemia	Transcriptional profiles from leukemias - ALL and AML Results of C1 GSEA analysis of this dataset	Leukemia_hgu95av2.gct Leukemia_collapsed.gct Leukemia.cls	Armstrong et al. (2002) Nat Genet 30(1): 41-7.
Lung cancer	Transcriptional profiles from two independent lung cancer outcome datasets	Lung_Michigan_hu6800.gct Lung_Michigan_collapsed.gct Lung_Mich_collapsed_common_Mich_Bost.gct Lung_Michigan.cls Lung_Boston_hgu95av2.gct Lung_Boston_collapsed.gct Lung_Bost_collapsed_common_Mich_Bost.gct Lung_Boston.cls	Beer et al. (2002) Nat Med 8(8): 816-24. Bhattacharjee et al. (2001) Proc Natl Acad Sci U S A 98(24): 13790-5.
Gene sets	Archived gene sets from the GSEA PNAS 2005 publication.	C1.symbols.gmt (positional) C2.symbols.gmt (curated)	Subramanian and Tamayo PNAS 2005

Fig. 4.23 GSEA sample data download page

The MCODE plug-in adopts a Molecular Complex Detection algorithm, which is used to detect the closely connected subnet structure (highly inter-connected local network structures) in the network. This closely connected subnet is also known as community. Communities usually have different practical meanings in different networks. The communities in protein interaction networks are usually part of protein complexes and molecular pathways, whereas the communities in similar networks of protein structures usually represent the protein family. With respect to community extraction, MCODE also supports visualization analysis of the community structure. A simple operation demonstration of MCODE is shown in Fig. 4.31.

Launch the Cytoscape software and import the network. Select the MCODE plug-in from the Apps menu bar. Then select and set the relevant parameters, such as degree coefficient, etc. Click clustering; the corresponding clustering results are displayed in the right panel. Click the appropriate category to display the specific community analysis results in the graph.

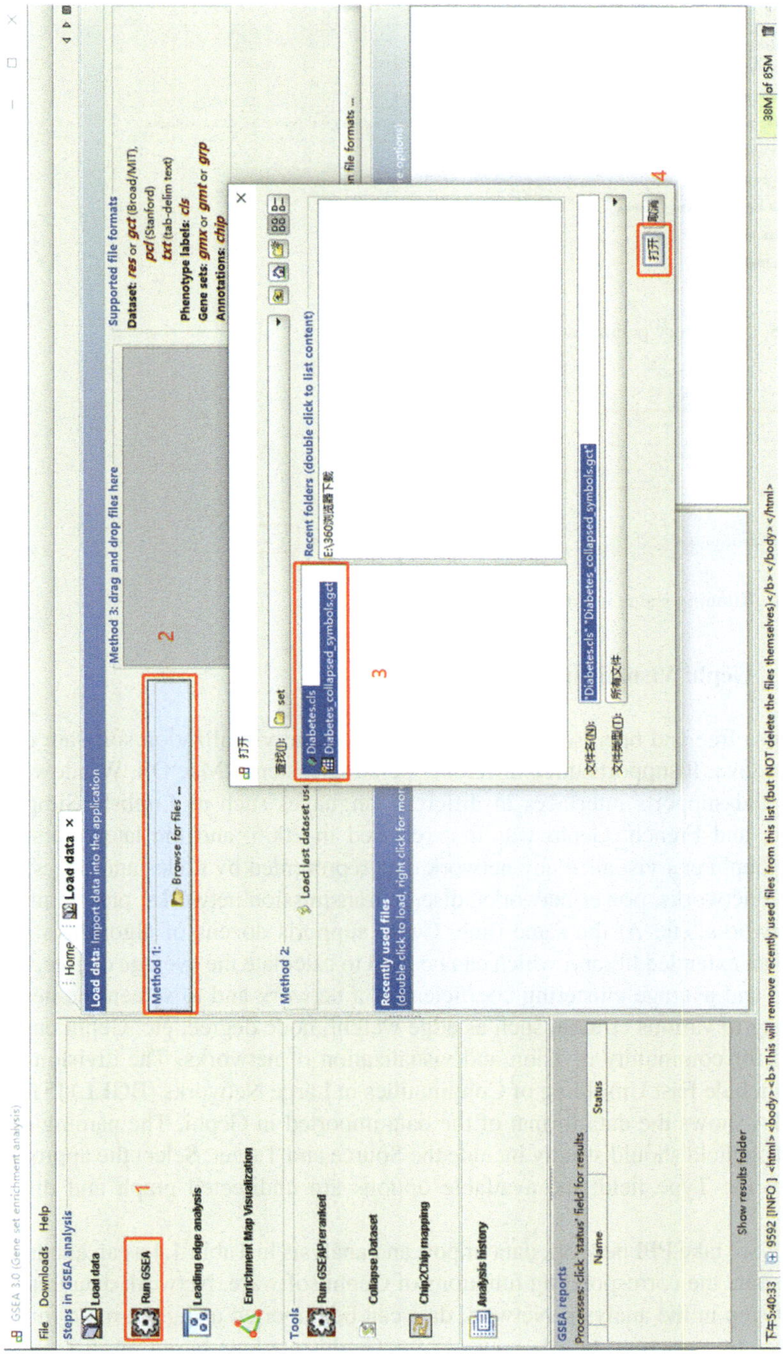

Fig. 4.24 Import data interface

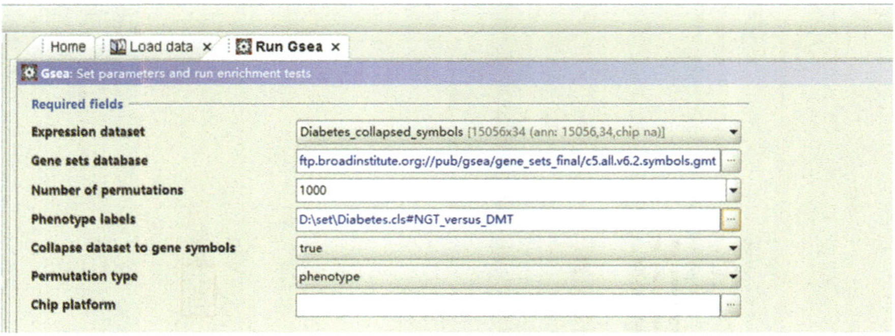

Fig. 4.25 Mandatory parameter setting interface

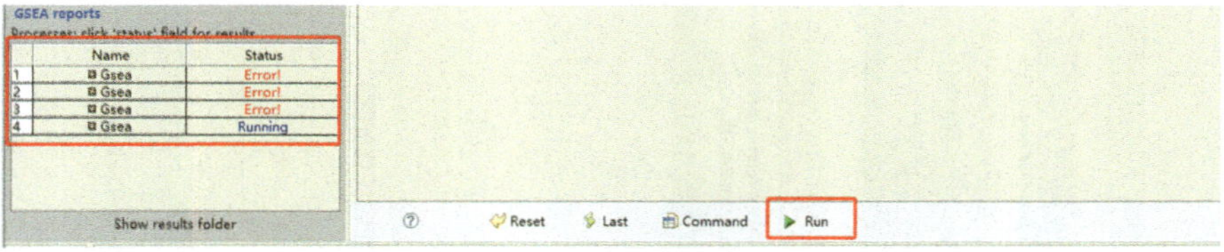

Fig. 4.26 Running status interface

4.3.2.2 Gephi Visualization Software

Gephi is a free and open source network analysis and visualization software developed on Java. It supports three different operating systems, Mac OS, Windows, and Linux, and supports interfaces in different languages such as English, Simplified Chinese, and French. Gephi was first released in 2006, and the latest version is V0.92. Gephi can visualize any network data represented by nodes and edges, such as social networks, power networks, disease transmission networks, protein interaction networks, etc. At the same time, Gephi supports dozens of algorithms in the form of an extended library, which can be used to calculate the average degree, graph density, and average clustering coefficient of a network and to screen the network according to various criteria, such as edge weight, node degree, etc. Gephi can also be used for community division and visualization of networks. The division algorithms include Fast Unfolding of Communities in Large Networks (BGLL) [51], etc. Table 4.4 shows the data format of the data imported in Gephi. The naming of the node name field should strictly include the Source and Target. Select the appropriate value in the Type field; the available options are undirected graph and directed graph.

Next, we take PPI network data import and analysis in Table 4.4 as an example to demonstrate the corresponding functions of Gephi software. Network data import is the first step in the analysis. Network data can be imported using the main function interfaces by selecting the file menu in the Gephi interface based on different file formats (the data format is shown in Table 4.4 and Fig. 4.32). After the data is

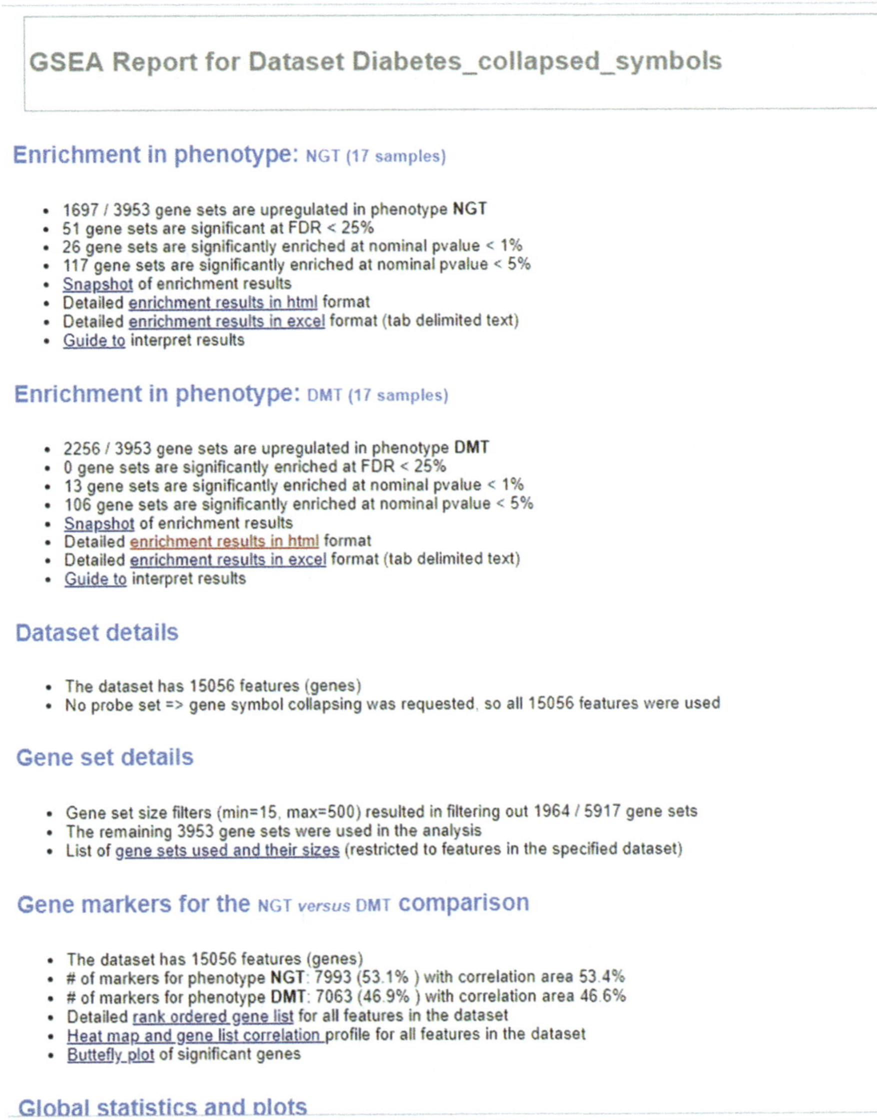
GSEA Report for Dataset Diabetes_collapsed_symbols

Enrichment in phenotype: NGT (17 samples)

- 1697 / 3953 gene sets are upregulated in phenotype **NGT**
- 51 gene sets are significant at FDR < 25%
- 26 gene sets are significantly enriched at nominal pvalue < 1%
- 117 gene sets are significantly enriched at nominal pvalue < 5%
- Snapshot of enrichment results
- Detailed enrichment results in html format
- Detailed enrichment results in excel format (tab delimited text)
- Guide to interpret results

Enrichment in phenotype: DMT (17 samples)

- 2256 / 3953 gene sets are upregulated in phenotype **DMT**
- 0 gene sets are significantly enriched at FDR < 25%
- 13 gene sets are significantly enriched at nominal pvalue < 1%
- 106 gene sets are significantly enriched at nominal pvalue < 5%
- Snapshot of enrichment results
- Detailed enrichment results in html format
- Detailed enrichment results in excel format (tab delimited text)
- Guide to interpret results

Dataset details

- The dataset has 15056 features (genes)
- No probe set => gene symbol collapsing was requested, so all 15056 features were used

Gene set details

- Gene set size filters (min=15, max=500) resulted in filtering out 1964 / 5917 gene sets
- The remaining 3953 gene sets were used in the analysis
- List of gene sets used and their sizes (restricted to features in the specified dataset)

Gene markers for the NGT *versus* DMT comparison

- The dataset has 15056 features (genes)
- # of markers for phenotype **NGT**: 7993 (53.1%) with correlation area 53.4%
- # of markers for phenotype **DMT**: 7063 (46.9%) with correlation area 46.6%
- Detailed rank ordered gene list for all features in the dataset
- Heat map and gene list correlation profile for all features in the dataset
- Buttefly plot of significant genes

Global statistics and plots

Fig. 4.27 Analysis result page

imported, the main interface can be selected through the corresponding properties to flexibly view the network diagram. For example, multiple network layouts and styles can be selected (such as Fruchterman Reingold), and then the corresponding visualization effect can be obtained by running the operation. In addition, the color and size of nodes in the network and the color and size of edges can be adjusted and processed accordingly (as shown in Fig. 4.33). Various topological statistical

Table 4.1 Network analysis software

Three commonly used visualization software			
Directory	Cytoscape	Gephi	Pajek [48]
Developer	UCSD	Mathieu Jacomy, Sebastien Heymann	eytanAdar
Development language	Java	Java	Java
Supported Platforms	Mac OS, Windows, Linux	Mac OS, Windows, Linux	Mac OS, Windows, Linux
Supported languages	English	English, Simplified Chinese, etc.	English
Open source and free	Yes	Yes	Yes

Table 4.2 Examples of PPI network data

Source	Target	Weight
FKBP4	HSP90AA1	1
CFTR	HSPA8	1
CFTR	SLC9A3R1	1
CFTR	UBC	1
CYP51A1	LSS	1
USH1C	CDH23	1
RALA	RALBP1	1
RALA	EXOC2	1
RALA	EXOC8	1
CX3CL1	CX3CR1	1

features of the network, such as average degree, network diameter, and betweenness, can be conveniently calculated and displayed (as shown in Fig. 4.34). Community analysis is an important algorithm for complex network analysis and is also one of the basic functions. Gephi integrates the classic community analysis method into a toolbar called "statistics." After clicking and running, the results of the community structure analysis in the network are displayed. The visualization of specific community structure can be classified and displayed (as shown in Fig. 4.35) through the color rendering mode (the selection is based on modules) of nodes in the menu on the left side of the main interface. It is worth noting that several other Gephi analysis functions are integrated in the form of plug-ins; users can load the corresponding plug-ins through the menu to obtain new analysis functions.

4.3.2.3 Pajek Complex Network Visualization Software

Among the more complex network analysis software, Pajek is a free large-scale complex network analysis tool with a more than two decade-long research and development history (since 1996). Compared with other software, most network

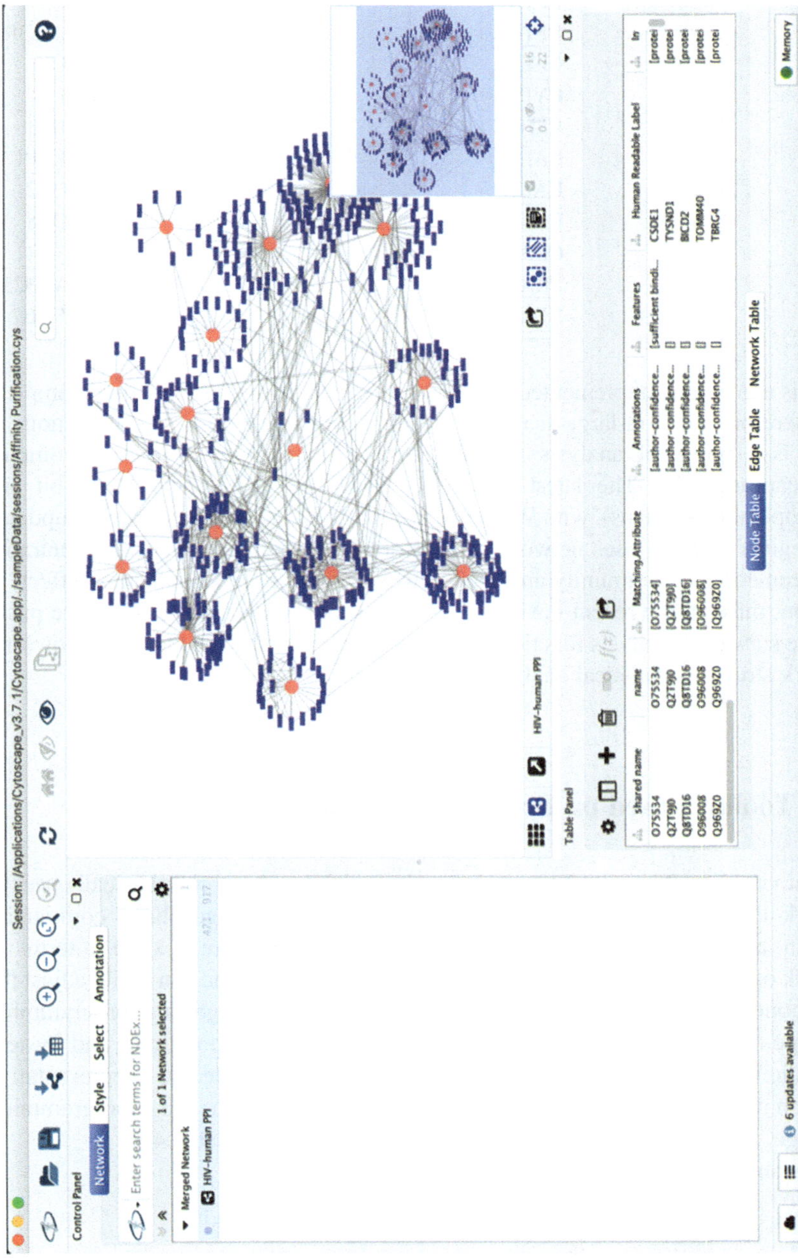

Fig. 4.28 Cytoscape software homepage

Table 4.3 Import data format of cytoscape

source	interaction	target
FKBP4	Pp	HSP90AA1
CFTR	pp	HSPA8
CFTR	pp	SLC9A3R1
CFTR	pp	UBC
CYP51A1	pp	LSS
USH1C	pp	CDH23
RALA	pp	RALBP1
RALA	pp	EXOC2
RALA	pp	EXOC8
CX3CL1	pp	CX3CR1
TRAPPC6A	pp	TRAPPC3
NDUFAB1	pp	NDUFB7

analysis algorithms implemented in Pajek have a low computational time complexity. Therefore, an ultra-large-scale network that can handle hundreds of millions of nodes is a powerful analysis tool for developing various large-scale complex nonlinear networks. The latest version of Pajek is V5.08 (supports 32-bit and 64-bit operating systems), with Windows, Linux, and Mac versions. Pajek is updated on a regular basis. It uses network exploratory analysis methods such as centrality measurement and community analysis; however, it has poor visualization effect. In addition, through the recent development (2019) of the R language interface package, the statistical analysis function of the R language can be used to create powerful network structure statistical analysis capability.

4.4 Toolkit Based on Programming Languages

Current visualization toolkits based on programming language calls basically use the network topology statistical measurement, classic graph algorithms, community division, and link prediction analysis methods. They are more flexible in terms of network operations, can accurately control nodes and edges, and can easily adjust the corresponding calculation functions as required. However, in general, programming language-call-based tools are suitable for backend batch computing and system integration. Based on the programming language, we have selected a representative common network visualization package for C++, Java, Python, and R programming language. Some common visualization toolkits are listed in Table 4.5.

C++ and Java toolkits are briefly introduced below:

1. Boost Graph Library: A C++ Network Visualization Toolkit

The Boost Graph Library (BGL) is a C++ visualization toolkit that provides generic interfaces that can access the internal structure of a graph while hiding implementation details. It has an open interface and the graph library that

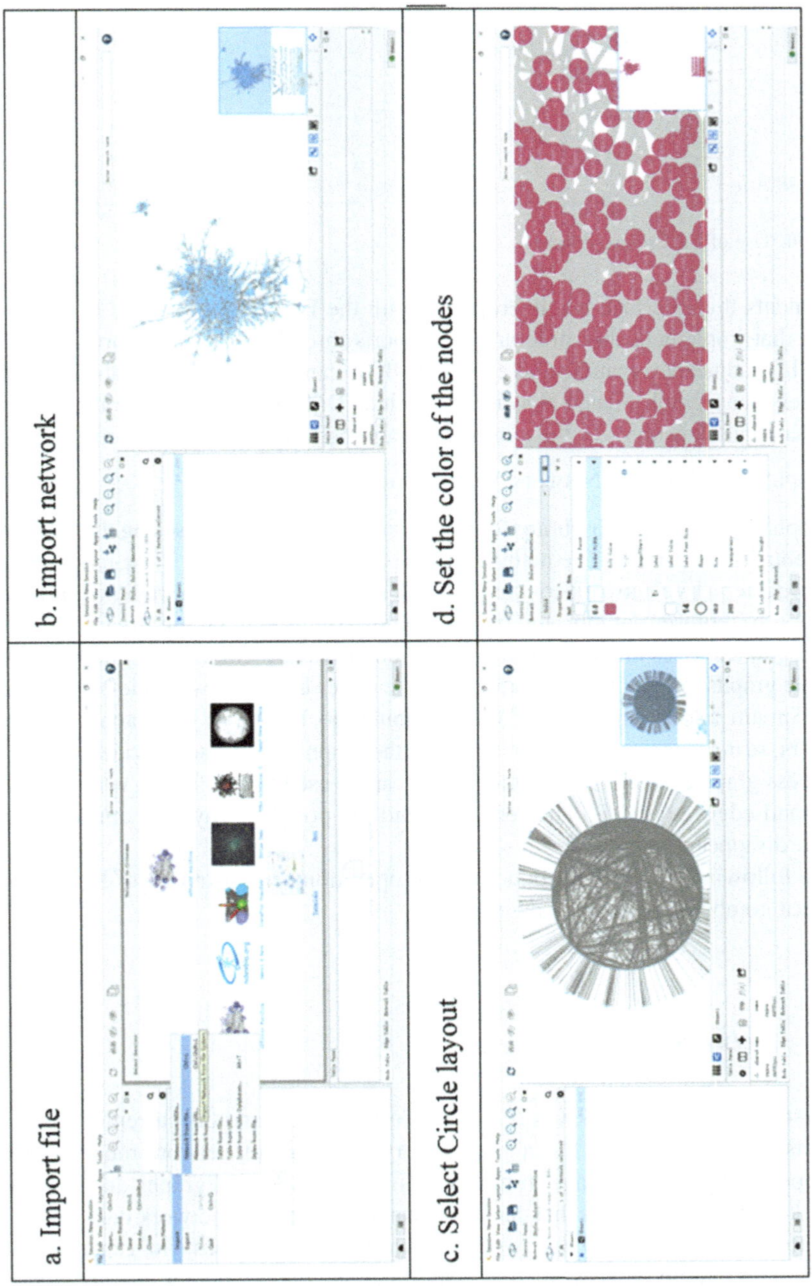

Fig. 4.29 Cytoscape visualization network

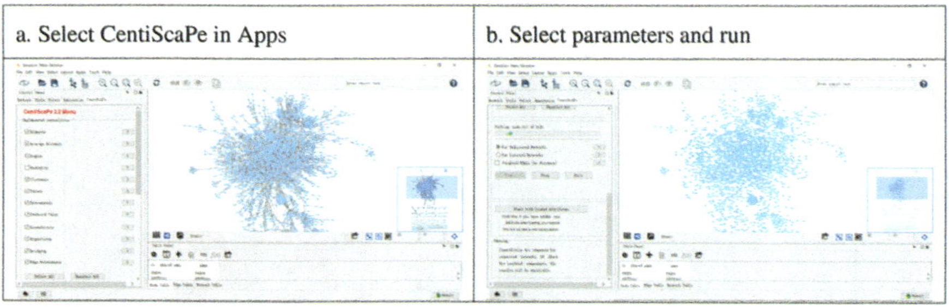

Fig. 4.30 Use of Centiscape plug-in

implements this interface can interoperate with the BGL algorithm and other algorithms that implement this structure. It supports three kinds of data format—adjacency list, adjacency matrix, and edge list. BGL can be used for visualization and provides many graph-related algorithms, such as Dijkstra algorithm for the shortest path, Kruskal algorithm for the minimum spanning tree, topological sorting, etc.

2. GraphStream: A Java Network Visualization Toolkit

GraphStream is a graph library for processing Java which focuses on the dynamic representation of graphs. The main research object of this library is the modeling of dynamic interactive networks of various scales. The goal of this library is to provide a method to represent graphs and process them. To this end, GraphStream provides several graph classes that allow directed and undirected, 1-graph, or P-graph (that is, multiple graphs, graphs that can have multiple edges between two nodes) modeling. GraphStream allows any type of data attributes to be stored on graph elements: numbers, strings, or any objects. In addition, the graphic flow also provides a method to process graph evolution over time, which can be used to display the way in which nodes and edges are added and removed, and the possible way data attributes can appear, disappear, and evolve.

The following is a brief introduction and operation demonstration of Python and R toolkit combined with some cases.

4.4.1 NetworkX

The first version of NetworkX was released in May 2002, and the current number of citations has reached 2149. It is a graph theory and complex network modeling tool developed in Python language. It has built-in commonly used graphs and complex network analysis algorithms that can easily carry out complex network data analysis, simulation modeling, and other work. NetworkX makes it easy to generate both classical and random graphs, such as scale-free networks (where a few nodes have several), which is convenient for carrying out some network analysis without data. NetworkX supports the creation of simple undirected graphs, directed graphs, and

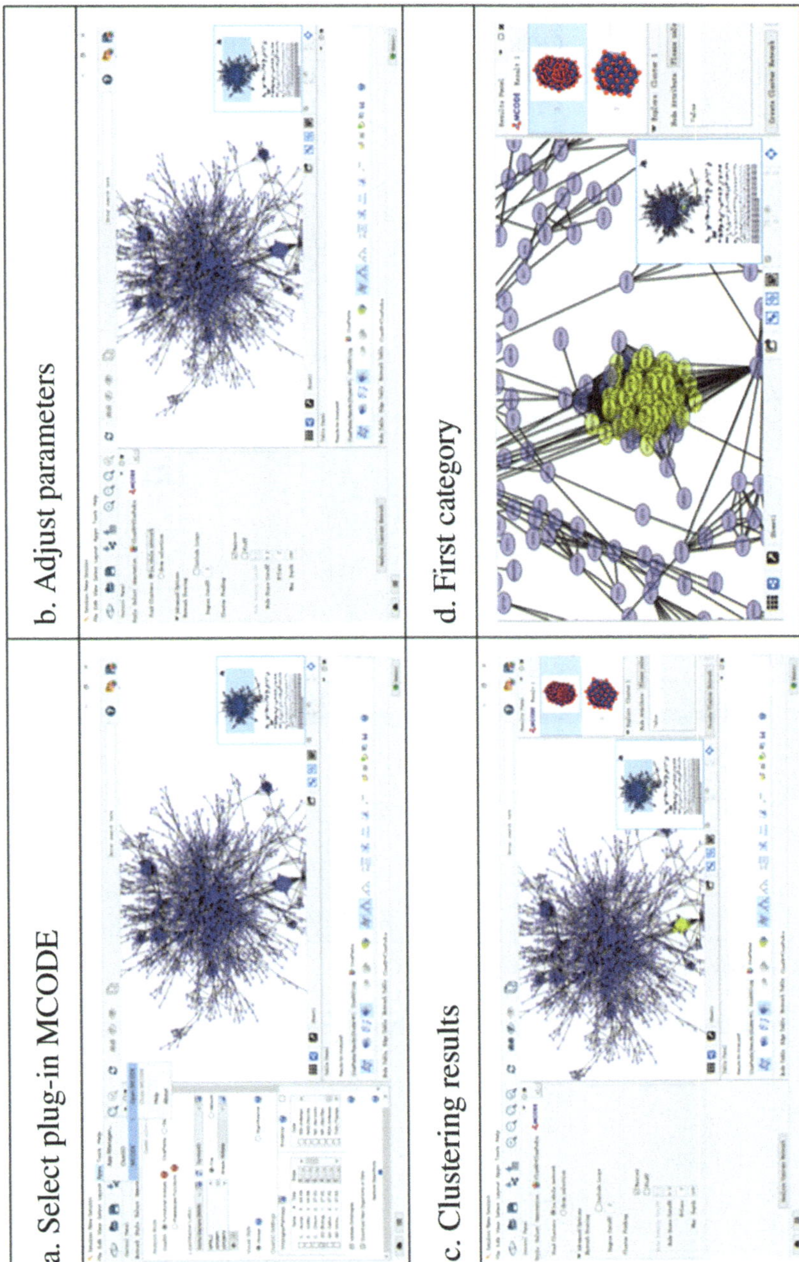

Fig. 4.31 MCODE plug-in use

Table 4.4 Gehpi data format

Source	Target	Weight
FKBP4	HSP90AA1	1
CFTR	HSPA8	1
CFTR	SLC9A3R1	1
CFTR	UBC	1
CYP51A1	LSS	1
USH1C	CDH23	1
RALA	RALBP1	1
RALA	EXOC2	1
RALA	EXOC8	1
CX3CL1	CX3CR1	1

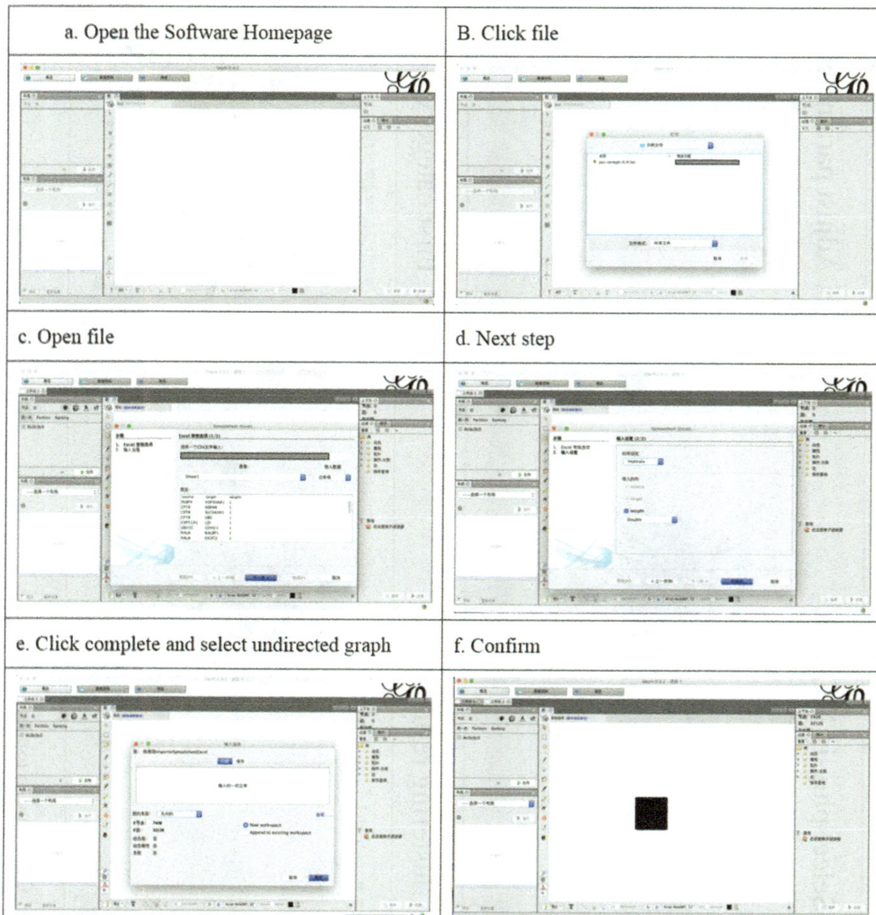

Fig. 4.32 Gephi import network

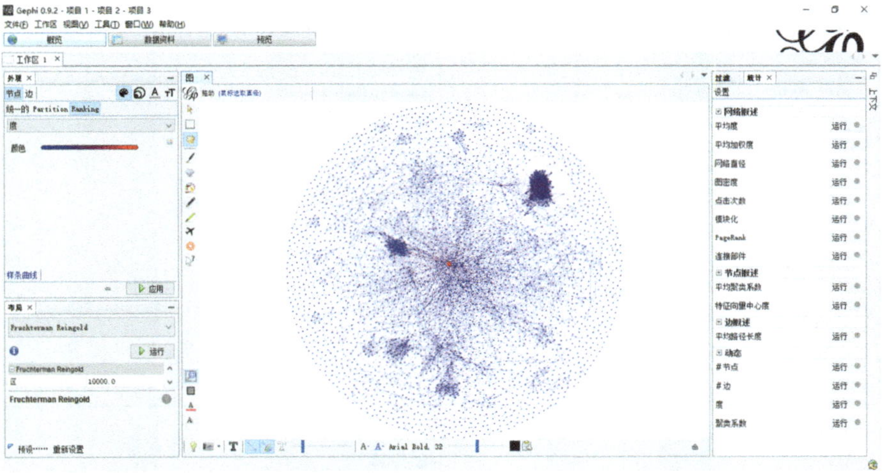

Fig. 4.33 Network layout and node edge settings

multiple graphs. It has many standard graph theory algorithms built-in, and the nodes can be any data. It has rich functions and is easy to use. For programmers who are familiar with Python, the NetworkX visualization Python package is a very convenient tool with simple and efficient operation. Table 4.6 shows some basic functions of NetworkX in the Python environment. For detailed functions, please check the documents on the official website.

To more vividly demonstrate the visualization effect of NetworkX, this chapter uses an exemplary small amount of clinical disease merger relational data and uses Python code to generate a visualized network diagram. The disease merger relational network data contains 51 disease nodes and 150 disease merger relational edges (as shown in Table 4.7). The core codes are shown in Table 4.8. The visualization result is shown in Fig. 4.36. The case diagram uses a circular layout. The larger the node degree in the network, the larger the node. The color is also set according to the node degree. The larger the node degree, the closer the node color is to blue. The greater the weight of the edge between the two nodes, the wider the line of the edge; the width of the edge between hypertension and renal insufficiency in the merger disease network is the widest, as hypertension and renal insufficiency are more likely to occur as co-morbidity.

4.4.2 igraph

igraph is a simple and easy-to-use network analysis tool. Several of its functions are developed using C language. It has high computing efficiency and is highly suitable for solving large and complex network problems. R, Python, and C/C++ can be used to call the corresponding packages for visualization. The latest version is V1.0.0. In

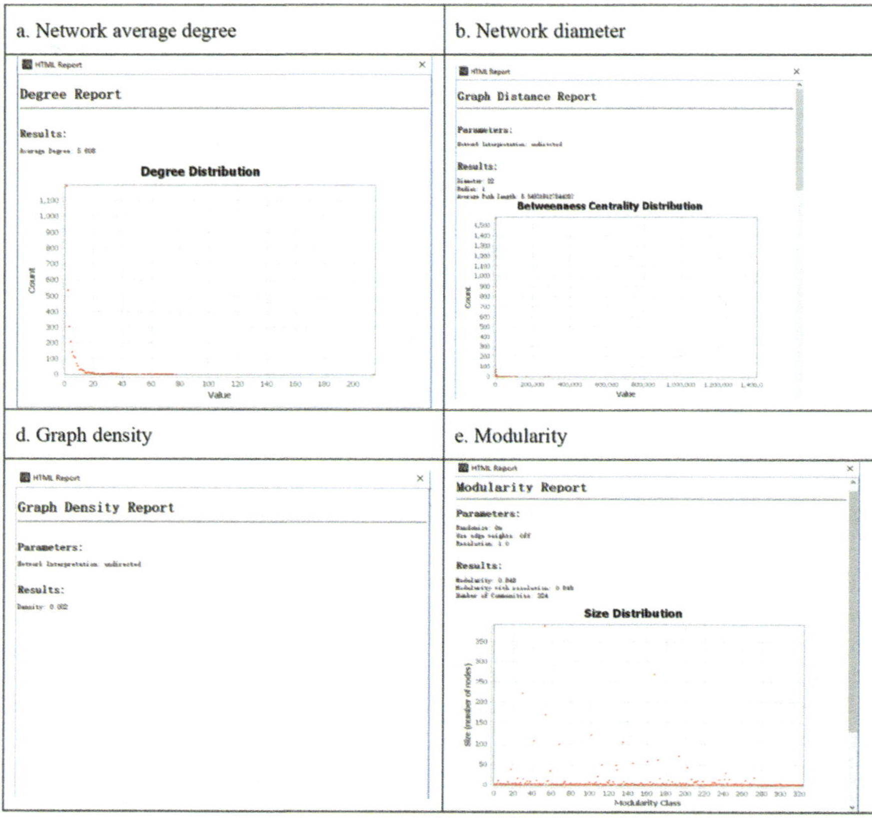

Fig. 4.34 Statistical index of the Gephi diagram

the igraph network graph we can set the node color and calculate node degree, edge density, clustering coefficient, and other statistics and their distribution and can also cluster the network and visualize each category. In this section, we first call the igraph R language package with the R language to create a visualization example. Table 4.9 lists the basic functions of the igraph R package.

To show the visualization effect of igraph, we perform a simple operation demonstration using the disease network dataset. First, install RStudio, and then install the igraph R package. Table 4.10 shows the core codes of the case (based on R language), and Fig. 4.37 shows the visualization effect of the case. Different colors in the figure represent different communities, and each community represents a set of closely related diseases.

Taking into account the wide range of network pharmacology applications, this chapter only provides a high-level introduction to the main network pharmacology methods and software. It focuses on introducing common software and methods such as common complex network analysis and visualization, molecular and network function analysis, drug-target prediction, and drug indication prediction that

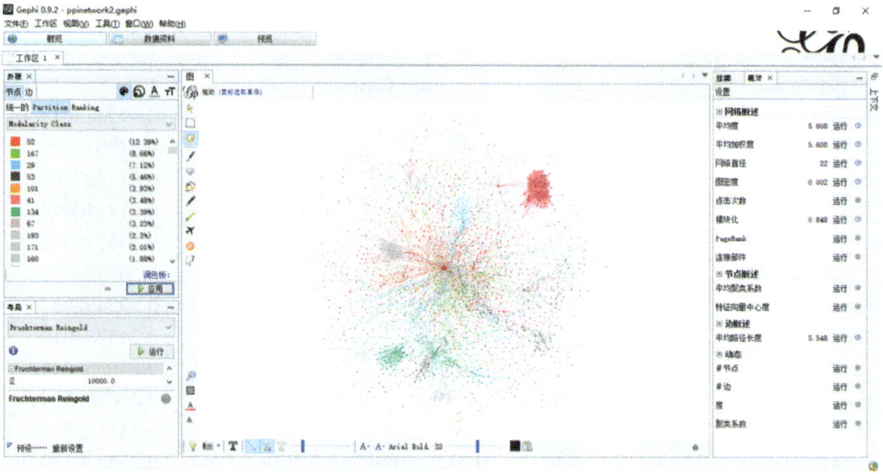

Fig. 4.35 Gephi module rendering

Table 4.5 Common web visualization toolkits

Name	NetworkX [52]	igraph [53]	Boost Graph Library [54]	GraphStream [55]
Developers	Aric Hagberg, Pieter J. Swart	Szabolcs Horvát	Douglas Gregor Andrew Lumsdaine	Julien Baudry Antoine Dutot
Programming languages	Python	R, Python, C/C++	C++	Java
Open source and free	Yes	Yes	Yes	Yes
Latest versions	2.3	1.0.0	1.70.0	1.3

Table 4.6 NetworkX functions

Functions	Description
add_node(node)	Add node to graph
get_node_attributes(G, name)	Get node attributes from graph
all_neighbors(G, node)	Return to neighboring node of the node
common_neighbors(G, u, v)	Return to common neighbor of the two nodes
is_directed(G)	Judge whether graph is a directed graph
nodes(G)	Return to nodes of the graph
number_of_nodes(G)	Find the number of graph nodes of the graph
add_edge(node1, node2)	Add edge
get_edge_attributes(G, name)	Get edge attributes
number_of_edges(G)	Return to number of edges
clear()	Delete nodes and edges in the graph

Table 4.7 Dataset of diabetes with combination of diseases

Disease 1 (node 1)	Disease 2(node 2)	Weight (Weight)
Hypertension	Renal insufficiency	1
Lipid metabolism disorder	Hypertension	0.995283019
Hypertension	Heart disease	0.872641509
Cerebral infarction	Hypertension	0.613207547
Hypertension	Hepatic disease	0.514150943
Lipid metabolism disorder	Hepatic disease	0.504716981
Lipid metabolism disorder	Renal insufficiency	0.367924528
Gastrointestinal lesions	Hypertension	0.29245283
Lipid metabolism disorder	Cerebral infarction	0.245283019
Retinopathy	Renal insufficiency	0.240566038
Hypertension	Cervical spondylosis	0.240566038
Heart disease	Renal insufficiency	0.231132075
Neuropathy	Hypertension	0.202830189
Cerebral infarction	Heart disease	0.202830189

Table 4.8 NetworkX drawing core codes

Core Codes of NetworkX Drawing Network Diagram

import networkx as nx # Import networkx package
import matplotlib.pyplot as plt # Import drawing kit
G = nx.Graph() # Create a graph

G.add_nodes_from(nodes) #Add nodes to graph, nodes are edge list of the graph
G.add_weighted_edges_from(edges)# Add edges to graph, edges are edge list of the graph
de = G.degree() # Calculate degree of graph
node_color = [convert_to_hex(de[i]) for i in nodes]#Set node color according to degree
node_size = [de[i]*30 for i in nodes]#Set node size according to degree
widths = [int(line[2])/50 for line in data]#Set width of edge according to weight of edge
nx.draw(G,pos=nx.spring_layout(nodes), with_labels = True,font_size=10, node_size=node_size,width=widths,node_color=node_color)
plt.rcParams['font.sans-serif'] = ['SimHei'] #Display Chinese tag
plt.savefig("ba.png") #Save figure
plt.show() #Display

are unique to network pharmacology. Traditional computational pharmacology software such as virtual screening (Docking) software is not involved [56]. At the same time, this chapter provides some further details from the perspective of network pharmacology technology and application scope including the construction methods of network pharmacology-related resources, such as the information extraction method of drug-target and drug side effect relationship [57], the transformation network pharmacology method combining clinical and basic medicine [58], the network pharmacology prediction method based on deep learning, etc., which have become new and key research topics [59]. This chapter does not elaborate much on the above aspects. Particularly, there are several important studies in the

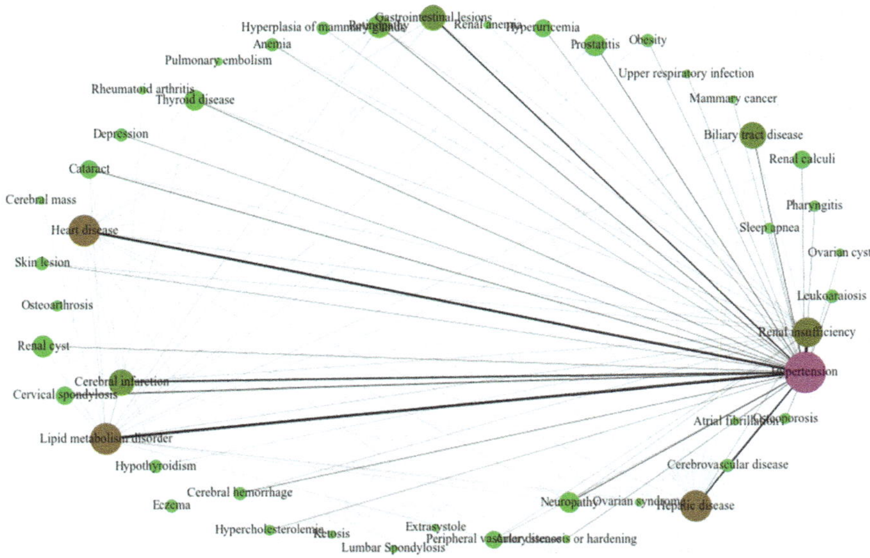

Fig. 4.36 NetworkX graph visualization display

Table 4.9 igraph basic functions

Functions	Description
nodes<-read.table("nodes.txt")	Read information of the node
links<-read.table("links.txt")	Read information of the edge
net<-graph_from_data_frame(d = links, vertices = nodes, directed = F)	Create network
E(net)$color<- "red"	Designate node color
plot(net,vertex.color="gray50",edge.color = E(net) $color)	Graph visualization
plot(net, layout = layout_in_circle)	Layout
degree(g, mode="all")	Compute all node degrees in the graph
edge_density(net)	Calculate edge density
transitivity(g, type="global")	Calculate clustering coefficient
cfg <- cluster_fast_greedy(net)	Clustering, mining community in the network

prediction and analysis of adverse drug reactions and drug side effects, as well as the prediction method of drug interaction relationship. The related research plays a vital role in network pharmacology research. However, this chapter does not cover the methods and software information from this aspect. Readers who are interested can refer to other research works [60, 61].

Conversely, current network pharmacology software and analysis processing algorithms are focused on the functions of independent technical links, such as

Table 4.10 igraph visualization core codes

Core codes: igraph visualization
library(igraph)#load igraph package
net <- graph_from_data_frame(relation, directed=FALSE)#Create graph
cfg <- cluster_fast_greedy(net)#Community division algorithm
plot(cfg, net)#visualization
Degree(net)#Add up node degree
edge_density(net)#Calculate edge density
transitivity(net, type="global")#Calculate clustering coefficient

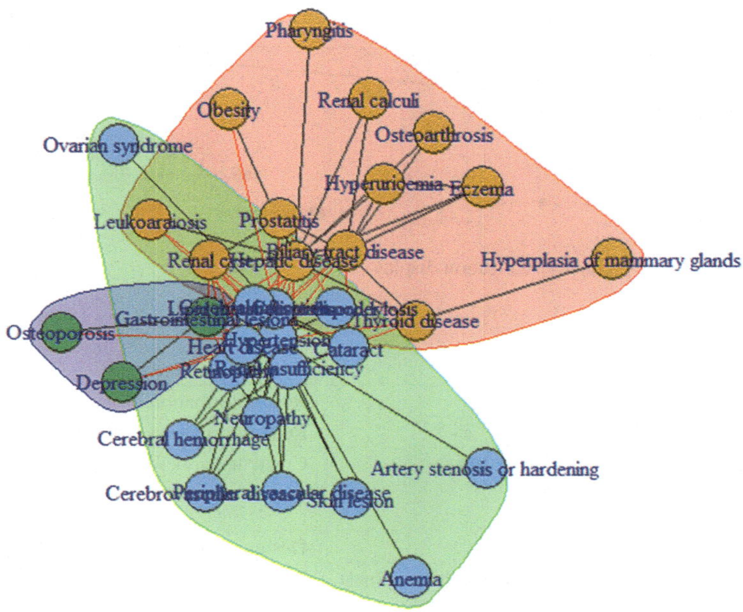

Fig. 4.37 igraph disease network visualization

network analysis and visualization, drug-target relationship prediction, etc. However, as network pharmacology research involves many upstream and downstream technologies and functional links, researchers need to combine and apply different software and algorithms to generate corresponding research results. To this end, in order to improve the effectiveness of network pharmacology research, there is an urgent need to develop an integrated, high-performance, and service-oriented network pharmacology software platform. The platform needs to include network data integration, network analysis and prediction, visualization processing, functional enrichment analysis, and related literature validation, to support the integrated network pharmacology research process.

References

1. Hopkins AL. Network pharmacology: the next paradigm in drug discovery. Nat Chem Biol. 2008;4(11):682–90.
2. Newman MEJ. Networks: An Introduction. Astronomische Nachrichten. 2010;327(8):741–3.
3. Barabasi AL. Network science: Luck or reason. Nature. 2012;489(7417):507–8.
4. Barabasi AL, Gullbahce N, Loscalzo J. Network medicine: a network-based approach to human disease. Nat Rev Genet. 2011;12(1):56–68.
5. Lu LY. Link Prediction on Complex Networks. J Univ Electron Sci Technol China. 2010;39 (5):651–61.
6. Watts DJ. Identity and Search in Social Networks. Science. 2002;296(5571):1302–5.
7. Barabasi AL, Albert R. Emergence of scaling in random networks. Science. 1999;286 (5439):509–12.
8. Watts DJ, Strogatz SH. Collective Dynamics of Small World Networks. Nature. 1998;393 (6684):440–2.
9. Barabasi AL. Scale-Free Networks: A Decade and Beyond. Science. 2009;325(5939):412–3.
10. Menche J, Harma A, Kitsak M. Uncovering disease-disease relationships through the incomplete interactome. Science. 2015;347(6224):1257601.
11. Zhou ZH. Machine learning [M]. Beijing: Tsinghua University Press; 2016.
12. Duan H, Zhai CX. Mining coordinated intent representation for entity search and recommendation[C]. New York: ACM; 2015.
13. Deng J, Yuan Q, Mamitsuka H, et al. DrugE-rank: predicting drug-target interactions by learning to rank. Data Mining Syst Biol. 2018;1807:195–202.
14. Juurlink DN, Mamdani M, Kopp A, et al. Drug-Drug Interactions Among Elderly Patients Hospitalized for Drug Toxicity. JAMA. 2003;289(13):1652.
15. Cheng FX, Kovacs IA, Barabasi AL. Network-based prediction of drug combinations. Nat Commun. 2019;10(1):1197.
16. Govindaraj RG, Naderi M, Singha M, et al. Large-scale computational drug repositioning to find treatments for rare diseases. NPJ Syst Biol Appl. 2018;4(1):13.
17. Law V, Knox C, Djoumbou Y, et al. DrugBank 4.0: shedding new light on drug metabolism. Nucleic Acids Res. 2014;42(D1):D1091–7.
18. Kuhn M, Von MC, Campillos M, et al. STITCH: interaction networks of chemicals and proteins. Nucleic Acids Res. 2007;36(Database issue):D684–8.
19. Kuhn M, Letunic I, Jensen LJ, et al. The SIDER database of drugs and side effects. Nucleic Acids Res. 2016;44(D1):D1075–9.
20. Yamanishi Y, Kotera M, Moriya Y, et al. Dinies: drug–target interaction network inference engine based on supervised analysis. Nucleic Acids Res. 2014;42(W1):W39–45.
21. Nickel J, Gohlke BO, Erehman J, et al. SuperPred: update on drug classification and target prediction. Nucleic Acids Res. 2014;42(W1):W26–31.
22. Gfeller D, Grosdidier A, Wirth M, et al. SwissTargetPrediction: a web server for target prediction of bioactive small molecules. Nucleic Acids Res. 2014;42(W1):W32–8.
23. Vanhaelen Q. Computational methods for drug repurposing[M]. New York: Springer Science Business Media; 2018.
24. Xie DF, Li P, Li F, et al. Computational Approaches to Analyze the Strategies of Drug Repositioning. Prog Biochem Biophys. 2012;39(11):1029–36.
25. Brown AS, Patel CJ. meshdd: literature-based drug-drug similarity for drug repositioning. J Am Med Inform Assoc. 2016;24(3):614–8.
26. Moosavinasab S, Patterson J, Strouse R, et al. RE: fine drugs: an interactive dashboard to access drug repurposing opportunities. Database. 2016; pii: baw083
27. Wang X, Yin TS, Li BY, et al. Progress in Gene Functional Enrichment Analysis. Scientia Sinica(Vitae). 2016;46(4):363.
28. Huang DW, Sherman BT, Lempicki RA. Bioinformatics enrichment tools: paths toward the comprehensive functional analysis of large gene lists. Nucleic Acids Res. 2009;37(1):1–13.

29. Wu J, Mao X, Cai T, et al. KOBAS server: a web-based platform for automated annotation and pathway identification. Nucleic Acids Res. 2006;34:W720–4.
30. Szklarczyk D, Gable AL, Lyon D, et al. STRING v11: protein-protein association networks with increased coverage, supporting functional discovery in genome-wide experimental datasets. Nucleic Acids Res. 2018;47(D1):D607–13.
31. Wang J. Protein-protein Interaction Databases. Chin J Biochem Mol Biol. 2017;2017(33):767.
32. Gao JR. Molecular Biology [M]. Chemical Industry Press; 2011.
33. Licata L, Briganti L, Peluso D, et al. MINT, the molecular interaction database: 2012 update. Nucleic Acids Res. 2012;40(Database issue):D857–61.
34. Stark C, Breitkreutz BJ, Reguly T, et al. BioGRID: a general repository for interaction datasets. Nucleic Acids Res. 2006;34(Database issue):D535–9.
35. Stelzl U, Worm U, Lalowski M, et al. A human protein-protein interaction network: a resource for annotating the proteome. Cell. 2005;122(6):957–68.
36. Goh KI, Cusick ME, Valle D, et al. The human disease network. PNAS. 2007;104 (21):8685–90.
37. Scott J. Trend report social network analysis. Sociology. 1988;22(1):109–27.
38. Dholakia UM, Baggozzi RP, Pearo LK. A social influence model of consumer participation in network- and small-group-based virtual communities. Int J Res Mark. 2004;21(3):241–63.
39. Cha M, Mislove A, Gummadi KP. A measurement-driven analysis of information propagation in the flickr social network[C]//. In: Proceedings of the 18th International Conference on World Wide Web; 2009. p. 721–30.
40. Johnell K, Klarin I. The Relationship between Number of Drugs and Potential Drug-Drug Interactions in the Elderly. Drug Saf. 2007;30(10):911–8.
41. Muhammed AY, Kwang G, Michael EC, et al. Drug-target network. Nat Biotechnol. 2007;25 (10):1119–26.
42. Subramanian A, Kuehn H, Gould J, et al. GSEA-P: A desktop application for Gene Set Enrichment Analysis. Bioinformatics. 2007;23(23):3251–3.
43. Bastian M, Heymann S, Jacomy M. Gephi: an open source software for exploring and manipulating networks[C]. In: International AAAI Conference on Weblogs and Social Media; 2009.
44. Shannon P, Markiel A, Ozier O, et al. Cytoscape: A Software Environment for Integrated Models of Biomolecular Interaction Networks. Genome Res. 2003;13(11):2498–504.
45. Ley RE, Hamady M, Lozupone C, et al. Evolution of mammals and their gut microbes. Science. 2008;320(5883):1647–51.
46. Krogan NJ, Cagney G, Yu H, et al. Global landscape of protein complexes in the yeast Saccharomyces cerevisiae. Nature. 2006;440(7084):637–43.
47. Barberan A, Bates ST, Casamayor EO, et al. Using network analysis to explore co-occurrence patterns in soil microbial communities. ISME J. 2012;6(2):343–51.
48. Batagelj V, Mrvar A. Pajek - Analysis and Visualization of Large Networks. In: Lecture Notes in Computer Science. Berlin: Springer; 2004. p. 77–103.
49. Scardoni G, Tosadori G, Faizan M, et al. Biological network analysis with CentiScaPe: centralities and experimental dataset integration. F1000research. 2014;3:139.
50. Bader GD, Hogue CW. An automated method for finding molecular complexes in large protein interaction networks. BMC Bioinform. 2003;4(1):1–27.
51. Blondel VD, Guillaume JL, Lambiotte R, et al. Fast unfolding of community hierarchies in large networks. J Statistical Mech Theory Exper. 2008;2008(10):P10008.
52. Hagberg A, Schult D, Swart P, et al. Exploring Network Structure, Dynamics, and Function using NetworkX[C]//. In: Proceedings of the 7th Python in Science Conference (SciPy); 2008. p. 11–5.
53. Csardi G, Nepusz T. The igraph software package for complex network research. Inter J Complex Syst. 2006;2006:1695.
54. Gregor D, Lumsdaine A. The Parallel BGL: A Generic Library for Distributed Graph Computations. Parallel Object-Oriented Scientific Computing (POOSC). 2005;2:1–18.

55. Antoine D, Frederic G, Damien O, et al. GraphStream: A Tool for bridging the gap between Complex Systems and Dynamic Graphs. 2008.
56. Pagadala NS, Syed K, Jack T. Software for molecular docking: a review. Biophys Rev. 2017;9 (2):91–102.
57. Xue H, Li J, Xie H, et al. Review of Drug Repositioning Approaches and Resources. Int J Biol Sci. 2018;14(10):1232–44.
58. Messinis DE, Melas IN, Hur J, et al. Translational systems pharmacology-based predictive assessment of drug-induced cardiomyopathy. Cpt Pharmacometrics Syst Pharmacol. 2018;7 (3):166–74.
59. Geoffrey H. Deep learning-a technology with the potential to transform health care. JAMA. 2018;320(11):1101–2.
60. Lounkine E, Keiser MJ, Whitebread S, et al. Large-scale prediction and testing of drug activity on side-effect targets. Nature. 2012;486(7403):361.
61. Zitnik M, Agrawal M, Leskovec J. Modeling polypharmacy side effects with graph convolutional networks. Bioinformatics. 2018;34(13):i457–66.

Chapter 5
Case Study of Network Pharmacology and Modernization of Traditional Chinese Medicine

Shibing Su, Yuanjia Hu, and Huali Zuo

5.1 Guide to this Chapter

Pioneering work in the early stages [1, 2] on network pharmacology and integration of TCM theory and modern chemistry, systems biology, and information science has resulted in modernization of TCM. Network pharmacology has developed rapidly in the past 10 years and is on the rise. As a result several high quality academic achievements have emerged.

Network pharmacology combines system and reduction theories, macro and micro research, and in vivo and in vitro research. The basic research concepts are consistent with the TCM philosophy. Gauging by the current research, network pharmacology will undoubtedly herald new opportunities in the development of TCM [3], especially in the research of syndromes, TCM prescriptions (compatibility, efficacy), new drug discovery, national and international traditional medicine research, etc. This chapter explores relevant studies in recent years, and also summarizes and concludes results, thus helping readers to get familiar with network pharmacology. This chapter also covers major aspects of TCM modernization research and hopes to enhance readers' understanding of TCM science, based on network analysis and by reviewing specific application examples. For each achievement, this chapter analyzes the research purpose, data sources, network construction and visualization, analysis index and algorithm, experimental verification, and conclusions, to facilitate a clearer and structured understanding of the case, as well as to highlight the comparison between cases.

S. Su
Shanghai University of Traditional Chinese Medicine, Shanghai, China

Y. Hu (✉) · H. Zuo
State Key Laboratory of Quality Research in Chinese Medicine, Institute of Chinese Medical Sciences, University of Macau, Macau, China
e-mail: yuanjiahu@umac.mo

S. Li (ed.), *Network Pharmacology*, https://doi.org/10.1007/978-981-16-0753-0_5

5.2 Study of Network Pharmacology and TCM syndromes

The clinical manifestations of diseases are ever-changing and complicated. Syndrome is a certain stage in the process of disease occurrence and evolution. Based on the "Four Diagnostic Methods" of TCM, the etiology, pathogenesis, disease location, and disease progress are revealed in varying degrees, thus providing a rationale for treatment [4]. In long-term clinical practice, TCM doctors have summarized a methodology: Eight Principal Syndromes, namely, data obtained from the four diagnostic methods (observation, auscultation and olfaction, inquiry, pulse diagnosis). Based on the rise and fall of healthy qi, the nature of pathogens, and position and progress of disease, comprehensive analysis can be summarized into eight syndromes: yin, yang, external, internal, cold, heat, deficiency, and excess. Yin and yang can be used to determine the type of disease and nature of cold and heat to illustrate the nature of the disease. Disease location and progress can be reflected externally and internally. The strengths and weaknesses of vital qi and pathogens can be explained by deficiency and excess.

The core idea of TCM lies in its holistic view and treatment, based on syndrome differentiation. The main objective of TCM intervention is syndrome management, which is characterized by an integrated diagnosis and treatment of "disease-syndrome-prescription," which is a combination of disease and syndrome and the corresponding prescription. Syndrome forms the core of the diagnosis and treatment system of TCM, and is the summary of disease complexity and long-term clinical practice in TCM. Understanding the biological basis for syndrome is the key to explaining traditional concepts and efficacy of TCM, and integrating it with modern medicinal practices. Since long, the clinical practice of TCM lacked scientific and objective standards and basis. TCM research often follows the reductionism thinking approach of western medicinal research and ignores its holistic features. A prescription is often characterized by a few simple index models, due to which, it is difficult to reflect the holistic characteristics of TCM. Due to the complex characteristics of diseases and TCM, the scientific interpretation of syndrome theory, material basis of prescriptions, and the mechanism of action have become key problems restricting the modernization of TCM.

Unclear biological mechanism of syndrome hinders the understanding of efficacy of TCM prescriptions, as well as the expansion and application of TCM prescriptions in the modern medical system. At a molecular level and considering the complex biological systems, the biomolecular network is an important system in maintaining body homeostasis. However, the theory of nonspecific holistic regulation of TCM is similar to the regulation of biomolecular networks in modern medicine. Therefore, it is a new research strategy [5], in line with the holistic characteristics of TCM, which helps in carrying out syndrome research, and analyzes the association of "disease-syndrome-prescription" by using network analysis method.

In November 2002, the National Natural Science Foundation of China launched a major plan for research on TCM—"Modern Research on Several Key Scientific

Issues in Traditional Chinese Medicine." A key funding project is the "Research on Syndrome Genomics and Syndrome Proteomics," which indicates that systems biology research based on syndrome genomics and syndrome proteomics is set to enter a new phase [6]. With the development of network pharmacology supported by systems biology, complex network analysis methods can be applied in TCM research.

The development of systems biology, bioinformatics, and network pharmacology provides feasible options for the study of complex systems in TCM. A complex network is an abstract model with objective systems. It is essentially a big data set with systematic characteristics that can bridge TCM with modern science. In recent years, network analysis has been widely used in the study of TCM syndromes and some progress has been made. Li et al. [7, 8] used network pharmacology to carry out syndrome-related research. The biomolecular network of cold and hot syndromes is constructed and network analysis is conducted based on the Neuro-Endocrine-Immune (NEI) system. Research results indicate that the cold syndrome mainly manifests in the hormone function module, the hot syndrome manifests in the cytokine function module, and the neurotransmitter function module is distributed simultaneously in both cold and hot networks. Also, network topology analysis shows that there is a scale-free attribute in the biomolecular network of cold and hot syndromes, that is, the functions of the network depend on some key nodes, which are expected to become the syndrome classification markers of the biological molecular network. Wutou Decoction (WTD) has good therapeutic effects on the Rheumatoid Arthritis (RA) cold syndrome model. It is a mechanism used to regulate the thermogenesis pathway of PPAR-γ co-activator, which reflects the principle of "cold syndrome hot treatment" in TCM theory. Su et al. [9] studied HBV Causing Cirrhosis (HBC) as a research topic based on the network pharmacology and clinical transcriptome data. They found that some miRNAs are related to deficiency and excess, resulting in chronic hepatitis B, which laid the foundation for "same disease with different treatment" for HBC. By analyzing the drug target network and biomolecular network related to RA hot syndrome, Lv et al. [10] discovered common biological pathways involved in the molecular network of RA hot syndrome and TCM targets: GM-CSF signaling pathway, CTLA4 signaling pathway, T cell receptor signaling pathway, and CD28 signaling pathway in helper T cells, may be molecular biological mechanisms of "drug-syndrome correspondence" in the TCM treatment of RA hot syndrome. They may also be the molecular biological mechanisms of "drug-syndrome correspondence" treatment for RA hot syndrome. Network pharmacology has also made some progress in the study of syndrome of other diseases, such as RA deficiency syndrome [11], liver cancer deficiency syndrome [12], etc. The biomolecular network and drug target network are predictive studies based on several databases and algorithms, which provide a new channel for basic TCM syndrome research differentiation, treatment, and "drug-syndrome correspondence."

A brief summary of some related studies is shown in Table 5.1:

Network pharmacology in TCM syndrome research elaborates conventional TCM theories from a modern science perspective, by exploring syndrome

Table 5.1 Network pharmacology research on typical TCM syndromes

TCM syndrome	Corresponding TCM/prescription	Corresponding disease	Data resource	Research method	Research conclusion	Literature
Cold/Hot syndrome	Wenluo prescription/Qingluo prescription	RA	Literature	The network is constructed based on the protein interrelation of network co-occurrence literature mining and the results of network analysis are verified by experiments	Hormones play a dominant role in the cold syndrome network, while immune factors play a dominant role in the hot syndrome network. The two networks are connected by neurotransmitters. In addition, the genes related to hot syndrome are mainly involved in the cytokine–cytokine receptor interaction pathway, while genes related to cold and hot syndromes are all related to the neural active ligand–receptor interaction pathway	[7]
Cold syndrome	Wutou decoction (WTD)	RA	Chinese Medicine Chemistry Database drugCIPHER-CS	PPI network, topology analysis of "WTD Chinese medicine-target" network and "traditional Chinese medicine-target-RA pathway" network, animal pharmacology experiment, WB verification of important targets	WTD has a good therapeutic effect on cold syndrome RA model. Its possible mechanism is to regulate the thermogenesis pathway of PPAR-γ co-activator, which reflects the principle of "cold syndrome hot treatment" in TCM theory	[8]

Cold/hot syndrome		Chronic superficial gastritis/ chronic atrophic gastritis	Literature clinical data	The network is constructed based on the protein interrelation of network co-occurrence literature mining and gene chip expression profile mining, ELISA, and immunohistochemistry	In patients with cold syndrome gastritis, Leptin is used as a marker, indicating that the energy metabolism level of cold syndrome patients is low; in patients with hot syndrome gastritis, CCL2/ MCP1 is used as the marker, indicating that the immune regulation of patients with hot syndrome is intensified	[13]
Deficiency of spleen Qi	Astragalus membranaceus	–	Literature drug CIPHER CIPHER clinical GEO database	PPI network, Macrophage proliferation experiment, animal experiment	The biological molecules related to spleen Qi deficiency syndrome are closely related to immune and metabolic biological processes. Astragalus membranaceus is a TCM for tonifying qi deficiency. Its compounds promote macrophage proliferation and lymphocyte proliferation in tumor-bearing mice	[14]
Deficiency syndrome	–	RA	Clinical data	Gene chip expression profile, PPI network.	Toll-like receptor activation of NF-κ B regulatory gene transcription pathway and apoptosis and nucleotide metabolism related apoptosis pathway may be related to patients with RA deficiency syndrome, which may have a close relationship with face	[11]

(continued)

Table 5.1 (continued)

TCM syndrome	Corresponding TCM/prescription	Corresponding disease	Data resource	Research method	Research conclusion	Literature
Liver and gallbladder damp heat syndrome (LGDHS)/liver and kidney yin deficiency syndrome (LKYDS)/liver depression and spleen deficiency syndrome (LDSDS)	–	Liver cancer	Clinical data	Gene chip expression profile, "miRNA-target" network, SVM.	The miRNA expression profiles of liver and gallbladder damp heat syndrome (LGDHS), liver and kidney yin deficiency syndrome (LKYDS) and liver depression and spleen deficiency syndrome (LDSDS) are different; the miRNA expression profiles of LDSDS and LKYDS with the same deficiency syndrome are similar	[12]
Liver and gallbladder damp heat syndrome (LGDHS)/liver and kidney yin deficiency syndrome (LKYDS)/liver depression and spleen deficiency syndrome (LDSDS)	–	HBC	Clinical data	Gene chip expression profile, "miRNA-target" network	Study on the same disease with different syndromes: LDSDS is an important link in the development of chronic hepatitis B liver fibrosis. Under certain conditions, LDSDS can transform into LGDHS or LKYDS. Based on significant statistical analysis results, four important miRNAs are found in the process of LKYDS conversion to LDSDS, including hsa-miR-17-3p,	[9]

					-377-3p, -410-3p, and -495; five important miRNAs in the process of LDSDS developing into LKYDS, including hsa-miR-377-3p, -410-3p, -149-5p, 27a-3p, and -940	
Damp heat stasis syndrome (DHAS)/liver depression and spleen deficiency syndrome (LDSDS)	–	HBC	Clinical data	Gene chip expression profile	Study on the same disease with different syndromes: the transcription profile, gene co-expression characteristics and functional characteristics of samples from patients with chronic hepatitis B liver fibrosis damp heat accumulation syndrome (DHAS) and liver depression and spleen deficiency syndrome (LDSDS) are different; PNP, AQP7, PSMD2 are significantly different, and can provide a reference for the clinical differentiation of DHAS and LDSDS	[15]
Blood stasis syndrome	–	Acute Ischemic Stroke Angina pectoris	Clinical data	Gene chip expression profile	Mir-146b-5p, -199a-5p and their related 23 mRNA can be used as diagnostic markers of blood stasis syndrome	[16]

(continued)

Table 5.1 (continued)

TCM syndrome	Corresponding TCM/prescription	Corresponding disease	Data resource	Research method	Research conclusion	Literature
Blood stasis syndrome	–	Angina pectoris	Clinical data	Gene chip expression profile	The up-regulation of miR-146b-5p may lead to the down-regulation of CALR and decrease in inflammatory reaction. The up-regulation of miR-199a-5p may lead to the down-regulation of TP53, thus inhibiting cell apoptosis	[17]

differences at the molecular level. It is possible to clarify the scientific rationale for TCM Syndrome Differentiation Treatment at multiple levels by establishing characteristic gene expression profiles or functional gene regulatory networks of different syndromes, and combining the identification of differential proteomics and key functional proteins of different syndrome types with traditional TCM theories. Also, it is possible to find the specific gene and functional protein markers corresponding to the syndrome, to further provide the scientific basis for the clinical syndrome differentiation in TCM and the establishment of the TCM "prescription-syndrome correspondence" model.

The following two specific research cases were selected for analysis.

5.2.1 Case Analysis of Network Pharmacology Research on Cold and Hot Syndromes and Corresponding Prescriptions

In clinical practice using TCM, treatment of the same disease requires the use of different TCM prescriptions based on different syndromes. For example, for the cold syndrome, hot-type Chinese medicine is used for treatment, while for the hot-type syndrome, cold-type Chinese medicine is used for treatment, namely as described in TCM theories: cold syndrome hot treatment, hot syndrome cold treatment. The differentiation of cold and hot syndromes mainly reflects the different nature of the disease. Although long-term clinical experience with TCM can help to accurately distinguish between the two syndromes, however, this experience-based method is difficult to be understood by modern science.

Currently, there are a lot of studies on cold and hot syndromes, and these studies are still growing. Most of these research results are isolated results, for example, functions of a single gene or a few interactions. Literature mining technology combined with network analysis can discover the potential holistic and common characteristics hidden in isolated studies. Based on the above research foundation, Li et al. [7] studied the molecular characteristics of cold and hot syndromes based on the background of the Neuro-Endocrine-Immune (NEI) system by using co-occurrence literature mining method and network analysis method.

5.2.1.1 Research Objective

Cold and hot syndromes are two common clinical syndromes. From the perspective of Western medicine, most diseases such as inflammation, infection, stress, and autoimmune diseases are related to interactions between NEI systems. The NEI system plays an important role in the occurrence and development of various diseases, and its abnormality is an important cause of related diseases. Therefore, the NEI system can provide a breakthrough in modern medicine to explore the syndrome mechanism and to communicate the concept of TCM and modern medicine.

Previous studies have shown that the NEI system of patients with cold and hot syndromes exhibits abnormal functions. In the TCM diagnosis and treatment process, most RA patients can be divided into cold and hot syndrome types, and correspondingly, hot or cold Chinese medicine is used for treatment. Therefore, the purpose of this study is to explore the molecular characteristics of cold and hot syndromes using the NEI system based on network analysis, to provide reference for modern research of cold and hot syndromes.

5.2.1.2 Data Source

Chemical Messengers (CMs) such as hormones, cytokines, and neurotransmitters in the NEI system act as hubs for host regulation during their complex interaction processes, thereby maintaining the stability of the NEI system and health of the organism. If CMs are regarded as a component of the NEI system, the genes that encode CMs (directly or indirectly) can be considered as related genes. These genes and CMs are the basis of network construction in this study. The data acquisition and processing methods are as follows:

(1) The synonyms of NEI determined by searching Medical Subject Headings (MeSH), and the relevant abstracts retrieved and downloaded from the PubMed database were used as the literature summary pool of the NEI PubMed; NEI-related genes in the HUGO database were retrieved, to obtain the interrelationship between genes. In addition, the CMs related to the NEI system were manually collected from English literature (published from September 30, 2000 to September 30, 2005), with keywords including "hormone", "cytokine", and "neuro-transmitter"; as well by using the keyword "disease" to search relevant CMs in the literature abstract pool of NEI PubMed. Comprehensive database HUGO and NEI-related genes and CMs in literature were also searched.
(2) Related literature on cold and hot syndromes was searched in the abstract pool of NEI PubMed based on keywords of cold and hot syndromes, and the literature pools for cold and hot syndromes were established.
(3) Syndrome-related disease data sets and syndrome-related NEI pathways were obtained using the TCM online database (containing more than 4,000 kinds of disease information) established by the China Academy of Chinese Medical Sciences. This research selection was usually diagnosed as a typical disease with cold or hot syndromes. Genes related to cold and hot syndrome-related diseases were obtained from the OMIM database; these genes were enriched through DAVID and the NEI-related KEGG pathway information was screened (In the DAVID gene annotation system, Fisher's test is used to measure whether the proportion of genes in a specific pathway in the enrichment result is significantly higher than the background genes of the human genome).

5.2.1.3 Network Construction and Visualization

The NEI-related gene/CMs network was constructed based on the literature co-occurrence mining method. The nodes are biomolecules (genes or CMs) and the edges are the connections based on the literature co-occurrence relationships. If two biomolecules appear in the same literature at the same time, then they are related. Graphviz software was used for network visualization.

5.2.1.4 Analysis Index and Algorithm

The network constructed using the above method was analyzed. The topological structure feature of node i in the network is represented by the topological vector in formula (5.1):

$$v_{i(W)} = [c_{i1}, c_{i2}, \ldots, c_{in}]^{\mathrm{T}} \tag{5.1}$$

In formula (5.1), n represents the sum of the special nodes of the cold and hot syndromes; $W = \{C, H\}$ represents the network of the cold and hot syndromes, c_{ij} is the indicator variable between node i and node j (if $c_{ij} = 1, \quad i \neq j$, it means there is a connection between i and j, and $c_{ij} = 0, \quad i \neq j$ means there is no connection between i and j).

The topological distance between the cold and hot syndromes is defined as follows:

$$d_i = \left(v_{i(H)} - v_{i(C)}\right)^T \cdot e \tag{5.2}$$

In formula (5.2), v_i is the topological vector of node i, and e is the unit vector. The topological distance is standardized by the following formula, so that its value range is $[-1, 1]$.

$$\overline{d_i} = \frac{d_i}{\left(v_{i(\mathrm{H})} + v_{i(\mathrm{C})}\right)^{\mathrm{T}} \cdot e} = \frac{\left(v_{i(\mathrm{H})} - v_{i(\mathrm{C})}\right)^{\mathrm{T}} \cdot e}{\left(v_{i(\mathrm{H})} + v_{i(\mathrm{C})}\right)^{\mathrm{T}} \cdot e} \tag{5.3}$$

In formula (5.3), if $\overline{d_i} > 0$, node i is classified as a hot syndrome node; if $\overline{d_i} < 0$, then node i is classified as a cold syndrome node. Then, the proportion of cold and hot syndrome nodes observed under each NEI category was analyzed by using cumulative binomial distribution:

$$P(c \leq c_0) = \sum_{c=0}^{c_0} \binom{N}{c} \left(\frac{1}{2}\right)^N \tag{5.4}$$

In formula (5.4), N is the number of nodes in the cold and hot syndromes, excluding nodes with $\overline{d_i} = 0$, c_0 is the smaller of the node number of the cold and hot syndromes.

5.2.1.5 Experimental Verification

RA was selected as the disease model as it has been widely studied in Chinese and Western medicine and exhibits typical cold and hot syndromes. Experiments were carried out on CIA rat models (most widely used RA model) to study the therapeutic effects of Wenluo decoction (HCHF is composed of aconite, Atractylodes macrocephala, cassia twig, and Selaginella) and Qingluo decoction (CWHF is composed of radix sophorae flavescentis, cortex phellodendri, caulis sinomenii, and rhizoma dioscoreae) on the central nodes of the NEI network.

Therapeutic effects of CWHF and HCHF were explored on prescriptions for syndrome, by observing the effects of CWHF and HCHF (two prescriptions that have proven to be effective for RA) on the central node of the NEI network for cold and hot syndromes, respectively. The experiment involved rats that were randomly divided into four groups: normal group, CIA model group, HCHF treatment group, and CWHF treatment group. Radioimmunoassay was used to determine the concentration levels of important CMs in both the cold and hot syndrome networks in the four groups of mice, every 6 h from 0:00 (midnight) to 24:00. Unilateral analysis of variance was used to analyze the differences between CIA rat and normal rat, and CIA rat and the two other groups of treatment rats. Bonferroni post-hoc test was carried out later, where $p < 0.05$ was regarded as significant difference.

5.2.1.6 Conclusion

(1) Analysis of the network topology structure shows that the biological molecular network of cold and hot syndromes has scale-free properties, that is, the functional realization of the network is mainly dependent on some central nodes, thought to be the syndrome classification markers of the biomolecular network.
(2) Compared to the cold syndrome, hot syndrome-related biomolecules exhibit significant cytokine–cytokine receptor interaction in the pathway. Overall, the cold syndrome is characterized by the hormone function module, hot syndrome is characterized by the cytokine function module, and neurotransmitter function module is distributed in both cold and hot networks at the same time.

5.2.2 *Case Study and Analysis of "Same Disease with Varying Syndromes" in Hepatic Fibrosis Caused by Chronic Hepatitis B*

HBC is a common stage in chronic hepatitis B development before progressing into liver cirrhosis or even liver cancer, and an important link that seriously affects the prognosis of chronic hepatitis B disease. The 5-year survival rate of patients with severe HBC is only 50%, and Hepatocellular Carcinoma (HCC) occurs in almost all HBC patients. In the past few decades, there has been a lack of clinically effective methods for the treatment of HBC in Western medicine. TCM has shown adequate therapeutic benefits in the treatment of HBC. In the preliminary study of this research group, it was found that PNP (Purine Nucleoside Phosphorylase), AQP7 (Aquaporin-7), and PSMD2 (26S Proteasome non-ATPase Regulatory Subunit 2) correlated with HBC's TCM syndrome differentiation. However, the characteristics of TCM syndrome development in HBC are not clear, especially from liver and gallbladder damp heat syndrome (LGDHS) progression to liver depression and spleen deficiency syndrome (LDSDS), and LDSDS progression into liver kidney yin deficiency syndrome (LKYDS).

miRNA is associated with several liver diseases, including liver metabolism, fibrosis, regeneration, and HCC. miRNA has excellent stability in serum or plasma, making it valuable in clinical research. For example, it can be used as a biomarker to distinguish chronic hepatitis B, liver cirrhosis, and HCC. This section introduces the related network analysis research carried out by Su et al. [9] based on different syndromes of HBC.

5.2.2.1 Research Objective

In the clinical diagnosis and treatment of HBC, syndromes are helpful to understand the homeostasis of the human body and guide individualized treatment. However, the scientific rationale for syndrome classification of chronic hepatitis B and the mechanism of "treating the same disease with different methods" are still unclear. This study analyzes the expression levels of miRNA transcription profiles of different syndrome samples during the development of chronic hepatitis B, and then explores the biological basis of TCM syndrome differentiation in chronic hepatitis B-induced hepatic fibrosis, and consequent progression to chronic hepatitis B syndrome.

5.2.2.2 Data Source

One hundred and sixty-two clinical serum samples were collected from a hospital, including LGDHS ($n = 36$), LDSDS ($n = 62$), LKYDS ($n = 34$), and normal controls ($n = 30$). The diagnostic criteria of HBC in Western medicine follow the guiding principles formulated by the Chinese Association of Hepatology and Chinese Society of Infectious Diseases in 2005. To study miRNA profiles, miRNA microarray analysis was performed on nine HBC serum samples (LGDHS, $n = 3$; LDSDS, $n = 3$; LKYDS, $n = 3$) and 7 healthy samples. Further, human miRNA microarray V3 was used for differential expression analysis.

miRNA targets were predicted using TarBase (v7.0), miRecords, and miRTarBase databases. In addition, miRanda, miRDB, miRWalk, and RNAhybrid programs were used to predict non-experimental targets. The gene ontology, pathway, and disease information of target-related genes were obtained by David online enrichment analysis.

5.2.2.3 Network Construction and Visualization

The relationship between differentially expressed miRNAs and their predicted targets was used to construct a "miRNA target" network. miRNAs were then weighted by difference multiple (|log2|), and target genes were weighted based on degree distribution. Then, all nodes were sorted based on the weight. Similarity was tested and the nodes obtained were used to reconstruct the network. In the new network, nodes represented miRNAs or targets, and edges represented connection strength.

5.2.2.4 Analysis Index and Algorithm

Network Analysis

The common network was knocked out from the original network (common network refers to the same part of the "miRNA-target" network of LGDHS, LDSDS, and LKYDS), and the stability of the network with robustness was evaluated, as shown in the following formula (5.5):

$$R = \frac{C}{(N - N_\tau)} \quad (5.5)$$

In formula (5.5), C is the maximum connectivity after network knockout, N is the number of original network nodes, and $N\tau$ is the number of knockout nodes. In addition, continuous parameters of the network such as betweenness centrality (BC), compactness centrality (CC), and degree centrality (DC) were discussed. During network analysis, the core nodes in the network were defined as the nodes of $\mathrm{BC} \geq \overline{\mathrm{BC}}$, $\mathrm{CC} \geq \overline{\mathrm{CC}}$, and $\mathrm{DC} \geq \overline{\mathrm{DC}}$. The core node miRNAs are important miRNAs and play an important role in different HBC syndromes.

Analysis of Clinical Experimental Data

RT-qPCR was used to detect co-expression miRNAs and important miRNAs in 162 serum samples. The stepwise logistic regression model was used to screen for the diagnosis of the miRNA group (which is considered as a potential marker in the development of HBC syndrome).

5.2.2.5 Main Conclusion

(1) The "miRNA-target" network (referred to as "original network") of LGDHS, LDSDS, and LKYDS of different syndromes of HBC is shown in Fig. 5.1a–c [9]. The common network of the three syndromes is shown in Fig. 5.1d. The original network in the three syndromes replaced by the common network is shown in Fig. 5.1f, g. The three syndromes (network centralization (NC), characteristic path length (CPL), and network heterogeneity (NH)) were compared before and after the original network replaced the common network. Results show that in LGDHS and LKYDS networks, the change rate of NC is 30.57% and 38.52%, CPL is 3.79% and 4.58%, NH is 8.26% and 8.30%, respectively. Relevant parameters of LDSDS network are only 1.50%, 0.17%, and 0.26%, as shown in Fig. 5.1h. In addition, robustness calculation results show that LDSDS network ($R = 0.87$) is more stable than LGDHS ($R = 0.68$) and LKYDS network ($R = 0.64$), as shown in Fig. 5.1i. The results show that the co-expression of miRNA in the three syndromes may be closely related to LGDHS and LKYDS, in the development of HBC syndromes.

(2) The signal pathway that regulates the pluripotency of stem cells and the Transforming Growth Factor-β (TGF-β) signal pathway is closely related to the development of HBC syndromes (LGDHS, LDSDS, and LKYDS). Previous studies have shown that as a central regulator, TGF-β is involved in the progression of many diseases of chronic liver disease, from initial liver injury to inflammation/fibrosis, to liver cirrhosis or hepatocellular carcinoma. Overexpression of TGF-β is also associated with tumor development, metastasis, angiogenesis, and poor prognosis, suggesting that these pathways are important for understanding the mechanisms of HBC syndrome development.

(3) In HBC syndrome, six co-expressed miRNAs including LGDHS, LDSDS, and LKYDS may have a greater relationship with the HBC syndrome development.

(4) LDSDS is an important link in the development of chronic hepatitis B liver fibrosis. LDSDS can be mutually converted to LGDHS or LKYDS under certain conditions. Based on significant statistical analysis results, four important miRNAs are found in the process of LKYDS developing into LDSDS, including: hsa-miR-17-3p, -377-3p, -410-3p, and -495; and five important miRNAs are found in the process of LDSDS developing into LKYDS, including hsa-miR-377-3p, - 410-3p, -149-5p, 27a-3p, and -940.

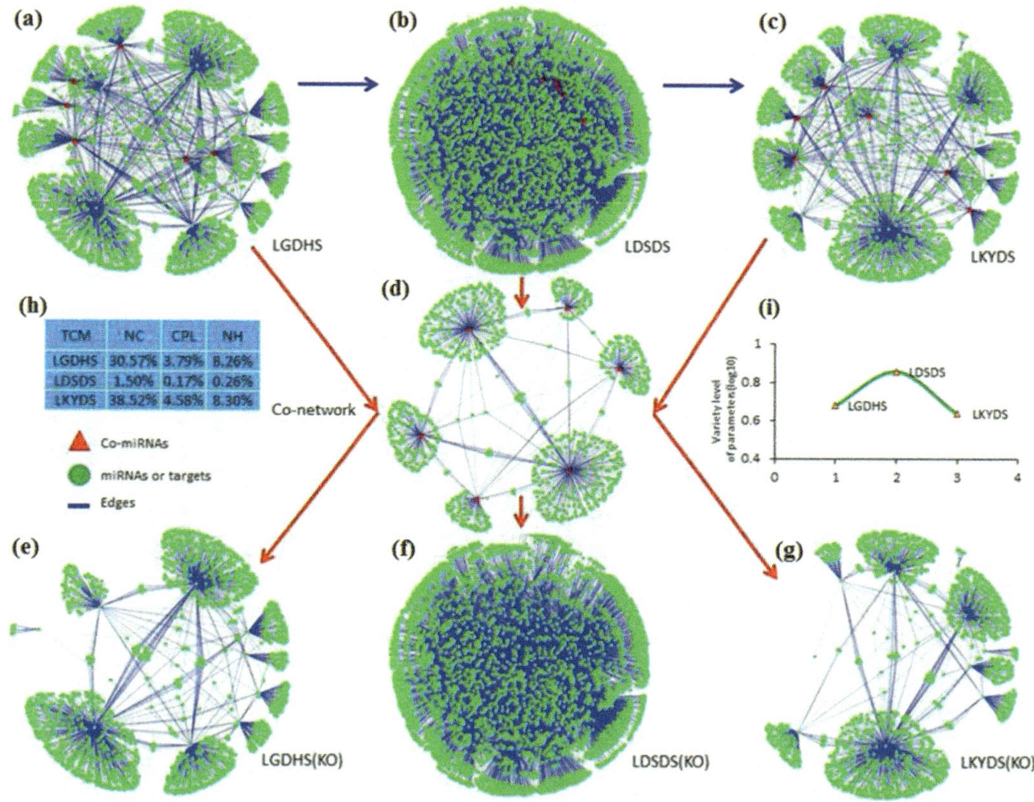

TCM	NC	CPL	NH
LGDHS	30.57%	3.79%	8.26%
LDSDS	1.50%	0.17%	0.26%
LKYDS	38.52%	4.58%	8.30%

Fig. 5.1 "miRNA-target" Network of Chronic Hepatitis Syndromes [9]. (**a**) LGDHS global network; (**b**) LDSDS global network; (**c**) LKYDS global network; (**d**) common network; (**e**) LGDHS network after common network knockout; (**f**) LDSDS network after common network knockout; (**g**) LKYDS network after common network knockout; (**h**) change rate of network parameters before and after knockout; (**i**) robustness of network

5.3 Case Study of Network Pharmacology and TCM Prescriptions

TCM prescriptions are used to prevent and treat diseases. They are based on conventional theories (for example: TCM medicinal properties, prescription compatibility, etc.) of TCM, and composed of various kinds of Chinese herbs with specific therapeutic effects. TCM prescriptions have definite curative effects and less side effects in the treatment of complex diseases. However, compared to Western medicine, TCM prescriptions contain various ingredients and interactions. There also exists a problem of unclear drug targets and mechanisms. Therefore, clarifying the scientific basis of compatibility in TCM prescriptions is a key issue in the modernization of TCM. TCM prescriptions are characterized by personalized treatment and overall regulation of patients' organ functions, analysis of interactions between networks by medicinal substances in the prescriptions, and the biological molecules in the organism while exploring the comprehensive effects and holistic regulation mechanisms of the respective prescriptions. Designing new principles for formulating drugs from network regulation perspective is a key issue and difficulty in this field. Clarifying the mechanism of action of TCM under the background of modern science remains a huge challenge.

In recent years and with the rise of multi-target drug discovery concepts, network pharmacology has gradually become a popular research model that may have a profound impact on contemporary TCM research. The quantity, proportion of the constituent substances in the prescriptions, and their relationship with patients' organs are highly complex. It is imperative to understand this complex relationship from a network perspective. Network ideas and analysis are being applied to the study of TCM prescriptions, to understand the compatibility of Chinese medicines using multi-target synergy and to study the action mechanisms of TCM prescriptions at the molecular level. Several research breakthroughs have been made in this process.

The compatibility principles of TCM, such as "Traditional Chinese Medicine Formulation", "Qiqing Hehe" etc., reflect regulating patient health holistically, which is consistent with the research ideology of systems biology and network pharmacology. Prescriptions provide fodder for the study of the relevant theories in Chinese medicine for network analysis. Based on TCM research, Li first proposed the concepts of "network target" and "TCM Network Pharmacology," and studied the molecular mechanism of compound action based on this concept [18, 19]. "Network target" considers the core link of "disease-syndrome" biological molecular network as the main target. Medicinal substances and the mechanism of action of TCM prescriptions are found by measuring the relationship between the target spectrum of prescription ingredients and the key links of the disease-syndrome molecular network. This paper explores the network characteristics of "Traditional Chinese Medicine Formulation" by analyzing the distribution of targets contained in prescriptions, on the network. Furthermore, this network feature is used to predict clinical biomarkers of prescription drugs, and this knowledge is used to rationally formulate prescription drugs. At present, network targets are being explored in TCM prescriptions. For example, Li et al. [20] analyzed the compatibility of TCM prescriptions by analyzing the joint module of "TCM network-target network-disease network." In this study, a DMIM model (Distance-based Mutual Information Model) of TCM was established. The model combined the average amount of interactive information and the spacing between TCM formulation in the TCM prescription to identify TCM combinations with similar efficacy across other prescriptions. DMIM method was used to analyze the TCM network of 3865 traditional prescriptions, drug pair compatibility, and its therapeutic characteristics. At the same time, new drug pairs with synergistic or incompatible effects were also found [20]. Furthermore, considering Liuwei Dihuang Decoction (LWDH) as an example, a novel "Co-module" was proposed, that is, the compatibility mechanism of TCM prescriptions was explored using multi-layer network joint module analysis of "TCM-target-disease." In the disease phenotype analysis of LWDH prescription and LWDH treatment, it was found that diseases treated by LWDH have statistically significant similar phenotypes, and these co-modules were enriched in multiple pathways such as metabolism and immunity, thus providing a new explanation on the traditional efficacy of LWDH for nourishing yin and the clinical mechanism of "homotherapy for heteropathy." [21]

Bai et al analyzed the main chemical components of Qingfei Xiaoyan Pill by UPLC-MS, then simulated and predicted its acting target based on the database, and then observed its effect on the expression of pneumonia-related genes through animal model and cell model experiments [22]. Research results showed that some representative components of Qingfei Xiaoyan Pill have anti-inflammatory effects by participating in Fc epsilon RI signaling pathway, toll-like receptor signaling pathway, NK cell (natural killer cell) mediated cytotoxicity, and ERK/MAPK signaling pathway. Hu et al. explored the possibility of establishing the chemical composition inter-relationship based on the prescription compatibility frequency. A chemical composition network of prescription was constructed for coronary heart disease, to provide a basis for further optimizing the complex network of "component-target-effect." [23] At the same time, the network mode conversion was applied to transform the two-mode network into the one-mode network, and then the deep connotation of TCM-related data was mined through the new network. For example, take Xuefu Zhuyu Decoction (XZD) and Gualou Xiebai Banxia Decoction (GXBD), which are commonly used clinical prescriptions for coronary heart disease "treating the same disease with different methods," as examples. Constructing a model network with the target as the network node component, and using the approved drug target for the treatment of coronary heart disease as a reference, it is more likely to result in the discovery of a common target in the two prescriptions [24]. Using Yu ping feng San (YPF) as an example, a target network was constructed with targets as nodes and the common pathway relationship between targets as edges. After dividing the network modules, a scoring algorithm was established to evaluate the strength of the relationship between each module and the disease, to find out the target modules that are closely related to the immune-related effects of Yu ping feng San [25].

In recent years, some concepts similar to network pharmacology have been proposed, such as network toxicology [26], network formulaology [27], integrated pharmacology [28], and modular pharmacology [29], all of which are characterized by adopting the idea and method of network analysis. These are combined with other methods, to carry out grid and systematic integrated research, and to study the biological effects and efficacy mechanism of TCM prescriptions. The application of network pharmacology in the relevant research of TCM prescriptions can effectively combine macro-integration and micro-mechanisms, to help reveal the scientific connotation of prescriptions, provide a scientific basis for the clinical rational use of Chinese medicines, and to conduct the research and development of innovative Chinese medicines. It is also beneficial to enrich TCM prescription research, promote solutions to key scientific problems of prescriptions, and cultivate ideas of modern drug research and development.

A brief summary of some relevant studies is shown in Table 5.2:

There are abundant studies on network pharmacology in the field of TCM prescription that explore active ingredients, potential drug targets, mechanism of action, and compatibility of the prescriptions, which effectively combine macro-integration and micro-mechanisms. This paper attempts to use the network analysis method to explain the complex system of TCM and its modernization, which will ultimately help to reveal the scientific basis of prescriptions, clinical application, and the creation of new Chinese medicines. It is also conducive to enriching the research on TCM prescriptions, thereby promoting solutions to key scientific problems while using these prescriptions, and thus expanding modern drug research and development.

The following two specific research cases are selected for analysis.

5.3.1 Research and Analysis of DMIM: An Interactive Information Model Based on the Spacing of TCM Compound Prescriptions

The long-term clinical practice of TCM has proved that there are potential interactions, both beneficial and detrimental, between TCM and their components. In the conventional application of TCM prescriptions, different TCM prescriptions play different roles in terms of compatibility: principle drug, assistant drug, adjuvant drug, and envoy drug. Understanding the compatibility mechanism of TCM is not only conducive to the modernization of TCM, but also contributes to the development of modern drugs.

Based on long-term application of TCM, it has been found that some Chinese medicine have been clearly effective in inhibiting angiogenesis. This pathological angiogenesis is closely related to various diseases, especially cancer and rheumatoid arthritis. More than 60% of cancer chemotherapeutic agents are natural products or small molecules based on natural products. Many pro-angiogenic and anti-

Table 5.2 Application of typical network pharmacology in the study of TCM prescriptions

TCM prescription	Corresponding disease	Data resource	Research method	Research conclusion	Literature
3865 prescription, Liuwei Dihuang	–	SIRC-TCM traditional chinese medicine information system established by Shanghai traditional Chinese medicine data center	DMIM	DMIM is an effective method to explore the compatibility of traditional Chinese medicine. Using LWDH prescription as an example, through a multi-layer network co-module of "TCM—target—disease," and the disease phenotype analysis of LWDH treatment; diseases treated by LWDH have statistically significant phenotypes that are similar. These co-modules are enriched in multiple pathways such as metabolism and immunity, thus providing a new interpretation of the traditional efficacy of LWDH and its effects on Yin and the clinical mechanism of "homotherapy for heteropathy."	[20]
Qingluo Yin (QLY)	RA	Database drugCIPHER	DMIM; Principal ingredient analysis, "compound-target" network analysis, enrichment analysis, etc.	QLY anti-RA target network and related mechanisms, including angiogenesis, inflammatory response, and immune response. Activities, synergetic composition, and compatibility of QLY are predicted. Principle drug radix	[30]

				sophorae flavescentis plays a major role in the treatment of RA (mainly reflected in the inflammatory reaction, immune response, and angiogenesis). Caulis sinomenii is conducive to enhancing the anti-inflammatory and anti-angiogenesis effects of the principal medicine. Adjuvant drug cortex phellodendri and rhizoma dioscoreae mainly regulate the therapeutic effect of principal and synergistic drugs, and to a certain extent inhibit the side effects caused by the off-target effect of radix sophorae flavescentis	
Liuwei Dihuang (LWDH)	–	Database drug CIPHER	LWDH target prediction is conducted through drugCIPHER, network analysis based on "drug-target-pathway-disease" and protein–protein interaction (PPI) network, and experimental verification of analysis results	Network analysis results show that LWDH acts mainly on the endocrine and immune systems and related pathways. For example, PPAR signaling pathway is used to treat osteoporosis, arthritis, and other diseases related to yin deficiency. It can also treat other types of diseases such as esophageal cancer and colon cancer. This study not only explains the molecular mechanism of traditional medicinal	[21]

(continued)

Table 5.2 (continued)

TCM prescription	Corresponding disease	Data resource	Research method	Research conclusion	Literature
				functions of LWDH, but also provides insights into new usage of old drugs	
Guizhi Shaoyao Zhimus decoction (GSZD)	RA	Database	Analysis of “TCM-pathway/pharmacological effect” network, “drug-target” network, and “central target-pathway” network; Experimental verification	GSZD can alleviate RA symptoms by reversing inflammatory-immune system imbalance and regulating the HDAC1-HSP90AA1-NFKB2-IKBKB-TNF-α signaling axis	[31]
Compound danshen dripping pills (CDF)	CVD	Database Molecular simulation	“Compound-target” network, “compound-pathway” network, “target-disease” network analysis	Based on the chemical composition, there are 101 active compounds in CDF, 56 of which are from principle drug Salvia miltiorrhiza, 29 active molecules in assistant drug pseudo-ginseng, and only 9 active molecules in adjuvant drug borneol. CDF inhibits inflammation and prevents inflammatory factors from damaging blood vessels and myocardium through the targets eNOS, CYP2C9, HSP90s, PPARα/γ, and MIF. CDF can also regulate ACE, chymase, VDR, VEGFR2, and other targets, and plays a certain therapeutic role on	[32]

				cardiovascular diseases; Network analysis of compounds and pathways suggests: CDF may treat cardiovascular disease by participating in glucocorticoids and inflammatory signaling and L-arginine/NO signaling pathways. The results of target-disease network analysis suggest a diversity of CDF applications	
Eight prescriptions for the treatment of coronary heart disease	Coronary heart disease (CHD)	Database	Chemical composition network analysis based on compatibility relationship of TCM	In this study, a method of chemical composition and its cluster division based on compatibility frequency of TCM was established. 1588 chemical components were obtained from 36 herbs of 8 main prescriptions, for treating CHD. Ingredients were used as nodes to build a chemical composition network based on the compatibility of prescriptions. Through network analysis, it was found that there are 9 clusters that are significantly related to 14 chemical structures, and they are closely related. The important components, component groups, and TCM determined by network analysis are worthy of further	[23]

(continued)

Table 5.2 (continued)

TCM prescription	Corresponding disease	Data resource	Research method	Research conclusion	Literature
				pharmacological research. For example, 3α-O-acetyl paclitaxel in frankincense	
Xuefu Zhuyu Decoction (XZD), Gualou Xiebai Banxia Decoction (GXBD)	CHD	Database	Construction and analysis of "compound-compound" network based on common target relationship	XZD and GXBD, as the TCM prescriptions for the "same disease with different treatment" of CHD, are quite different from each other in terms of chemical composition level but have high similarities in terms of target level. Using the approved drug targets for coronary heart disease as a reference and statistical analysis, results indicate that the common target of the two prescriptions is more likely to be a drug target, including: NOS3, PTPN1, GABRA1, etc.	[24]
YupingfengSan (YPF)	Autoimmune diseases	Database	Functional tendentiousness analysis of "target-target" network construction and its cluster based on common pathway relationship	By constructing the "target-target" network with common pathway relationship and dividing into network clusters, the statistical analysis shows that each target cluster has a certain functional tendentiousness. Using YPF (treatment of immune-related diseases) as a reference point, targets with	[25]

				high network centrality among clusters that contribute the most to immune-related diseases are screened out as potential therapeutic targets for YPF, including: PRKCA, MAPK3, PRKACA, etc.	

angiogenic plant components may be used to treat angiogenesis disorders and are well tolerated. In particular, the "activating collaterals" in TCM have been found to be effective for angiogenesis disorders [33]. Based on these studies, Li et al. [20] applied complex networks combined with mutual information-based DMIM methods to screen effective TCM combinations for the angiogenesis activity. The following is the detailed introduction of relevant studies.

5.3.1.1 Research Objective

TCM prescription is an empirical system of multi-component therapy. Complex Chinese medicine can be used in combination under certain compatibility rules to meet the needs of the treatment of complex diseases. To explore the relationship between TCM prescriptions and complex diseases, it is important to establish a method to bridge the conventional understanding of TCM and modern science. In this study, the research team established a DMIM model to extract the compatibility relationship among different traditional Chinese medicines from a large repository of TCM prescriptions. Taking the classic prescription Liuwei Dihuang (LWDH) as an example, a network analysis was conducted, followed by in vitro experiments, to evaluate the pharmacological and synergistic effects of LWDH prescription, which is closely related to the compatibility network on angiogenesis. Furthermore, a new concept of "co-module" was proposed, and network analysis was carried out to explore the potential synergistic mechanism of networked TCM prescriptions.

5.3.1.2 Data Source

DMIM Analysis-Related Data

The SIRC-TCM Chinese medicine information system established by Shanghai TCM Data Center was searched using "collateral" (Luo) as the keyword. A total of 3865 TCM prescriptions with names, functions, and "meridian tropism" information were collected. All polysemous words, synonyms, and acronyms of Chinese medicines were replaced in the data set by using a standardized list of Chinese medicine names. After the names of Chinese medicines were standardized, 3,865 prescriptions containing a total of 737 Chinese medicines were sorted.

Related LWDH Data

The target sources affected by several Chinese medicines for LWDH were obtained from PubMed and CNKI, and then the PPI network of these targets was obtained through the HPRD database. There were a total of 146 LWDH-related targets, 127 of which have interaction relationships.

5.3.1.3 Network Construction and Visualization

1. The DMIM algorithm was used to calculate the Chinese drug pairs with "close spacing" (closely related), and the network was built according to the connections between these pairs.
2. Multi-layer Network of "Chinese medicine-target-disease" taking LWDH as an example.

To further explore the mechanism of prescription combination predicted by DMIM, the concept of "joint module" was proposed. Based on the fact that the prescription combinations may have consistent or common biological patterns, they can be used as "joint modules," and can be used as the basis for interpreting TCM and treating diseases at the same time. After DMIM analysis, six Chinese medicines (Cornus officinalis, Alisma orientalis, Cortex Moutan, Rehmannia glutinosa, Poria cocos, and yam) for LWDH were found to be closely related, thus LWDH was selected for joint module analysis.

Chinese medicine joint module: If two Chinese medicines have a common acting target, there is a connection between the two medicines, forming a "joint module"; Disease module: Indicates common related genes between the two diseases; Chinese medicine-related targets and disease genes were revealed through the PPI network. The "Traditional Chinese Medicine-Target-Disease" multi-layer network was visualized based on the inter-relationship between TCM, target, and disease.

5.3.1.4 Analysis Index and Algorithm

1) Mathematical Expression of TCM Prescriptions

Firstly, the prescription was expressed in matrix. Suppose there are n kinds of traditional Chinese medicine and m kinds of prescription, which can be expressed in matrix form. $A = (a_{ij})_{m \times n}$ represents the entire matrix. The serial number of TCM is from $1 \sim n$, the serial number of the prescription is from $1 \sim m$, i stands for a specific prescription, j stands for a specific TCM, a_{ij} stands for the ordinal position of TCM j in prescription i, $a_{ij} = 0$ means that TCM j is not included in prescription i. In order to eliminate the influence of the amount of TCM in the prescription, set matrix $B = (b_{ij})$, $b_{ij} = \frac{a_{ij}}{\max\limits_{1 \le k \le n} a_{ik}}$, k represents the amount of TCM in the prescription. Here b_{ij} represents the relative spacing of Chinese medicine j in prescription i. In actual research, these data form a 3865×737 matrix.

The following examples are provided for ease of understanding. As shown in Table 5.3, the matrix contains ten Chinese medicines: Chinese medicine$_1$, Chinese medicine$_2$...Chinese medicine$_{10}$ ($j = 1, 2..., 10$), three kinds of prescriptions: prescription$_1$, prescription$_2$, and prescription$_3$ ($i = 1, 2, 3$). Their compatibility is in the following Chinese medicine order: prescription$_1$ (TCM$_4$, TCM$_2$, TCM$_9$, and TCM$_6$; $k = 4$); prescription$_2$: (TCM$_4$, TCM$_8$, TCM$_1$, TCM$_{10}$, TCM$_2$, TCM$_5$, TCM$_3$,

Table 5.3 Examples of mathematical expression of TCM prescriptions

b_{ij}	TCM_1	TCM_2	TCM_3	TCM_4	TCM_5	TCM_6	TCM_7	TCM_8	TCM_9	TCM_{10}
$Prescription_1$	0	0.5	0	0.25	0	1	0	0	0.75	0
$Prescription_2$	0.375	0.625	0.875	0.125	0.75	0	1	0.25	0	0.5
$Prescription_3$	0.5	0	0	0	0	1	0	0	0	0

and TCM_7; $k = 8$); $prescription_3$: (TCM_1 and TCM_6; $k = 2$). In $prescription_1$, TCM_4 ranks as 1, $a_{14} = 1$, there are 4 TCMs in total, so $b_{14} = 0.25$, i.e., the spacing of TCM_4 in $prescription_1$ is 0.25. Similarly, the spacing of TCM in prescriptions 1, 2, and 3 were calculated.

For the given two kinds of TCM *x* and *y*, it is inferred that the trend of forming drug pair of *x* and *y* depends on two factors: mutual information entropy characteristics and the average spacing between TCM.

Mutual Information Entropy

The mutual information entropy of TCM *x* and *y* is calculated as follows:

$$MI(x,y) = P(x,y) \cdot \log\left(\frac{P(x,y)}{P(x) \cdot P(y)}\right) \tag{5.6}$$

In formula (5.6), $P(x,y) = \frac{\sum_{i=1}^{m} I(x,y,i)}{m}$ represents the occurrence frequency of TCM *x* and *y*, the function $I(x,y,i) = 1$ means that *x* and *y* appear in prescription *i* at the same time, otherwise it means that *x* and *y* do not appear at the same time. $P(x) = \frac{\sum_{i=1}^{m} I(x,i)}{m}$ represents the occurrence frequency of TCM*x*; similarly, $P(y) = \frac{\sum_{i=1}^{m} I(y,i)}{m}$ represents the occurrence frequency of TCMy. The higher the value of $MI(x,y)$, the closer the connection between TCM*x* and TCM*y*.

Spacing of Chinese Medicine Between Prescriptions

According to the TCM formulation compatibility law, in the TCM prescriptions composed of multiple herbs, the lower the order of Chinese medicine, the less importance it has. Therefore, it is assumed that the farther the spacing between the two herbs in the prescription, the less likely they are related. Hence, the TCM spacing between prescriptions is defined as follows: $d(x,y,i) = |B(x,i) - B(y,i)|$, in the formula, where *x* and *y* appear at the same time; their average spacing is shown in formula (5.7):

$$d(x,y) = \frac{\sum_{i=1}^{m} I(x,y,i) \cdot d(x,y,i)}{\sum_{i=1}^{m} I(x,y,i)} \tag{5.7}$$

DMIM Scoring System

The DMIM score integrates two important scores—the mutual information entropy score and the spacing score of TCM between prescriptions: $\text{score}(x,y) = \frac{MI(x,y)}{d(x,y)}$; DMIM score reflects the tendency level of x and y to form a drug pair.

5.3.1.5 Experimental Verification

The Angiogenesis Activity of Chinese Medicines Screened by DMIM System was Evaluated Through In Vitro Experiments

According to the scoring results of DMIM, the ingredients of main Chinese medicines were selected to evaluate angiogenesis activity. Two endothelial cell proliferation tests, with or without VEGF stimulation, were used to evaluate the anti-angiogenesis or pro-angiogenesis activity of Chinese herbal medicine ingredients, respectively.

Experiment of Traditional Chinese Drug Pairs Predicted by DMIM

To verify whether the drug pair predicted by DMIM produces a synergistic effect, the highest single compound model [34] was used as an experimental reference model to determine the interaction of TCM, such as synergy or incompatibility.

5.3.1.6 Main Conclusion

(1) The DMIM algorithm established in this study considers and balances the frequency, relative independence, and spacing between prescriptions in the process of TCM prescription compatibility, which is an effective method to explore the compatibility rules of TCM.
(2) Through DMIM analysis of 3865 kinds of TCM prescriptions related to "activating collaterals" the drug pairs with greater connection were selected and a network was built. The constructed network can reproduce the traditional application of drug pairs or prescriptions, as shown in Fig. 5.2 [20]. The TCM network in the figure was constructed from the first 100 traditional Chinese drug pairs extracted by DMIM, showing Chinese medicines with different medicinal properties (chilly, cold, smooth, warm, hot) and composed of six classical compound prescriptions. New drug pairs with synergistic or incompatible effects were also found.
(3) Taking LWDH prescription as an example, through the joint module analysis of "TCM-target disease" multi-layer network (as shown in Fig. 5.3 [20]) and the disease phenotype analysis of LWDH treatment, it was found that the diseases

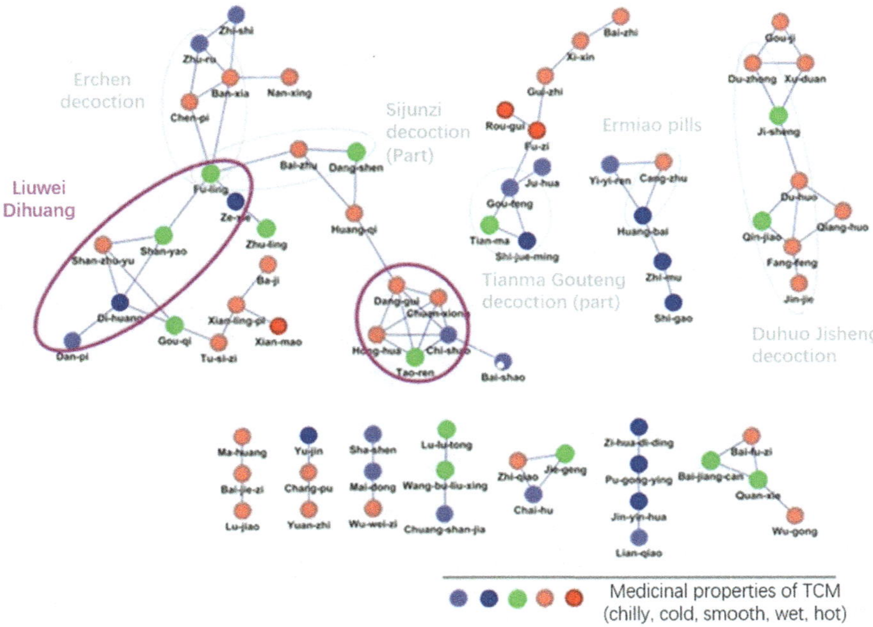

Fig. 5.2 TCM network based on DMIM extraction of 3865 TCM prescriptions [20]

treated with LWDH have statistically significant similar phenotypes, and these joint modules are enriched in multiple pathways such as metabolic and immune pathways, thus providing a new interpretation of LWDH's traditional Yin nourishing effect and the clinical mechanism of "treating the same disease with different methods."

In the TCM module, if the traditional Chinese medicine shares a common target, then the two kinds of traditional Chinese medicine of Liuwei Dihuang are interrelated. For the disease module, if there is a common disease target between diseases, then there is a link between the two diseases. The width of the solid line reflects the number of the same target or disease target between TCM. All Chinese medicine targets and disease targets are mapped to the protein-protein interaction network. The part connected by dotted line is the common network target module associated with the TCM module and disease module.

5.3.2 Network Pharmacology Analysis of Liuwei Dihuang Prescription

The LWDH prescription is a classic prescription for "tonifying Yin deficiency" in TCM theory and practice. In modern clinical treatment, LWDH mainly treats a variety of complex diseases, such as hypertension and esophageal cancer. In

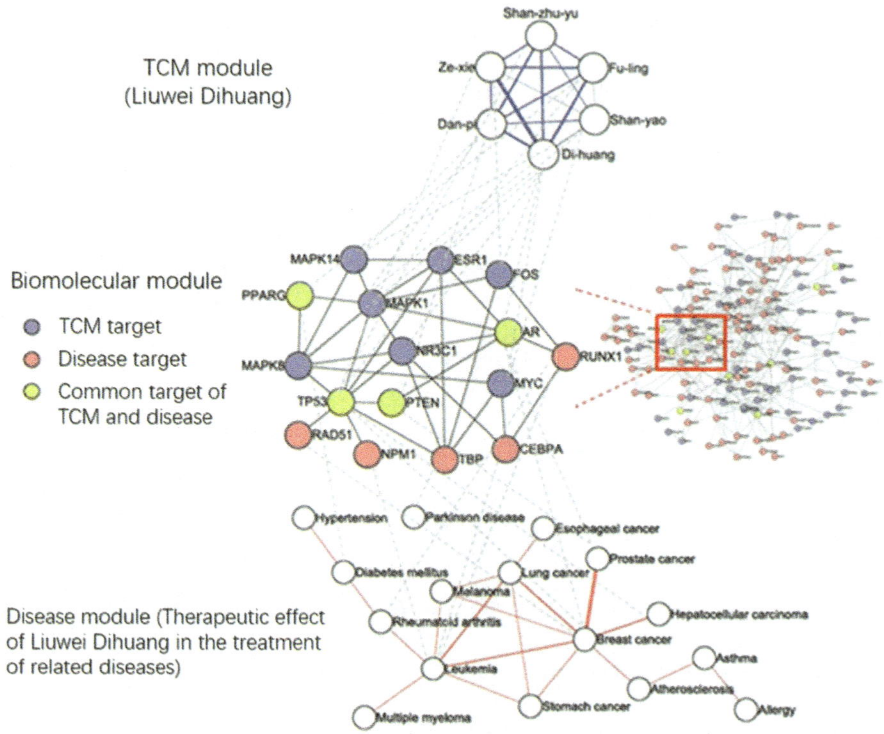

Fig. 5.3 Joint module of Liuwei Dihuang prescription and disease [20]

previous studies, we explained the traditional efficacy of LWDH for nourishing Yin through multi-layer "TCM–target–disease" network analysis. In this study [21], the mechanism of action of LWDH was further analyzed based on network pharmacology.

5.3.2.1 Research Objective

To better understand the therapeutic mechanism of the LWDH prescription.

5.3.2.2 Data Source

The compound data of LWDH were obtained from HerBioMap, TCM Database@Taiwan, and relevant literature. The target information source of LWDH comes from the predication of drugCIPHER; target-related pathways and related biological processes and disease data of LWDH were from the DAVID online tool.

5.3.2.3 Network Construction and Visualization

(1) "Compound-Target-Disease" Network
Based on the compound and target of LWDH and the relationship between target and disease, a multi-layer network of "compound-target-disease" was constructed. The establishment of "compound-target" link was based on DrugCIPHER and optimized through relevant algorithms (Please refer to the following "4. Analysis Index and Algorithm"). The "target-disease" link was derived from the DAVID online analysis tool.
(2) PPI network
(3) "Compound-biological process-disease" network
The biological process information of the LWDH target set was obtained through the DAVID online analysis tool, and the "compound-biological process" link was established through the "compound-target" link and the "target-biological process" link. Then, the "biological process-disease" link was established through the "disease-related target-disease" and "target-biological process" link, i.e., if the biological process and the disease have a common target, they were linked. Thus the "compound-biological process-disease" network was constructed.
(4) Analysis index and algorithm

a. Target screening
Assumptions: Some targets may be acted on by many ingredients in TCM prescriptions. It is assumed that this kind of target protein is likely to be the key point of pharmacological action of TCM prescriptions, and there may be synergistic effect of ingredients of TCM prescriptions on these targets.
After DrugCIPHER predicted targets of LWDH ingredients, to assess the probability that the target is associated with the pharmacological effects of LWDH, we compared the number of occurrences of each target protein in the target set of all ingredients in LWDH with a purely random process, represented by the Poisson binomial statistical model.

$$\Pr(K = k) = \sum_{A \in F_k} \prod_{i \in A} p_i \prod_{j \in A^c} (1 - p_j) \qquad (5.8)$$

In formula (5.8), $\Pr(K = k)$ is the probability of the target appearing in the target set of the k ingredient, F_k is the set of all target subsets of the k ingredient, A is a specific target subset of the k ingredient, A^c is the complement set of A. p_i and p_j are the probability that the target is contained in a set of ingredient targets. In random cases, the value of p is m/n, wherein m is the number of targets of the prescription ingredients, n is the total number of targets in the drugCIPHER database. After adjustment using the Bonferroni method, under random conditions, P value, $Pr(K > k)$ represents the probability of target occurrence in a target set with more than k ingredients. The P value indicates the relative importance of the target protein to LWDH (significant when $p < 0.01$).

b. Ingredient score

To evaluate the effectiveness of ingredients in LWDH, the ingredient scores were defined as follows:

$$\text{Score}_{\text{ingredient } i} = \frac{1}{N_i} \sum_{j=1}^{N_i} -\frac{1}{r_{ij}} \log_{10}\left[P(k)_j\right] \cdot I_j \tag{5.9}$$

In formula (5.9), N_i is the number of targets in ingredient i, r_{ij} is the grade of the target j of ingredient i in all targets, $Pr(k)_j$ is the P value of the target calculated using the Poisson binomial model. k is the number of ingredients that can act on target j, and I_j is an indicator function that shows whether target j is in the selected target set:

$$I_j = \begin{cases} 1, & \text{The } j_{\text{th}} \text{target is in the set of selected targets} \\ 0, & \text{The } j_{\text{th}} \text{target is not in the set of selected targets} \end{cases}$$

This score considers the specificity of ingredients and their relationship with important target proteins. The ingredients were ranked according to the scoring results, and it was found that the top 25% of the ingredients can cover 90% of the selected targets. Therefore, these chemical ingredients were subsequently selected as representative ingredients for network construction in LWDH.

5.3.2.4 Experimental Verification

The effect of compounds on the expression levels of related proteins was analyzed by using Western blot method. Based on the results of network analysis, four proteins were selected for experimental verification: including PPARG (Peroxisome Proliferator-Activated Receptor Gamma), RARA (Retinoic Acid Receptor Alpha), CCR2 (C-C Chemokine Receptor type 2), and ESR1 (estrogen receptor). The reason for choosing PPARG, RARA, and CCR2 is that they have different functions, are acted on by different groups of compounds, and are associated with esophageal cancer, esophagitis, and colon cancer (these diseases are potential and special therapeutic indications for LWDH). ESR1 is the hub node of the network. According to the related compounds of the selected target, 6 compounds were selected for experimental verification through their composition score. Their effects on the same kind of protein were analyzed based on the distribution of the compounds in the network cluster and the sources of different Chinese medicines.

5.3.2.5 Main Conclusion

(1) The selected targets of LWDH can be found to be closely related to each other through the PPI network, which means that the selected targets reflect the core molecular basis of the LWDH effect.
(2) WB experiments show that coumarin can reduce the expression of RARA, while caffeic acid increases the expression of RARA; caffeic acid increases the expression of PPARG; betulin, α-amylase, β-amino acid, and fucitol all down-regulate the expression of CCR2; Betulin, fucitol, and caffeic acid down-regulate the expression of ESR1. The results also show that there are complex interactions between the effects of different ingredients of TCM prescriptions.
(3) The network analysis results show that LWDH mainly acts on the pathways related to the endocrine and immune system, for example, PPAR signaling pathway, which is used to treat osteoporosis. This study not only explains the molecular mechanism of the traditional medicinal function of LWDH, but also provides the basis for the new use of old drugs. Arthritis and other diseases related to Yin deficiency, and esophageal cancer, colon cancer, and other types of diseases can all be treated.

5.4 Research Case on Network Pharmacology and TCM Formulation

From 1981 to 2014, among the 1211 small molecule new drugs approved by the FDA in the USA, 6% were natural products and 26% were derived from natural products. In addition, most anti-cancer drugs and anti-infective drugs are derived from natural products [35, 36]. As an important source of natural products, TCM can provide an abundant material basis for the research and development of new drugs.

At present, there are two main R&D models for new TCM drugs, one is the reduction analysis model based on the Western drug R&D model, and the other is the holistic development model. Artemisinin, Ginkgo biloba extract, tea polyphenols, and PHY906 (a new drug researched and developed on the basis of Classical TCM prescription Huangqin Decoction for the treatment of toxic reactions of chemotherapy drugs) developed by these two models have been internationally recognized. Taking the discovery of artemisinin as a typical case, the reduction analysis method aims at screening out monomer compounds with specific activity from several traditional Chinese medicines. This research model is characterized by heavy workload, low success rate, and low replicability. Therefore, this R&D model has become increasingly challenging in the current research stage, especially for TCM prescriptions with more herbal medicines.

As a holistic research and development model, network pharmacology differs from the conventional holistic research and development model. It focuses more on using computational methods to mine valuable information from existing data and provides reference for further traditional holistic research and development, as well as explores the complex mechanisms of drug action based on sorting. At present, research in this field mainly involves the interaction of compounds (synergism, incompatibility, etc.), the exploration of the pharmacodynamic mechanism, the screening of active ingredients, new prescriptions, drug repositioning, and other studies. In clinical practice, TCM is mainly used to achieve therapeutic effect through the compatibility of multiple traditional Chinese medicines. Exploring the compatibility relationship of "Traditional Chinese medicine formulation" between traditional Chinese medicines is conducive to explaining the concept of TCM from the perspective of modern medicine. The exploration of network pharmacology with respect to compound interaction is highlighted by Li et al. [19] based on the NIMS identification method, which can screen and optimize the combination of multi-component synergistic effects in TCM or compound prescriptions on a large scale.

The exploration of the multi-target pharmacodynamic mechanism of TCM ingredients is represented by artemisinin. Artemisinin is extracted from Artemisia annua and is currently the most effective anti-malaria drug, which has significantly reduced the mortality rate of malaria patients. However, the mechanism by which artemisinin and its derivatives kill malaria parasites is not completely clear. Researchers from National University of Singapore and Nanjing University conducted in-depth research on this and found the important mechanism of artemisinin's action against plasmodium falciparum [37].

The identification of effective TCM ingredients is particularly important in the process of TCM modernization. Based on network pharmacology analysis and combined with composition content analysis and screening, Fan et al. [38] studied the therapeutic effect of Xuesaitong (XST) injection on myocardial infarction; they screened out part of the potential active ingredients and verified the same in a rat model for myocardial infarction.

There have been several studies on exploring new prescriptions based on TCM prescriptions such as based on a large number of pharmacological experimental studies, Zhou et al. [39] found that LW-AFC, a new Chinese medicine composed of LWDH active ingredients, can improve the behavior and pathological injury of AD model mice by overall regulating, restoring, and maintaining the balance of neuro-endocrine and immune regulatory network, suggesting that LW-AFC has potential clinical value and good development prospect in preventing and treating AD. Zhou et al. [40] integrated tendentious case matching, complex network analysis, and enrichment analysis of TCM sets, and proposed a multi-stage analysis method to screen effective Chinese medicine combinations for treating specific diseases.

The same TCM prescription has therapeutic effect on different diseases, i.e., "treating different diseases with the same treatment," and is a multi-component and multi-target holistic medical treatment. Therefore, TCM and TCM prescriptions are rich sources for multi-target drug R&D and drug repositioning. The R&D concept of highly selective single-target drugs has certain limitations in the R&D of new Chinese medicines. Therefore, repositioning drugs with reliable clinical efficacy can not only effectively reduce the cost and shorten the period of research and development, but also effectively control the safety and pharmacokinetics, which is a good drug R&D strategy with a relatively good risk/benefit ratio at present. Network pharmacology's multi-level research strategy is similar to the holistic treatment balance and coordination of TCM, which provides new hope for the exploration of new drug compatibility and targets for TCM prescriptions and Chinese patent medicines, with a view to implementing "new use of old medicine." For example, by integrating the "drug-target" network and the protein–protein interactions of known cardiovascular disease-related proteins, Cheng et al. [41] established a computational model to predict the potential association between approved drugs and natural products in cardiovascular diseases, and based on this, predicted the potential anti-cardiovascular mechanism of action of TCM compounds and the potential side effect targets of anti-cardiovascular drugs.

A brief summary of some relevant studies is shown in Table 5.4:

5.4.1 Multi-component Synergy Recognition Method Based on Network Target

There are potential interactions between TCM and TCM prescriptions, including synergism, incompatibility, and mutual restraint [47]. For example, a synergistic effect occurs when the efficacy of a combination of Chinese medicines (or ingredients) is greater than the sum response of separate individuals. The combination of TCM ingredients can effectively reduce side effects, improve adaptability, and reduce drug resistance, thus increasing the possibility of treating complex diseases in a synergistic manner. TCM is a typical representative of a multi-component complex system, and its multi-component synergistic therapy provides hope for the treatment of complex diseases. How to screen a combination of compounds with potential therapeutic effects from several compounds continues to remain a challenging research direction.

The evaluation of multi-component synergy is usually carried out through experiments in case studies. However, such a method is suitable for in-depth verification research on the ingredients with synergistic effect. For complex systems like TCM, even in the case of a small number of compounds, a large number of possible composition combinations are formed, which increases the workload of experimental methods. Therefore, the high-throughput evaluation of compound synergies by system-based network pharmacology method is a research area that needs further attention. Li et al. [19] established a NIMS scoring algorithm based on a large amount of data and rapid accumulation of calculation methods, which provides a more promising method for multi-component drug research.

5.4.1.1 Research Objective

The NIMS method established in this study aims to provide a method for evaluating the synergistic effect of multi-component therapy and drug combination, to

Table 5.4 Application of typical network pharmacology in new drug formulation

Research object	Corresponding diseases/ function	Data source	Research method	Research conclusion	Literature
Synergistic effect of drugs	Anti-angiogenesis	Literature Database	NIMS cooperative coefficient algorithm based on network.	Based on the concept of network target and biomolecular network, NIMS predicts the synergistic drug combination from many drug molecules, and quantitatively represents the synergistic effect of drug combination. At the same time, the molecular mechanism of its synergistic effect is explained at the molecular level, which can effectively reduce the cost of screening effective drug combinations	[19]
Fuzheng TCM	Tumor	Database Drug CIPHER Literature	Gene expression high-throughput detection technology HTS2 of high-throughput sequencing, molecular map of tumor and immune-related biological networks regulated by TCM ingredients	The targets of Fuzheng TCM ingredients are mainly enriched in natural killer cell-mediated cytotoxicity, antigen presentation, and other immune-related pathways. The components of ginseng, Astragalus membranaceus, and Liuwei Dihuang can significantly up-regulate the gene expression of immune-related pathways such as natural killer cells, T cells, etc. Some ingredients of Fuzheng TCM can inhibit the	[42]

				gene expression of tumor signal pathways such as cell cycle and apoptosis. This study revealed the mechanism of action of Fuzheng TCM to a certain extent, suggesting that it has great R&D value in tumor prevention and tumor immune regulation, and provides a direction for the modernization of TCM	
Artemisinin	Malaria	Screening of potential targets of artemisinin by covalent binding method	No preference chemical proteomics analysis	The study combined artemisinin labeled by alkynes with a fluorescent dye to monitor the binding of artemisinin to proteins, and found 124 covalently bound artemisinin proteins that were analyzed through the network, many of which are involved in the basic life pathway of the Plasmodium falciparum. In addition, the results suggest that haem is the main cause of artemisinin activation, not free iron. Haem is mainly derived from the haem biosynthesis pathway of Plasmodium falciparum (the early ring stage) and later hemoglobin digestion	[37]
Xuesaitong (XST)	CVD		HPLC conducts ingredient identification and	The study takes the therapeutic effect of Xuesaitong (XST)	[38]

(continued)

Table 5.4 (continued)

Research object	Corresponding diseases/ function	Data source	Research method	Research conclusion	Literature
		Experiment Literature PharmMapper	quantification, PharMapper predicts the target of the ingredient, ingredient content-weighted "compound-target" network and network efficiency analysis, animal experiments	injection on myocardial infarction as an example to determine the content of ingredients, and applies the results to network analysis to screen out some potential active ingredients: notoginsenoside R1, ginsenoside Rg1, Rb1, Rd, and Re. The activity of these ingredients was verified in a rat model for myocardial infarction	
Clinical prescription of TCM	Insomnia	Clinical prescription	Tendentious case matching, core TCM network extraction, TCM enrichment analysis, and efficacy-based interactive information algorithm for identifying the relationship between TCM and symptoms	The research results show that compared with the original prescription, the optimized TCM prescription has higher efficiency. At the same time, the study also identified a specific group of patients with symptoms, which is conducive to subsequent research on the indications of effective Chinese medicine prescriptions	[40]
Approved anti coronary heart disease (CAD) drugs and Chinese medicines for the treatment of CAD	CAD	Database	"Drug/compound–target" network, drug repositioning algorithm based on network	By integrating the drug-target network with known CAD protein-protein interactions, a computational model was established to predict the potential association between	[41]

				approved drugs and natural products on CAD, and based on this model, the potential mechanism of action of TCM compounds and potential side effect targets of anti-CAD drugs were predicted. Key points include-mechanism of action of approved drugs (fasudil, parecoxib, and dexamethasone) and natural products (resveratrol, luteolin, daidzein, and caffeic acid) in the treatment of CAD	
Qijian decoction (Astragalus, Guijianyu, Coptis, Pueraria lobata) (QJM)	Type 2 diabetes	CNKI Database	Metabonomics, system pharmacology, animal experiments	The new compound prescription QJM is obtained by Epidata 3.1 analysis of the TCM prescription with T2D therapeutic effect. Results of animal experiments show that QJM could safely and effectively regulate blood glucose level. Although the effect of QJM is not as good as metformin hydrochloride, both show a similar trend of reducing blood glucose. Metabolites with deep changes in QJM treatment group were identified based on metabonomics studies. There are 55 proteins and 4 signaling pathways related to QJM,	[43]

(continued)

Table 5.4 (continued)

Research object	Corresponding diseases/ function	Data source	Research method	Research conclusion	Literature
				including galactose metabolism, valine, leucine, and isoleucine degradation metabolism, aminoacyl tRNA biosynthesis and alanine, aspartic acid, and glutamic acid metabolic pathways. The results of PCoA analysis of intestinal microbiota show that the structure of intestinal microflora in QJM and metformin groups show similar trend. Systematic pharmacology QJM may act through TP53, AKT1, and PPARA proteins	
Yinchenhao Tang (YCHT)	Hepatic injury	Animal experiments IPA	Immunohistochemistry, biochemistry, metabolomics, and proteomics	DRG, the main active ingredient combination in YCHT, may play a more powerful therapeutic effect than any one or two of the three single compounds by acting on multiple targets in rat models with liver injury. The combination of DGR can cause strong dynamic changes of metabolic biomarkers and exert synergistic effect by regulating the molecular network of target proteins	[44]

Anticoagulant compounds	Blood coagulation	Literature Database Molecular docking	Tongluo network construction and network efficiency, network flux algorithm, in vitro coagulation experiment verification.	The coagulation Tongluo network is a scale-free network with strong robustness. The results of network analysis combined with experimental verification show that the antiplatelet aggregation activities of papaverine and silybin, which have great influence on network efficiency, require greater attention	[45]
Xiaochaihu Tang (XCHT)	Anti-cancer	Database Molecular docking	Network construction of "compound-compound" and "compound-target"	The "compound-target" network analysis results show that the potential active compounds of XCHT are diverse and have synergistic effects. The "compound-compound" network is divided into four clusters, and different clusters contain compound combinations that act on different targets. It shows that XCHT has a variety of pharmacological effects in the treatment of cancer	[46]

effectively identify the synergistic effect of multi-component therapy. The use of computational methods and the current research data can provide a more promising method for multi-component drug research. At present, computing-related research used to evaluate multi-component therapy mainly focuses on two directions. The first approach is to identify and optimize the influence of multiple targets by modeling signal pathways or specific biological processes, which are usually used to solve small-scale problems. The limitation is that cross-feedback, feedback, or interaction in the pathway widely exists in complex diseases and isolating the pathway may cause a certain degree of deviation. The other approach is to use network analysis to predict the efficacy of drugs, especially multi-target drugs.

5.4.1.2 Data Source

Forty-nine Chinese medicines with potential anti-inflammatory, anti-angiogenesis, or anti-tumor activities were selected from the Chinese Pharmacopoeia, along with 12 Chinese medicine-derived compounds, and 2 Western medicine ingredients: 5-fluorouracil and rapamycin, totaling 63 agents. The five drug pairs that have been reported to have a synergistic effect were used as the benchmark of the NIMS algorithm. Drug targets and phenotypes were manually collected from more than 2000 related literature on PubMed and CNKI.

5.4.1.3 Network Construction and Visualization

The angiogenesis network was constructed using the LMMA method [48] that was published by the team earlier. Using keywords such as "angiogenesis" or "neovascularization" we retrieved relevant literature from PubMed and 49,885 related abstracts (as of February 9, 2007), which involve 2707 genes. These genes act as network nodes; if any two genes are connected in the HPRD database or have a connection on a pathway, then an edge is formed in the network, from which a PPI network was established. In the study, three types of global networks, namely PPI network and two types of global pathway networks were used to evaluate the network robustness of NIMS. In KEGG, a node in KO (KEGG Orthology) can represent a group of genes/proteins, and a gene can belong to different KOs. For example, k01090 contains 26 human genes, and CDKN3 is classified as K01090 and K01104. Therefore, we constructed two different pathway networks: Keep Node Content Pathway Network (KNC) and Merge Node Content Pathway Network (MNC). The original nodes were consistent in the KNC network, whereas different KOs with one or more overlapping genes were merged into one node in the MNC network.

5.4.1.4 Analysis Index and Algorithm

Under the context of the biological network of a specific disease or pathological process, the concept of network targets and the basic principle of NIMS are related to transfer of the relationship between drugs to the interaction between targets or the gene products affected by the drugs. In NIMS, a group of genes or gene products acted upon by drugs are called drug targets; the biological network of a specific disease was used as the background network for NIMS evaluation. Therefore, two NIMS-based elements: Topology Score (TS) and Agent Score (AS) were proposed to evaluate the synergy of drugs.

TS mainly comes from the topological characteristics of background networks related to specific diseases and drug effects. From the perspective of network target, the "Achilles' heel" of a specific disease biological network is more likely to become the action site of drugs. Therefore, the more important the topological properties of drug-related targets as a network node in the network, the greater the impact of the drug. In order to determine the importance of drug targets as network nodes, a node importance score $IP(v)$ was proposed by integrating DC, BC, and CC of the network nodes, where v refers to the network node. In addition, it was assumed that if a pair of drugs have a synergistic effect, their drug targets are adjacent in the network. Therefore, for candidate drug pairs: drug 1 and drug 2, topological score TS was defined to evaluate the importance score ($IP(v)$) of drug 1 target and drug 2 target, and the network distance between the two target groups.

$$TS_{1,2} = \frac{1}{2} \times \left(\frac{\sum_i IP_1(i) \times \exp - \min\left(d_{i,j}\right)}{\sum_i IP_1(i)} + \frac{\sum_j IP_2(j) \times \exp - \min\left(d_{j,i}\right)}{\sum_j IP_2(j)} \right) \quad (5.10)$$

In formula (5.10), $IP_1(i)$ represents the importance of related targets of drug 1, $IP_2(j)$ represents the importance of the relevant targets of drug 2, $IP_1(i)$ and $IP_2(j)$ are calculated by principal ingredient analysis, combining BC, CC, and variation eigenvectors. The negative exponential function is used to measure the interaction between two drugs based on the shortest distance. $\min(d_{i,j})$ is the shortest path from the target of drug 1 to all targets of drug 2, and $\min(d_{j,i})$ is the shortest path from the target of drug 2 to all targets of drug 1.

Drugs that have independent mechanisms of action and treat similar diseases have a higher chance to produce synergistic effects. Therefore, the study also introduced *AS*, whose algorithm was inspired by the similarity of disease phenotypes. If a drug target is included in the target set of an OMIM phenotype, the phenotype is called a drug phenotype, and the similarity between the two drug phenotypes quantifies the overlap of their OMIM descriptions. AS was calculated by referring to the study by Van Driel et al. [49], the formula is as follows:

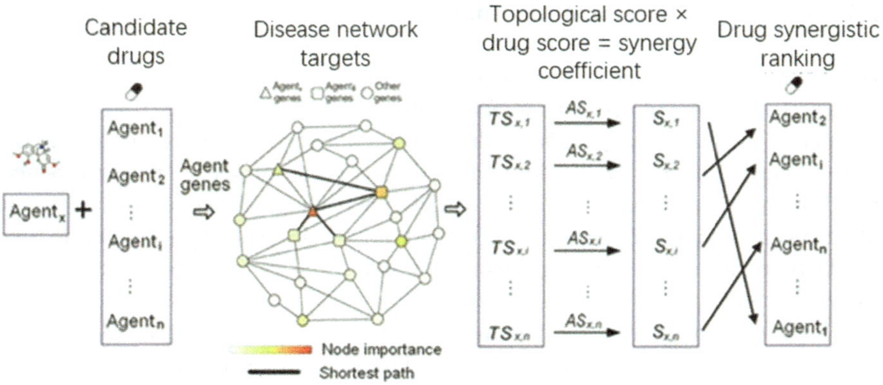

Fig. 5.4 Schematic diagram of multi-component synergetic identification method based on network targets [19]

$$AS_{1,2} = \frac{\sum_{i,j} P_{i,j}}{N} \tag{5.11}$$

In formula (5.11), $P_{i,j}$ represents the similarity between phenotype i of drug 1 and phenotype j of drug 2, and N represents the number of phenotype pairs.

Finally, the synergy coefficient between network-based drug 1 and drug 2 is calculated by NIMS algorithm, as shown in formula (5.12) below:

$$S_{1,2} = TS_{1,2} \times AS_{1,2} \tag{5.12}$$

The algorithm takes into account the importance of drug 1 and drug 2 targets in the network, the distance between adjacent network nodes, and the functional similarity of drug 1 and drug 2 targets. In general, the synergy coefficient S is 0–0.9. The higher the score, the greater the synergistic potential between the two drugs.

NIMS schematic diagram is shown in Fig. 5.4 [19].

5.4.1.5 Experimental Verification

The study used the endothelial cell proliferation test to verify the synergistic effect of the drug combination predicted by NIMS on angiogenesis. Endothelial cell division and proliferation are the material basis for tumor angiogenesis. The research used the HUVEC model.

5.4.1.6 Main Conclusion

(1) NIMS is a method for predicting synergistic drug combinations from several drug molecules based on the concept of network targets and biomolecular networks, and for quantitatively expressing the synergistic effects of drug combinations. In this study, NIMS was applied to evaluate the synergistic effect scores of 63 drugs. Based on the evaluation results, firstly, the synergy coefficients of five drug pairs with known synergistic effects were ranked; the synergy coefficients of 5-fluorouracil (5-FU) and vinblastine, and 5-FU and rapamycin are among the top three; the other three are vinblastine and camptothecin, genistein and camptothecin, and genistein and rapamycin. The synergy coefficient score ranks first in NIMS algorithm. Then, the synergy coefficient was calculated in three global background networks, including global PPI network, KNC, and MNC. The results show that in these cases, NIMS calculation results are relatively reliable and robust under different background networks.

(2) Based on the angiogenesis network target, NIMS was used to calculate the synergy scores of three groups of drugs. The three groups of drugs include: 5-FU and vinblastine, sinomenine and matrine, and sinomenine and paeoniflorin; NIMS calculation results show that the three groups of drugs exhibit different synergistic effects. From the perspective of ingredient action targets: 5-FU and vinblastine act on the interaction between the KDR protein complex, AKT1 and MAPK1 pathways, the PTEN feedback loop, the two biological processes of endothelial cell proliferation and apoptosis, and the four central nodes (KDR, MAPK1, JUN, and TP53). The network targets affected by sinomenine and matrine include interactions with EGFR, KDR, and TNFRSF1A pathways, PTEN feedback loop, four biological processes, and two central nodes (Jun and TP53) closely related to angiogenesis. However, sinomenine and paeoniflorin with lower scores of synergistic effects could only affect two biological processes and one central node (TP53).

    The detailed results are shown in Fig. 5.5a–c:

(3) The mechanism of multi-component synergy was evaluated from the perspective of network targets. First of all, in the NIMS scoring algorithm, the shortest path distance of two targets for drug/TCM ingredients is one of the key factors, as shown in Fig. 5.6a [19], the two drugs/TCM ingredients acting on the protein complex in the left figure have a smaller shortest path distance in the network, and vice versa, as shown in the right figure; under the same conditions, the combination of drugs/TCM ingredients with the action characteristics shown in the left picture has a higher NIMS score. Secondly, the two drugs/TCM ingredients acting on the central node or high-density centrality node may produce higher synergistic effect than the combination acting on the peripheral nodes, as shown in Fig. 5.6b [19]. In addition, two drugs/TCM ingredients acting on two complementary modules related to the same disease or similar disease produce higher synergistic effects than two drugs/TCM ingredients acting on two unrelated modules unrelated to any diseases, as shown in Fig. 5.6c [19].

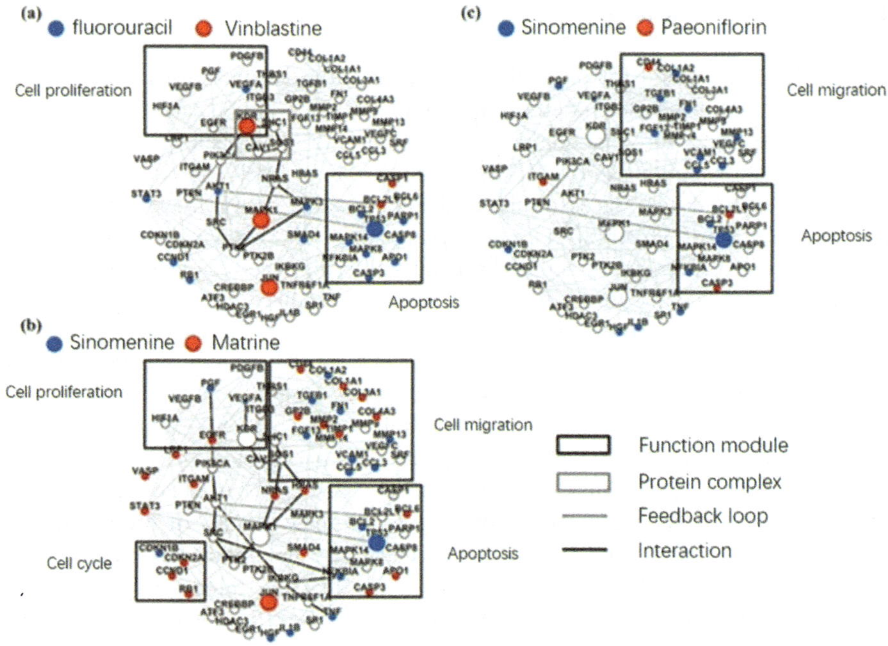

Fig. 5.5 Synergistic drug combination characteristics based on angiogenesis network targets [19]. (**a**) 5-FU and vincristine with synergistic effect; (**b**) Sinomenine and matrine with a higher NIMS synergy score; (**c**) Sinomenine and paeoniflorin with low NIMS synergy score. The nodes in red and blue represent targets with different drug and TCM ingredients, respectively

(4) The synergic intensity of sinomenine, luteolin, quercetin, magnolol, matrine, and paeoniflorin decreased successively in the HUVEC model, which is consistent with the results predicted by NIMS. The background network of NIMS also provides molecular-level explanations for the mechanism of synergistic drugs.

5.4.2 *Study on the Multi-target Mechanism of Artemisinin Against Plasmodium Falciparum*

Plasmodium falciparum infection is a serious public health threat. To deal with this problem, the most effective treatment at present is the antimalarial drug artemisinin and its derivatives. Artemisinin is a sesquiterpene lactone in terms of its structure, and has an endoperoxide bridge. The activation of artemisinin is marked by the production of highly reactive free radicals in the carbon center through the cleavage of endoperoxides. Over the past several decades of research, two key issues concerning the mechanism of action of artemisinin remain unresolved: (1) The source of iron needed for the activation of artemisinin. Studies have suggested that free ferrous iron and haem may be the main source of iron for its activation.

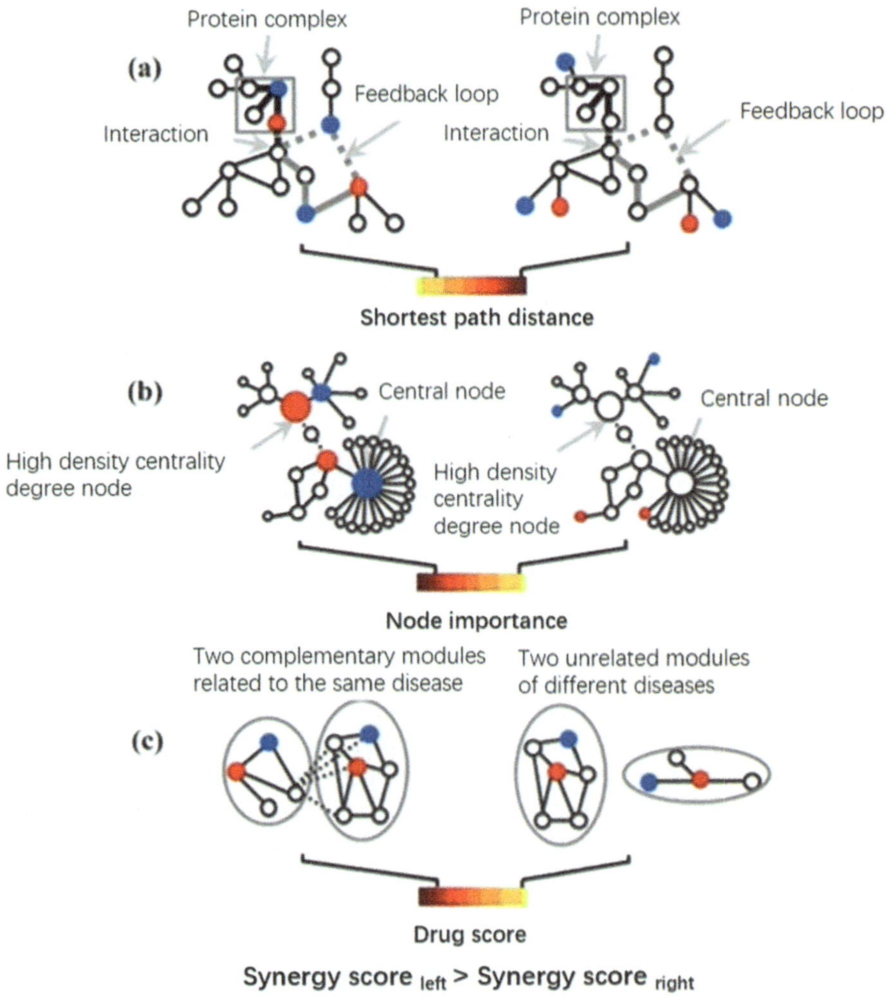

Fig. 5.6 Understanding the mechanism of multi-component synergy from the perspective of network targets [19]. (**a**) The two drugs/TCM ingredients acting on the protein complex in the left figure have a smaller shortest path distance in the network, and vice versa, as shown in the right figure; (**b**) The two drugs/TCM ingredients acting on the central node or high-density centrality node (left figure) may produce higher synergistic effect than the combination acting on the peripheral nodes (right figure). (**c**) The two drugs/TCM ingredients (left figure) acting on two complementary modules related to the same disease or similar disease produce higher synergistic effects (right figure) than the two drugs/TCM ingredients acting on two unrelated modules unrelated to any diseases. The dotted line indicates the direct or indirect connection in the network; the blue and red nodes indicate the targets of the two drugs and TCM ingredients, respectively

(2) Acting target for activation of artemisinin. Several proteins have been reported as potential acting targets of artemisinin, but none of them can explain its rapid and highly efficient pharmacological action. Due to the complexity of free radicals,

activated artemisinin may have many other direct targets. This section introduces the multi-target characteristics of artemisinin explored by Lin et al. and Wang et al. based on network pharmacology combination experiments [37].

5.4.2.1 Research Objective

To explore and explain the sources of iron required for activation of artemisinin and the action targets of artemisinin activation. This is of great significance to clarify the mechanism of action of artemisinin.

5.4.2.2 Data Source

To explore the potential acting proteins of artemisinin, an alkyne-labeled artemisinin activity probe (AP1) was designed and synthesized, and further combined with a fluorescent dye or biotin, so that the AP1 covalent binding target can be observed on SDS-PAGE, or affinity purified, for mass spectrometry identification.

Firstly, it was confirmed that the activity of AP1 is consistent with that of the unmodified artemisinin, and then AP1 was used to replace the unmodified artemisinin to identify the target protein that could covalently bind to it. Live parasites were incubated with 500 nM AP1 (a clinically achievable dose of artemisinin) for 4 hours to prepare a crude protein extract, and then labeled with alkyne biotin. Through Streptomyces avidinii protein beads, the AP1 target protein was affinity purified and identified by using tandem mass spectrometry. A total of 124 parasite proteins were identified as direct targets of artemisinin in three separate experiments, including a reported artemisinin target, SERCA/PfATP6 (Calcium-Transporting ATPase).

5.4.2.3 Network Construction and Visualization

Based on 124 related target proteins found in the study, the ClueGO plug-in of Cytoscape was used for relevant functional enrichment analysis and network visualization.

5.4.2.4 Analysis Index and Algorithm

In the network diagram constructed by the ClueGO plug-in, each node represents a functional group, and the Kappa statistics based on the same target protein between functional groups was taken as the index and as the assigned value of the lines between nodes. According to the functional groups that the nodes belong to, the enrichment and classification of nodes were analyzed and represented by different colors of nodes.

5.4.2.5 Experimental Verification

(1) Western Blot (WB) was used to verify the potential acting targets of AP1: OAT (Ornithine Aminotransferase), PyrK (Pyruvate Kinase), LDH (L-Lactate Dehydrogenase), SpdSyn (Spermidine Synthase), and SAMS (S-Adenosylmethionine Synthetase).
(2) GO functional enrichment analysis revealed that the target protein of AP1 is involved in many basic biological processes of the parasite, including hemoglobin catabolism. In addition, through cell location analysis, it was found that hemoglobin digestion provides a source of amino acids needed to maintain intracellular osmotic pressure during the rapid growth of parasites. Through experiments, it was found that haem has a greater contribution in the activation of artemisinin, hence, the HCT116 model was used to further verify the main role of haem in the activation of artemisinin.

5.4.2.6 Main Conclusion

(1) In this study, alkyne-labeled artemisinin was combined with fluorescent dyes to monitor the binding of artemisinin to proteins. One hundred and twenty-four proteins covalently bound to artemisinin were found. Through network analysis, many of them were found to be involved in the basic biological processes of Plasmodium falciparum, including carboxylic acid metabolism, cellular bioamines metabolism, nucleoside metabolism, ribonucleoside biosynthesis, and hemoglobin catabolism process. The combination of experiments and network analysis provides a more complete picture of the mechanism of action of artemisinin and its derivatives.
(2) In addition, the results suggest that haem is the main cause of artemisinin activation and not free iron. Haem mainly comes from the haem biosynthesis pathway of Plasmodium (the early ring stage), or from hemoglobin digestion at a later stage.

5.5 Network Pharmacology and Ethnic Medicine Research Cases

Ethnic medicine is an important component of the country's traditional medicine, and has unique curative advantages in the prevention and treatment of difficult and frequently occurring diseases. The current network pharmacology research cases in ethnic medicine mainly include the anti-cancer activity mechanism of Hedyotis diffusa, prediction of its potential active ingredients and targets by network analysis, and verification of its effect on activity related pathways through in vitro cell experiments by Wang et al. [50]. In addition, the potential active ingredients of galleon were predicted through network analysis, the active part containing active ingredients was used for experimental verification, and the mechanism of its treatment for ulcerative colitis was explored [51]. Hu and Yu also used network analysis combined with in vitro cell experiments to compare the chemical composition and biological mechanism of anti-rheumatoid arthritis of Siegesbeckiae (including Siegesbeckia orientalis, Siegesbeckia pubescens, and Siegesbeckia glabrescens) from different plant origins [52]. The summary of application cases is shown in Table 5.5:

The research on ethnic drugs through network pharmacology can on the one hand promote the development of ethnic drugs, which are an integral component of TCM and an important source of new drug innovation, on the other hand, it can provide certain reference for quality control. For example, the Siegesbeckia orientalis included in *Chinese Pharmacopoeia* (2015 Edition) contains three kinds of plant origins. Although their therapeutic effects are similar, research has revealed that there are some differences in composition and mechanism of action between Siegesbeckia orientalis with different plant origins.

The following two specific research cases are selected for analysis.

5.5.1 Comparative Study and Analysis on Chemical Components and Pharmacological Effects of Three Species of Siegesbeckia

First published in *Xinxiu Bencao*, Siegesbeckia Herba (SH) is a traditional Chinese herbal medicine prescribed for rheumatoid arthritis. It has anti-inflammatory, hypotensive, vasodilatory, and other pharmacological effects, and is often used to treat rheumatic arthralgia. Plant sources of Siegesbeckia Herba included in the Chinese pharmacopoeia include SO (*Siegesbeckia orientalis* L.), SP (*S. pubescens Markino*), and SG (*S. glabrescens* Markino). Although the therapeutic effects of these Siegesbeckia species on RA are similar, their differences in chemical composition suggest that their anti-rheumatoid mechanisms may be different. This section introduces the comparative study of Hu and Yu on network pharmacology of these three species of Siegesbeckia, combined with experimental verification [52].

5.5.1.1 Research Objective

This study aims to compare the chemical and biological similarities and differences between Siegesbeckiae (SO, SP, and SG) with different plant origins in the treatment of RA through the combination of computational prediction and biological experimental research.

Table 5.5 Research and application of network pharmacology in ethnic medicine

Ethnic medicine	Corresponding disease/ function	Data source	Research method	Research conclusion	Literature
Hedyotis diffusa Willd (HDW)	Non-small cell liver cancer	Database	Analysis of "compound–target" network, "target–pathway" network, in vivo animal experiment, in vitro cell experiment.	Studies in mouse models have shown that HDW significantly inhibits tumor growth, improves tumor microenvironment, and activates immune response, thereby prolongating survival. Quercetin and kaempferol have higher node degrees in the "compound-target" network, and are predicted to be key compounds. The "target-pathway" network suggests that HDW may act on a variety of signaling pathways to inhibit inflammation, enhance immune response, and inhibit angiogenesis. Using kaempferol for in vitro cell experiments, kaempferol inhibits the proliferation of tumor cells by regulating the PI3K/AKT, MAPK, and VEGF pathways, while downregulating the inflammatory factors iNOS, COX2, and inhibiting the inflammatory response	[50]
Siegesbeckia orientalis (SO), Siegesbeckia pubescens (SP), Siegesbeckia glabrescens (SG)	Rheumatoid arthritis	Database	"Compound–target" network analysis, in vitro cell experiment	SO, SP, and SG differ significantly in chemical composition levels. The results of cellular experiments based on the potential protein targets predicted by network analysis	[52]

(continued)

Table 5.5 (continued)

Ethnic medicine	Corresponding disease/ function	Data source	Research method	Research conclusion	Literature
				show that although the therapeutic effects of SO, SP, and SG are very similar in the treatment of rheumatoid arthritis, the potential biological mechanisms of different types of Siegesbeckia orientalis are quite different	
Nutgall	Ulcerative colitis	Experiment database	Liquid chromatography-mass spectrometry (LC-MS), "Compound–target–pathway" network analysis, in vitro cell experiment, in vivo animal experiment	Through virtual computer simulation research and network analysis, it was found that the active ingredients may show therapeutic effect on ulcerative colitis (UC) by acting on multiple targets and regulating multiple pathways. Relevant targets mainly involved in the NF-κB pathway were selected for verification. By comparing the cytotoxicity and detecting the levels of pro-inflammatory factors of nine kinds of ingredients through in vitro studies, five types of ingredients were finally screened as active ingredients. In vivo, the active ingredients show a significant improvement in UC mice induced by dextran sulfate sodium (DSS). The results show that the active part containing gallicin, oxalic acid,	[51]

				di-O-galloyl-β-D-glucose, and tri-O-galloyl-β-D-glucose mainly contributed to the treatment of UC. In addition, the active ingredients also inhibit the phosphorylation level of IKKβ, thereby inhibiting the downstream NF-κB signaling pathway	

5.5.1.2 Data Source

The compound information of the three SH plants was obtained from SciFinder, CCD V2009, DNP, and chemical database of Chinese Academy of Sciences. Furthermore, proteins associated with NF-κB, oxidative stress, and autophagy, as well as RA-related proteins from KEGG and Biocarta databases were collected.

5.5.1.3 Network Construction and Visualization

The connection between the compound and the target protein was established through molecular docking, and the "compound-target protein" network was constructed; the network visualization was carried out using Cytoscape.

5.5.1.4 Analysis Index and Algorithm

Compound similarity algorithm

Tanimoto similarity coefficient (T_c) was used to evaluate the level of similarity between any two Siegesbeckiae species.

$$T_c = \frac{c}{a + b - c} \tag{5.13}$$

wherein a and b represent the number of set A and set B (in this study, it refers to the number of compounds of the two Siegesbeckiae species), and c represents the intersection of set A and set B (in this study, it refers to the number of the same compounds of the two Siegesbeckiae species). The T_c value ranges from 0 to 1. The higher the value, the higher the similarity, while the lower the value, the lower similarity, i.e., higher the difference.

Network Analysis

The topological structure (node degree) analysis of the network assumes that compounds with high node degree or RA-related protein nodes in different SO, SP, and SG, are of great significance for further experimental study.

5.5.1.5 Experimental Verification

Through network analysis, protein targets with higher centrality were selected: BTK (Tyrosine-Protein Kinase BTK), SYK (Tyrosine-Protein Kinase SYK), MAPK8 (Mitogen-Activated Protein Kinase 8), PIK3C3 (Phosphatidylinositol 3-Kinase

Catalytic Subunit Type 3), and KEAP1 (Kelch-like ECH-associated Protein 1) were selected for experimental verification. The effects of 50% ethanol extracts of SO, SP, and SG on the predicted target proteins were studied by WB on RAW264.7 macrophages induced by lipopolysaccharide (LPS).

5.5.1.6 Main Conclusion

(1) Based on the study of reported compounds of the three Siegesbeckiae varieties, there are 112, 130, and 23 compounds in SO, SP, and SG, respectively. The T_c values of the three siegesbeckiae varieties between SG/SO, SO/SP, and SP/SG are 0.0714, 0.0614, and 0.0625, respectively. This indicates that there are large differences among the compounds of the three Siegesbeckiae species.
(2) Although all three Siegesbeckiae species are used to treat RA clinically, this study found that their potential mechanisms of action are somewhat different. Compared with the control group, LPS (200 ng/mL) significantly induces phosphorylation of BTK, SYK, MAPK8, and PIK3C3, and decreases the expression of BTK and KEAP1, but does not affect the expression of PIK3C3 in RAW 264.7 cells. However, after being treated with SO, SP or SG extracts, a series of protein changes occurred: SO restores the lPS-induced decrease in KEAP1 expression in a dose-dependent manner, but does not affect the phosphorylation or expression of BTK and PIK3C3; SP inhibits the phosphorylation of PIK3C3 induced by LPS in a dose-dependent manner, and has no significant effect on the phosphorylation or expression of BTK and KEAP1. In addition, SG inhibits LPS-induced MAPK8 phosphorylation in a dose-dependent manner but has no effect on the phosphorylation or expression of BTK and SYK.

5.5.2 Study and Analysis on the Mechanism of Hedyotis Diffusa Willd against Non-small Cell Lung Cancer

First published in the *Guangxi Journal of Traditional Chinese Medicine*, Hedyotis Diffusa Wild (HDW) is an important ethnic medicine. It has functions of clearing heat and detoxifying, promoting blood circulation and relieving pain, and antibacterial, anti-inflammatory, and anti-tumor effects. It is mainly used for the clinical treatment of malignant tumors. However, the underlying mechanism of action remains unclear. It has been reported that HDW has anti-tumor effects on a variety of cancers. It has been reported that the extract of HDW shows effective inhibition on human lung cancer cells by inhibiting cell proliferation and reducing cell activity in a concentration-dependent manner. This section introduces the research of Wang et al. [50] on the application of network pharmacology to explore the pharmacological mechanism of HDW.

5.5.2.1 Research Objective

This study aims to systematically reveal the pharmacological mechanism of HDW in the treatment of non-small cell lung cancer (NSCLC) at the molecular, target, and pathway levels, using the systemic pharmacology platform.

5.5.2.2 Data Source

The compound information source of HDW is the TCMSP database, and computer models were used to predict the absorption, distribution, metabolism, and excretion of compounds (ADME). Two indicators were selected—Oral Bioavailability (OB) and Druglikeness (DL), which were used to evaluate the pharmacokinetics and drug properties of HDW compounds. The following two factors were considered: (1) The related compounds were comprehensively studied by using as few compounds as possible; (2) The reported pharmacological data was used to explain and establish the model more reasonably. In addition to screening candidate compounds, compounds with OB $> 26\%$ and DL ≥ 0.18 (Drugbank drug DL average value) can continue to be used as candidate compounds for subsequent studies.

After the candidate compound was selected, the study used the System Drug Targeting Tool (SysDT) and the Weighted Set Similarity (WES) algorithm to predict the target of the compound. In addition, NSCLC-related proteins were obtained from the TTD database, CTD database, and PharmGKB database.

The biological functions of potential targets were analyzed by GO and the biological processes of several genes were analyzed by the GlueGO plug-in of Cytoscape.

5.5.2.3 Network Construction and Visualization

Two networks were constructed in this study: "compound–target" network and "target–pathway" network. In these two networks, the nodes are compounds, targets, and pathways, and the edges represent their interactions.

5.5.2.4 Analysis Index and Algorithm

The CentiScaPe 1.2 plug-in of Cytoscape was used to analyze the topological properties of the network.

5.5.2.5 Experimental Verification

Animal Experiments

Firstly, in order to evaluate whether HDW has anti-tumor effect, C57BL/6 tumor-bearing mice model[1] was constructed. The tumor-bearing mice were divided into two groups: the blank control group and the HDW administration group. The changes in tumor size, weight, and survival rate of the tumor-bearing mice after HDW administration were observed. Secondly, in order to detect whether HDW affects the tumor microenvironment, flow cytometry was used to detect the tumor microenvironment after HDW treatment. The tumor tissues of the mice in the blank group or HDW treatment group were cut into thin slices, and the tumor dissociation kit was used to lyse the tumor tissues, which were then filtered on a 70 μm nylon mesh filter, and the cell suspension was collected. TILs (Tumor Infiltrating Lymphocytes) from tumors were isolated using percoll (GE, 17-0891-02) prior to detection of CD8 (T Cell Surface Glycoprotein CD8) and Treg (Regulatory Cells) cells. Then, MDSC (Myeloid-Derived Suppressor Cell), NK, and TAM (Tumor-Associated Macrophage) were tested by fluorescence-labeled antibody staining.

Cell Experiments

The effects of the main active compounds of HDW on the main proteins of related pathways verified at the cellular level. Mouse macrophages RAW264.7 and human NSCLC cell line H1975 were cultured by treating RAW264.7 cells with kaempferol at different concentrations, then incubated with 0.1μg/mL LPS; the cells were collected for WB analysis to detect the inflammatory mediators at the end of the culture and to explore their effects on PI3K/AKT signaling pathway. As mentioned above, H1975 cells were treated with kaempferol at different concentrations, and the expression of related proteins was detected by WB analysis to explore its effects on PI3K/AKT and VEGF pathways.

5.5.2.6 Main Conclusion

(1) The anti-tumor effect of HDW on C57BL/6 mice was analyzed. Compared with the blank control, the HDW extract significantly reduced tumor growth, the tumor weight of tumor-bearing mice in the HDW treatment group was lower than that of the blank control group, and the tumor growth in the treatment group was significantly reduced. Compared with the blank control tumor-bearing mice,

[1]C57BL/6 is often called "C57 black 6," "C57," or "black 6" (standard abbreviated as B6) and is a common inbred strain of laboratory mice. It is a commonly used strain in oncology, physiology, immunology, and genetics research.

the mice in the HDW treatment group showed a significant increase in the proportion of intracellular cytotoxic $CD8^+$ T cells, and the average fluorescence intensity of $IFN\gamma^+$ $CD8^+$ T cells also significantly increased. In addition, the expression of NK cells in the tumors of HDW-treated mice significantly increased, indicating the activation of innate immunity. In conclusion, the study showed that HDW has anti-tumor activity and prolongs the life cycle of tumor-bearing mice. At the same time, it affects the tumor microenvironment and can activate immunity.

(2) Through node degree analysis of the "compound–target" network, the study assumes that compounds with higher nodes in the network are more likely to play a key role in the mechanism of HDW. The compounds with higher degree of nodes in the network are quercetin ($DC = 73$), kaempferol ($DC = 47$), and 2-hydroxy-1-methoxyanthraquinone ($DC = 40$). According to the hypothesis, the first two components may be the key compounds in the treatment of NSCLC. The "target-pathway" network suggests that HDW may act on a variety of signaling pathways to inhibit inflammation, enhance immune response, and inhibit angiogenesis.

(3) The results of the cell experiment show that the levels of Bcl2 (Antiapoptotic B Cell Lymphoma 2), p-Akt (Activated Akt), and CDK2 (Cyclin-Dependent Kinase 2) in H1975 cells treated with kaempferol are significantly decreased, suggesting that kaempferol may regulate H1975 cell growth inhibition through the PI3/AKT pathway; kaempferol can significantly reduce the inflammatory factors of RAW264.7 macrophages cells stimulated by LPS: COX-2 (Prosta-glandin G/H Synthase 2), iNOS (Nitric Oxide Synthase), and IKK (IκB Kinase Complex). It is speculated that it may reduce the expression of inflammatory mediators induced by RAW264.7 cells mainly through the PI3/AKT pathway. Compared with the control group, the kaempferol treatment group has fewer expressions of p-STAT3, p-p38, and eNOS (Endothelial Nitric Oxide Synthase) in the cells, STAT3-mediated inflammatory factor expressions, and corresponding immune responses, and also plays an important role in tumor cell migration. It is inferred that kaempferol may inhibit cell migration by inhibiting VEGF pathway and related downstream protein kinase activity.

5.6 Network Pharmacology and International Traditional Medicine Research Cases

Traditional medicine is not fully recognized in many countries due to the great challenge of providing a comprehensive and scientific explanation for the material basis and pharmacological mechanism of traditional medicine using existing methods. The emergence of network pharmacology provides technical support for the modernization of traditional medicine by establishing a multi-dimensional data network, and enabling the study of traditional medicine from a systematic perspective and effectively explaining its "ingredient-target" relationship and pharmacological mechanism with modern scientific thinking. At present, there has been increasing influence of TCM internationally, and the world has gradually begun to pay attention to traditional medicine. In November 2017, the *Journal of the National Cancer Institute* published a special issue with the theme "Advancing the Global Impact of Integrated Oncology," and published a white paper issued by the National Institutes of Health (NIH)/National Cancer Institute (NCI) on complementary and alternative cancer medicine research, which emphasized the importance [3] of computational methods such as network pharmacology and data analysis methods for revealing the complex mechanism of traditional drugs and designing effective clinical schemes. At present, relevant studies include the study by Gómez-Verjan et al. [53] on the coumarin compounds in *Calophyllum brasiliense* leaf extract using network pharmacology and experimental research to carry out an in-depth explanation of the compounds' anti-cancer mechanism; the study by Jin et al. [54] on the effectiveness of Peucedanum Japonicum extract for the treatment of Osteoarthritis (OA) on an animal model, and their study of the potential active ingredients and acting targets of the extracts' efficacy through network pharmacology research; the study by Wang et al. [55] on potential types of active components (terpene lactones and flavonoids) through network analysis, and verification of the role of ginkgolide A (GA), ginkgolide B (GB), and ginkgolide C (GC), as well as the combination of these compounds GDJ, on a mouse model. Detailed contents are summarized, as shown in Table 5.6:

At present, although the application of network pharmacology in countries around the world other than in China is not as prevalent, the application difficulty of the network analysis algorithm and methodology are relatively basic. With the gradual recognition of traditional medicine, network pharmacology will gradually penetrate all aspects of medicinal research. The research on the material basis and pharmacological mechanism of traditional medicine will be increased, and their therapeutic effect will be accepted and promoted further.

The following two specific research cases are selected for analysis.

5.6.1 Study and Analysis on Anti-cancer Activity of Calophyllum Brasiliense

Coumarins contain a large group of secondary metabolites with a phenolic structure, and are composed of molten benzene and α-pyrrolidone. Mammea-type coumarin is a special type of secondary metabolite bio-synthesized by the tropical rainforest tree *Calophyllum Brasiliense*, mainly distributed in South America and Mexico. Some studies have shown that coumarin compounds have a wide range of pharmacological properties, including anticoagulant, anti-inflammatory, antiviral, and anti-cancer. In particular, mammea A/BA and A/BB (either alone or as a mixture) have strong anti-tumor activity. However, most of their molecular targets remain unknown. This section introduces the network pharmacology study and

Table 5.6 Research and application of network pharmacology in international traditional medicine

Research object	Corresponding disease/ function	Data source	Research method	Research conclusion	Literature
Mammea coumarin compounds in *Calophyllum brasiliense* leaves (Mammea A/BA and A/BB)	Cancer	Experiment database	Network analysis, in vitro cell experiment, computer simulation	Network pharmacology analysis shows that mammea A/BA and A/BB have an effect on the apoptosis, PI3K/AKT, MAPK, Ras, and cancer pathways. In vitro cell model studies show that mammea A/BA and A/BB induce apoptosis and destroy autophagy flux by expressing pro-apoptotic proteins Bax and Bak. As shown by the accumulation of cytosolic manifestations in LC3-II and p62, they destroy mitochondrial ultrastructure and simultaneously increase intracellular calcium concentration. In addition, this study was the first to report that mammea A/BA and A/BB coumarin may inhibit autophagy flux and induce apoptosis by interacting with mTOR	[53]
Peucedanum Japonicum Extract (PJE)	Arthritis	Literature database	In vivo animal experiments, "compound–target" network analysis	Animal experiments indicate that PJE could relieve the joint discomfort in arthritis (OA) rats and reverse the cartilage damage caused by MIA injection; the levels of IL-6 and LTB4 in OA model rats in the PJE treatment group are lower, while TNF-α and	[54]

				5-LOX are slightly lower; The mRNA expression levels of inflammatory factors and the levels of the five inflammatory factors in MIA group significantly increased, while the mRNA expression levels of IL-1β, IL-6, COX-2, and iNOS in the PJE treatment group are significantly lower. The results of network analysis indicate that the main active compounds of PJE may be rutin, inositol, chlorogenic acid, and methoxypsoralen. In addition, the major targets are CASP3 (acts with rutin, chlorogenic acid, and isoquercetin), CASP7 (acts with rutin and chlorogenic acid), and CYP2D6 (acts with methoxypsoralen and alloisoimperarorin). These major compounds and targets may play an important role in the progression of OA	
Ginkgo biloba leaves (GBLs)	Cardiovascular disease	Database	In vivo animal experiments, "compound–target" network and "compound–target–pathway" network analysis	Through network analysis, it was found that two types of compounds in GBLs are relatively important: terpene lactones and flavonoids; GA, GB, and GC were selected for the experiment, and the results show that they could improve the middle cerebral artery	[55]

(continued)

Table 5.6 (continued)

Research object	Corresponding disease/ function	Data source	Research method	Research conclusion	Literature
				occlusion. GDJ, a combination of GA, GB, and GC, may play a neuroprotective role by inhibiting the NF-κB signaling pathway, and GDJ has shown that it can significantly block and inhibit the increase in COX-2 and c-myc expression induced by I/R; in addition, GDJ can also improve cerebral ischemia by regulating the PI3K-Akt pathway	

experimental verification of coumarin components in *Calophyllum brasiliense* leaves conducted by Reyes-Chilpa et al. [53].

5.6.1.1 Research Objective

Explore the acting target of mammea-type coumarin of *Calophyllum brasiliense* leaves based on network pharmacology, and verify the relevant network prediction results through K562 cancer cell in vitro experiments.

5.6.1.2 Data Source

Coumarin-type compounds (MABB) from the extracts of *Calophyllum brasiliense* leaves were separated and structural identification was conducted by ^{1}H-NMR. Target prediction of compounds was based on the following methods: DRAR-CPI, SEA, SwissTarget, and STITCH. CTD, GSEAPY software package of Python and DAVID were then used for enrichment analysis of potential acting targets (the first 50 related targets interacting with each compound).

5.6.1.3 Network Construction and Visualization

GeneMania plug-in of Cytoscape was used to construct the target protein interaction network. The nodes are the first 50 related target proteins that interact with each compound of MABB through prediction, and the edges represent the connections between the nodes.

5.6.1.4 Analysis Index and Algorithm

The target protein interaction constructed using the GeneMania plug-in of Cytoscape essentially reflects the interaction between target proteins. In this study, the associations between nodes (different colored edges) include physical interactions between nodes, predicted interactions, and interactions based on common signal pathways. The different colored edges between the target proteins reflect different interrelationships.

5.6.1.5 Experimental Verification

Cell Experiment Verification

A K562 cell model was used to study the role of MABB in apoptosis, by fluorescence analysis of Bcl-2, Bax (Apoptosis Regulator BAX), and Bak (Bcl-2

Homologous Antagonist/Killer) proteins in K562 cells; Transmission electron microscope was used to further explore whether MABB produces mitochondrial damage concurrently. WB was used to detect the expression of LC3-II and p62 to verify the effect of MABB on the related pathways.

Virtual Docking

According to literature reports, several synthetic coumarins exert anti-cancer effects by inhibiting the PI3K-AKT-mTOR pathway or act as inhibitors of mTOR. mTOR is the central protein in the signal transduction pathway. In addition, some of these compounds have been patented, such as CN103254203, therefore, the study explores whether MABB might interact with mTOR through virtual docking. ICM software was used to predict the interaction between coumarin and its related allosteric binding sites.

5.6.1.6 Main Conclusion

(1) In this study, the network pharmacology approach was used to predict the MABB targets and to identify unknown signal transduction pathways that interact with compounds. Research data shows that MABB interacts with apoptosis and the PI3K/AKT, MAPK, Ras, and Erb pathways, most of which have tyrosine kinase characteristics; the PI3K/AKT pathway is related to autophagy. Disease enrichment analysis indicates that MABB may be related to cancer pathways, indicating its potential as an anti-tumor compound.
(2) Immunofluorescence studies show that MABB treatment-induced overexpression of Bax and Bak significantly reduces the fluorescence of Bcl-2. These results indicate that MABB can induce apoptosis through the expression of pro-apoptotic proteins Bax and Bak; by detecting the expression of LC3-II and p62 proteins, acidic vesicle accumulation and autophagy volume aggregation can be observed, suggesting that MABB can induce apoptosis by destroying autophagy flux.
(3) The analysis of docking results suggests that MABB could inhibit autophagy flux and induce apoptosis by interacting with mTOR.

5.6.2 Protective Effect of Peucedanum Japonicum Extracts on Osteoarthritis

Osteoarthritis (OA) is a common degenerative inflammatory arthritis, characterized by articular cartilage degeneration, subchondral osteosclerosis, osteophyte formation, and joint tissue inflammation. The pathogenesis of OA has not been fully elucidated. There are related therapies for OA to relieve joint pain and stiffness, reduce inflammation, and prevent joint injury, but there is no cure for OA. As a chronic and complex disease, people are increasingly pay more attention to the use of Chinese herbal medicine to treat or alleviate OA symptoms. Many studies have reported that Peucedanum Japonicum, a kind of Chinese herbal medicine used to treat neuralgia, rheumatoid arthritis, and inflammation related diseases, has the potential to treat OA. This section introduces the discussion on the mechanism of Peucedanum Japonicum in the treatment of OA based on network pharmacology conducted by Chun et al. [54].

5.6.2.1 Research Objective

Although there have been studies on the chemical components and effects of peucedanum japonicum, there is no network pharmacology analysis on its effect on OA from a holistic perspective. Therefore, in this study, pharmacological network analysis was used to comprehensively evaluate the regulatory mechanism of peucedanum japonicum extracts, to identify potential active compounds and OA-related target genes. In addition, the pharmacological effects of peucedanum japonicum extract (PJE) by its inhibitory effect in model rats induced by monosodium iodoacetic acid (MIA) were also studied.

5.6.2.2 Data Source

For network pharmacology research, the chemical components of peucedanum japonicum were collected by retrieving literature, PubMed database, and the KTKP database. The ADME properties of the compounds were predicted by the TCMSP database. The compounds with Oral Bioavailability (OB) $>30\%$ and Druglikeness (DL) >0.18 were selected as the potential active components of peucedanum japonicum for subsequent studies. The potential acting targets of the compound were obtained from the STITCH database, and then the TTD database was used to determine whether the targets are related to OA.

5.6.2.3 Network Construction and Visualization

A "compound-target" network was constructed by using Cytoscape (node: compound or target, edge: inter-relationship between compound and target). Then, the enrichment analysis was performed by using the DAVID database.

5.6.2.4 Analysis Index and Algorithm

Topological (degree) analysis of "compound-target" network.

5.6.2.5 Experimental Verification

An MIA-induced OA rat model was constructed, and the load-bearing level of hind paw of the mice between the PJE treatment group and the control group was compared, as a measure of OA progression and a reflection of the efficacy of anti-inflammatory compounds. Histopathological analysis: the cartilage degeneration of OA rats was observed to verify whether PJE plays a therapeutic role in the MIA-induced OA rat model; measurement of serum cytokines and inflammatory mediator level: various inflammatory mediators in OA may participate in the pathogenesis. Therefore, this study determined the effects of PJE on serum levels of TNF-α (Tumor Necrosis Factor), IL-6 (Interleukin-6), LTB4 (Leukotriene B4), and 5-LOX (5-Lipoxygenase) in MIA-induced OA model rats. OA is a chronic disease affecting joints. It can promote the emergence of various inflammatory mediators and it is known that cytokine interaction plays a vital role. Therefore, this study determines the effect of PJE on the mRNA expression levels of inflammatory mediators (IL-1β, IL-6, TNF-α, COX-2, and iNOS).

5.6.2.6 Main Conclusion

(1) Through hind paw load-bearing experiments, it was found that on the 7th day after MIA injection, the MIA group showed a significantly lower load-bearing distribution and maintained at this level for at least 21 days. However, in the PJE administration group, load-bearing levels of mice gradually increased and recovered 21 days after MIA injection. The results show that PJE therapy could restore balance and relieve joint discomfort. In addition, histological features show that PJE can reverse cartilage damage caused by MIA injection. In contrast, the levels of IL-6 and LTB4 in the PJE treatment group were lower, and TNF-α and 5-LOX were slightly lower; the mRNA expression levels of inflammatory factors and levels of 5 kinds of inflammatory factors in the MIA group were significantly increased, while the mRNA expression levels of IL-1β, IL-6, COX-2, and iNOS in the PJE treatment group were significantly lower.
(2) To explore the potential active components and targets of PJE, the main ($DC \geq 6$) compound nodes were found through network analysis: Rutin ($DC = 20$), inositol ($DC = 7$), chlorogenic acid ($DC = 6$), and methoxypsoralen ($DC = 6$). In addition, the major targets are CASP3 (Caspase-3, acts with rutin, chlorogenic acid, and isoquercetin), CASP7 (Caspase-3, acts with rutin and chlorogenic acid), and CYP2D6 (Cytochrome P450 Proteins 2D6, acts with methoxypsoralen and alloisoimperarorin). These major compounds and targets may play an important role in the progression of OA.

TCM network pharmacology breaks through the current mainstream R&D thinking of Western medicine, tries to interpret the therapeutic mechanism of TCM from the perspective of system and molecular network balance, and explores the occurrence and development process of complex diseases, to understand the interaction between

TCM ingredients and the organism and guide the discovery of new drugs. TCM network pharmacology represents philosophical ideas and research model transformation in the modernization of TCM, and has made remarkable progress in the above five aspects. Based on existing research, we can find that the direction that is more closely integrated with clinical research is research on TCM syndromes, such as discovering syndrome markers, and the biological basis of "treating the same disease with different methods." The growing trend in research is the exploration of active ingredients and potential mechanism of action of Chinese medicine prescriptions. The research in the direction of new drug development based on TCM can be better integrated with the development of modern new drugs, and at the same time, the R&D of new Chinese medicine is also the fundamental driving force of TCM research. Compared with the first three directions, the research of network pharmacology in ethnic medicine and international traditional medicine is still relatively poor, but it is believed that with the growing recognition of traditional medicine and the in-depth application of modern omics research and complex system research, research in these two directions will continue to grow.

In the past few decades, TCM has focused on the separation of chemical components and the activity detection of chemical components, and has accumulated a lot of information for the development of network pharmacology. Moreover, with the rapid development of modern medicine, people have a more in-depth understanding of single molecular targets and their relationship with diseases and drugs. In addition, the continuous development of high-throughput omics data analysis, computer virtual computing, and artificial intelligence provides support for the in-depth study of the scientific connotation of Chinese medicine from a system perspective.

As an emerging subject integrating multi-disciplinary knowledge and methods, network pharmacology in TCM reveals more complex and systematic scientific laws and modern expression of TCM philosophies, ideas, and laws, rather than just the "single compound-single target-single effect." Both, the research on the mechanism of action of TCM based on network and the R&D of new drugs based on network target represent the new research mode in the modernization of TCM. Network pharmacology in TCM is consistently moving forward with a steady accumulation of relevant data such as diseases and TCM, and with the ongoing development and improvement of network analysis and software, artificial intelligence, machine learning, and other technologies, it will definitely provide more valuable information to reveal the complex disease mechanism and R&D of new TCM drugs. This new model of drug and pharmacology research based on network analysis and network target is going to provide a major breakthrough in the modernization of TCM.

References

1. Li S. Possible association between TCM syndromes and regulatory mechanisms of molecular networks. In: Scientific and technological progress and social and economic development facing the 21st century. Beijing: China Science and Technology Press; 1999. p. 442.
2. Hopkins AL. Network pharmacology. Nat Biotechnol. 2007;25(10):1110–1.
3. Xi D, Bao T, Chen Q, et al. State of the science: cancer complementary and alternative medicine therapeutics research—NCI strategic workshop highlights of discussion report. J Natl Cancer Inst Monogr. 2017;2017(52):62–7.
4. Guo L, Qiao ZL. Interpretation the connotation of the syndrome from the concept of 'state'. Chin J Trad Chin Med Pharm. 2015;30(4):1086–8.
5. Li S, Wang YY, Ji L, et al. A discussion and case study of complexities in traditional Chinese medicine. J Syst Simul. 2002;11:23–5.
6. Xie SP, Zuo G. Thinking of using systems biology to study TCM syndromes. World Chin Med. 2011;6(5):369–71.
7. Li S, Zhang ZQ, Wu LJ, et al. Understanding ZHENG in traditional Chinese medicine in the context of neuro-endocrine-immune network. IET Syst Biol. 2007;1(1):51–60.
8. Zhang YQ, Mao X, Guo QY, et al. Pathway of PPAR-gamma coactivators in thermogenesis: a pivotal traditional Chinese medicine-associated target for individualized treatment of rheumatoid arthritis. Oncotarget. 2016;7(13):15885–900.
9. Liu YM, Wang M, Luo YQ, et al. miRNA-target network analysis identifies potential biomarkers for traditional Chinese medicine (TCM) syndrome development evaluation in hepatitis B caused liver cirrhosis. Sci Rep. 2017;7:11054.
10. Xiu XY, Li J, Lu C, et al. The molecular mechanism of 'herbs-pattern correspondence' in RA with heat pattern based on network pharmacology. Chin J Exp Tradit Med Formulae. 2012;18 (8):299–303.
11. Wang MZ, Chen G, Lu C, et al. Rheumatoid arthritis with deficiency pattern in traditional Chinese medicine shows correlation with cold and hot patterns in gene expression profiles. Evid Based Complement Alternat Med. 2013;2013:248650.
12. Chen QL, Lu YY, Zhang GB, et al. Characteristic analysis from excessive to deficient syndromes in hepatocarcinoma underlying miRNA array data. Evid Based Complement Alternat Med. 2013;2013:324636.
13. Li R, Ma T, Gu J, et al. Imbalanced network biomarkers for traditional Chinese medicine Syndrome in gastritis patients. Sci Rep. 2013;3:1543.
14. Wang X, Wu M, Zheng J, et al. Unveiling the molecular network underlying the Spleen-Qi deficiency syndrome in traditional Chinese medicine and immune functions. Cell Physiol Biochem. 2019;128:724–31.
15. Lu YY, Chen QL, Guan Y, et al. Study of Zheng differentiation in Hepatitis B-caused cirrhosis: a transcriptional profiling analysis. BMC Complement Altern Med. 2014;14:371.
16. Liao JQ, Liu YM, Wang J. Identification of more objective biomarkers for blood-stasis syndrome diagnosis. BMC Complement Altern Med. 2016;16:371.
17. Wang J, Yu G. A systems biology approach to characterize biomarkers for blood stasis syndrome of unstable angina patients by integrating MicroRNA and messenger RNA expression profiling. Evid Based Complement Alternat Med. 2013;2013:510208.
18. Li S. Network targets: an entry point for the network pharmacology research of TCM prescriptions. Chin J Chin Mater Med. 2011;36(15):2017–20.
19. Li S, Zhang B, Zhang N. Network target for screening synergistic drug combinations with application to traditional Chinese medicine. BMC Syst Biol. 2011;5(Suppl 1):S10.
20. Li S, Zhang B, Jiang D, et al. Herb network construction and co-module analysis for uncovering the combination rule of traditional Chinese herbal formulae. BMC Bioinf. 2010;11(Suppl 11):1–12.
21. Liang XJ, Li HY, Li S. A novel network pharmacology approach to analyse traditional herbal formulae: the Liu-Wei-Di-Huang pill as a case study. Mol BioSyst. 2014;10(5):1014–22.

22. Cheng BF, Hou YY, Jiang M, et al. Anti-inflammatory mechanism of Qingfei Xiaoyan Wan studied with network pharmacology. Acta Pharm Sin. 2013;48(5):686–93.
23. Ding F, Zhang QR, Col U, et al. An analysis of chemical ingredients network of Chinese herbal formulae for the treatment of coronary heart disease. PLoS One. 2015;10(2):e0116441.
24. Zhang QR, Yu H, Qi J, et al. Natural formulas and the nature of formulas: exploring potential therapeutic targets based on traditional Chinese herbal formulas. PLoS One. 2017;12(2): e0171628.
25. Zuo HL, Zhang QR, Su SB, et al. A network pharmacology-based approach to analyse potential targets of traditional herbal formulas: an example of Yu Ping Feng decoction. Sci Rep. 2018;8:11418.
26. Fan XH, Zhao XP, Jin YC, et al. Network toxicology and its application to traditional Chinese medicine. Chin J Chin Mater Med. 2011;36(21):2920–2.
27. Fan XH, Cheng YY, Zhang BL. Network formulaology: a new strategy for modern research of traditional Chinese medicine formulae. Chin J Chin Mater Med. 2015;40(1):1–6.
28. Xu HY, Yang HJ. Integrative pharmacology: a new model of modern research on traditional Chinese medicine. Chin J Chin Mater Med. 2014;39(3):357–62.
29. Wang Z, Wang YY. Modular pharmacology: deciphering the interacting structural organization of the targeted networks. Drug Discov Today. 2013;18(11):560–6.
30. Zhang B, Wang X, Li S. An integrative platform of TCM network pharmacology and its application on a herbal formula. Evid Based Complement Alternat Med. 2013;2013:456747.
31. Guo QY, Mao X, Zhang YQ, et al. Guizhi-Shaoyao-Zhimu decoction attenuates rheumatoid arthritis partially by reversing inflammation-immune system imbalance. J Transl Med. 2016;14 (1):1–16.
32. Li XX, Xu X, Wang JN, et al. A system-level investigation into the mechanisms of Chinese traditional medicine: compound danshen formula for cardiovascular disease treatment. PLoS One. 2012;7(9):e43918.
33. Li S, Lu AP, Wang YY, et al. Suppressive effects of a Chinese herbal medicine qing-luo-yin extract on the angiogenesis of collagen-induced arthritis in rats. Am J Chin Med. 2003;31 (5):713–20.
34. Borisy AA, Elliott PJ, Hurst NW, et al. Systematic discovery of multicomponent therapeutics. Proc Natl Acad Sci U S A. 2003;100(13):7977–82.
35. Newman DJ, Cragg GM. Natural products as sources of new drugs over the 30 years from 1981 to 2010. J Nat Prod. 2012;75(3):311–35.
36. Newman DJ, Cragg GM. Natural products as sources of new drugs from 1981 to 2014. J Nat Prod. 2016;79(3):629–61.
37. Wang JG, Zhang CJ, Chia WN, et al. Haem-activated promiscuous targeting of artemisinin in Plasmodium falciparum. Nat Commun. 2015;6:10111.
38. Wang LL, Li Z, Shao Q, et al. Dissecting active ingredients of Chinese medicine by content-weighted ingredient–target network. Mol BioSyst. 2014;10(7):1905–11.
39. Wang JH, Lei X, Cheng XR, et al. LW-AFC, a new formula derived from Liuwei Dihuang decoction, ameliorates behavioral and pathological deterioration via modulating the neuroendocrine-immune system in PrP-hA beta PPswe/PS1(Delta E9) transgenic mice. Alzheimers Res Ther. 2016;8:15.
40. Yang K, Zhang RS, He LY, et al. Multistage analysis method for detection of effective herb prescription from clinical data. Front Med. 2018;12(2):206–17.
41. Fang JS, Cai CP, Chai YT, et al. Quantitative and systems pharmacology 4. Network-based analysis of drug pleiotropy on coronary artery disease. Eur J Med Chem. 2019;161:192–204.
42. Zheng JH, Wu M, Wang HY, et al. Network pharmacology to unveil the biological basis of health-strengthening herbal medicine in cancer treatment. Cancer. 2018;10(11):1–23.
43. Gao K, Yang R, Zhang P, et al. Effects of Qijian mixture on type 2 diabetes assessed by metabonomics, gut microbiota and network pharmacology. Pharmacol Res. 2018;130:93–109.

44. Wang XJ, Zhang AH, Wang P, et al. Metabolomics coupled with proteomics advancing drug discovery toward more agile development of targeted combination therapies. Mol Cell Proteomics. 2013;12(5):1226–38.
45. Gu JY, Li Q, Chen LR, et al. Platelet aggregation pathway network-based approach for evaluating compounds efficacy. Evid Based Complement Alternat Med. 2013;2013:425707.
46. Zheng CS, Wu YS, Bao HJ, et al. Understanding the polypharmacological anticancer effects of Xiao Chai Hu Tang via a computational pharmacological model. Exp Ther Med. 2014;7 (6):1777–83.
47. Patwardhan B, Gautam M. Botanical immunodrugs: scope and opportunities. Drug Discov Today. 2005;10(7):495–502.
48. Li S, WU L J, Zhang Z Q. Constructing biological networks through combined literature mining and microarray analysis: a LMMA approach. Bioinformatics. 2006;22:2143–50.
49. van Driel MA, Bruggeman J, Vriend G, et al. A text-mining analysis of the human phenome. Eur J Hum Genet. 2006;14(5):535–42.
50. Su X, Li YP, Jiang M, et al. Systems pharmacology uncover the mechanism of anti-non-small cell lung cancer for Hedyotis diffusa Willd. Biomed Pharmacother. 2019;109:969–84.
51. Zang J, Ma SZ, Wang CZ, et al. Screening for active constituents in Turkish galls against ulcerative colitis by mass spectrometry guided preparative chromatography strategy: in silico, in vitro and in vivo study. Food Funct. 2018;9(10):5124–38.
52. Zhang QR, Zhong ZF, Sang W, et al. Comparative comprehension on the anti-rheumatic Chinese herbal medicine Siegesbeckiae Herba: Combined computational predictions and experimental investigations. J Ethnopharmacol. 2019;228:200–9.
53. Gómez-Verjan JC, Rivero-Segura NA, Estrella-Parra E, et al. Network pharmacology uncovers anticancer activity of mammea-type coumarins from calophyllum brasiliense. Planta Med. 2018;85(01):14–23.
54. Chun MJ, Lee YA, Kim SJ, et al. Protective effects of peucedanum japonicum extract against osteoarthritis in an animal model using a combined systems approach for compound-target prediction. Nutrients. 2018;10(6):754.
55. Yang YF, Li Y, Wang JH, et al. Systematic investigation of Ginkgo biloba leaves for treating cardio-cerebrovascular diseases in an animal model. ACS Chem Biol. 2017;12(5):1363–72.

Chapter 6
Network Pharmacology and Modern Drug R&D Cases

Weidong Zhang and Jing Zhao

6.1 Guide to this Chapter

Drug discovery has predominantly followed the concept of "one drug, one target, one disease" for an extended period, case in point, to design chemical entities that can specifically bind to one key target related to a specific disease [1]. Collateral pharmacology aims to develop drugs that earmark multiple proteins or networks connected to diseases. It also demonstrates the possibility of finding multi-target and multi-component drugs that earmark disease-related networks at the system level [2]. Network pharmacology research integrates the data of various public databases, high-throughput screening (HTS), genome-wide association studies (GWAS), and large-scale omics (such as genomics, transcriptomics, metabonomics, and proteomics) to construct a network prediction or inference model. The analysis of the complex biological pathways influenced by drug therapy at different biological levels (molecules, cells, tissues, organs, and phenotypes) has given a boost to cognition of the biological mechanisms of complex diseases, the systemic mechanism of the impact of drugs, and the development of multi-target, multi-component drugs. This chapter selects some exceptional results of network pharmacology in the R&D and application of modern drugs in recent years, and analyzes the results from the dimensions of research purpose, data source, analysis index and algorithm, analysis results, experimental verification, and main conclusion, as a means to introduce the principal research contents, ideas, and procedures of frontier research in network pharmacology, for readers.

W. Zhang (✉)
The Second Military Medical University, Shanghai, China

J. Zhao
Shanghai University of Traditional Chinese Medicine, Shanghai, China

S. Li (ed.), *Network Pharmacology*, https://doi.org/10.1007/978-981-16-0753-0_6

6.2 Internal Mechanism and Intervention Targets of Complex Diseases

The incidence and progress of complex diseases are not only caused by changes in a single gene or protein, but are related to a series of interacting genes or proteins. Therefore, in their research and treatment, one must not only consider the function of a single gene, but also the interactions between genes or gene products. The network pharmacology method has inevitably become a powerful tool for the study of complex diseases and their intervention targets. These methods are chiefly based on the "Guilt-by-Association" principle [3], particularly the pathogenic genes of the same or related diseases are interrelated in function, hence their positions in biological networks are adjacent and close, and they are similar in network topology.

One of the most important aspects of the research of complex diseases is the prediction of disease-related genes. The local similarity and global similarity between candidate genes and known disease genes on the network, functional similarity between genes, and phenotypic similarity between diseases are all employed in the design of prediction algorithms. For example, the CIPHER algorithm proposed by Wu et al. defined phenotypic similarity vector and gene proximity vector, and utilized the consistency score of these two vectors to predict the disease genes [4]; Lin et al. integrated phenotypic similarity information with PPI background network to construct a phenotypic-specific network as the background network for prediction, and then the topological similarity and functional similarity of the network between genes were combined using the gravity-similar indexes to predict disease genes [5].

A variety of data that constitute genome, transcriptome, and proteome are integrated with several diverse mathematical models and calculation procedures. The establishment of regulatory networks related to complex diseases and the identification of key regulatory genes are important to deduce the mechanism of complex diseases and to subsequently develop corresponding drugs. For example, Zhang et al. constructed a molecular network of LOAD by using the genome-wide gene expression profile and genotyping data obtained from hundreds of patients with Late-Onset Alzheimer's Disease (LOAD) and 1647 autopsy brain tissue samples from non-dementia subjects. This resulted in the discovery of several distinct functional categories and cell-specific modules, many of which displayed an enormous reconstruction effect on LOAD brains. They applied a comprehensive network-based procedure to grade the correlation between these modules and LOAD pathology, and used Bayesian inference to identify the key causal regulators in these networks [6]. Mani et al. proposed the Interactome Dysregulation Enrichment Analysis (IDEA) algorithm [7] to identify the carcinogenic lesions of lymphoma. This procedure initially integrated different types of experimental and predicted molecular interactions to construct a "priori" network model of B cells. Subsequently, the gene expression profiles of B cell populations from patients with lymphoma and B cell populations from normal people were used to calculate the differences in gene co-regulation between the two expression profile data sets.

Mutual information indicators were used to identify ill-adjusted signal pathways in the disease.

Diseases are typically classified according to the physiological system they affect and the phenotypic symptoms they exhibit. At the molecular level, on account of possessing identical disease-causing genes, their mutual association, or their involvement in common biological processes, diseases with distinct phenotypes may lead to comorbidities. Network-based disease research helps to ascertain the interconnection between different diseases at the molecular level, understand the relationship between diseases at the molecular level, improve the level of disease diagnosis and treatment, and accelerate the progress of drug development. For example, Menche et al. used the method of network analysis to find that the network position of the disease module determines its pathobiological relationship with other diseases. Diseases with network module overlap show significant symptom similarities and comorbidities, while diseases separated by network module are clinically different types of diseases [8].

The following two specific research cases are selected for analysis.

6.2.1 Transcription Factor POU3F2 Regulates the Gene Co-expression Networks in the Brain Tissues of Patients With Mental Disorders

Schizophrenia (SCZ) and Bipolar Disorder (BD) are complex mental disorders and are associated with the dysfunctions of multiple gene expressions. However, the related procurable facts are minimal. Precursory research has reported anomalies in the gene expression network in brain tissue of postmortem patients with SCZ or BD. However, this research is predominantly related to networks with single dimension, which cannot analyze the driving nodes in the network module, or the regulatory relationship. A majority of the research results are expressed as the correlation between genes rather than the causal relationship of gene regulation.

In this research, multi-dimensional data sets were integrated to construct a genome-wide co-expression network comprising microRNA (miRNA), and a co-expression module with differential expression in the brain tissue of patients was identified [9]. The module comprised genes that are primarily involved in the generation of glial and nerve cells and the differentiation of glial cells, which incorporates schizophrenia-risk genes that carry atypical mutations. By means of network analysis and experimental verification, it was established that POU3F2 is the primary regulatory factor of the co-expression network module, which plays a crucial role in the incidence and progress of psychiatric disorders.

6.2.1.1 Research Objective

Based on the hypothesis that co-expression means co-regulation and that the hub genes in the co-expression module are likely to be the key regulating factors of gene co-expression, this study integrated the genotype, mRNA, and miRNA data from brain tissue samples from patients with SCZ and BD, searched transcription factors and miRNAs as hub nodes in disease-related co-expression modules, and substantiated the predicted regulatory relationship by virtue of experimental verification.

6.2.1.2 Data Source

Data Set Discovery

The tissue samples of Parietal Cortex (PC) were from the Stanley Medical Research Institute (SMRI) and Neuropathology Consortium and Array Collections [10], containing SCZ, BD, and control samples. Excluding the non-European, duplicate, the missing mRNA, miRNA, or genotyping data samples, a total of 75 samples were procured, including 51 disease samples and 24 control samples.

Duplicate Data Set

A total of 2 duplicate data sets: the gene chip data GSE15745 in GEO, including 138 samples of Frontal Cortex Tissue (FCTX) from normal nervous system in Caucasians, and RNA-seq data from BrainGVEX dataset of PsychENCODE [11], including samples from SMRI, were used. After removing duplicate samples, 70 SCZ, 48 BD, and 63 control samples were procured.

6.2.1.3 Analysis Index and Algorithm

Module Construction and Maintaining Statistics

Weighted gene co-expression network analysis (WGCNA) method was used to identify mRNA and miRNA with related expression patterns [12]. The correlation matrix was calculated for all possible node pairs (mRNA and miRNA), and the power value was 6, so that the network constructed by the correlation matrix had a scale-free network topology. The minimum module size was set to 30 and a co-expression network with double-weighted median correlation was constructed. The dynamic tree cutting algorithm was used to identify the network module, in which the parameter mergeCutHeight was 0.05, and deepSplit was 2. WGCNA and dynamic tree cutting algorithm were executed using the corresponding packages of R language. The unsigned network was used to represent the negative regulatory relationship between miRNA and mRNA. The Cytoscape software was used for network visualization.

As the sample size was relatively small, two other duplicate data sets were used to evaluate the module retention. The verification dataset contained samples from BrainGVEX and GSE15745. $Z_{summary}$ was used to test and evaluate the module retention between expression profile datasets. The recommended threshold value is: $Z_{summary} < 2$ is no proof of module retention; $2 < Z_{summary} < 10$ is weak to moderate evidence; $Z_{summary} > 10$ is strong evidence of module retention.

Network Edge Orienting (NEO) Analysis of miRNA Interactions of Transcriptional Factors

In addition to combining information, the modified NEO analysis was used to investigate the causal relationship between transcriptional factors and miRNAs [13]. The input data were the expression data of transcriptional factors and miRNAs, as well as genotype data. NEO analysis uses the likelihood degree of local structural equation model to integrate selected features and markers, to evaluate the causal relationship between related variables. The output was the edge orientation score of the local structure. Genotype data of eQTL containing transcriptional factors and miRNAs from the analysis of SMRI samples, GTEx portal site, CommonMind Consortium, and UK Brain Expression Consortium were selected. A total of 901 SNPs were included in the NEO analysis. The CPA model was used to test the edge orientation of a single marker, and the OCA model was used to test multiple genetic markers. The likelihood-based CPA score was used to evaluate whether the selected model produces a higher likelihood than the alternative model. According to the software, the threshold value is 0.8, which means that the model likelihood score of the causal model is $10^{0.8} = 6.3$ times higher than that of the next best model. For the OCA score, the threshold value is 0.3 according to the software, which means that the model likelihood score of the causal model is $10^{0.3} = 2$ times higher than that of the next best model.

6.2.1.4 Analysis Result

Identify Disease-Related miRNA and mRNA Co-expression Network Modules

First, mRNA and miRNA expression in PC tissue samples from SMRI were analyzed using WGCNA. Diseases (including SCZ and BD) were combined with control samples to construct a co-expression network, and a total of 46 co-expression modules were found. After correcting for the influence of gender, age, brain tissue pH, RNA integrity number, and death interval, a disease-associated module (daM) was found. The module contained 5 miRNAs and 545 genes. DAVID enrichment analysis revealed that these genes were enriched in three biological processes: glial formation, glial cell differentiation, and neurogenesis.

Module Retention in an Independent Data Set

Two independent duplicate data sets were used to test the module retention of daM. $Z_{summary} = 36.8$ between the daM of SMRI's PC tissue sample data and the FCTX sample data of GSE15745, and $Z_{summary} = 10.9$ between the FCTX sample data of the BrainGVEX database. The results show that the genes and connection relationships in daM were well maintained in different data sets.

Enrichment of Genetic Variation Associated with SCZ or BD in daM

Whether the genes in daM are genetically related to SCZ or BD was tested. For genetic variation, the test focused on the common or rare single nucleotide variation and copy number variation (CNV). For common variations, MAGMA [14] and INRICH [15] were used to detect the enrichment of genes in daM in Genome-Wide Association Study (GWAS) of SCZ or BD, but no significant enrichment was detected. For rare variations, based on the data from two exome sequencing studies [16, 17] and data from the NPdenovo database [18], using hypergeometric method, it was found that the genes in daM were significantly enriched in these three data sets. When the data of the three data sets are merged, the gene enrichment in daM is more significant.

Potential Key Regulatory Factors and Their Roles in daM

This section involved the research on the transcriptional factors and miRNAs that may be major regulatory factors in daM and involved the study of their functional roles. There were five miRNAs in daM: hsa-miR-585, hsa-miR-320b, hsa-miR-320c, hsa-miR-320d, and hsamiR-320e, as well as 6 transcriptional factors: POU3F2, EPAS1, PAX6, ZNF423, SOX5, and SOX9 (as shown in Fig. 6.1).

This network shows all mRNA, miRNAs and their co-expression in daM. Six transcriptional factors (POU3F2, PAX6, EPAS1, ZNF423, SOX5, and SOX9), their targets, and the names of five miRNAs are shown in the figure. The other genes are represented by dots. Six transcriptional factors and their corresponding targets are shown in six boxes with different colors.

In this module, 87.3% of the mRNA expression was negatively correlated with the miRNA in it, indicating that the regulation of miRNA on transcription was achieved by directly downregulating their mRNA target genes. The most connected node in the module is miR-320e, which connects 68 nodes.

Using the transcriptional factor binding information provided by the studies done by Fuxman [19] and Kheradpour [20], it was found that the six transcriptional factors

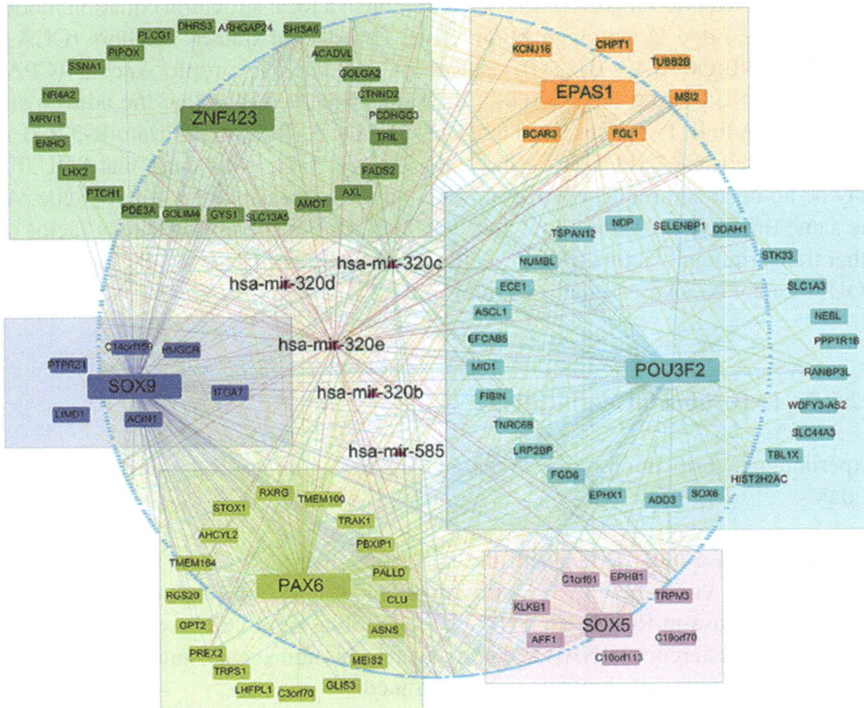

Fig. 6.1 Transcriptional factors and their targets in daM [9]

in daM have a total of 101 targets in the module, among which POU3F2 has the most potential targets in the module, a total of 26, including transcriptional factors PAX6 and SOX9. Other transcriptional factors EPAS1, PAX6, ZNF423, and SOX9 have 9, 21, 24, 10, and 11 potential targets, respectively, in the module.

Causal Relationship Between Key Regulatory Factors in daM

Whether transcriptional factors are the upstream or downstream regulators of miRNA, or whether they are regulated by other transcriptional factors was detected by integrating genetic markers. The NEO method was used to infer the causal relationship between the related nodes (i.e., miRNA, transcriptional factors, and their targets). As the main interest lies in the causal relationship between five miRNAs and six transcriptional factors, only miRNA Quantitative Trait Locus (miQTL) signals associated with five miRNAs and expression QTLs (eQTL) signals associated with six transcriptional factors were used here. Among the five miRNAs, only hsamiR-320e had significant miQTL signals ($P < 0.05$, FDR $q < 0.05$), hence, this miRNA and six transcriptional factors were selected to identify the regulatory direction.

An improved NEO method was used to establish a local structural equation model to obtain the Edge Orienting fraction. If the Orthogonal Causal Anchors (OCAs) meet LEO.NB.OCA(A→B) > 0.3 and the Candidate Pleiotropic Anchor (CPA) meets LEO.NB.CPA(A→B) > 0.8 at the same time, it means that the adjustment direction is A to B. If it is observed that LEO.NB.OCA (POU3F2→hsamiR-320e) = 0.526, LEO.NB.CPA (POU3F2→hsa-miR-320e) = 1.55, it indicates that POU3F2 may be an upstream regulatory factor affecting the expression of hsa-miR-320e. At the same time, NEO results show that POU3F2 is an upstream regulatory factor of other transcriptional factors (PAX6, ZNF423, and SOX9). These results suggest that POU3F2 may be a key regulatory factor in daM.

6.2.1.5 Experimental Verification

Experimental Verification of the Potential Causal Regulatory Relationship in daM

POU3F2 and hsa-miR-320e are in the hub position in daM. Here, this suggested relationship is confirmed by in vitro experiments. The expression changes of POU3F2 and hsa-miR-320e in SH-SY5Y neuroblastoma cells were induced by using RNA interference (RNAi) and gene overexpression agents, and the expression changes of their predicted targets were examined.

After conducting RNA interference in SH-SY5Y, the expression of POU3F2 decreased by 41%, while the expression of hsa-miR-320e increased by 170%. In the overexpression experiment, the expression of POU3F2 increased nearly 10 times ($P < 0.001$), while the expression of hsa-miR-320e decreased significantly by 33%. In the case where hsa-miR-320e was knocked out, the expression of hsa-miR-320e reduced by 33%, but the expression of POU3F2 was not affected; overexpression of hsa-miR-320e (increased by 120%) did not change the expression of POU3F2. These in vitro experiment results confirm that POU3F2 is an upstream regulatory factor of hsa-miR-320e.

Effects of POU3F2 on Proliferation and Differentiation of Neural Progenitor Cells

After knocking out POU3F2 in human neural progenitor cells (NPC), it was found that the proliferation rate from EdU+ cells (5-ethynyl-2′-deoxyuridine; a marker of proliferating cells) to DAPI+ cells (4′,6-Diamidino-2-phenylindole; a live cell marker) significantly increased. Next, the differentiation of NPC to neurons was analyzed, and it was found that the ratio of Tuj1+ cells (a marker of immature neurons) and MAP2+ cells (a marker of mature neurons) significantly reduced. These results indicate that knocking out POU3F2 can promote the proliferation ability of NPC and inhibit NPC differentiation into neurons.

To study how POU3F2 affects the cell proliferation and differentiation abilities, the expression changes of POU3F2 in six predicted targets (SOX9, PAX6, ZNF423, NOTCH2, CLU, and TRIM8) in daM were examined after POU3F2 was knocked out or overexpressed. It was found that the expression of SOX9, ZNF423, NOTCH2, CLU, and TRIM8 decreased significantly after POU3F2 knockout; and their expression increased significantly after POU3F2 was overexpressed. The expression of PAX6 did not increase significantly after overexpression of POU3F2, indicating that it may not be regulated by POU3F2 in the NPC model.

6.2.1.6 Main Conclusion

Starting from the transcriptome data of neurological diseases, this study constructed a gene co-expression network. A disease-related module containing 5 miRNAs and 545 mRNAs was identified from the network, among which 6 transcriptional factors were the central genes of the module. The genes in the module were enriched in the three biological processes: glial formation, glial cell differentiation, and neurogenesis. Integrating a variety of data, and through network analysis, it was found that the central node in this module—the transcriptional factor POU3F2—can regulate miRNA hsa-miR-320e and other predicted target mRNAs. In vitro experiments and gene knockout verified the regulatory effects of POU3F2 on hsa-miR-320e and the other five predicted targets, and confirmed the influence of POU3F2 on the proliferation and differentiation of neural progenitor cells. These results indicate that POU3F2 plays a key role in the occurrence and development of neurological diseases.

6.2.2 *Network-Based CRISPR-Cas9 Combinatorial Screening and Recognition of Synergistic Modules in Human Cells*

Tumorigenesis is a complex biological process driven by a series of genes and environmental factors. Inflammation-induced tumorigenesis (IIT), i.e. inflammation-mediated cancer transformation, is the main driving factor of tumorigenesis. It is rarely caused by a single gene mutation, but by the disturbance of a complex gene network. A thorough understanding of the functional network of IIT is essential for preventing the occurrence of inflammation-mediated cancer transformation, especially for early diagnosis. However, so far there have not been any effective methods to do so.

In this study, Li et al. proposed a comprehensive network-based strategy to systematically discover the functional synergistic modules [21] that play a decisive role in IIT. This method first integrated experimental and computational methods to predict candidate genes related to IIT in the whole genome. On this basis, a differential gene interaction network of IIT was constructed using TGFβ1-induced colon epithelial cell transformation model, combined with a new combination CRISPR-Cas9 screening strategy. In addition, the differential gene interaction of opposite IIT in the network was identified—synergistic promotion and inhibition. The synergistic promotion is mainly caused by the loss of immune and metabolic modules, and the synergistic inhibition is mainly induced by the loss of proliferation and immune modules or proliferation and metabolism modules. These results help to understand the possible early combination targets and biomarkers of IIT, especially the synergistic effects among immune, proliferative, and metabolic modules.

6.2.2.1 Research Objective

Identifying the functional networks that drive IIT, especially the transformation from inflammation to cancer associated with colitis, is the main focus of current cancer research. This study combines the experimental method with the network-based computing method to systematically discover the functional synergistic modules that plays a decisive role in IIT.

6.2.2.2 Data Source

Collection of Genes Associated with IIT:

(1) Using the CIPHER method [4], the top 100 candidate disease genes of inflammatory bowel disease (Inflammatory Bowel Disease 1, IBD1; OMIM ID 266600) and colorectal cancer (Colorectal Cancer, CRC; OMIM ID 114500) were predicted.
(2) Among the candidate genes selected using CIPHER, 59 genes were selected in the following 12 KEGG signaling pathways linking inflammation and cancer: [1] Inflammatory bowel disease [IBD]; [2] RAS signaling pathway; [3] Toll-like receptor signaling pathway; [4] NF-kappa B signaling pathway; [5] JAK-STAT signaling pathway; [6] HIF-1 signaling pathway; [7] PPAR signaling pathway; [8] MAPK signaling pathway; [9] TGF-beta signaling pathway; [10] mTOR signaling pathway; [11] TNF signaling pathway; and [12] PI3K-Akt signaling pathway.
(3) Thirty candidate genes were manually collected from the literature.
(4) From the gene expression data set GSE4183 of the GEO (Gene Expression Omnibus) database, a total of 38 differentially expressed genes were collected from IBD compared to normal tissues, and CRC compared to normal tissues.

Combining the genes collected from (1) to (4), a total of 84 non-repetitive genes were collected, which are the candidate genes related to IIT.

Design and Synthesis of sgRNA

For each of the 84 candidate genes associated with inflammation-mediated cancer transformation, three sgRNA targets were designed to target inflammation-mediated cancer transformation by using the CRISPR-era sgRNA design tool. At the same time, 20 negative control sgRNA without targeting human genomic loci were designed.

6.2.2.3 Analysis Index and Network Construction

Research Process

As shown in Fig. 6.2.

Construction of Gene Co-expression Network

The GEO database was searched to obtain gene expression data of three tissues (colon, stomach, and liver), and these expression data were used to construct a gene co-expression network among 84 candidate genes related to IIT.

Then, enrichment analysis of GO and KEGG pathways was conducted. Significant overexpression pathways include signal transduction and immune system-related signaling pathways, such as sphingolipid signaling pathway and chemokine

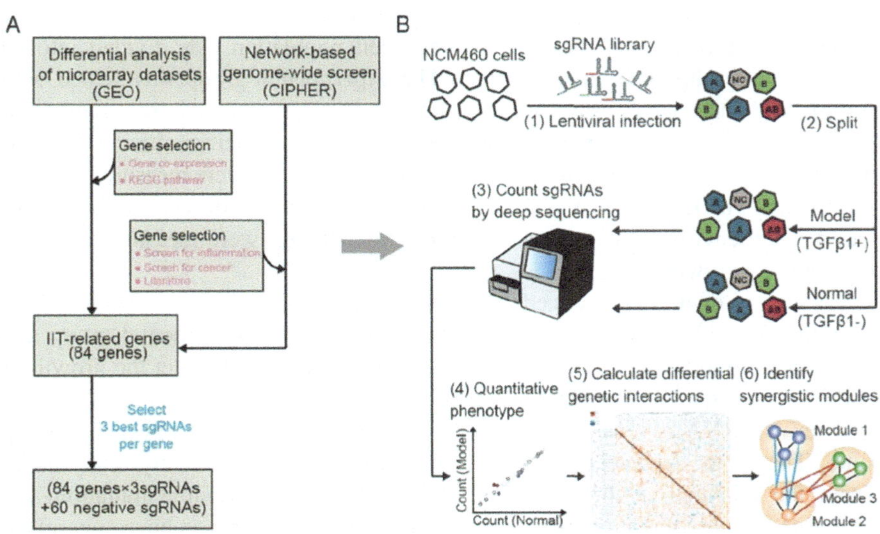

Fig. 6.2 Process of identifying system policies for synergistic modules [21]. (**a**) Prediction of genes related to IIT based on data and network; (**b**) a new CRISPR-Cas9 combination screening strategy for identifying synergistic modules

signaling pathway. Enriched GO items include cell cycle related items, such as positive regulation of cell proliferation, programmed cell death, cell differentiation, and metabolic and immune related items, such as positive regulation of cell metabolism process, positive regulation of cytokine production, positive regulation of immune response, inflammatory response. To sum up, there were two significantly enriched modules in the gene co-expression network of the colon, namely immune process and metabolic process. Here, the module identified using Pearson's correlation coefficient analysis corresponds to the function-related gene clusters.

Determining the Differential Gene Interaction Network by Using Double Knockout Technique Based on CRISPR

To study the 84 kinds of candidate genes that are crucial to IIT, a differential gene interaction network (Genetic Interaction Network) was established using the CRISPR-based double knockout method.

To determine the new genes involved in IIT and their functional relationships, a CRISPR-based double knockout method was used to perform functional screening of the NCM460 cell line, and an inflammation-related cancer cell model was used to simulate the cell transformation phenomenon of colonic epithelial cell malignant proliferation caused by IBD [22]. This screening measured all possible interactions among 104 genes (including 84 candidate genes and 20 negative control genes). To confirm the role of 84 candidate genes in IIT, a double sgRNA was used to knock out all possible interactions in NCM460 cells, and a differential Genetic Interaction map (dGImap) of these genes was constructed to reveal their functional relationship. The sgRNA lentivirus library was used to infect a modified NCM460 cell line, to stably express cas9 protein, and then the obtained cell population was divided into an experimental group and a control group. The experimental group was treated with TGFβ1, and the control group was not treated. After the cells were cultured for 10 days, two groups of cell populations were collected, and their genomic DNA was extracted. Next, the counts of different sgRNA combinations were measured by deep sequencing. The number of viable cells under normal condition and in the inflammatory microenvironment induced by TGFβ1 for 10 days were measured to determine the cell growth rate.

The cell growth rate induced by TGFβ1 was evaluated by ρ value, which quantifies the difference of cell growth rate between the experimental group and the control group [23, 24]. If the presence of TGFβ1 does not affect the growth of sgRNA, its ρ value is 0; if sgRNA gives TGFβ1-induced cell growth, it has a positive ρ value; if sgRNA is sensitive to TGFβ1-induced cell growth, it has a negative ρ value. Then, the sequencing data was standardized and statistically analyzed to obtain the quantitative difference GI score (DGI) of the double mutation. An accelerated double mutation growth rate shows that the two genes have synergistic effect, and the dGI score is positive; on the contrary, the inhibition of growth rate after double mutation shows that the two genes have antagonistic effect, and their dGI score is negative. The differential genetic interaction network of the 84 genes contains the quantitative DGI scores of a total of 7056 gene pairs. By analyzing the distribution of dGI scores, the gene pairs satisfying $dGI < -0.84$ or $dGI > 1.11$ were selected as having extremely significant interactions, and 39 positive gene pairs and 45 negative gene pairs with significant differences were identified, which revealed the significant differences between TGFβ1-induced and normal colon epithelial cells.

Exploring Specific Mechanisms of IIT Through Different Interaction Modes

To identify significantly different gene interaction patterns (as shown in Fig. 6.3a), the authors constructed a significantly different gene interaction network (as shown in Fig. 6.3b) based on the previously determined differential genetic interaction relationships. The network consists of 63 gene interactions among 84 candidate genes. To determine the correlation between different interaction patterns and the specific mechanisms of IIT, functional enrichment analysis of the 63 genes was performed. It was found that these genes were mainly enriched in three pathways of IIT: namely immune related pathways (such as innate immune response, positive regulation of immune response, immune system development), metabolic pathways (such as positive regulation of cellular metabolic process, positive regulation of macromolecular metabolism, positive regulation of nitrogen compound metabolism), and proliferation related pathways (such as positive regulation of cell proliferation).

There are reports in literature that the possibility of differential genetic interaction between genes in different modules is greater than that between genes in the same

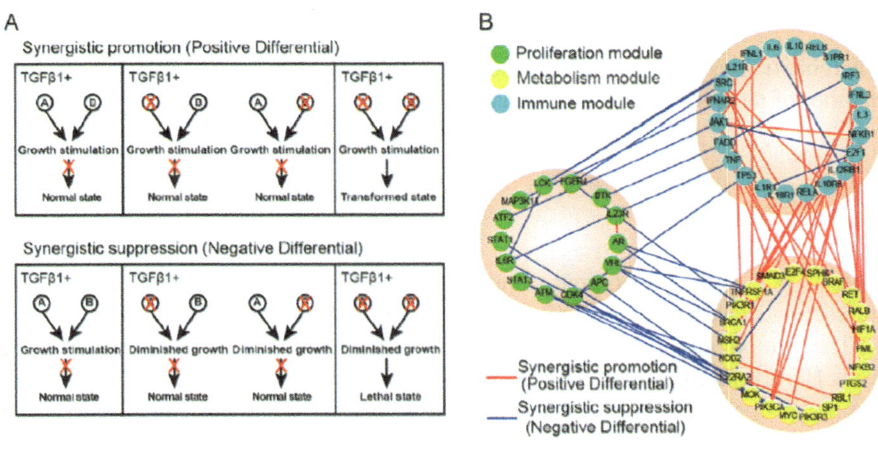

Fig. 6.3 Modularization of differential genetic interaction network [21]. (**a**) The differential genetic interaction network was constructed by analyzing the differences of cell growth rate between single mutation and double mutation. (**b**) Differential genetic interaction network. The network includes positive interaction (red edge) and negative interaction (blue edge) of differences, in which the modules are divided according to the biological processes involved by genes in the network

module [25]. Therefore, the authors carried out a correlation analysis between biological processes and differential genetic interactions, and found that the differential genetic interactions are enriched among modules, indicating that the differential genetic interactions between these biological functional modules are reprogrammed after inflammatory stimulation (as shown in Fig. 6.3b). Based on this analysis, a functional network was constructed to show the differential genetic interactions among biological functional modules after inflammatory stimulation (as shown in Fig. 6.3b). This network shows that there are three kinds of module combinations that strongly affect IIT, i.e., the synergistic effects between proliferation and immune modules or between proliferation and metabolism modules can inhibit the process of IIT, and the synergistic effects between the metabolic and immune modules can promote the occurrence of IIT. Therefore, the interactions between immune and proliferation modules, or between metabolism and proliferation modules, provide possible targets for the occurrence of early IIT, whereas the interactions between immune and metabolic modules may be an early biomarker for the risk of IIT (as shown in Fig. 6.3b).

Prediction of Drugs Intervening in IIT Based on Synergistic Module

Given compound *k*, the following formula was used to calculate the drug score *DS* for the differential Genetic Interaction of IIT:

$$DS(k) = \sum_{i=1}^{N} K(i)S(i,k)$$

wherein *S(i, k)* is the drug CIPHER score of compound *k* to target *i*, and *N* is the total number of targets. *K(i)* is calculated as follows:

$$K(i) = \sum_{j=1}^{M} \rho(j) dGI(i,j)$$

wherein $\rho(j)$ is the phenotypic value of gene *j*, *dGI(i, j)* is the differential Genetic Interaction score between gene *i* and gene *j*, and *M* is the total number of genes.

The compounds in Liuwei Dihuang pill compound prescription were obtained from HerbBioMap, a Chinese medicine database. For each compound, the target profile was predicted with drugCIPHER, and its drug score was calculated for the differential genetic interaction of IIT. The drug scores were sorted from high to low, and the top four compounds quercetin, isorhamnetin, kaempferol, and resveratrol, which are the predicted drugs used for intervention in IIT, were selected.

6.2.2.4 Experimental Verification

Experimental Verification of the Differential Genetic Interaction Relationships

To assess the quality of differential genetic interactions determined by sgRNA, RNA interference (shRNA) was used to confirm the phenotype based on screening. Experiments confirmed that when used in combination with corresponding sgRNA pairs, three specific shRNA pairs targeting MYC-CDK4, IL6R-TNF, and PIK3CA-NFKB1 lead to synergistic changes in cell growth. Similarly, sgRNA pairs and shRNA pairs that simultaneously target these three specific gene pairs show similar synergistic or antagonistic effects. These results indicate that the differential genetic interactions detected in this study indeed capture the underlying molecular basis of IIT.

Experimental Verification of Drugs that Intervene in IIT

Cell viability analysis (MTT assay) was used to evaluate the inhibitory effects of the four compounds that are predicted for TGFβ1-induced colonic epithelial cells (NCM460). Four compounds (quercetin, kaempferol, isorhamnetin, and resveratrol) were observed to inhibit the occurrence of IIT, with IC50 values of 64.79, 139.9, 232.4, and 464 μM, respectively. These results indicate that the computational analysis of this study can predict the compounds that mitigate IIT.

6.2.2.5 Main Conclusion

This study first integrated a variety of data sources and prediction methods to obtain 84 candidate genes related to IIT. Then, the differential genetic interaction network among 63 candidate genes was constructed using the TGFβ1-induced cell transformation model and combined CRISPR-Cas9 screening strategy. It was found that these 63 genes are mainly enriched in three biological pathways: immunity, proliferation, and metabolism, and the interaction between genes was mainly enriched between different modules: the interactions between proliferation and immune modules or between proliferation and metabolism modules were mainly negative, that is, the interaction that inhibits IIT; and the interactions between metabolism and immunity modules were mainly positive, that is, the interaction that promotes IIT. On this basis, it is predicted that quercetin, kaempferol, isorhamnetin, and resveratrol in the compound prescription of Liuwei Dihuang pills can inhibit the occurrence of IIT, and the prediction is confirmed with cell survival rate analysis. This work has deepened the understanding of the potential mechanism by which inflammation increases the risk of malignant transformation of cells and has important significance for the identification of related biomarkers and the development of related drugs.

6.3 Systemic Mechanism of Action of Drugs

Network pharmacology studies the effects of small molecules on molecular networks by using the network method to elucidate the mechanism of action and determine new therapies. In addition to the targets that directly interact with drugs, known as on-target, and are direct targets for drug indications, there are also off-targets, since other unforeseen targets exist that interact directly with drugs. When the drug acts on these direct targets, its effects on target proteins spread to other proteins through intracellular signal transmission, resulting in a series of physiological reactions. Due to the complex interactions between disease-related genes and proteins, the effects of drugs on targets spread to other proteins through signal transmission and interaction between genes and proteins. These molecular networks have thus become a powerful tool for studying the mechanism of action of drugs on the human body.

In studies, various molecular networks (such as transcriptional regulatory network, gene co-expression network, protein interaction network, signal network, drug association network, etc.) have been constructed based on experimental data, databases, and literature mining. Then corresponding algorithms are designed to analyze the effects of diseases and drugs on molecular networks and signal pathways, as well as the relationship between drug targets and disease genes in molecular networks. This helps in inferring the effects of drugs on diseases and the mechanisms of drug action. The CMAP (Connectivity Map) online platform is widely used for network-based drug research [26, 27]. This platform searches for disease–gene–drug relationships based on the similarity of gene expression profiles. The CMAP database contains several gene expression profiles of human cell lines treated with drugs or bioactive compounds. Users can compare gene expression profiles after drug treatment in the database, and find compounds with similar effects at the transcriptional level to infer the effects of the drug under study, using the online software tool provided by CMAP. For example, Iwata et al. proposed a strategy to study the mechanism of action (MoA) of small bioactive molecules based on gene expression profiles and identified the signal pathways of activation and inhibition of small molecules based on the gene expression profile of 16,268 small molecules acting on 68 human cell lines. Targets and new indications of small molecules were predicted based on the latest version of CMap, namely L1000 v1 [27]. Some of the predicted results were verified using in vitro cell tests [28].

The following two specific research cases are selected for analysis.

6.3.1 Network-Based Computational Drug Efficacy Screening

Currently, drug development is expensive and the number of new drug approvals has decreased significantly. Drug development tends to shift from focusing on individual genes that carry diseases, to changes in disease mechanisms at the network level. Therefore, there is a greater demand for developing newer low-cost and higher efficiency methods based on networks, for drug-target identification and drug efficacy prediction.

In this study, Barabasi et al. developed a network-based method. In the human protein–protein interaction network, a network proximity index was used to quantify the distance relationship between drug targets and disease proteins. This index is helpful to reveal therapeutic effects of drugs and distinguish palliative treatment from effective drugs [29].

6.3.1.1 Research Objectives

Recent studies have shown that genes associated with the same disease cluster in the same region of the network to form a disease module. Thus, for a drug to be effective against a disease, it should target proteins inside or next to the corresponding disease module. To verify this hypothesis, integrating protein–protein interaction, drug-disease association, and drug-target association data were used to analyze the topological relationship between drug targets and disease proteins in the network. A drug-disease network proximity index was proposed to quantify the therapeutic effects of drugs, thus distinguishing the non-etiological palliative treatment from effective treatment method based on etiology.

6.3.1.2 Data Sources

Disease-Gene Association

Disease-gene association relationship comes from the group's previous work [8]. In other words, OMIM and GWAS data were obtained from UniProtKB and PheGenI, respectively, and only data with genome-wide significance meeting $p < 5.0 \times 10^{-8}$ were extracted from PheGenI. The Medical Subject Headings (MeSH) hierarchical tree organization was used to organize and standardize the disease names, thus combining data from the two databases. Only diseases corresponding to at least 20 disease genes in the protein interactome were retained.

Drug-Disease Data

For each disease, the corresponding FDA-approved drug was searched in the DrugBank database. Using MEDI-HPS [30] (using the file MEDI_01212013_UMLS.csv)and Metab2Mesh [31], 79 diseases were obtained, where each disease was associated with at least one drug, with a total of 402 drug-disease associations. MEDI-HPS contains drug–disease relationships integrated from RxNorm, MedlinePlus, SIDER, and Wikipedia. Only data with drug-disease association that strongly correlated in the Metab2Mesh text mining were accepted, of which 337 drugs were obtained. A total of 99 drugs that have no known targets in the interaction group or have the same target of another drug for the same disease were removed, and finally 238 different drugs and 384 targets were obtained. Only pharmacological targets have been considered here (the "Targets" chapter in DrugBank), also excluding drug metabolism enzymes, carriers, and transporters. To ensure accuracy of the drug-disease association, the information of these drugs were downloaded from DailyMed and the indications were checked to remove any inconsistent information. To calculate the enrichment of neighboring drug-disease pairs in clinical trials, information about these drugs and the diseases they act on in various trials were extracted from clinicaltrials.gov.

Classification of Known Drug-Disease Pairs

Three data sets were constructed: (1) Label: for the known 402 drug-disease pairs, the labeling information was extracted from DailyMed, and the corresponding diseases were fetched from the indication column. Two hundred and sixty-nine drug-disease associations were found and considered as labeled pairs. The remaining 133 drug-disease associations were considered as unlabeled pairs. (2) Palliative treatment: for each labeled pair, the indication column of DailyMed was reviewed for any statement of non-etiological use of the drug in the disease (e.g., management, remission, palliation, etc.), resulting in 50 palliative drug-diseases. The remaining 219 drug-disease pairs were classified as non-palliative. (3) Drug efficacy: side effects and efficacy report were gleaned from the FDA's adverse event reporting system. The report listed patients' responses to a given drug-disease, including "pain," "nausea," "drug failure," etc. 204 drug-disease pairs involving at least 10 reports were obtained from the open FDA application interface to extract the corresponding information. The relative effectiveness score *RE* is defined as:

$$\mathrm{RE} = 1 - \frac{n_{\mathrm{inefficient}}}{n_{\mathrm{top}}}$$

where $n_{\mathrm{inefficient}}$ and n_{top} are the number of the drug-disease pairs containing "drug failure" reports and the total number of reports, respectively.

Human Protein–Protein Interaction Network

Human protein–protein interaction network data is from the previous work of this team [8]. This data was integrated from TRANSFAC, IntAct, MINT, BioGRID, HPRD, KEGG, BIGG, CORUM, and PhosphoSitePlus, with experimental evidence from a large-scale signal network. The largest branch of this interaction group was used here, which contains 141,150 pairs of interactions among 13,329 proteins.

6.3.1.3 Analysis Index and Algorithm

Network Proximity Between Drugs and Diseases

Suppose *S* and *T* are the disease gene set and drug-target set, respectively, and *d(s, t)* is the shortest distance between nodes *s* and *t* in the PPI network. Different network distances are defined as follows:

$$\text{Closest distance}: d_c(S,T) = \frac{1}{\|T\|}\sum_{t\in T} \min{}_{s\in S} d(s,t)$$

$$\text{Shortest distance}: d_s(S,T) = \frac{1}{\|T\|}\sum_{t\in T}\frac{1}{\|S\|}\sum_{s\in S} d(s,t)$$

$$\text{Kernel distance}: d_k(S,T) = \frac{-1}{\|T\|}\sum_{t\in T}\ln\sum_{s\in S}\frac{e^{-(d(s,t)+1)}}{\|S\|}$$

$$\text{Centre distance}: d_{cc}(S,T) = \frac{1}{\|T\|} d(centre_s, t)$$

wherein center$_s$ is the topological center of *S*, which is defined as: $centre_s = \arg\min{}_{u\in S}\sum_{s\in S} d(s,u)$

When center$_s$ is not unique, all nodes are used to define center$_s$, and the shortest path length to these nodes is averaged.

$$\text{Separation distance}: d_{ss}(S,T) = \text{dispersion}(S,T) - \frac{d'_c(S,S) + d'_c(T,T)}{2}$$

wherein $dispersion(S,T) = \frac{\|T\|d_c(S,T)+\|S\|d_c(T,S)}{\|T\|+\|S\|}$, d'_c is the nearest correction distance, where the shortest distance from a node to itself is set to infinity.

To evaluate the statistical significance of the network proximity between drugs and diseases, 1000 sets of random nodes with the same number of disease genes and drug targets, and the same node connectivity distribution were constructed, and the distance between them was calculated. Thus, the mean value $\mu_{d(S,T)}$ and standard deviation $\sigma_{d(S,T)}$ of the randomized control proximity could be obtained. The Z-score of the distance between the disease protein and drug target set can then be calculated as a measure of the network proximity between the disease and drug:

$$z(S,T) = \frac{d(S,T) - \mu_{d(S,T)}}{\sigma_{d(S,T)}}$$

Threshold Analysis of the Area Under the ROC Curve and the Optimal Proximity

The Area Under ROC Curve (AUC) was used to evaluate the network proximity between known and unknown drug-disease pairs. For a set of known positive drug-disease associations (i.e., drugs that are known to be effective against the disease) and a set of negative drug-disease associations (i.e., drugs that have no effect on the disease), the true positive rate and false positive rate can be calculated at different thresholds to draw the ROC curve and calculate the AUC. Here, the corresponding relationship between drugs and diseases other than known drug-disease association is considered as the negative control. Due to the imbalance in the scale of known and unknown drug-disease associations, 402 pairs of unknown drug-disease associations were randomly selected as negative controls in the calculation of AUC. This process was repeated 100 times and the average AUC value was used to compare different network proximity values. Also, all unknown drug-disease associations were used as negative controls to calculate AUC. The results of the two methods were consistent and the network proximity z_c was defined by the closest distance that can best distinguish positive from the negative samples.

The optimal threshold ($z_c^{\text{threshold}}$) of network proximity was discovered, such that when the network proximity of a drug to a disease is less than this threshold, the drug has a very high probability of acting on the disease by using Sensitivity and Specificity curves of proximity. Sensitivity refers to the proportion of positive drug-disease association having proximity in all positive drug-disease pairs. Specificity refers to the proportion of negative drug-disease association that does not meet proximity in all negative drug-disease pairs. Thus, the network proximity threshold $z_c^{\text{threshold}}$ that can result in a high coverage rate (evaluated by Sensitivity) and a low false positive rate (evaluated by 1-specificity) was defined as the z_c value at the intersection of the Sensitivity and Specificity curves. Through analysis, the threshold value was set as $z_c^{\text{threshold}} = -0.15$.

6.3.1.4 Analysis Results

Proximity Analysis of Drugs and Diseases in the PPI Network

A total of 238 drugs were collected in this study, corresponding to 78 indications. There were a total of 18,564 possible drug-disease association pairs among them, of which 402 were known drug-disease association pairs, and the remaining 18,162 drug-disease association pairs were unknown.

The 402 known drug-disease association pairs and the 18,162 unknown pairs were treated as positive and negative groups, respectively, and the ability of network proximity defined by five distances (d_c, d_s, d_k, d_{cc}, d_{ss}) were compared to distinguish between the two groups. It was found that the performance of network proximity defined by the nearest distance d_c has the best distinguishing ability ($AUC_{z_c} = 0.66$), which is better than that defined by the shortest distance ($AUC_{z_s} = 0.58$), core distance ($AUC_{z_k} = 0.61$), centre distance ($AUC_{z_k} = 0.61$) and separation distance ($AUC_{z_{cc}} = 0.58$).

If the network proximity between the target proteins of a drug and the disease protein of a disease satisfies: $z_c \leq -0.15$, the drug is defined to be close to the disease. The findings are as follows:

(1) Known drugs are closer to their indications: 237 pairs of 402 known drug-disease associations are close (59%); of 18,162 unknown drug-disease associations, 7276 pairs are close (40%), which contain several potential candidates for drug repositioning.
(2) Drug-disease pairs that tend to be closer in clinical trials: Compared with distant unknown drug-disease pairs, close and currently unknown drug-disease pairs are significantly enriched in clinical trials.
(3) Most known drugs are not specific (exclusive): Among the drug-disease pairs significantly close to each other ($z_c \leq -2$), there are more known drug-disease pairs than unknown ones. However, of 402 known drug-disease pairs, only 79 are significantly close. Thus, known drugs are sufficiently high in selectivity (i.e., close to disease), but not necessarily specific (i.e., significantly close to disease).
(4) Proximity can emphasize non-trivial associations: Among 402 pairs of known drug-disease associations, 18 pairs of drug targets are disease proteins. Among the 44 pairs of drug targets, there are non-disease proteins but at least one of them is a disease protein, and only one drug is not close to the corresponding disease (disopyramide-arrhythmia). Of the remaining 340 pairs, 176 of the drug targets are not the same as the disease protein of the corresponding disease (as shown in Fig. 6.4). This shows that the network method can find non-trivial drug-disease association, that is, the situation where the drug does not target any related disease protein.

Determining Palliative Treatment with Network Proximity

The distribution of RE values of palliative drug-disease pairs was observed and from the remaining known drug-disease pairs, it was found that the RE values of palliative drug-disease pairs was significantly smaller. RE, the value of the drug's relative efficacy score, ranges from 0 to 1, with 0 and 1 representing the worst and best relative efficacy, respectively. It shows that palliative drugs are less effective in treating diseases.

Next, the network proximity of different types of known drug-disease pairs was compared, and it was observed that the network proximity of non-palliative drug-disease pairs and unlabeled drug-disease pairs was smaller than that of palliative drug-disease pairs. It suggests that network proximity can distinguish palliative from non-palliative drug-disease pairs, and that unlabeled drug-disease pairs may contain drugs that are more effective than the palliative ones.

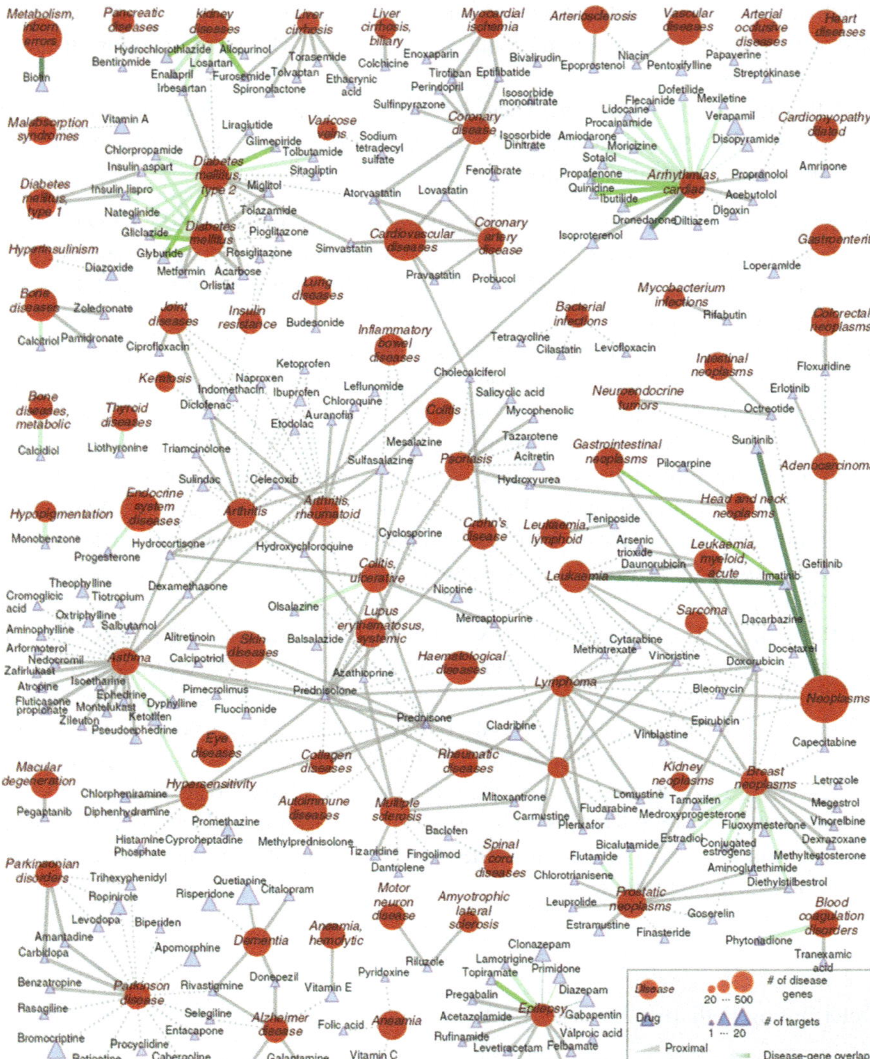

Fig. 6.4 Known drug-disease association [29]. The triangular and circular nodes represent drugs and diseases, respectively, and the node size is proportional to the number of corresponding drug targets and disease proteins. The connecting edge represents the relationship between drugs and diseases, and the solid line and the dashed line indicate that the drug and the disease are close and distant, respectively. The color of the line represents the number of overlapped drug targets and disease proteins (0, gray; 6, dark green)

Finally, the distribution of RE scores for the close and distant drug-disease pairs was examined and it was found that the close drug-disease pairs had significantly higher RE scores.

These results indicate that network proximity is a good index to measure the efficacy of drugs.

Treatment Bottleneck

Drugs of diseases that met the network proximity index were observed and it was found that:

(1) Most of the drugs used for asthma, Alzheimer's disease, heart disease, arrhythmia, cardiovascular disease, diabetes, epilepsy, allergy, kidney disease, liver cirrhosis, systemic lupus erythematosus, and ulcerative colitis have low network proximity to their indications. Similarly, among the antineoplastic drugs, drugs for treating prostate cancer, breast cancer, and lymphoma tend to be close to their indications.
(2) For inflammatory diseases such as Crohn's disease, psoriasis, and rheumatoid arthritis, the network proximity of current drugs to diseases is high. It shows that most of the drugs used in these immune system-related diseases are inflammation management or symptom relief drugs. Similarly, most drugs for Parkinson's disease are usually away from the disease on the network.

By examining the Anatomical Therapeutic Chemical Classification (ATC) of these drugs, it was found that drugs that are close to diseases tend to involve more intervention mechanisms on the endocrine system and metabolic process, while drugs for distant diseases are richer in anti-inflammatory and analgesic categories.

6.3.1.5 Main Conclusion

In this study, a network-based algorithm was proposed to calculate the proximity between drug targets, and between drug targets and disease genes on the network. Accordingly, six network modes of drug-drug-disease combination were obtained. By using a statistical method, it is inferred that two of the modes are related to the positive effects and side effects of the drug combination, respectively, hence predicting an effective drug combination.

The results of this study suggest that network-based drug and disease proximity provide an unbiased evaluation of drug treatment effects, and can be used as an effective tool to identify an effective treatment and palliative regimen. Although proximity can provide system level quantitative indexes to explain the effects of drugs, understanding therapeutic effects of drugs on individuals (that is, patients with different genetic predispositions) needs to incorporate large-scale patient-level data, such as electronic health records and personal genomes, which is still the goal of future work in this field.

6.3.2 Discovery of Mechanism of Drug Action and Drug Repositioning Through Transcriptional Response

One of the bottlenecks in drug discovery is to recognize the molecular target and off-target effects of compounds, i.e. Mode of Action (MoA). Methods to elucidate drug MoA include analyzing chemical structure of compounds, transcriptional response after treatment, and text mining. Among them, the transcriptional response-based method needs the least amount of information and can be quickly applied to new compounds. However, there is a lack of good algorithms and tools to make effective use of transcriptional data for drug discovery.

In this study, Iorio et al. developed a method to predict the effects and mechanisms of drugs by using the similarity of gene expression profiles after drug treatment [32]. Based on the transcriptional profile data in CMap [26], they constructed a drug network composed of 1302 drugs based on the similarities between their transcriptional profiles. These were then decomposed into communities, and compounds with similar MoA or action effects were found to be significantly enriched in the same community. They integrated the new compounds into the drug network to predict its treatment and off-target effects, while also predicting drug repositioning in the network.

6.3.2.1 Research Objectives

CMap database is useful for predicting the MoA and drug repositioning of new compounds based on expression profiles. The Build 02 version of the database contains expression profile data obtained from 1309 drugs with different doses acting on 5 different cell lines. By comparing the "Gene Signatures" (i.e., the list of differentially expressed genes) of the sample after treatment with the new compound, similar expression profiles were found in the database, which infers the MoA of the new compound. Problems affecting the accuracy of gene signature methods are choosing genes that constitute the signature and proper processing of multiple expression profiles obtained from the same drug intervention in different cell lines from the database. Choosing the wrong genetic signature will result in capturing similarities in the experimental setting (such as same cell lines) rather than the similarities in drug MoA.

They integrated the expression profiles of the same drug in the same cell line and/or different doses into a "consensus" transcriptional response profile, constructed a drug network based on the similarity of the consensus response profile of the drug, and then used the network analysis method to predict the MoA of the new compound.

6.3.2.2 Data Sources

CMap Data

Downloaded from the CMap website, it includes a total of 6100 expression profile data obtained from 1309 drugs with different doses acting on 5 different human cell lines.

Drug Information

The ATC codes and target genes of 1309 drugs in CMap were extracted from DrugBank and ChemBank databases, from which the ATC codes of 768 drugs and target gene information of 535 drugs were obtained.

Transcriptome Data of the Test Drug

Nine types of anti-cancer compounds (HSP90 inhibitor Tanespimycin, NVP-AUY922, NMS-E973; topoisomerase inhibitor SN-38, and doxorubicin; Cyclin-dependent kinases (CDKs), inhibitors such as Flavopiridol, PHA-848125, PHA-690509, and PHA-793887, were used to treat MCF7 and A2780 cell lines, respectively. Transcriptome experiments were performed in the treatment and the control groups; data is stored in the GEO database with GSE18552 as the ID. In the nine drugs used, some (e.g. Tanespimycin) were included in CMap as controls.

6.3.2.3 Analysis Index and Algorithm

Overview of Methods

As shown in Fig. 6.5.

Calculation of Prototype Ranked List (PRL)

Since the same drug in CMap was used to treat different cell lines at different concentrations, multiple sorting sequences of gene expression profiles were generated (that is, genes are ordered from high to low expression levels). Here, the Kruskal algorithm [33] was used to obtain a final PRL according to multiple sorting sequences of the same drug. The algorithm steps are as follows: firstly, the Spearman's Footrule Distance [34] was calculated between every neighboring pairs of all sorting sequences of the same drug; then, the Borda combination method [35] was used by merging the two sequences that are closest to each other into a new

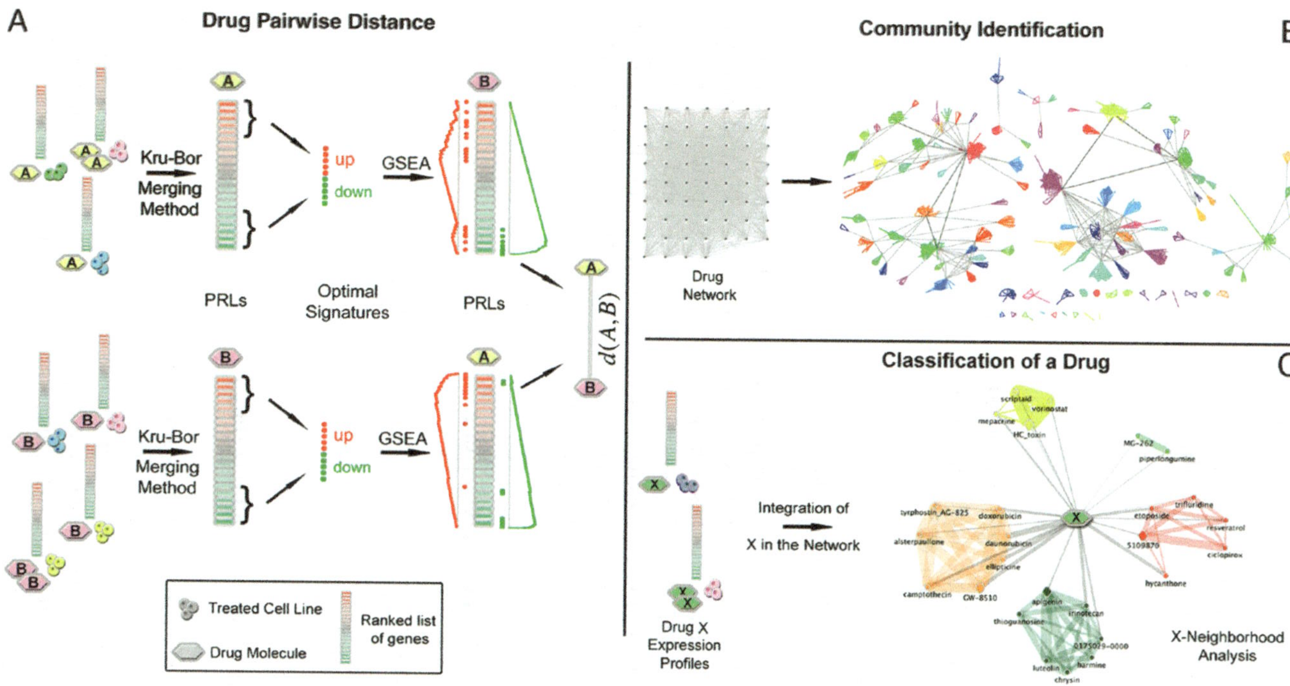

Fig. 6.5 Overview of methods [32]. (**a**) Calculate the distance value of each pair of drugs. (**b**) Construct a drug network and identify network communities. Among them, the network node is a medicine, and the medicines whose distance is less than the threshold are connected to the edges, and the weight of the edges is proportional to the distance between the medicines. (**c**) Incorporate drug X of unknown mechanism into the network and classify it. Calculate the distance d(X, Y) between X and each drug Y in CMap, and connect X to Y whose distance is less than a certain significant threshold

sequence. Then the new sequence was used to replace the original two sequences, and Spearman's Footrule Distance was recalculated between every neighboring pair of sequences. This process was repeated until all the sequences merged into one.

Calculation of the Distance Between Drugs

For the PRL of each drug, the top and last 250 genes (i.e., 250 genes with the highest expression and 250 genes with the lowest expression) were selected as p and q, respectively, and $\{p, q\}$ were used as the gene marker of the corresponding drug.

Suppose the gene marker of drug d be $\{p, q\}$, $p = \{p_1, \ldots, p_n\}$, $q=\{q_1, \ldots, q_n\}$, the Inverse Total Enrichment Score (TES) of drug d marker relative to the PRL of drug x is defined as follows:

$$TES_{d,x} = 1 - \frac{ES_x^p - ES_x^q}{2}$$

Here ES_x^r (r is p or q) is the calculated enrichment score of r marker of d relative to PRL of x based on Kolmogorov–Smirnov statistics. It measures whether a group of genes are distributed at the top of a gene sequence, and its value is within $[-1, 1]$. A value close to 1 indicates that these genes are close to the top of the sequence, and close to -1 indicates that these genes are close to the bottom of the sequence. $TES_{d,x}$ measures the degree to which the p set of drug d are placed at the top of the PRL of drug x, and the degree to which the q set of d are placed at the bottom of PRL of x. the values are within [0, 2].

The distance between drug A and drug B is defined as follows:

Average enrichment score distance: $D(A, B) = \frac{TES_{A,B}+TES_{B,A}}{2}$

Maximum enrichment score distance: $D(A, B) = \frac{\min(TES_{A,B}, TES_{B,A})}{2}$

Threshold for estimating the significance of drug distance

The distance between every neighboring pairs of all 1309 drugs in CMap was calculated—a total of 856,086 distances. Using a 5% quantile as the significant truncation, the corresponding average enrichment score distance and maximum enrichment score distance thresholds were 0.8339 and 0.8056, respectively. That is, if the distance between two drugs is less than the threshold, they are similar.

Network Community Identification

Affinity propagation algorithm was used to identify communities [36] in drug networks.

Distance Between Drugs and Community

Suppose x is a test drug, C is a network community, C_x is a subset of C, C_x contains at least two drugs and they are both connected to x through a significant edge (that is, an edge whose weight is lower than the significance threshold), the distance between x and C is defined as:

$$\sqrt[|C_x|]{\prod_{d \in C_x} D(d,x)/|C_x|}$$

where $D(d,x)$ is the maximum enrichment score distance between drug d and x. If $|C_x| < 2$, set the distance between x and C as ∞.

6.3.2.4 Analysis Result

Drug Network and Community

By calculating the pairwise distances of 1309 drugs in CMap, edges of drug pairs were connected whose distances were less than the significance threshold, and a drug network was constructed with 1309 drugs and 41,047 edges. The largest connected component contains 1302 drugs. The affinity propagation algorithm was used to decompose the drug network and [106] network communities were identified.

To determine whether the drugs in the same community have the same MoA, the ATC codes and target genes of drugs were mapped to the drugs of each community. A total of 804 drugs have known MoA (i.e., there are known ATC codes or target genes). For each community, the number of drugs with the same MoA was calculated and the statistical significance was analyzed. It was found that among 92 evaluable communities (in which at least 2 drugs have known MoA), 52 communities significantly enriched drugs with similar MoA, and 3 communities enriched the same target gene. Twenty-eight communities enriched the same ATC code, and 21 communities simultaneously enriched the same target gene and ATC code. In addition, literature reveals that 43 communities contain several drugs with the same MoA, and none of the drugs in 9 communities has known ATC codes or target genes. Therefore, 61 communities are significantly enriched in drugs with the same MoA.

Predicting MoA of Drugs

Nine types of anti-cancer drugs not included in CMap were used as test drugs. For each drug tested, its PRL and the distance from each of the 1039 drugs were calculated in CMap. If the distance between the tested drug and the drug in CMap is less than the significance threshold, they are edged; this method integrates the

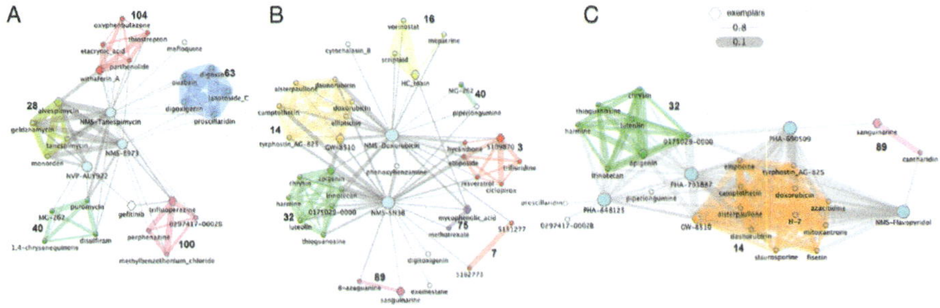

Fig. 6.6 Classifying test drugs with drug network [32]. According to the distance between drugs, the tested drugs relate to the drugs in the original network, and the tested drugs (cyan nodes) are integrated into the drug network. The color represents the community and the thickness of the edge is inversely proportional to the distance between the drugs. For clarity, only drugs with a distance of less than 0.8 ((**a**, **c**)) or 0.72 (**b**) from the drug under test are included. (**a**) HSP90 inhibitor; (**b**) Topo inhibitor; (**c**) CDK inhibitor

tested drug into the drug network. Then, the distance from each test drug to each community was calculated. The results are shown in Fig. 6.6.

Figure 6.6a shows the position of three HSP90 inhibitors in the drug network. The closest community to the three drugs is No. 28, which contains HSP90 inhibitor in cMap and antiestrogenic drug fulvestrant (this drug is known to bind to estrogen receptors, dissociate HSP90, and initiate intracellular degradation). These three drugs can be identified as HSP90 inhibitors.

Figure 6.6c shows that the closest community of the four CDK inhibitors is No. 14, followed by No. 32. These two communities contain many CDK inhibitors and topoisomerase inhibitors, wherein these two inhibitors account for about 80% of the total in No. 14 community. Figure 6.6b also shows that the closest communities of the two topoisomerase inhibitors are No. 14 and No. 32. This suggests that although the CDK inhibitor and topoisomerase inhibitor may have similar effects at the transcriptional level, they have different intracellular protein targets. To confirm this, CMap's own transcriptional profiles of SN-38 (the active metabolite of irinotecan, a Topo I inhibitor) and doxorubicin (Topo II inhibitor) were used to analyze the drug network. It was found that the transcriptional profiles of SN-38 and doxorubicin are close to those of community No. 14 and No. 32 in the network.

Predicting Unique Clinical Application of Known Drugs

Drug network method can be used to find candidates for drug repositioning, that is, to determine the unique clinical application of known drugs. Here we focus on identifying drugs that can enhance autophagy. Autophagy is a key biological process involved in cancer, infectious diseases, and neurodegenerative diseases.

To this end, drugs similar to drug 2-deoxy-D-glucose (2DOG) that induce molecular autophagy were retrieved from the drug network. 2DOG was positioned in the No. 1 community. Its neighboring drugs in the community were arranged in ascending order of distance, including fasudil, sodium phenylbutyrate, tamoxifen, arachidyl trifluoromethane, and novobiocin. In the No. 1 community, two drugs (2DOG and tamoxifen) were known autophagy inducers, and fasudil was the closest drug to 2DOG. In addition, the compounds closest to 2DOG in the whole network, in ascending order of distance, are fasudil, tazarotene, trifluoperazine, and gossypol. Among them, tazarotene, trifluoperazine, and gossypol are well-known autophagy inducible factors, but the relationship between fasudil and autophagy has not been reported. Therefore, it has been predicted that fasudil can induce autophagy.

6.3.2.5 Experimental Verification

Verifying that the CDK Inhibitor and Topoisomerase Inhibitor Have Similar Effects at the Transcriptional Level

Firstly, it has been verified that the topoisomerase inhibitor SN-38 (the active metabolite of Topo I inhibitor irinotecan) and adriamycin (Topo II inhibitor) have no direct inhibitory effects on CDK. The CDK inhibitor flavopiridol could not interfere with the ATPase activity of Topo II. MCF7 cells were treated with PHA-793887 (CDK inhibitor), adriamycin, or SN-38 for 6h, respectively, and protein cell lysates were analyzed by Western Blot. The experimental results indicate that the observed transcriptional effects induced by Topo I and Topo II inhibitors are mediated by (indirect) inhibition of CDK2 (and other possible CDK, i.e. CDK4) through p21 induction. These results explain the reason why the topoisomerase inhibitor and CDK inhibitor have similar effects at the transcriptional level.

Experimental Verification of Fasudil Induced Autophagy

Western Blot (WB) test with anti-LC3 antibody was used to evaluate the level of LC3-II in wild-type human fibroblasts treated with fasudil. Measurements show that treatment with fasudil, trifluoperazine, and two well-known autophagy inducers, 2DOG and rapamycin, all significantly increase the LC3-II levels of fibroblasts. The results of WB analysis were further confirmed by immunostaining with LC3 antibody. The effects of fasudil on autophagy enhancement were further confirmed using HeLa cells.

6.3.2.6 Main Conclusion

In this study, a general computational method was developed to predict the molecular effects and MoA of new compounds, and to identify previously unknown applications of well-known drugs. This method uses information hidden in the gene expression profile after drug treatment to capture the similarity of drug MoA.

When using gene expression profiles of mammalian cells after drug treatment, previous studies did not consider the changes in the transcriptional response to drugs under different cell lines, different doses, and different experimental settings. Moreover, previous studies did not fully mine the global structural information of drug similarity networks. The method proposed in this study captures the "consensus" transcriptional reactions of compounds in various cell lines and doses, automatically extracts the gene signature of each compound, and calculates the similarity between neighboring pairs of all compounds based on the gene signature. The MoA of new compounds and repositioning information of well-known drugs were successfully predicted by network community analysis.

6.4 R&D of Multi-target Drugs

Drug discovery usually follows the concept of "one drug, one target, one disease," that is, to search for the "pathogenic gene" of the disease, and to design a "Magic Bullet" that can specifically combine with the target protein corresponding to the gene. The drawback of a single target drug is that it ignores the complexity and robustness of the disease as a system, that is, the disease network has redundancy and alternative compensation signal pathways like other molecular networks. In many cases, inhibition of a target protein does not cause phenotypic changes and may even activate other related proteins in the disease system to protect the stability of system functions, resulting in the drug's loss of efficacy or toxic side effects. Studies have shown that in most cases, inhibition of a single protein has little effect on the disease network, while the regulation of multiple proteins at the same time will have an effect on the robust phenotype of the disease [37]. The drug discovery concept of multi-target drugs has gradually become a new trend [2, 37–39].

There are two ways to achieve multi-target therapy: one is to use existing drugs to act on different targets at the same time to produce a combination effect, called drug combination research and development; the other is to design a new chemical entity, using a small molecule to simultaneously block multiple targets related to the disease, to achieve better therapeutic effects. Ramsay et al. systematically analyzed the categories of 101 new molecular entities approved by FDA from 2015 to 2017 [40]. It was found that the proportion of small molecule single targets, multi-targets, and drug combinations are 34%, 21%, and 10% respectively. The proportion of newly approved multi-ingredient and multi-target small molecule drugs (31%) is equivalent to that of single target small molecule drugs. This indicates the developmental trend of the multi-target drug strategy.

However, whether in terms of target selection or discovery of targeted small molecules, finding multi-target drugs remains a great challenge. To select a target combination for a certain disease, we need to deeply understand the relationship of target-disease, pathway-target-drug-disease, and the side effects of drugs. We also need to consider whether the selected target combination can produce synergistic effects. These problems are easier to solve in molecular networks; hence, network pharmacology plays an increasingly important role in multi-target drug discovery. For example, in order to discover multi-target anti-inflammatory drugs, Meng et al. constructed a metabolism network of arachidonic acid and established a Multi-Target Optimal Intervention (MTOI) method to search and identify an effective and safe anti-inflammatory multi-target combination in the network [41]. Keane et al. constructed a protein–protein interaction network related to mitochondrial dysfunction and autophagy disorder, and predicted the proteins P62, GABARAP, GBRL1, and GBRL2 corresponding to the four nodes with the largest betweenness centrality in the network as key proteins of MPP^+ cytotoxicity, in Parkinson's disease. Experimental verification confirmed that high expressions of multiple combinations (rather than a single) of these four proteins would lead to a decrease of MPP^+ cytotoxin [42].

The following two specific research cases are selected for analysis.

6.4.1 Ischemic Stroke: From Single Drug Target to Synergistic Network Pharmacology

In order to develop multi-target drugs, this study used the treatment of ischemic stroke as an example, and establishes a set of systematic methods combining computational prediction with experimental verification [43]. First, starting from the known single target, the network pharmacology method was used to predict multiple targets, then a single drug corresponding to the predicted target was used for combination therapy, and both in vivo and in vitro experiments were carried out to verify the curative effect of multi-target drugs.

6.4.1.1 Research Objectives

In the past, the developmental strategies of multi-target drugs were mainly based on directly studying different drug combinations and the results of many ab initio prediction methods, which were not verified by experiments. This study aimed to develop a target-based method. Firstly, network pharmacology method was used to predict reliable target combinations, and then existing drugs that act on these targets were combined and experimentally verified.

6.4.1.2 Data Sources

(1) Protein–protein interaction: the integrated interactions database (IID) [44]; only the interactions detected in the experiments were extracted.
(2) Protein-metabolite interactions: the human metabolome database (HMDB) [45]
(3) Drug target proteins: the therapeutic target database (TTD) [46]

6.4.1.3 Algorithm and Results

The analysis process is shown in Fig. 6.7.

The algorithm process considers NOX4 as the initial target protein related to stroke. The goal is to identify more relevant target proteins using the public database. The calculation is based on the Guilt-by-Association algorithm. This process consists of three interdependent modules. Steps for calculation are as follows:

(1) Starting from seed NOX_4, a total of three metabolites were extracted from module one that interact with protein NOX_4 from the HMDB database [47]. Then, two main substrate oxygen (O_2) and product hydrogen peroxide (H_2O_2) of NOX_4 were obtained using methods described in literature, and a total of five metabolites related to NOX_4 were obtained. 537 proteins associated with these five metabolites were extracted from the HMDB database. From the intersections of these 537 proteins and the target proteins in TTD, a total of 166 proteins were obtained.
(2) The IID database was used in module 2 to extract the interactions between 166 proteins produced by module 1, and a PPI network was constructed; 166 proteins with protein-metabolites and protein–protein association relationships of five metabolites were integrated, to construct a double-layer network. In this network, the proximity of connection between proteins in the network and NOX4 was scored by using the Guilt-by-Association algorithm.
(3) GOSim in R-package was used in module 3 to calculate the semantic similarity scores based on GO molecular function (MF) between 166 proteins and NOX4, and the proteins were ranked from high to low according to similarity score.

The nine proteins with the highest scores obtained from modules 2 and 3 were extracted. Four proteins were obtained after getting intersection: CYBB, NOS2, NOS3, and NOS1. These four proteins are the predicted potential therapeutic targets for stroke.

6.4.1.4 Network Construction and Visualization

The association between NOX4 and 5 metabolites, the association between 5 metabolites and 166 target proteins, and the association between 166 proteins were integrated to construct a double-layer molecular network (as shown in Fig. 6.8).

6.4.1.5 Experimental Verification

In Vitro Experimental Verification

Two models are used: organotypic Hippocampal Culture (OHC) and the blood–brain barrier model constructed by human brain microvascular endothelial cells. Oxygen

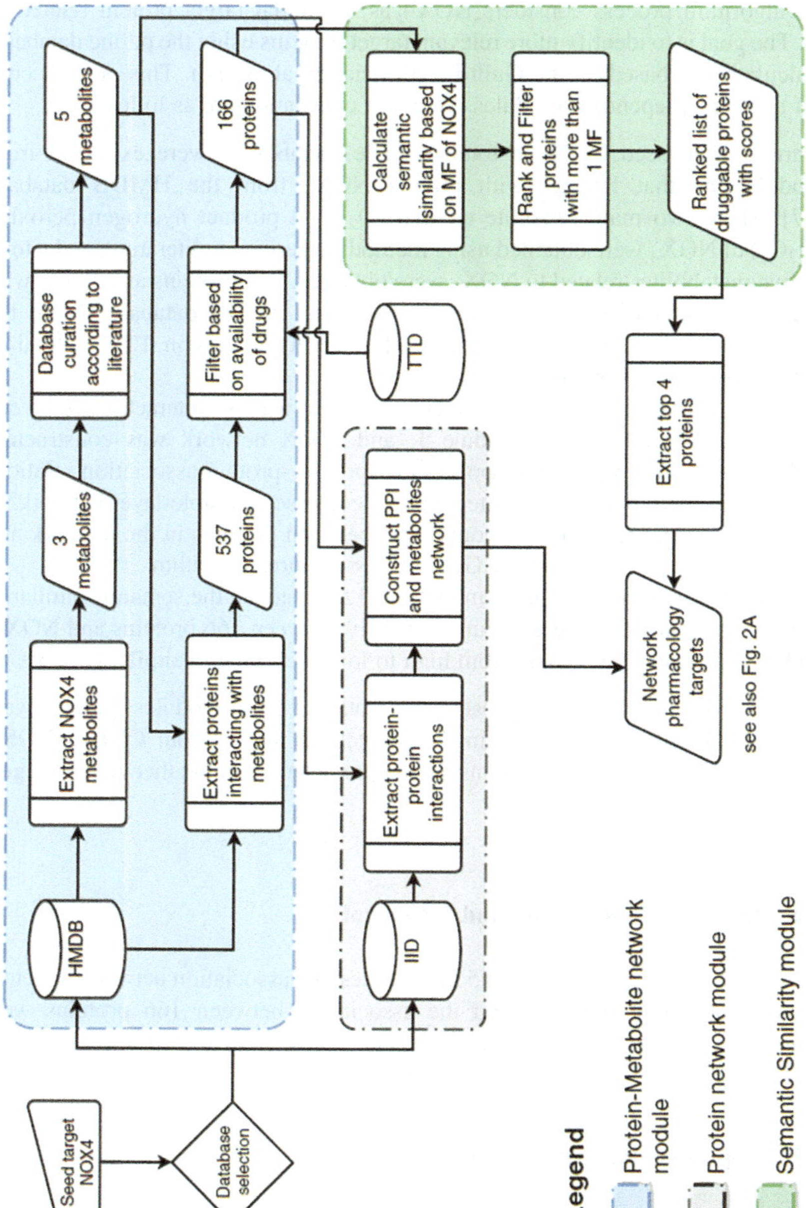

Fig. 6.7 Algorithm for optimizing targets through network pharmacology [43]

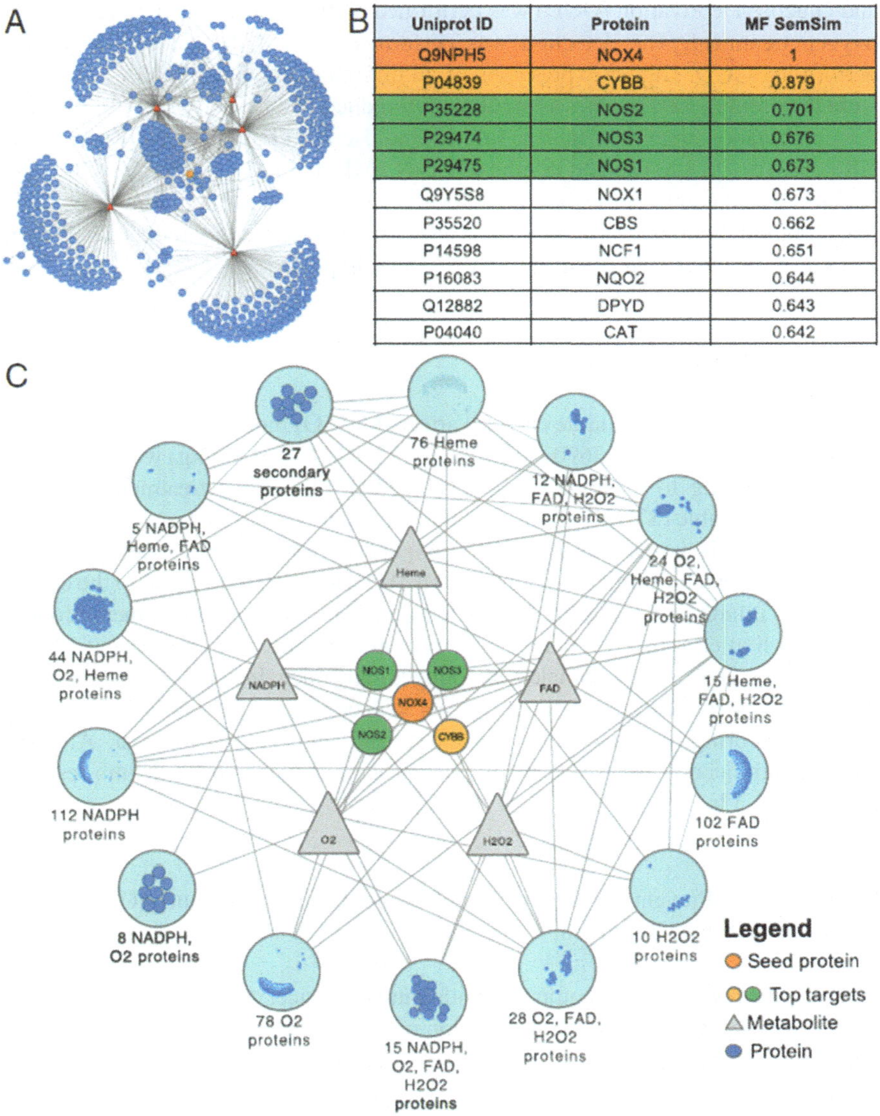

Uniprot ID	Protein	MF SemSim
Q9NPH5	NOX4	1
P04839	CYBB	0.879
P35228	NOS2	0.701
P29474	NOS3	0.676
P29475	NOS1	0.673
Q9Y5S8	NOX1	0.673
P35520	CBS	0.662
P14598	NCF1	0.651
P16083	NQO2	0.644
Q12882	DPYD	0.643
P04040	CAT	0.642

Fig. 6.8 Integrated multi-layer molecular interaction network using NOX4 as the seed for obtaining candidate target proteins [43]. (**a**) A double-layer network of integrin-metabolite and protein–protein interaction is constructed starting from seed NOX4. (**b**) The list of semantic similarity between protein and NOX4 based on GO molecular function. (**c**) Simplified network. Only seed protein, top 4 similar proteins, and related metabolites are shown separately, while the rest of the proteins and interactions are combined

and Glucose Deprivation (OGD) was performed on the OHC model before applying oxygen treatment. The detection was performed at 2, 4, 8, 12, and 24 h after performing OGD. Higher expressions of all different subtypes of NOX4 and NOS were thus found. Cell death was significantly reduced 24 h after OGD, followed by the combination treatment with a sub-threshold concentration of NOX4 inhibitor GKT136901 (0.1 μM) and NOS inhibitor L-NAME (0.3 μM), and Reactive Oxygen Species (ROS) and Reactive Nitrogen Species (RNS) were formed. Similarly, in the human blood–brain barrier model, the same combination therapy reduced cell death and prevented increased permeability caused by hypoxia.

In Vivo Experimental Verification

Mouse occlusion of the middle cerebral artery (MCAO) model was used to compare the treatment using GKT136901 (10 mg/kg) or L-NAME (3 mg/kg) with the control group. According to the guidelines developed by the stroke treatment academic industry roundtable (STAIR), transient and permanent, female and male, and old and young rat models were evaluated. Firstly, single drug sub-threshold treatment did not show neuroprotective effects on transient MCAO. However, compared to the control group, the infarct area was significantly reduced in the combined treatment group at 1 h and 3 h after stroke. Similar effects were also confirmed in permanent MCAO models, as well as in older female and younger male mice. In addition, in adult mice, three independent neuromotor function tests were conducted at 1 and 3 h after stroke: Bederson scoring, elevated body sway test, and limb suspension test. All three indexes significantly improved at 1 h post-stroke and Bederson and limb test also improved at 3 h.

Experiments to Prevent the Destruction of Blood–Brain Barrier and ROS Formation in Stroke Treatment

Experiments revealed that, compared with untreated mice, combined treatment after stroke significantly reduced the destruction of the blood–brain barrier. Next, oxidative stress and N-Tyr production were measured in brain tissue slices, and it was found that ROS and N-Tyr production were significantly reduced 24 h after combination treatment.

6.4.1.6 Main Conclusion

Considering the development of multi-target drugs for stroke as an example, this study developed a calculation method based on the initial target NADPH oxidase type 4 (NOX4) and predicted the related target-nitric oxide synthase (NOS) from the network pharmacological mechanism. In vivo and in vitro experiments confirm that NOX4 and NOS inhibition is highly synergistic, simultaneously inhibiting multiple related targets and leads to a significant reduction in infarct size. It also plays a direct role in neuroprotection and blood–brain barrier stabilization.

This network pharmacology method can develop multi-target drugs according to the mechanism-based synergy, which can improve the therapeutic effect, and reduce single drug dosage, side effects, and the risk of failure of drug development based on a single target. This method can be extended to the study of multi-target therapy for other complex diseases.

6.4.2 Combining Network Pharmacology and Phenotype Screening to Develop New Analgesic Drugs

Phenotypic drug screening is a method based on biological phenotypes. That is, drug screening and design are carried out based on phenotypic data of diseases, given that there are no clear disease targets and relevant mechanisms of action. When a certain small molecule is found to reverse the phenotype of a disease, the molecule may have potential therapeutic effects on the respective disease. Phenotypic drug screening provides a framework for identifying compounds that are effective for disease systems and has received extensive attention in the field of drug discovery. However, a certain small molecule obtained by phenotypic screening may regulate the disease system, but its mechanism is not clear. It is time-consuming and expensive to clarify the mechanism. In general, based on the transcription profile of the compound and the disease, the activity of the compound is linked with the biological process of the disease.

This study explored the combination of phenotypic screening and network pharmacology to develop analgesic drugs [48]. Firstly, a reasonable method was proposed to select and screen compounds with enough throughput and multiple pharmacological characteristics to improve screening ability of small molecules. This was for the phenotype of active molecules in complex diseases. Network pharmacology was used to construct the disease network of target disease, and related protein information of compounds obtained from the selected phenotype screening, which was added into the disease network. The network algorithm was then used to screen out compounds with significant influence on the disease. The mechanism of the compound on the disease obtained this way can be elucidated by network pharmacology.

6.4.2.1 Research Objective

Chronic pain is a complex disorder whose etiology involves many molecular mechanisms but is often characterized by neuronal hyperexcitability. Existing treatments still do not control pain well and have many side effects. The subjectivity of individual patients and the differences in pain sensitivity make the development of new therapies time-consuming, expensive, and prone to failure.

This study combines phenotypic screening with pain network to construct a new phenotype model of neuronal excitability for the discovery of new multi-target drugs for chronic pain.

6.4.2.2 Data Sources

(1) Pain network: The chronic pain-specific disease network [49] was constructed by the group in the past. Firstly, 765,692 pain-related papers were collected, and 93,271 pairs of different protein–protein interactions were obtained from the papers by literature mining. PPI was then sorted based on conditional correlation score value and literature evaluation and the first 3000 pairs were manually annotated and verified. Finally, a pain network consisting of 822 pairs of PPI between 583 different proteins was constructed.
(2) Normal network: constructed by extracting protein–protein interaction from the IRefIndex database [50].
(3) Compound-target information: High-throughput screening data for small molecule compound targets-specificity from Pfizer. A total of 2869 compounds and 2322 target specificity were analyzed. For each compound, analysis was conducted to obtain a target with IC50 < 10 μM. Among 583 proteins in the pain network, 233 such targets were found.

6.4.2.3 Algorithm and Results

In this study, a method was proposed to evaluate network integrity while screening compounds that have the greatest impact on the pain network. Network integrity is defined as the ratio of the number of edges left in the network after being attacked (i.e., removing some nodes and edges). The normal network was used as the control network of the pain network. The algorithm steps are as follows:

(1) For each compound, the targets with their $IC_{50} < 10$ μM in the pain and control networks were found, and all the targets and their associated edges were removed from the network.
(2) The number of edges remaining in the network and their integrity were calculated, to define the changes as the influence of drugs.

6.4.2.4 Results

Impact Prediction of Single Compound

Based on the calculation, the biggest impact of a single compound on the pain network was to reduce its integrity by 16.55%, and had comparatively little impact

Table 6.1 Ten compounds predicted to have the greatest impact on the pain network

Compound	No. targets	Pain network (% change)	Control network (% change)
Apomorphine	14	16.55	0.84
SNX2112	24	16.55	5.14
Chlorpromazine	31	15.09	0.78
Loperamide	24	13.5	0.3
Hypericin	14	13.26	1.89
Flunarizine	23	13.26	0.43
Ruboxistaurin	17	13.02	1.71
Haloperidol	29	12.9	0.38
Sertraline	21	12.77	0.41
Pimozide	22	12.65	0.44

on the normal network. Table 6.1 lists the 10 compounds predicted to have the greatest impact on the pain network. In contrast, Sutent, a single compound, had the greatest impact on the normal network, reducing its integrity by 6%.

Impact Prediction of Combining Two Compounds

Using calculation methods, it was predicted that the effects of drug combination pairs on the pain network are more than 30% and greater than that of any single drug in the combination.

Comparison of Prediction Results with Past Experimental Screening Results

Prediction results of 107 compounds were compared with the inhibition levels measured by neuron excitations in the past. It was found that these results were moderately positively correlated with the experimental results (Spearman's correlation coefficient for ranked data = 0.58), while the prediction results in the normal network had no correlation with the experimental results (Spearman's correlation coefficient for ranked data = 0.22).

6.4.2.5 Experimental Verification

Sixty-six compounds were selected from the predicted single compounds for phenotypic screening and verification. Firstly, 29 compounds, predicted to have an impact on the pain network greater than 10% and less than 1% on the normal network, were removed. Then 37 compounds with predicted activity greater than 3.8% and those that have chemical structural diversity were added.

Phenotypic analysis was carried out on the selected compounds (10 μM single target screening). It was found that 28 compounds had more than 75% inhibitory effects on neuronal excitability, that is, the accuracy of this group of compounds was 42%.

6.4.2.6 Main Conclusion

In this study, an algorithm based on network pharmacology was proposed to calculate the effects of compounds on the integrity of the pain network. This was done by establishing a compound-target relationship obtained by high-throughput phenotypic screening. Among the compounds predicted to have the greatest impact on the integrity of the pain network, D2 dopamine receptor antagonists and dopamine inhibitors were included, which are known pain-related drugs. 66 predicted single compounds were selected for phenotypic screening and verification and the correct rate was 42%. This indicates that the prediction based on network integrity algorithm is of great value for the development of multi-target drugs.

6.5 Drug Repositioning

Drug repositioning (drug repurposing, reprofiling, or re-tasking) is also called "new use of old drugs" or "drug reuse," which refers to the discovery of new uses of drugs already in the market or in the stage of clinical research. Since drugs for repositioning studies have been used in the clinic or have passed several stages of clinical trials, their safety risks have been significantly reduced, reducing R&D costs and shortening the R&D cycle. Therefore, drug repositioning is one of the best strategies with good risk/benefit ratio in drug development strategies. In the past, drug repositioning came largely from accidental discovery, and by far the most successful examples of drug reuse have not involved a systematic approach [51]. For example, reuse of the antihypertensive drug sildenafil citrate for treatment of erectile dysfunction relied on retrospective clinical studies. The reuse of sedative thalidomide for treatment of multiple myeloma was based on accidental discovery. At present, there are some technical platforms and methods specially established for drug repositioning R&D. One is the experimental screening method based on high-throughput technology, and the other is computational method based on computer virtual screening, computational biology, and bioinformatics.

In drug development, drugs that can be combined with multiple targets are called dirty drugs. Off-target proteins in dirty drugs, that is, proteins that are not the exact targets (on-target) for the current indications of the drug, are often considered to be associated with toxic side effects. From the perspective of drug repositioning, deviation from the target may lead to the treatment of other diseases. Network pharmacology is widely used in the study of drug repositioning due to its systematic analysis of multiple targets. This kind of research usually predicts drug repositioning by analyzing drug similarity, target similarity, and network similarity [52]. For example, based on the similarity of the 2D structure of drugs, gene sequence similarity of target, and structural similarity of drug-target bipartite network, Cheng et al. proposed methods of drug-based similarity inference (DBSI), target-based similarity inference (TBSI) and network-based inference (NBI), to predict unknown targets of drugs and drug reposition. Among them, NBI showed the best performance in all four test data sets [53]. Iorio et al. used CMap data to build a drug similarity network based on the "transcription label" of drugs, and predicted and verified the effects of fasudil on autophagy induction [54]. Luo et al. integrated drug-drug similarity, disease-disease similarity, and drug-disease association into a hybrid double-layer network. A "Bi-random Walk" algorithm was then used to predict the new drug-disease association relationship [55].

The following two specific research cases are selected for analysis.

6.5.1 Network-Based Drug Repositioning Prediction and Population-Based Verification

In drug repositioning studies, predicted new usage of known drugs must be strictly verified. Since drug repositioning studies mainly focus on drugs that have been approved and used in clinical practice, large-scale patient-level data accumulated in health care can be used for this kind of verification. Conventional medical health care data contains clinical diagnosis and treatment, combid conditions, demographics, public health monitoring, and other data from many patient groups. These enriched data sets make them an ideal choice for verifying network-based assumptions.

In this study, Barabasi et al. developed a method based on network pharmacology to quantify the relationship between disease proteins and drug targets in the human genome-wide protein–protein interaction for drug repositioning [56]. They used conventional health care data from more than 220 million patients to test the predictive effects, and conducted in vitro pharmacological experiments to test the potential mechanisms for repositioning drugs. They selected drug repositioning for cardiovascular diseases as an example of an approach to study the association between drugs for non-heart related disease and cardiovascular outcomes. Research results indicated the effectiveness of such comprehensive methods and can be extended to drug repositioning for other types of diseases.

6.5.1.1 Research Objectives

In the study of network pharmacology, the strength of the relationship between the subjects is usually measured by the distance in the genome-wide protein–protein interaction network of the subjects (such as diseases and drug-target genes). Large-scale health care data may be an ideal choice to verify the results based on the network.

In this study, a network-based algorithm was proposed to calculate the network proximity between drug targets and disease genes, to predict the repositioning of drugs and use the data from two large-scale health insurance claim databases in the US to verify the repositioning of the predicted cardiovascular drugs.

6.5.1.2 Data Sources

Human Protein–Protein Interaction Network

The human protein–protein interaction network was constructed by integrating data from 15 databases. Specifically, data resources were as follows:

1. Binary protein–protein interaction data from two high-quality Yeast-two-Hybrid (Y2H) high-throughput experiments [57, 58] and Barabasi laboratory website.
2. Kinase–substrate interaction data from low-and-high-throughput experiments recorded in the KinomeNetworkX [59], Human Protein Resource Database (HPRD) [60], PhosphoNetworks [61], PhosphositePlus [62], dbPTM 3.0 [63], and Phospho.ELM [64] database.
3. PPI data recorded by affinity purification and mass spectrometry (AP-MS) identification in literature as well as low-throughput experimental data reported in literature that are recorded in the BioGRID [65], PINA [66], HPRD [60], MINT [67], IntAct [68], and InnateDB [69] database.
4. High quality PPI obtained by analyzing the three-dimensional structure of proteins recorded in the Instruct database [70].
5. Signaling network obtained by low-throughput experiment reported in literature that are recorded in SignaLink database [71].

Data from evolutionary analysis, gene expression profiles, metabolic associations were deleted. Each ID of protein was mapped to the corresponding Entrez ID of the coding genes. The finally constructed PPI network contained 16,677 nodes and 243,603 edges.

Cardiovascular Disease Genes

Firstly, about 50 cardiovascular (CV) events were collected from Medline MeSH (Medical Subject Headings) and UMLS (Unified Medical Language System) databases [72]. For each CV event, disease-related genes from 8 data sources were collected: OMIM (Online Mendelian Inheritance in Man) [73], CTD (comparative toxicogenomics database) [74], HuGE Navigator [75], DisGeNET [76], ClinVar [77], GWAS Catalog [78], GWASdb [79], and PheWAS Catalog [80]. A total of 23 cardiovascular events were selected with at least 10 disease-related genes in the human protein–protein interaction network for subsequent research.

Drug-Target Network

Drug-target interaction data were obtained from DrugBank [81], TTD (the Therapeutic Target Database) [46], and PharmGKB [82] database. Drug-target binding affinity data are from ChEMBL [83], BindingDB [84], and IUPHAR/BPS Pharmacological guidelines [85]. Only drug-target pairs with affinity indexes K_i, K_d, IC_{50}, or EC_{50} not greater than 10 μM and the target was a human protein were retained.

Tissue-Specific Expression Genes

RNA-seq data (RPKM values) of 32 tissues were downloaded from the GTEx database [86]. For each tissue (e.g., blood vessel), genes with RPKM$\geq$1 in more than 80% of the samples were selected as the genes specifically expressed in the tissue.

Conventional Medical Health Care Data

Data comes from two large-scale health insurance claim databases in the USA: Truven MarketScan (2003–2014, containing data of 173 million patients) and Optum Clinformatics (2004–2013, containing data of 55 million patients) [87]. These data sources include demographic data of patients, comprehensive information on inpatient and outpatient diagnosis, and outpatient prescriptions, and medications. All personal identifications of the data included were removed and it was approved by the Institutional Review Board of Brigham and Women's Hospital in Boston, Massachusetts.

6.5.1.3 Analysis Index and Algorithm

Network Proximity

Let S and T be the set of disease protein and drug target, respectively. The closest distance of these two sets on human PPI network is defined as:

$$d(S,T) = \frac{1}{\|T\|}\sum_{t\in T} \min{}_{s\in S} d(s,t)$$

where $d(s, t)$ is the shortest path length between nodes s and t in the PPI network. To evaluate the statistical significance of the network proximity between drugs and diseases, 1000 random node sets with the same number of disease protein and drug targets and the same node degree distribution were constructed, and the nearest distance between them was calculated. Therefore, the Z-score of the nearest distance between the disease protein and the drug-target set can be calculated. This was used to represent the network proximity between the corresponding drug and disease.

Significance of Tissue-Specific Expression Genes

The significance of specific expression of gene *i* in tissue *t* is calculated as follows:

$$z_E(i,t) = \frac{E(i,t) - < E(i) >}{\delta_E(i)}$$

wherein $<E(i)>$ and $\delta_E(i)$ are the mean and standard deviations of the expression levels of gene *i* in all other tissues considered, respectively.

6.5.1.4 Network Construction and Visualization

In the constructed human protein–protein interaction network, the network proximity between 984 FDA-approved western drugs (including 177 cardiovascular drugs and 807 non-cardiovascular drugs) and 23 cardiovascular diseases (outcomes) was calculated. Proximity index Z-score < -0.4 was considered as highly reliable, hence it was predicted that 431 FDA-approved non-cardiovascular drugs can be repositioned as cardiovascular drugs. The network in Fig. 6.9 shows the predicted associations between these 431 drugs and 22 cardiovascular diseases.

To reveal the mechanism of action of the effect of anti-rheumatoid drug hydroxychloroquine on coronary artery disease, a sub-network was constructed by the following methods (as shown in Fig. 6.10):

(1) In the human protein–protein interaction network, proteins encoded by the genes specifically expressed in blood vessels and the edges between them were selected to construct a vascular specific sub-network.
(2) In the blood vessel-specific sub-network, the shortest paths from the targets TLR7 and TLR9 of hydroxychloroquine to other nodes was identified. On the shortest path, the protein that simultaneously satisfies conditions (3) and (4) was selected and a sub-network was established.
(3) Selected proteins were encoded by genes related to known coronary artery disease (CAD) or cardiovascular disease (CVD).
(4) Proteins that are supported by in vivo and in vitro experiments reported in literature were selected.

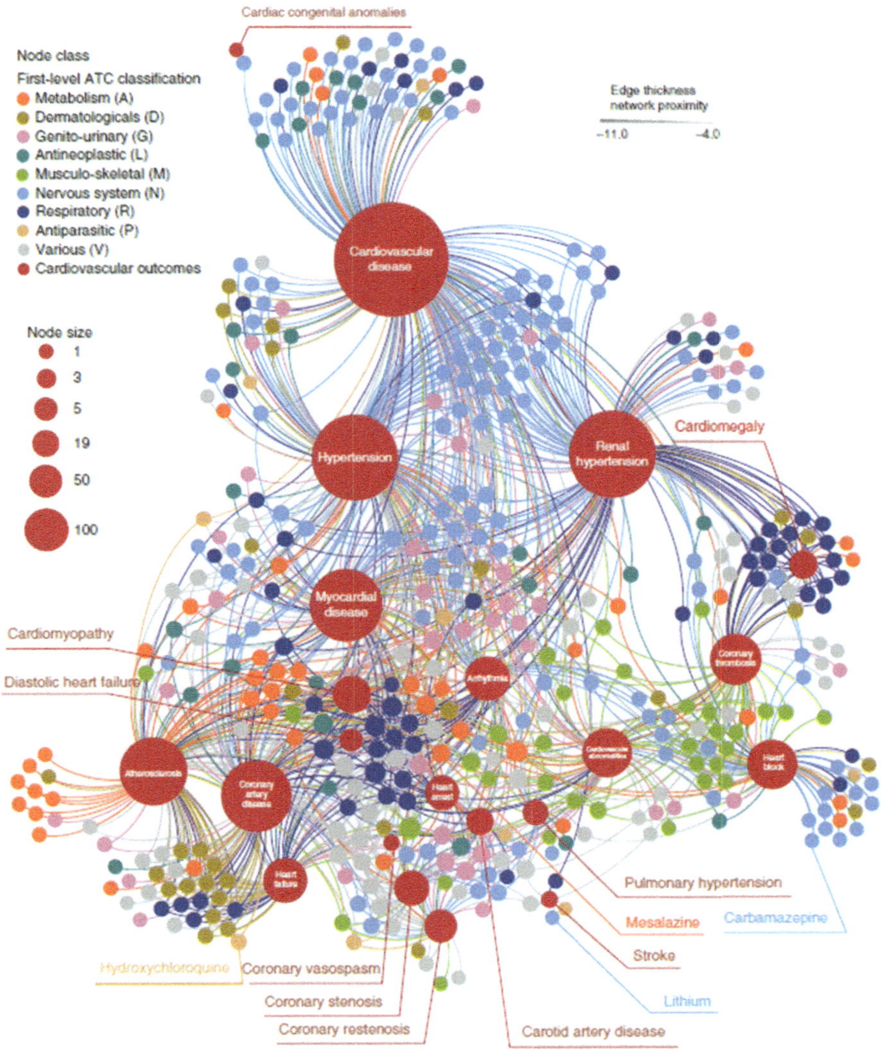

Fig. 6.9 Drug-disease association network between predicted outcomes of 22 cardiovascular diseases with high credibility and 431 non-cardiovascular drugs approved by the FDA [56]. The color of the drug node represents the first code of the ATC (Anatomical Therapeutic Chemical) drug classification system. The size of the node is proportional to its connection degree in the network. The thickness of the edge represents the network proximity between the drug and the disease (represented as Z-score)

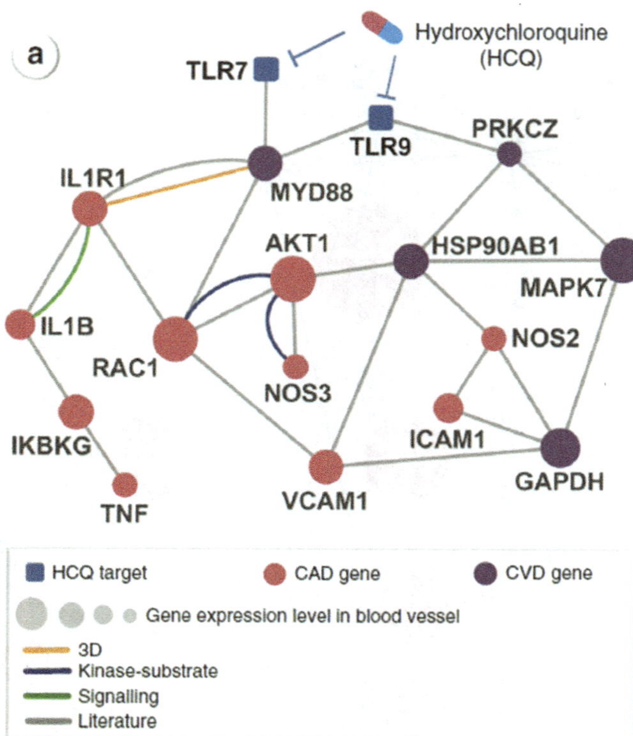

Fig. 6.10 The sub-network constructed by network analysis reveals the mechanism of action of anti-rheumatoid drug hydroxychloroquine on coronary artery disease [56]. Node size represents the blood vessel-specific expression level of the gene

6.5.1.5 Experimental Verification

Selection of Objects for Experimental Verification at a Later Stage

For the prediction results shown in Fig. 6.9, some individual results were selected based on the following five aspects for experimental verification:

(1) The strength of the associations predicted by the network-based method.
(2) After excluding non-cardiovascular drugs with known cardiovascular (CV) side effects, novel prediction results were selected.
(3) Sufficient patient data was obtained for verification (excluding infrequently used drugs).
(4) Availability of an appropiate comparative treatment data that is used for the same underlying (non-CV) indication as the drug of interest and predicted to have no association with the intended CV diseases by the network method.

(5) The fidelity with which the predicted CV outcomes were recorded in the insurance claims database.

Based on the above criteria, four groups of results were selected for subsequent verification:

(1) Correlation of epilepsy drug carbamazepine ($Z = -2.36$) and levetiracetam (comparator control, $Z = -0.07$) with CAD.
(2) Correlation of inflammatory colonic disease medication mesalazine ($Z = -6.10$) and azathioprine (comparator control, $Z = -0.09$) with CAD.
(3) Correlation of rheumatoid arthritis medication quinine ($Z = -3.85$) and methotrexate (comparator control, $Z = -1.87$) with CAD.
(4) Correlation of bipolar disorder medication lithium salt ($Z = -5.97$) and lamotrigine (comparator control, $Z = -0.19$) with CAD.

Verification of Pharmacoepidemiological Methods

Two large American commercial health insurance claim databases linked to Aetion evidence platform were used to carry out four cohort studies. The correlation between the four predicted drugs and cardiovascular events was assessed based on individual level longitudinal patient data and pharmacoepidemiological methods.

By studying large-scale patient data, two of the four predicted correlations were verified to be significantly associated with cardiovascular outcome, in which quinine was found to reduce CAD risk, while carbamazepine increased it. The verification results support the network-based prediction.

In Vitro Verification of the Mechanism of Action of Quinine

Based on the constructed sub-network of blood vessel-specific expression proteins related to quinine targets, the authors proposed a possible mechanism of action in the treatment of CAD as follows:

(1) The activation of ERK5, a protein encoded by MAPK7, further inhibited the expression of cell adhesion molecules VCAM-1 and ICAM-1, and prevented vascular endothelial inflammation.
(2) Inhibition of pro-inflammatory cytokines TNF-α and IL-1β.
(3) By activating endothelial nitric oxide synthase (NOS3), nitric oxide production increased, thus improving vascular endothelial dysfunction.

The authors conducted in vitro experiments to verify these mechanisms. The expression of VCAM1, IL1B, and NOS3 genes was monitored in the presence and absence of the cytokine TNF-α after treating human aortic endothelial cells with 10–50 μM quinine. It was found that TNF-α (5, 10, 20 ng/ml) caused a strong increase of VCAM1 and IL1B expression, and this pro-inflammatory effect was significantly reduced by all doses of hydroxychloroquine. TNF-α significantly inhibited the expression of NOS3, while 50 μM quinine significantly reversed the inhibition.

6.5.1.6 Main Conclusion

This study shows that the molecular network method combined with the pharmacoepidemiological method could identify drug repositioning and side effects. Using large-scale patient data, it was verified that quinine is associated with a 24% reduction in CAD risk compared to methotrexate, and this effect was also confirmed by subsequent in vitro experiments. At the same time, carbamazepine is associated with a 56% increased risk of CAD compared to levetiracetam. The widely used application of these methods proposed in this study is expected to promote the innovation of drug discovery and development.

6.5.2 Discovery of New Antidepressant Drugs by Drug Repositioning Based on Network Pharmacology

Depression is a serious and complex mental disease with high incidence, recurrence, and suicide rates, and has a serious family and social burden. Existing antidepressants have disadvantages such as late onset, high toxicity, and side effects; hence, the development of new antidepressants has high social value and economic benefits. However, the current target-oriented drug discovery model has repeatedly failed to develop new antidepressants, resulting in huge economic losses. Although there is a wealth of disease-related genes and drug targets, application of these resources to new drug discovery remains a huge challenge.

In this study, Li et al. proposed a new network-based drug repositioning method, and predicted the potential antidepressant drugs and their molecular targets from the drugs included in the DrugBank database [88]. This method firstly integrates chemical similarities, therapeutic similarities, and protein–protein interaction of drugs by using a network-based method, to predict the relationship between drugs and targets. Then, drugs related to known targets were screened for antidepressants. The potential antidepressant effects of six drugs were predicted using this method, and it was verified that the gastrointestinal antispasmodic drug alverine may be an effective antidepressant, as indicated in the experiments.

6.5.2.1 Research Objectives

Drug repositioning is one of the most economical strategies for new drug development as it can reduce costs and risk of failure due to adverse side effects. Traditionally, drug repositioning has been largely dependent on "happy surprises" that do not happen very often. The method based on network pharmacology provides a more rapid and effective method for drug repositioning by predicting the association between the drug and the target. At the same time, network-based drug repositioning is helpful for understanding the mechanism of action of drugs, and the drugs predicted by this method can reduce the risk caused by side effects.

In this study, the target prediction algorithm drugCIPHER [89] developed previously by the research group, was used to predict the targets of all small molecule drugs in DrugBank, and to establish connections between other types of drugs and known antidepressants through the targets, thereby predicting new antidepressant drugs.

6.5.2.2 Data Sources

All information related to all drugs from the DrugBank database was downloaded, totaling 3,817 drugs, among which 34 are FDA-approved antidepressants.

6.5.2.3 Analysis Index and Algorithm

(1) For 3817 downloaded drugs, the drug CIPHER algorithm developed by the research group in the past was used to predict the target of each drug, and the target list vector of each drug was obtained.
(2) For any pair of drugs, the consistency score of their biological activity similarity was calculated according to their target vectors.
(3) Hierarchical clustering analysis was carried out based on similarities in biological activity of drug pairs.

Two clusters containing 16 known antidepressants were obtained by clustering analysis (as shown in Fig. 6.11). The other 14 drugs in these two clusters may have had antidepressant effects. The pharmacological and toxicological information of these 14 drugs were extracted, and drugs that could not pass through the blood–brain barrier or induce serious side effects after long-term use were excluded. Six drugs were screened out for further experimental verification (red font in Fig. 6.11).

6.5.2.4 Network Construction and Visualization

To illustrate the antidepressant effects of the predicted drug alverine, the drug-target network of alverine and other similar antidepressants were constructed (as shown in Fig. 6.12). Figure 6.12a shows that the targets for antidepressants are also targets of alverine. Figure 6.12b shows that the predicted alverine target can directly or indirectly regulate depression-related molecules through protein–protein interactions or signal transduction pathways. From the network in Fig. 6.12b, four important targets of alverine-SLC6A2, SLC6A4, HTR1A, and HTR2A were selected, which

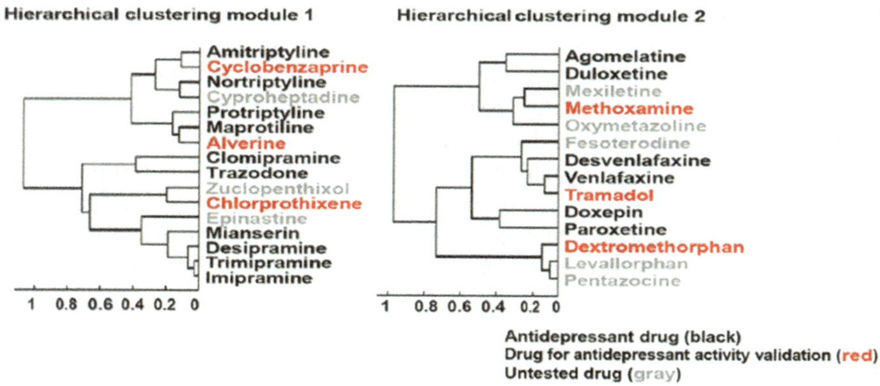

Fig. 6.11 Two clusters containing a large number of known antidepressants obtained by drug hierarchical clustering analysis [88]. Among them, the black font is known antidepressants, others are predicted potential antidepressants. The red font is for the drug selected for further experimental verification

are not only the disease genes related to depression, but also known targets for antidepressants. Also, they are in the top 100 in the prediction results. Experimental verification was further carried out on these four important targets.

6.5.2.5 Experimental Verification

(1) For the predicted six drugs, the results of tail suspension test (TST) and forced swimming test (FST) of mice verified that the six drugs have antidepressant effects.
(2) Alverine, a gastrointestinal antispasmodic drug was further used to verify its own antidepressant effects by using the learning helplessness model of depression and the chronic unpredictable stress model.
(3) Four important targets of alverine were verified by in vitro experiments, and the results show that avirin has medium-strength binding affinity with their encoded proteins.

6.5.2.6 Main Conclusion

This study used a network-based approach to predict potential antidepressants and verified their efficacy using a classic depression experimental model. It was observed that alverine, FDA-approved drug for irritable bowel syndrome, could be repositioned as an antidepressant. In addition, four predicted targets, namely SERT (SLC6A4), NET (SLC6A2), 5-HT1AR (HTR1A), and 5-HT2AR (HTR2A), were verified by biological experiments.

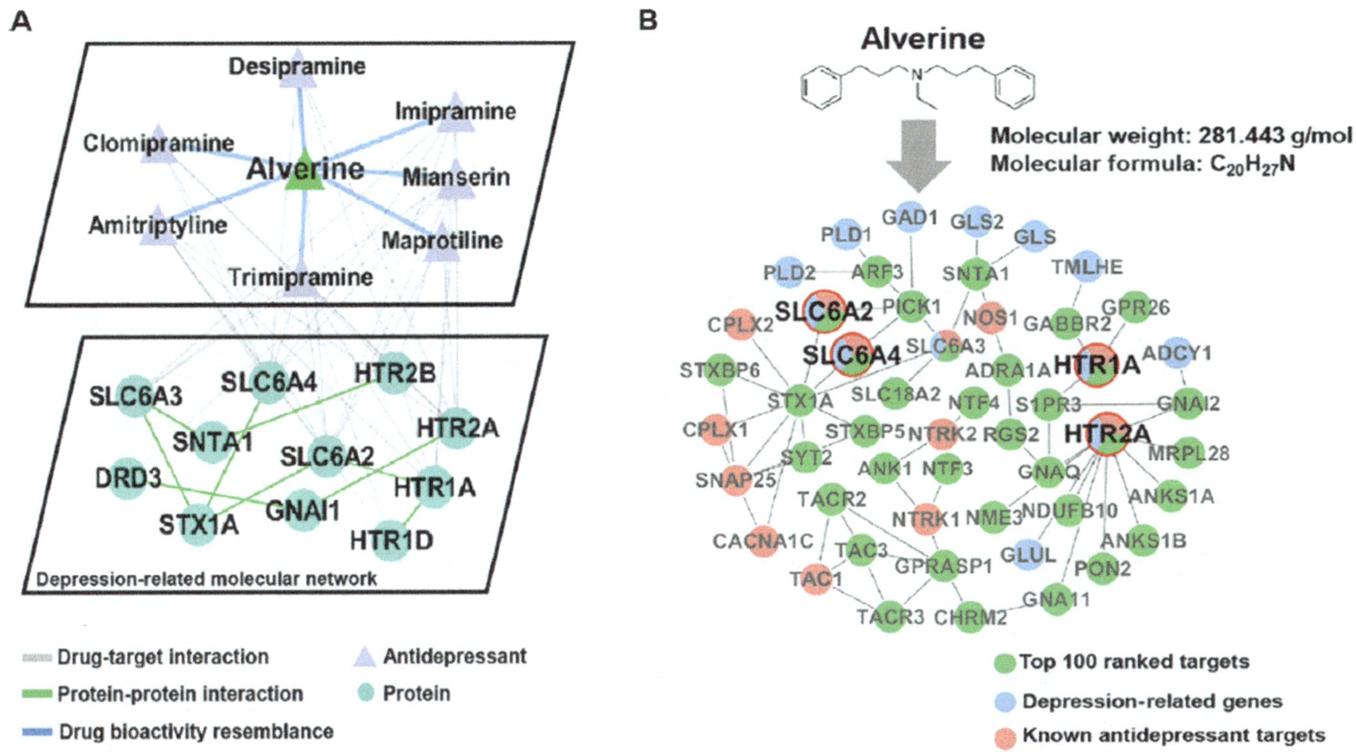

Fig. 6.12 Antidepressant related networks of the drug alverine [88]. (**a**) Drug-target network of alverine and other similar antidepressants. (**b**) Protein network targeted by alverine indicates the interaction between known antidepressant targets, depression-related disease genes, and the top 100 targets for alverine predicted by drugCIPHER

6.6 R&D of Drug Combination

Drug combination refers to a multi-ingredient, multi-targeted drug formed by combining two or more drugs with a clear mechanism of action and different targets, or after the effective ingredients are compatible in a reasonable dosage, for the treatment of diseases. As the human body can be regarded as a complex network system, the occurrence and development of diseases are the result of the comprehensive effects of multiple factors on the network of the human body. This complex mechanism makes the single target drug therapy model subject to certain limitations, which cannot comprehensively satisfy the treatment requirements of complex diseases. The development and application of drug combinations effectively make up for the defects of single target drugs. In recent years, the US Food and Drug Administration (FDA) has approved several drug combinations for clinical applications, especially for cardiovascular diseases, AIDS, neurodegenerative diseases, metabolic diseases, cancer, and other complex diseases. Clinical studies have shown that drug combinations are not a combination of single drug efficacy, but are based on a synergy of multiple drugs to achieve better efficacy and lower toxic side effects than single target drugs.

Most of the effective drug combinations used in clinical practice are driven by intuition and experience rather than by established principles. One method is to test pairwise drug combinations in a high-throughput, systematic manner, however, this method faces combinatorial challenges. For example, there are 499,500 possible pairwise combinations of 1,000 FDA-approved drugs, which require multiple dose combinations to be tested on about 3000 human diseases [90]. With the development of systems biology and network pharmacology, there are many network modeling methods for predicting drug combinations. These methods predict synergistic drug combinations based on drug-drug association, drug-target interaction, and multi-level drug–target–disease–gene interaction [91]. The method based on drug-drug association comprehensively takes advantage of multiple aspects of drug similarity information, including drug structure similarity, treatment spectrum similarity, target similarity, adverse reaction similarity, etc., to construct a similarity network between drugs and predict interactions between drugs, for example, the drug cocktail network method proposed by Wang et al. [92], the heterogeneous network-aided inference framework proposed by Cheng et al. [93], the prediction method of antibiotic drug combination based on chemical genomics data proposed by Chandrasekaran et al. [94], etc. Based on information such as drug-target correlation, topological structure similarity of target proteins, biological function of target, and position relationship on PPI network, the method based on drug–target interactions predicts drug interactions or infers the mode of action of drugs in the body. For example, the NIMS (Network Target-based Identification of Multicomponent Synergy) algorithm proposed by Li Shao et al. defines the agent score according to the relationship between the diseases treated by the drugs and the topology score according to the relationship of drug targets in the PPI network, and then integrates these two scores to predict the synergy of drug pairs [95]. TIMMA (Target Inhibition Interaction using

Maximization and Minimization Averaging) algorithm developed by He et al. combines the drug–target interaction network with a single drug sensitivity spectrum data from cell samples, to predict synergistic multi-target drug combinations [96]. Some other studies integrate the multi-dimensional relationship among drug-target-disease-gene to study the synergistic effect of drugs. For example, the DrugComboRanker algorithm developed by Huang et al. constructs the drug function association network and the disease-specific gene association network, decomposes the drug network into connected functional modules, and predicts the synergistic effect of drugs based on the inhibition of the drug function module on the disease network [97].

The following two specific research cases are selected for analysis.

6.6.1 Drug Combination Prediction Based on Network

Combination therapy is the co-use of multiple drugs, which has higher efficacy than single drug use. Also, by reducing the dose of single drug, the risk of adverse reactions can be reduced. However, there is still a lack of principles to systematically determine drug combinations with high efficacy and low toxicity.

In this study, Barabasi et al. developed a network-based method to quantify the relationships between drug targets and disease proteins in the human protein–protein interaction network, so as to design a reasonable and network-based drug combination discovery strategy [90].

6.6.1.1 Research Objectives

In network pharmacology research, the distance between research objects (such as diseases and drug target genes) in the whole genome protein–protein interaction network is usually used to measure the strength of the relationship between objects. In this study, the network proximity between drug targets and disease proteins is applied to the discovery of effective drug combinations.

6.6.1.2 Data Sources

Human Protein–Protein Interaction Network

By integrating the data construction of 15 databases, the same as Sect. 6.4.1.

Drug-Target Network

Drug-target interaction data was obtained from DrugBank, TTD (the Therapeutic Target Database) and PharmGKB Database [98]. Drug-target binding affinity data are from ChEMBL [99], BindingDB [100], and IUPHAR/BPS [101] Pharmacological guidelines. Only drug-target pairs with affinity indexes Ki, Kd, IC50, or EC50 no greater than 10 μM, in which the targets were human proteins were retained. A total of 15,051 high-quality interactions between 4428 drugs and 2256 human protein targets were obtained. Among them, 1978 drugs have at least two experimentally verified targets.

Gold Standard of Drug Combination Pairs

Clinical data were integrated from multiple data sources to obtain effective drug combination pairs. Each drug in the combination pair was required to have experimentally verified target information: EC_{50}, IC_{50}, K_i, or $K_d \leq 10$ μM. The drug name was standardized with MeSH and UMLS terms, and then converted into DrugBank ID. A total of 681 different drug combination pairs containing 362 drugs were obtained.

Adverse Drug–Drug Interactions

Clinically reported adverse Drug–Drug Interactions (DDIs) were collected from the DrugBank database. Only drugs with experimentally verified target information were collected. A total of 13,397 clinically reported adverse DDIs among 658 different drugs were obtained. In addition, cardiovascular event-specific adverse DDIs were collected from the TWOSIDE database [102]. TWOSIDE contains 59,220 drug combinations and 1301 adverse reaction events, totaling more than 868,221 significant adverse reaction related events. This study mainly focused on four cardiovascular events: arrhythmia (MeSH ID: D001145), heart failure (MeSH ID: D006333), myocardial infarction (MeSH ID: D009203), and hypertension (MeSH ID: D006973).

Disease-Related Genes

The disease-related genes were collected from 8 data sources and duplicate records were removed. The disease-related genes from 4 cardiovascular events were collected: arrhythmia (MeSH ID: D001145), heart failure (MeSH ID: D006333), myocardial infarction (MeSH ID: D009203), and hypertension (MeSH ID: D006973).

6.6.1.3 Analysis Index and Algorithm

Chemical Similarity of Drugs

The SMILES structural formula of each drug was downloaded from the DrugBank database and their MACCS fingerprints were calculated with Open Babel software. The Tanimoto coefficient was used to calculate the chemical similarity between a pair of drugs.

$$T = \frac{c}{a + b - c}$$

wherein a and b are the total number of digits in the fingerprints of the two drugs, and c is the same number of digits in their fingerprints.

Sequence Similarity of Target Proteins

The sequence of the target protein was downloaded from the UniProt database. The local sequence alignment algorithm, Smith–Waterman algorithm, was used to calculate the protein sequence similarity $S_P(a, b)$ between the two target proteins a and b. The sequence similarity of the targets of drugs A and B is defined as the average value of the similarities between their different target pairs:

$$< S_p >= \frac{1}{n_{pairs}} \sum_{\{a,b\}} S_p(a,b)$$

wherein $a \in A$, $b \in B$, $a \neq b$.

Gene Co-expression Similarity

RNA-seq data (RPKM values) for 32 tissues was obtained from the GTEx database. For each tissue, genes with RPKM$\geq$1 in more than 80% of the samples were selected as the genes specifically expressed in the tissue. The co-expression levels between two drug target encoding genes a and b were measured by the Pearson correlation coefficient $PCC(a,b)$ of their expression profiles. The co-expression similarity of targets of drug A and B is defined as the average value of the Pearson correlation coefficient between their target gene pairs:

$$< S_{co} >= \frac{1}{n_{pairs}} \sum_{\{a,b\}} PCC(a,b)$$

wherein $a \in A$, $b \in B$.

Gene Ontology (GO) Similarity

The GO information (Gene Ontology) of all drug target encoding genes was downloaded from the GO database and the GO annotation information predicted by the calculation was removed. The GO similarity $S_{GO}(a,b)$ between two drug target encoding genes a and b was calculated by using R-package GOSemSim. The GO similarity of the targets of drug A and B is defined as the average value of the GO similarity between their target gene pairs:

$$< S_{GO} >= \frac{1}{n_{pairs}} \sum_{\{a,b\}} S_{GO}(a,b)$$

wherein $a \in A$, $b \in B$.

6.6.1.4 Clinical Similarity of Drugs

The Anatomical Therapeutic Chemical codes (ATC) of all FDA-approved drugs in this study were downloaded from DrugBank. The k-level clinical similarity $S_k(A,B)$ of drugs A and B is defined as follows:

$$S_k(A,B) = \frac{ATC_k(A) \cap ATC_k(B)}{ATC_k(A) \cup ATC_k(B)}$$

wherein ATC_k represents all ATC codes at the kth level. The clinical similarity $S_{atc}(A,B)$ of drug A and B is defined as follows:

$$S_{atc}(A,B) = \frac{\sum_{k=1}^{n} S_k(A,B)}{n}$$

where n represents the five levels of ATC codes (ranging from 1 to 5). For drugs with multiple ATC codes, the similarity for each ATC code was calculated and then averaged.

Network Proximity Between Drugs

Suppose A and B are the drug-target sets of drug A and B, respectively (as shown in Fig. 6.13a). The separation of these two sets on the human PPI network can be divided into:

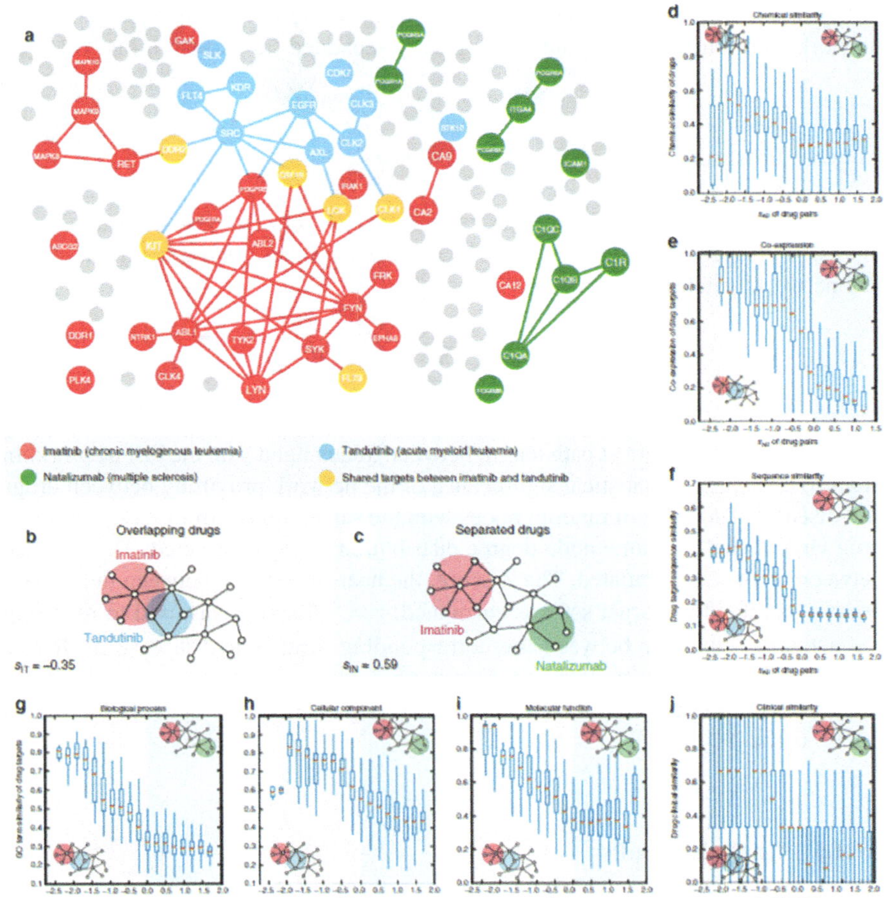

Fig. 6.13 Network model of relationship between drugs [90]. (**a**) The relationship between the target sets of the three drugs (imatinib [I], tandutinib [T], natalizumab [N]) in the human protein–protein interaction network. (**b, c**) are the definition of drug pairs with topological overlap ($s_{AB} < 0$) and topological separation ($s_{AB} \geq 0$). The correlation between the network proximity of (**d–j**) drug pairs and the similarity of five types of drugs: Drug-drug chemical similarity (**d**); Co-expression similarity of drug target genes in different human tissues (**e**); The sequence similarity of drug target protein (**f**); The GO similarity of drug target genes based on biological process similarity (**g**), cell component similarity (**h**), and molecular function similarity (**i**); as well as clinical similarity of drugs (**j**). In the graph, the background color of drug pair ($s_{AB} < 0$) with topological overlap is pink, and that of drug pair ($s_{AB} < 0$) with topological separation is blue

$$s_{AB} = < d_{AB} > - \frac{< d_{AA} > + < d_{BB} >}{2}$$

where $<d_{AB}>$ is the average shortest path length between targets in set A and B. It can be seen from this definition that if $s_{AB} < 0$, then the targets of drug A and drug B are adjacent on the network, and drug A and drug B topologically overlap (as shown in Fig. 6.13b). If $s_{AB} \geq 0$, then the targets of drugs A and B are separated in the network, and drugs A and B are topologically separated (as shown in Fig. 6.13c).

Network Proximity Between Drugs and Diseases

Suppose X and Y are the drug target and disease protein sets of drug X and disease Y, respectively. The nearest distance between these two sets on the human PPI network is defined as:

$$d(X, Y) = \frac{1}{\|Y\|} \sum_{y \in Y} \min_{x \in X} d(x, y)$$

where *d(x, y)* is the shortest path length between nodes *x* and *y* on the PPI network. In order to evaluate the statistical significance of the network proximity between drugs and diseases, 1000 sets of random nodes with the same number of disease genes and drug targets, and the same node degree distribution were constructed. The distance between them was calculated. The Z-score: the nearest distance between the disease protein and the drug-target set was calculated: $z = \frac{d-\mu}{\sigma}$ and it was used to represent the network proximity between the corresponding drug X and disease Y. If $z < 0$, then the drug-target module and disease module overlap on the network; If $z \geq 0$, then the drug target and disease modules are separated on the network (as shown in Fig. 6.13a–f).

6.6.1.5 Analysis Results

Correlation Between Network Proximity Index of Drugs and DRUG SIMILARITY

For every drug pair between the 1978 drugs with at least two experimentally verified targets, their network proximity, chemical similarity, clinical similarity, sequence similarity of target proteins, co-expression similarity of target protein encoding genes, and GO similarity were calculated. It was observed that the network proximity of the drug pairs has a negative correlation with the chemical, biological, functional, and clinical similarities of the drug pairs represented by the corresponding indexes (as shown in Fig. 6.13d–j). That is, drugs that are close to each other on the network have higher similarities in chemical, biological, functional, and clinical aspects. Therefore, the network proximity indexes of drugs can be used in the study of drug relationships.

Network Structure of Drug-Drug-Disease Combination

The network relationship between two drug target modules and one disease module (i.e. drug-drug-disease combination) was analyzed and it was found that this combination has six different network structure relationships:

(1) Overlapping exposure: two overlapping drug target modules simultaneously overlap with the disease module (P1 in Fig. 6.14a);
(2) Complementary exposure: two separated drug target modules overlap with the disease module (P2 in Fig. 6.14b);
(3) Indirect exposure: one of the two overlapping drug target modules overlaps with the disease module (P3 in Fig. 6.14c);
(4) Single exposure: two drug target modules are separated from each other, and one overlaps with the disease module (P4 in Fig. 6.14d);
(5) Non-exposure: two overlapping drug target modules are both separated from the disease module (P5 in Fig. 6.14e);
(6) Independent action: two drug target modules and one disease module are topologically separated from each other (P6 in Fig. 6.14f).

Through statistical analysis of the FDA-approved drug combination pairs for hypertension and cancer treatment (as shown in the bar graph on the right of Fig. 6.14), the following rules are found:

(1) Only when the two drug target modules overlap with the disease module, can the drug pair produce treatment-related effects.
(2) The therapeutic effect of overlapping exposure drug pairs (Fig. 6.14a) is not as good as that of single drug and has significant side effects.
(3) Only drug pairs with complementary exposure (Fig. 6.14b) have a significant therapeutic effect compared to the single drug.

6.6.1.6 Experimental Verification

For each pair between the 65 antihypertensive drugs approved by the FDA, its separation score S_{AB} was calculated and all the scores were then arranged in ascending order. Drug pair combinations with $S_{AB} < 0$ and complementary exposure to the hypertension disease module were identified. This method successfully predicted 24 antihypertensive drug combinations approved by the FDA, with an accuracy of 59%.

Next, the focus was on drug combinations involving hydrochlorothiazide. Hydrochlorothiazide is an FDA-approved antihypertensive sodium chloride co-transporter inhibitor. Drug combination pairs containing hydrochlorothiazide with complementary exposure to the hypertensive disease module were extracted. S_{AB} was ranked in ascending order and the top 30 combinations were considered. It was found that 21 cases (70% success rate) were supported by evidence, including FDA approval, clinical trial records, or reported preclinical data.

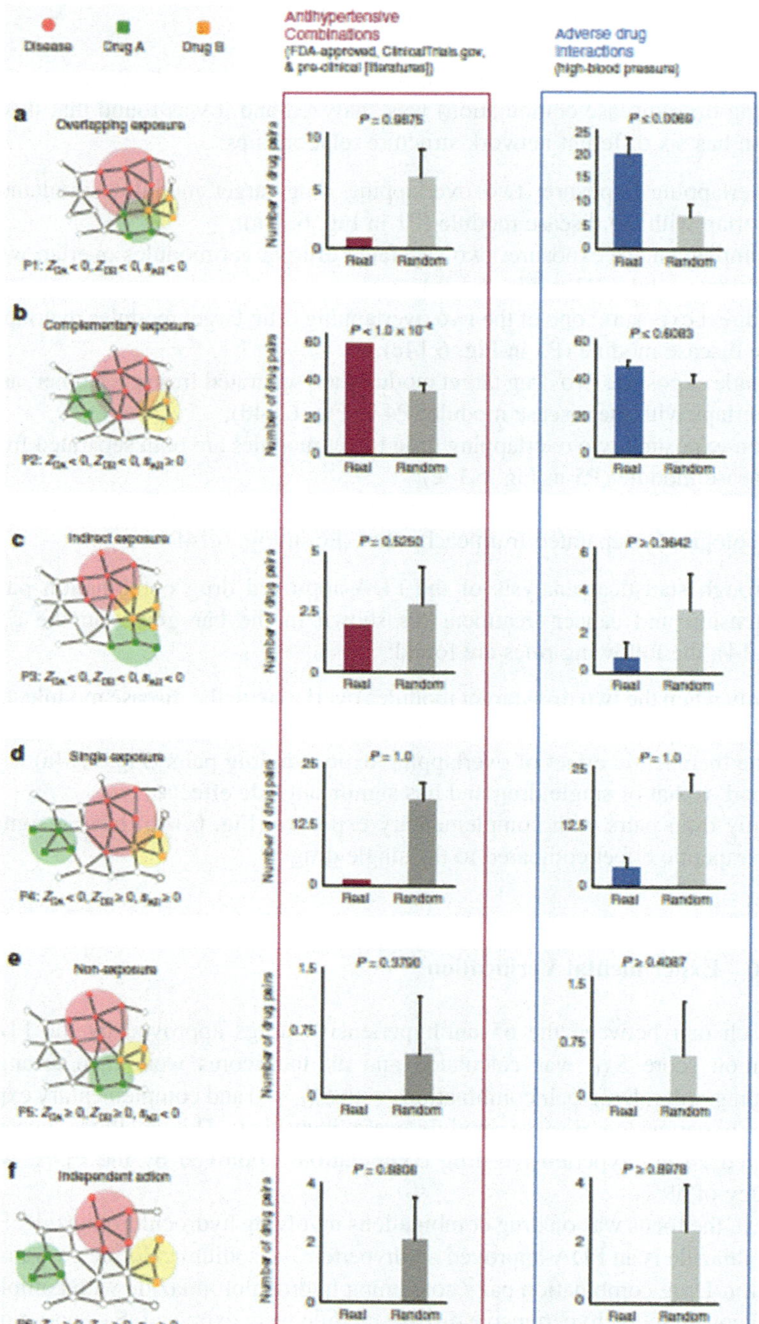

Fig. 6.14 Efficacy of hypertension drug interactions [90]. (**a**)–(**f**) Six different kinds of network structure relationships of drug-drug-disease combination. The purple and blue colored histogram represents the antihypertensive combinations and clinically reported adverse drug interactions on high blood pressure, respectively. The gray histogram shows the random control and the error bar represents the standard deviation

In this study, a total of 1455 kinds of potential drug combinations including 65 hypertensive drugs that meet the complementary exposure relationship were identified through calculations. In addition, an exhaustive list containing predicted drug combinations that were not used for hypertension and meet the complementary exposure relationship, as well as drug side effect combination pairs that meet the overlapping exposure relationship was also provided. This data provides potential drug combinations for hypertension for future experimental verification and prospective clinical trials.

6.6.1.7 Main Conclusion

In this study, a network-based algorithm was proposed to calculate the proximity between drug targets and disease genes on the network. Six network patterns of drug-drug-disease combination were obtained. By using the statistical method, two of them were inferred to be related to positive and negative side effects of drug combination, respectively, thus the effective drug combinations were predicted.

The relationship between drug targets and disease modules was explored in the human genome protein–protein interaction network. The method proposed in this study is useful in discovering effective drug combinations. If the network tools developed here can be widely used, they will help to develop novel and effective combination therapies for complex diseases.

6.6.2 Prediction of Synergistic Anti-cancer Drug Combinations Based on Genome and Network Characteristics

Cancer is a complex disease involving many factors and multiple biological processes. In clinical practice, single drug anti-cancer therapy is prone to drug resistance and side effects, while combination therapy has been widely considered as a better alternative. In recent years, synergistic drug combination has received special attention. It can achieve better curative effects than the sum of the effects of single drugs. Since each ingredient has a lower dose compared to a single therapy, side effects are greatly reduced. Some high-throughput screening platforms have been established to identify potential synergistic drug combinations. The calculation method is expected to provide more economical and rapid screening.

In this study, Cao et al. developed a computational model based on genome information and network characteristics, ranked the potential synergistic effects of drug pairs with unknown synergistic effects (unlabeled drug pairs) using drug pairs with known synergy (labeled drug pairs) as seeds, and predicted the synergistic combination of anti-cancer drugs [103].

6.6.2.1 Research Objectives

Currently, some known synergistic drug combinations have been recorded in databases or anti-cancer literature. Moreover, the molecular mechanisms underlying different aspects of existing synergistic drugs have been partially understood. For example, synergistic drugs may target multiple proteins in a pathway and its cross-talked pathways. In addition, compensatory pathway interactions, adaptive resistance, as well as molecular, pharmacological, and gene expression similarities were also related with drug synergy. Based on drug pairs with known synergistic effects, this study extracted the possible characteristics of synergistic drugs, constructed prediction models, and predicted more drug combinations with synergistic effects.

6.6.2.2 Data Source

Drug Pair Data

(1) A total of 41 kinds of synergistic anti-cancer agent combination pairs that have conducted clinical trials were obtained by using literature retrieval in Drug Combination Database (DCDB) [104] and PubMed. The drug pairs whose targets could not be mapped to KEGG signaling pathway were deleted, and the remaining 26 pairs were used as positive/marker samples for further modeling.
(2) 14 individual drugs or compounds were obtained from the NCI-DREAM consortium data set [105], of which only 13 have known protein targets. Seventy-eight kinds of paired combinations of these thirteen reagents were used as test data sets to interfere with human B cell lymphoma cell line OCI-LY3.
(3) 142 anti-cancer drugs that are approved by the FDA or have already entered clinical trials were obtained from DrugBank version 3.0, TTD, and PubMed. 118 anti-cancer drugs were obtained by deleting the drugs in which the target does not have the gene ontology (GO) annotation or KEGG information. These 118 drugs were combined to produce 6877 unlabeled drug pairs as test data sets for lung adenocarcinoma cell line A549 and ER positive breast cancer cell line MCF7. The target protein information of all research drugs was extracted from DrugBank version 3.0, TTD, and PubMed.

Network data

(1) Background protein–protein interaction network: the network was constructed with data from HPRD, MINT, Inact, BioGRID, DIP, and MIPS database, and the largest connected sub-network was obtained.
(2) Cancer Network (CN): Using all the genes in the "pathways in cancer" signaling in KEGG and cancer-related genes in literature, genes were connected in the

background, to construct a sub-network using protein–protein network interaction.

(3) Specific cancer signaling pathway (take breast cancer MCF7 as an example): The gene expression profile of MCF7 cancer cell line was obtained from CCLE (Cancer Cell Line Encyclopedia) [106]. Expression data of all other cell lines in the database was used as the control group, and differential expression genes of MCF7 were obtained based on the standards of $|\log2foldchange| > 0.5$. These differential expression genes were connected through the background network to form the breast cancer pathway.

Gene Expression Data

(1) Array data of labeled drugs: Gene expression profiles of each single drug in the labeled drug pairs were searched from CMAP, ArrayExpress, and GEO. Since these synergistic drug combinations are applicable to different cancer types, gene expression profiles on the same cell line of the specified cancer type were searched for each drug pair. Finally, the gene expression profiles of 9 pairs of labeled drug pairs (including 11 drugs) were found.
(2) Array data of cell line Ly3 of β-cell lymphoma: the expression profile data of this cell line treated with single drug was downloaded from the DREAM website [105].
(3) Array data of lung adenocarcinoma cell line A549 and ER positive breast cancer cell line MCF7: The expression profile data of the test drug acting on these two cell lines were also obtained from CMAP, ArrayExpress, and GEO.

6.6.2.3 Analysis Index and Algorithm

In this study, a semi-supervised learning model, which is called ranking system of anti-cancer synergy (RACS), was constructed, and its workflow is shown in Fig. 6.15.

Characteristics of the primary ranking model: Originally, 14 characteristics describing drug synergy were proposed. Then, the Z-score test was carried out to select the following seven characteristics ($|Z\text{-score}| > 3$), which make a significant difference between synergistic drug pairs and unlabeled drug pairs.

(1) Mutual information entropy (MI) based on GO: this characteristic represents the similarity between biological processes (BP) regulated by the target of two drugs. The calculation method is as follows:

    a. All the genes in the "Pathways in cancer" signaling pathway in KEGG were input into DAVID to conduct GO enrichment analysis, and 1,006 GO BP entries with significant enrichment ($P < 0.05$) were obtained, which are cancer-related BP.

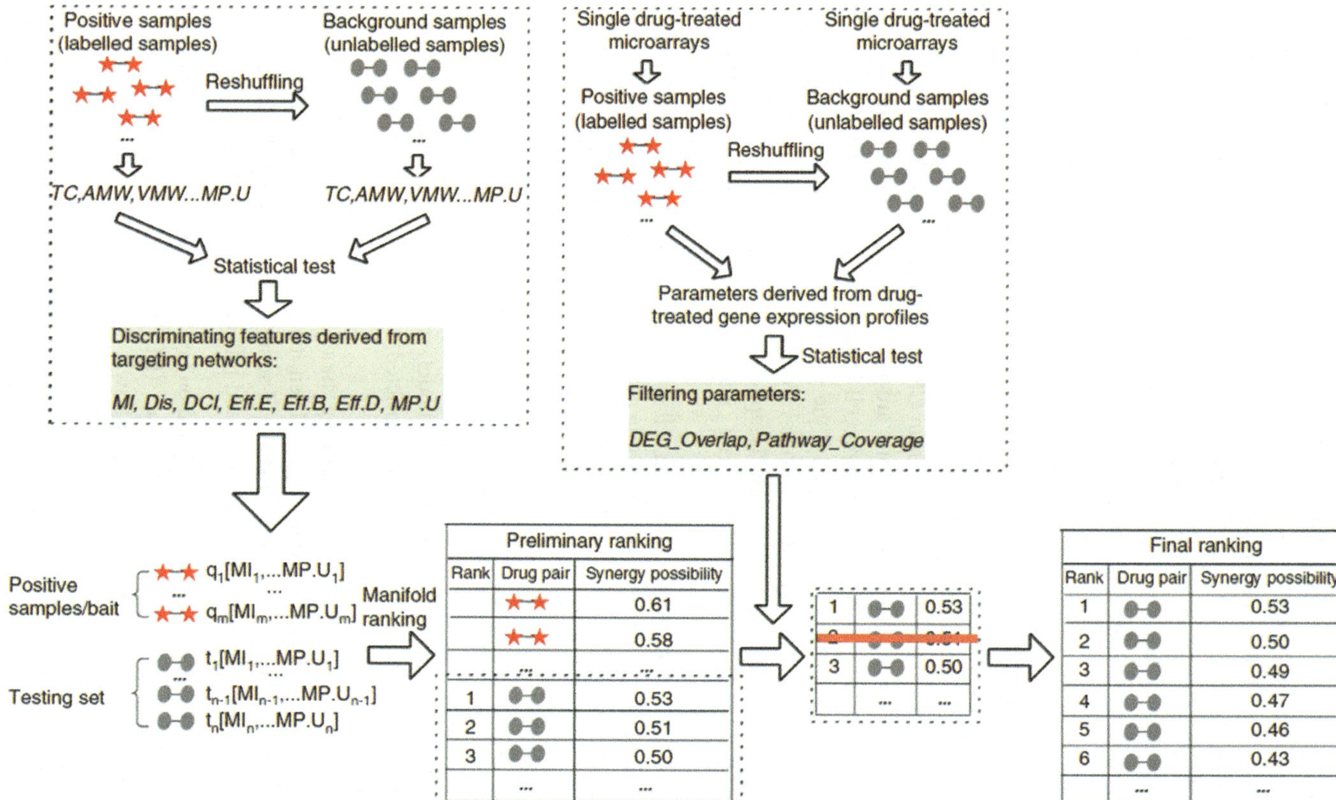

Fig. 6.15 Workflow of RACS system [103]. Red star pairs represent known synergistic drug pairs (labeled pairs), and gray ball pairs represent unknown synergistic drug pairs (unlabeled pairs). By using the manifold ranking algorithm, all marked and unlabeled pairs are sorted in multi-dimensional eigenvector space. After the marked pairs are excluded, the gene expression profile is further filtered to optimize the ranking of unlabeled pairs

b. A 0–1 binary vector was constructed with 1006 dimensions for each drug. If the drug target is in a certain BP, the corresponding component is 1.
c. Mutual information entropy was used to calculate the similarity between cancer-related BP vectors of drug pair (*x*, *y*):

$$MI(x,y) = P(x,y) \times \log \frac{P(x,y)}{P(x) \times P(y)}$$

wherein *P(x)* is the ratio of mapped GO terms in cancer-related BPs for agent *x*, and *P(x, y)* is the ratio of the common GO terms mapped to cancer-related BPs between *x* and *y*.

(2) Distance (Dis) describes the average distance between the target proteins of the two drugs in the protein–protein interaction network.

$$Dis(x,y) = \frac{\sum_{i=1}^{M}\sum_{j=1}^{N} dis(i,j)}{M \times N}$$

wherein *dis(i, j)* is the shortest distance between the *i*-th target of drug *x* and the *j*-th target of drug *y* in the background protein–protein interaction network. *M* and *N* are the number of targets of drug *x* and *y*, respectively.

(3) Drug combination interference (DCI) describes the variance of the effect of the combination of drugs and single drugs on the efficiency of network information transmission.

$$DCI(x,y) = \Delta E_{x+y} - (\Delta E_x + \Delta E_y)$$

wherein $\Delta E_x = \frac{E-E_x}{E}$, *E* represents the information transfer efficiency of the cancer network in the absence of drug disturbance, and is the average shortest path between node pairs in the network. E_x is the network information transmission efficiency calculated after removing all targets of drug *x* from the cancer network.

(4) Efficacy (Eff.D, Eff.B, and Eff.E): these characteristics represent the efficacy of drug combination pairs when both efficacy and additional efficacy are considered. The calculation of Eff.D, Eff.B, and Eff.E is based on the degree, betweenness, eigenvector centrality of the drug targets in the network, respectively. The design of the three characteristics follows the assumption that a good combination produces the greatest therapeutic effect and the least additional impact. The design concept of Efficacy (Eff) is that the drug combination should hit the key target of the cancer network and avoid hitting the target in the non-cancer network.

$$Eff = \lambda \frac{\sum_{i \in CN} W_i}{\sum_{i \in BD} W_i} - (1 - \lambda) \frac{\sum_{i \in NCN} W_i}{\sum_{i \in V} W_i} Eff = \lambda \frac{\sum_{i \in CN} W_i}{\sum_{i \in BD} W_i} - (1 - \lambda) \frac{\sum_{i \in NCN} W_i}{\sum_{i \in V} W_i}$$

The first and second parts of the formula represent the therapeutic effect and the additional effect, respectively. The parameter $\lambda \in [0, 1]$ is used to balance the two parts of the formula, here it is taken as 0.1. For three different kinds of efficacy—Eff. D, Eff.B, and Eff.E, the weight W_i of node i takes the degree, betweenness, and eigenvector centrality of the node in the corresponding network, respectively.

CN: Target proteins in cancer networks.

BD: Target proteins in background PPI network, including CN.

NCN: Target proteins in BD but outside of CN.

V: All nodes in the background PPI network, including CN.

(5) Mapped unrelated pathway pairs (MP.U): first, all genes in the "Pathways in cancer" signaling pathway in KEGG were input into DAVID for KEGG pathway enrichment analysis, and 132 pathways with significant enrichment ($P < 0.05$) were obtained, which are cancer-related pathways. Then, the target of a drug was mapped to 132 cancer-related pathways; the pathways on the target map constitute the pathway set of the drug. One pathway was taken from the pathway sets of drug pairs x, y, respectively, to form a pathway pair; the pathway pair has the following four types:

a. Identical pathway pair.
b. Cross-talking pathway pair: two different pathways share at least one gene in common.
c. Interaction pathway pair: the two pathways are neither identical nor intersecting, but there is interaction between the genes in the two pathways on the PPI network.
d. Unrelated path pair: a path pair that does not fall into any of the above three categories.

MP.U is defined as the proportion of unrelated path pairs to the total path pairs of x and y.

Primary ranking system: Each drug pair (including positive and unlabeled drug pairs) is represented by the 7-dimensional eigenvectors of the above-mentioned seven characteristics, and all drug pairs were arranged into a list:

$$X = \{x_1, \ldots, x_q, x_{q+1}, \ldots, x_n\}$$

wherein $x_1, \ldots, x_q$ are labeled drug pairs, followed by the unlabeled drug pairs. Then the drug pairs were sorted by Manifold Ranking, a semi-supervised learning algorithm. The steps are as follows:

(1) The Euclidean distance $d(x_i, x_j)$ of every neighboring pair of drugs was calculated, the distances were arranged in descending order, and the drug pairs were connected in order, until a connected network formed.
(2) The edge weight of the network is defined as: $W_{ij} = 1/d(x_i, x_j)$.
(3) The scoring function is defined as: $f(t + 1) = \alpha Sf(t) + (1 - \alpha)y$.

Wherein: $S = D^{-\frac{1}{2}}WD^{-\frac{1}{2}}$, y is the initial vector, whose first q components are 1, and the following components are 0.

The scoring function iterates to convergence, and each component is the score of the corresponding drug pair.

Secondary filtering system: Two indexes—DEG_Overlap and Pathway_Coverage, derived from the gene expression profile were used to further filter the ranking obtained by the primary ranking system.

$$\text{DEG\_Overlap}(x, y) = \frac{|A \cap B|}{\sqrt{|A| \times |B|}}$$

$$\text{Pathway\_Coverage}(x, y) = \frac{|(A \cup B) \cap N|}{|N|}$$

wherein A and B represent the differentially expressed gene (DEG) set caused by drug x and y intervention, respectively, and N represents all genes in the specific cancer signaling pathway.

These two indexes were calculated for each drug pair, and the drug pair with a p value of less than 0.05 for both indexes was retained.

6.6.2.4 Analysis Result

RACS System Significantly Improves DREAM Data on DLBCL Cells

To assess the predictive ability, RACS was applied to the standard data obtained from the DREAM Consortium. This experimental data uses a binary combination of 14 different drugs/compounds in the human Diffuse Large B-Cell Lymphoma (DLBCL) cell line OCI-LY3 to detect the activity of the combination and gene expression profile. As the target of the DNA cross-linker mitomycin C is as yet unclear, 78 drug pairs formed by combining the remaining 13 drugs as unlabeled combinations were tested using RACS and compared with the peering methods. The comparative methods include DIGRE (the best performing method in the DREAM Report), SynGen (the method proposed by the DREAM Organizer), DrugComboRanker [97], and Zhao [107]. The comparison indexes are area under ROC curve (AUC) value, true positive rate, and PC-index. The results show that the RACS system performs best on these three indexes; at the same time, based on the primary ranking, the secondary filtering based on the transcriptional profile data significantly improves the performance of the RACS system.

The RACS System has a Significant Ranking Ability to the Drug Pairs Acting on Breast Cancer and Lung Cancer Cells

The RACS system was further evaluated using the ER positive breast cancer cell line MCF7. A total of 118 anti-cancer drugs were combined into binary pairs, 26 known synergistic pairs were deleted, and the remaining 6877 pairs were unlabeled combinations. RACS was run 30 times using a different number of labeled pairs. For the combination that consistently appeared in the top 1% of the ranking, the consensus ranking containing 41 drug pairs was obtained by Spearman's Footrule Distance, which is the preliminary ranking list. After secondary filtering of drug-interfered transcriptional profile data based on cell line MCF7, 33 of the 41 drug pairs remained in the final ranking list. Literature search shows that there are five kinds of drugs that have a synergistic combined anti-cancer effect, including combined intervention of curcumin and resveratrol for colorectal cancer, trastuzumab and erlotinib in the treatment of breast cancer, topotecan and vorinostat in the treatment of small cell lung cancer, estramustine and docetaxel in the treatment of breast cancer, and bleomycin and etoposide in the treatment of endometrial carcinoma. From the remaining 28 combinations, the combinations containing antibody drugs and non-commercial drugs were removed, and subsequent in vitro experimental verification was conducted on the remaining 17 drug pairs.

Then, the RACS system was further verified using human lung adenocarcinoma cell line A549. Based on gene expression profiles and target information, 55 combinations of 11 drugs were analyzed, and these 55 drug pairs were ranked by the same procedure and criteria. The top 10% and bottom 10% of the drug pairs were verified through experiments.

6.6.2.5 Experimental Verification

Verifying the Synergistic Effect of Drug Pairs Through in vitro Experiments

For the remaining 17 pairs of drugs based on MCF7 cell line ranking, the corresponding drugs were purchased and verified by using human MCF7 cell line in vitro experiments. In this study, the synergestic effect was measured according to the Combination Index (CI) proposed by Chou and Talalay. Only when the CI values of a pair of drugs in the four combination concentrations are less than 0.9, they can be accepted as synergistic effects. Based on this criterion, 9 out of 17 pairs (52.94%) were newly identified as having synergistic effects of inhibiting MCF7 cell proliferation.

In vitro experimental verification was conducted on the top 10% and bottom 10% drug pairs obtained based on A549 cell line ranking. The results show that the top 10% of the two drug pairs (33.33%), namely gefitinib and quinacrine, and erlotinib and quinacrine, have synergistic effects of inhibiting A549 cell proliferation ($CI < 0.3$). In contrast, none of the six pairs ranked at the bottom showed synergy.

Verifying the Synergistic Effect and Potential Toxicity of Drug Pairs Through In Vivo Experiments

As anti-cancer effects usually involve cytotoxicity, further screening needs to be conducted to determine whether strong synergistic combinations are less toxic to normal cells or organs and have fewer side effects. To verify the results obtained in vivo, four drugs were selected, namely gefitinib, erlotinib, sorafenib, and tamoxifen, and a zebrafish-based toxicity model of human cancer cell xenografts was used to evaluate the synergistic effects and potential toxicity of the drugs. It was observed that the tolerance of zebrafish to the individual treatment of gefitinib or erlotinib alone was the same as the concentration used in cell experiments; however, the combined use of tamoxifen and sorafenib in the zebrafish model showed severe toxicity. The combination of erlotinib and sorafenib showed significant synergistic effect on inhibiting the proliferation of xenografted MCF-7 cells in zebrafish and had no obvious side effects; on the contrary, single drug treatment had no effect on tumors.

6.6.2.6 Main Conclusion

In this study, a set of characteristics related to the synergistic effects of anti-cancer drugs were proposed, and an effective model RACS was constructed to predict the synergistic effects of the drug combinations for cancer treatment. By verifying the predicted synergistic effects on three cancer cell lines and a zebrafish model, it is shown that RACS has a good effect in ranking drug combinations with potential synergistic anti-cancer effects.

At present, it is becoming increasingly difficult to find new single drugs. The combination use of existing drugs provides new opportunities for the treatment of cancer. With the accumulation of growing amounts of TCGA data and xenotransplantation (PDX) models, the process of predicting drug combinations from RACS, then using cell line for verification, and further screening with in vivo models proposed in this study is expected to accelerate the development of personalized combination therapy.

From the perspective of systems biology, a life form can be seen as a complex network formed by the interaction of various molecules, while drugs can change their functional state by acting on some nodes of the network, thereby intervening in the occurrence and development of diseases and achieve curative effects. Network pharmacology studies complex diseases and drug development at the genome-wide system level, and studies the role and relationship between multiple genes and drug targets of diseases under the context of various regulatory networks at different biological levels, to systematically predict and explain the role of drugs, discover the factors affecting the efficacy and safety of drugs, and propose new strategies for treatment of complex diseases. Network pharmacology is a transformation in the philosophy and research model of drug development, and has made significant progress in the five aspects introduced in this chapter. With the further improvement of various biological databases, a deeper understanding of molecular networks and signaling pathways involved in disease processes, as well as the introduction of pioneering experimental technologies (such as single cell sequencing, gene knock-out, etc.) and computational technologies (such as artificial intelligence, machine learning, etc.) into network biology research, network pharmacology is expected to make greater progress in the understanding and treatment of complex diseases.

References

1. Kaufmann SH. Paul Ehrlich: founder of chemotherapy. Nat Rev Drug Discov. 2008;7(5):373.
2. Hopkins AL. Network pharmacology: the next paradigm in drug discovery. Nat Chem Biol. 2008;4(11):682.
3. Oliver S. Guilt-by-association goes global. Nature. 2000;403(6770):601–2.
4. Wu X, Jiang R, Zhang MQ, et al. Network-based global inference of human disease genes. Mol Syst Biol. 2008;4:1.
5. Lin L, Yang T, Fang L, et al. Gene gravity-like algorithm for disease gene prediction based on phenotype-specific network. BMC Syst Biol. 2017;11(1):121.
6. Zhang B, Gaiteri C, Bodea L-G, et al. Integrated systems approach identifies genetic nodes and networks in late-onset Alzheimer's disease. Cell. 2013;153(3):707–20.
7. Mani KM, Lefebvre C, Wang K, et al. A systems biology approach to prediction of oncogenes and molecular perturbation targets in B-cell lymphomas. Mol Syst Biol. 2008;4:1.
8. Menche J, Sharma A, Kitsak M, et al. Uncovering disease-disease relationships through the incomplete interactome. Science. 2015;347(6224):1257601.
9. Chen C, Meng Q, Xia Y, et al. The transcription factor POU3F2 regulates a gene coexpression network in brain tissue from patients with psychiatric disorders. Sci Transl Med. 2018;10 (472):eaat8178.
10. Torrey EF, Webster M, Knable M, et al. The stanley foundation brain collection and neuro-pathology consortium. Schizophr Res. 2000;44(2):151–5.
11. Gibbs JR, van der Brug MP, Hernandez DG, et al. Abundant quantitative trait loci exist for DNA methylation and gene expression in human brain. PLoS Genet. 2010;6:5.
12. Langfelder P, Horvath S. WGCNA: an R package for weighted correlation network analysis. BMC Bioinf. 2008;9(1):559.
13. Aten JE, Fuller TF, Lusis AJ, et al. Using genetic markers to orient the edges in quantitative trait networks: the NEO software. BMC Syst Biol. 2008;2(1):34.
14. de Leeuw CA, Mooij JM, Heskes T, et al. MAGMA: generalized gene-set analysis of GWAS data. PLoS Comput Biol. 2015;11:4.
15. Lee PH, O'dushlaine C, Thomas B, et al. INRICH: interval-based enrichment analysis for genome-wide association studies. Bioinformatics. 2012;28(13):1797–9.
16. Purcell SM, Moran JL, Fromer M, et al. A polygenic burden of rare disruptive mutations in schizophrenia. Nature. 2014;506(7487):185–90.
17. Genovese G, Fromer M, Stahl EA, et al. Increased burden of ultra-rare protein-altering variants among 4,877 individuals with schizophrenia. Nat Neurosci. 2016;19(11):1433.
18. Li J, Cai T, Jiang Y, et al. Genes with de novo mutations are shared by four neuropsychiatric disorders discovered from NPdenovo database. Mol Psychiatry. 2016;21(2):290–7.
19. Bass JIF, Sahni N, Shrestha S, et al. Human gene-centered transcription factor networks for enhancers and disease variants. Cell. 2015;161(3):661–73.
20. Kheradpour P, Kellis M. Systematic discovery and characterization of regulatory motifs in ENCODE TF binding experiments. Nucleic Acids Res. 2014;42(5):2976–87.

21. Guo Y, Bao C, Ma D, et al. Network-based combinatorial crispr-cas9 screens identify synergistic modules in human cells. ACS Synth Biol. 2019;8(3):482–90.
22. Schäfer H, Struck B, Feldmann E, et al. TGF-β1-dependent L1CAM expression has an essential role in macrophage-induced apoptosis resistance and cell migration of human intestinal epithelial cells. Oncogene. 2013;32(2):180–9.
23. Bassik MC, Kampmann M, Lebbink RJ, et al. A systematic mammalian genetic interaction map reveals pathways underlying ricin susceptibility. Cell. 2013;152(4):909–22.
24. Kampmann M, Bassik MC, Weissman JS. Integrated platform for genome-wide screening and construction of high-density genetic interaction maps in mammalian cells. Proc Natl Acad Sci. 2013;110(25):E2317–26.
25. Bandyopadhyay S, Mehta M, Kuo D, et al. Rewiring of genetic networks in response to DNA daMage. Science. 2010;330(6009):1385–9.
26. Lamb J, Crawford ED, Peck D, et al. The Connectivity Map: using gene-expression signatures to connect small molecules, genes, and disease. Science. 2006;313(5795):1929–35.
27. Subramanian A, Narayan R, Corsello SM, et al. A Next generation connectivity map: l1000 platform and the first 1,000,000 profiles. Cell. 2017;171(6):1437–52.
28. Iwata M, Sawada R, Iwata H, et al. Elucidating the modes of action for bioactive compounds in a cell-specific manner by large-scale chemically-induced transcriptomics. Sci Rep. 2017;7:40164.
29. Guney E, Menche J, Vidal M, et al. Network-based in silico drug efficacy screening. Nat Commun. 2016;7:10331.
30. Wei W-Q, Cronin RM, Xu H, et al. Development and evaluation of an ensemble resource linking medications to their indications. J Am Med Inform Assoc. 2013;20(5):954–61.
31. Sartor MA, Ade A, Wright Z, et al. Metab2MeSH: annotating compounds with medical subject headings. Bioinformatics. 2012;28(10):1408–10.
32. Iorio F, Bosotti R, Scacheri E, et al. Discovery of drug mode of action and drug repositioning from transcriptional responses. Proc Natl Acad Sci. 2010;107(33):14621–6.
33. Kruskal JB. On the shortest spanning subtree of a graph and the traveling salesman problem. Proc Am Math Soc. 1956;7(1):48–50.
34. Diaconis P, Graham RL. Spearman's footrule as a measure of disarray. J R Stat Soc. 1977;39 (2):262–8.
35. Lin S. Space oriented rank-based data integration. Stat Appl Genet Mol Biol. 2010;9:1.
36. Frey BJ, Dueck D. Clustering by passing messages between data points. Science. 2007;315 (5814):972–6.
37. Csermely P, Agoston V, Pongor S. The efficiency of multi-target drugs: the network approach might help drug design. Trends Pharmacol Sci. 2005;26(4):178–82.
38. Keith CT, Borisy AA, Stockwell BR. Multicomponent therapeutics for networked systems. Nat Rev Drug Discov. 2005;4(1):71–8.
39. Korcsmáros T, Szalay MS, Böde C, et al. How to design multi-target drugs: target search options in cellular networks. Expert Opin Drug Discovery. 2007;2(6):799–808.
40. Ramsay RR, Popovic-Nikolic MR, Nikolic K, et al. A perspective on multi-target drug discovery and design for complex diseases. Clin Transl Med. 2018;7(1):3.
41. Meng H, Liu Y, Lai L. Diverse ways of perturbing the human arachidonic acid metabolic network to control inflammation. Acc Chem Res. 2015;48(8):2242–50.
42. Keane H, Ryan BJ, Jackson B, et al. Protein-protein interaction networks identify targets which rescue the MPP+ cellular model of Parkinson's disease. Sci Rep. 2015;5(1):1–12.
43. Casas AI, Hassan AA, Larsen SJ, et al. From single drug targets to synergistic network pharmacology in ischemic stroke. Proc Natl Acad Sci. 2019;116(14):7129–36.
44. Kotlyar M, Pastrello C, Sheahan N, et al. Integrated interactions database: tissue-specific view of the human and model organism interactomes. Nucleic Acids Res. 2016;44(D1):D536–41.
45. Wishart DS, Feunang YD, Marcu A, et al. HMDB 4.0: the human metabolome database for. Nucleic Acids Res. 2018;46(D1):D608–17.

46. Li YH, Yu CY, Li XX, et al. Therapeutic target database update 2018: enriched resource for facilitating bench-to-clinic research of targeted therapeutics. Nucleic Acids Res. 2018;46(D1): D1121–7.
47. Wishart DS, Tzur D, Knox C, et al. HMDB: the human metabolome database. Nucleic Acids Res. 2007;35(suppl_1):D521–6.
48. Sidders B, Karlsson A, Kitching L, et al. Network-based drug discovery: coupling network pharmacology with phenotypic screening for neuronal excitability. J Mol Biol. 2018;430 (18):3005–15.
49. Jamieson DG, Moss A, Kennedy M, et al. The pain interactome: connecting pain-specific protein interactions. Pain. 2014;155(11):2243–52.
50. Razick S, Magklaras G, Donaldson IM. iRefIndex: a consolidated protein interaction database with provenance. BMC Bioinf. 2008;9(1):405.
51. Pushpakom S, Iorio F, Eyers PA, et al. Drug repurposing: progress, challenges and recommendations. Nat Rev Drug Discov. 2019;18(1):41–58.
52. Zhang Y, Cheng X, Zhou W. Drug reorientation: an important application field of network pharmacology. Chin J Pharmacol Toxicol. 2012;26(6):779–86.
53. Cheng F, Liu C, Jiang J, et al. Prediction of drug-target interactions and drug repositioning via network-based inference. PLoS Comput Biol. 2012;8(5):e1002503.
54. Iorio F, Isacchi A, di Bernardo D, et al. Identification of small molecules enhancing autophagic function from drug network analysis. Autophagy. 2010;6(8):1204–5.
55. Luo H, Wang J, Li M, et al. Drug repositioning based on comprehensive similarity measures and bi-random walk algorithm. Bioinformatics. 2016;32(17):2664–71.
56. Cheng F, Desai RJ, Handy DE, et al. Network-based approach to prediction and population-based validation of in silico drug repurposing. Nat Commun. 2018;9(1):1–12.
57. Rolland T, Taşan M, Charloteaux B, et al. A proteome-scale map of the human interactome network. Cell. 2014;159(5):1212–26.
58. Rual J-F, Venkatesan K, Hao T, et al. Towards a proteome-scale map of the human protein–protein interaction network. Nature. 2005;437(7062):1173–8.
59. Cheng F, Jia P, Wang Q, et al. Quantitative network mapping of the human kinome interactome reveals new clues for rational kinase inhibitor discovery and individualized cancer therapy. Oncotarget. 2014;5(11):3697.
60. Keshava Prasad T, Goel R, Kandasamy K, et al. Human protein reference database—2009 update. Nucleic Acids Res. 2009;37(suppl_1):D767–72.
61. Hu J, Rho H-S, Newman RH, et al. PhosphoNetworks: a database for human phosphorylation networks. Bioinformatics. 2014;30(1):141–2.
62. Hornbeck PV, Zhang B, Murray B, et al. PhosphoSitePlus, 2014: mutations, PTMs and recalibrations. Nucleic Acids Res. 2015;43(D1):D512–20.
63. Lu C-T, Huang K-Y, Su M-G, et al. DbPTM 3.0: an informative resource for investigating substrate site specificity and functional association of protein post-translational modifications. Nucleic Acids Res. 2013;41(D1):D295–305.
64. Dinkel H, Chica C, Via A, et al. Phospho. ELM: a database of phosphorylation sites—update 2011. Nucleic Acids Res. 2010;39(suppl_1):D261–7.
65. Oughtred R, Stark C, Breitkreutz B-J, et al. The BioGRID interaction database: 2019 update. Nucleic Acids Res. 2019;47(D1):D529–41.
66. Cowley MJ, Pinese M, Kassahn KS, et al. PINA v2. 0: mining interactome modules. Nucleic Acids Res. 2012;40(D1):D862–5.
67. Chatr-Aryamontri A, Ceol A, Palazzi LM, et al. MINT: the Molecular INTeraction database. Nucleic Acids Res. 2007;35(suppl_1):D572–4.
68. Orchard S, Ammari M, Aranda B, et al. The MIntAct project—IntAct as a common curation platform for 11 molecular interaction databases. Nucleic Acids Res. 2014;42(D1):D358–63.
69. Breuer K, Foroushani AK, Laird MR, et al. InnateDB: systems biology of innate immunity and beyond—recent updates and continuing curation. Nucleic Acids Res. 2013;41(D1): D1228–33.

70. Meyer MJ, Das J, Wang X, et al. INstruct: a database of high-quality 3D structurally resolved protein interactome networks. Bioinformatics. 2013;29(12):1577–9.
71. Fazekas D, Koltai M, Türei D, et al. SignaLink 2–a signaling pathway resource with multi-layered regulatory networks. BMC Syst Biol. 2013;7(1):7.
72. Bodenreider O. The unified medical language system (UMLS): integrating biomedical terminology. Nucleic Acids Res. 2004;32(suppl_1):D267–70.
73. Hamosh A, Scott AF, Amberger JS, et al. Online Mendelian Inheritance in Man (OMIM), a knowledgebase of human genes and genetic disorders. Nucleic Acids Res. 2005;33(suppl_1): D514–7.
74. Davis AP, Grondin CJ, Lennon-Hopkins K, et al. The comparative toxicogenomics database's 10th year anniversary: update 2015. Nucleic Acids Res. 2015;43(D1):D914–20.
75. Yu W, Gwinn M, Clyne M, et al. A navigator for human genome epidemiology. Nat Genet. 2008;40(2):124–5.
76. Piñero J, Bravo À, Queralt-Rosinach N, et al. DisGeNET: a comprehensive platform integrating information on human disease-associated genes and variants. Nucleic Acids Res. 2016;2016:gkw943.
77. Landrum MJ, Lee JM, Riley GR, et al. ClinVar: public archive of relationships among sequence variation and human phenotype. Nucleic Acids Res. 2014;42(D1):D980–5.
78. Welter D, Macarthur J, Morales J, et al. The NHGRI GWAS catalog, a curated resource of SNP-trait associations. Nucleic Acids Res. 2014;42(D1):D1001–6.
79. Li MJ, Liu Z, Wang P, et al. GWASdb v2: an update database for human genetic variants identified by genome-wide association studies. Nucleic Acids Res. 2016;44(D1):D869–76.
80. Denny JC, Bastarache L, Ritchie MD, et al. Systematic comparison of phenome-wide association study of electronic medical record data and genome-wide association study data. Nat Biotechnol. 2013;31(12):1102.
81. Wishart DS, Feunang YD, Guo AC, et al. DrugBank 5.0: a major update to the DrugBank database for 2018. Nucleic Acids Res. 2018;46(D1):D1074–82.
82. Hernandez-Boussard T, Whirl-Carrillo M, Hebert JM, et al. The pharmacogenetics and pharmacogenomics knowledge base: accentuating the knowledge. Nucleic Acids Res. 2007;36(suppl_1):D913–8.
83. Bento AP, Gaulton A, Hersey A, et al. The ChEMBL bioactivity database: an update. Nucleic Acids Res. 2014;42(D1):D1083–90.
84. Gilson MK, Liu T, Baitaluk M, et al. BindingDB in 2015: a public database for medicinal chemistry, computational chemistry and systems pharmacology. Nucleic Acids Res. 2016;44 (D1):D1045–53.
85. Pawson AJ, Sharman JL, Benson HE, et al. The IUPHAR/BPS Guide to pharmacology: an expert-driven knowledgebase of drug targets and their ligands. Nucleic Acids Res. 2014;42 (D1):D1098–106.
86. Consortium G. The genotype-tissue expression (GTEx) pilot analysis: multitissue gene regulation in humans. Science. 2015;348(6235):648–60.
87. Wang S, Verpillat P, Rassen J, et al. Transparency and reproducibility of observational cohort studies using large healthcare databases. Clin Pharmacol Therap. 2016;99(3):325–32.
88. Zhang T-T, Xue R, Wang X, et al. Network-based drug repositioning: a novel strategy for discovering potential antidepressants and their mode of action. Eur Neuropsychopharmacol. 2018;28(10):1137–50.
89. Zhao S, Li S. Network-based relating pharmacological and genomic spaces for drug target identification. PLoS One. 2010;5:7.
90. Cheng F, Kovács IA, Barabási A-L. Network-based prediction of drug combinations. Nat Commun. 2019;10(1):1–11.
91. Li W, Mao X, Guo Q, et al. Application of network pharmacology research strategy in combinatorial drug research. E-j Transl Med. 2018;5(3):3–16.
92. Wang Y-Y, Xu K-J, Song J, et al. Exploring drug combinations in genetic interaction network. BMC Bioinf. 2012;2017:S7.

93. Cheng F, Zhao Z. Machine learning-based prediction of drug–drug interactions by integrating drug phenotypic, therapeutic, chemical, and genomic properties. J Am Med Inform Assoc. 2014;21(e2):e278–86.
94. Chandrasekaran S, Cokol-Cakmak M, Sahin N, et al. Chemogenomics and orthology-based design of antibiotic combination therapies. Mol Syst Biol. 2016;12:5.
95. Li S, Zhang B, Zhang N. Network target for screening synergistic drug combinations with application to traditional Chinese medicine. BMC Syst Biol. 2011;5(S1):S10.
96. He L, Wennerberg K, Aittokallio T, et al. TIMMA-R: an R package for predicting synergistic multi-targeted drug combinations in cancer cell lines or patient-derived samples. Bioinformatics. 2015;31(11):1866–8.
97. Huang L, Li F, Sheng J, et al. DrugComboRanker: drug combination discovery based on target network analysis. Bioinformatics. 2014;30(12):i228–36.
98. Gaulton A, Bellis LJ, BENTO AP, et al. ChEMBL: a large-scale bioactivity database for drug discovery. Nucleic Acids Res. 2012;40(D1):D1100–7.
99. LIU T, LIN Y, WEN X, et al. BindingDB: a web-accessible database of experimentally determined protein–ligand binding affinities. Nucleic Acids Res. 2007;35(suppl_1): D198–201.
100. Tatonetti NP, Patrick PY, Daneshjou R, et al. Data-driven prediction of drug effects and interactions. Sci Transl Med. 2012;4(125):125ra131.
101. SUN Y, SHENG Z, MA C, et al. Combining genomic and network characteristics for extended capability in predicting synergistic drugs for cancer. Nat Commun. 2015;6(1):1–10.
102. Liu Y, Wei Q, Yu G, et al. DCDB 2.0: a major update of the drug combination database. Database. 2014;2014:124.
103. Sun Y, Sheng Z, Ma C, et al. Combining genomic and network characteristics for extended capability in predicting synergistic drugs for cancer. Nat Commun. 2015;28(6):8481.
104. Liu Y, Wei Q, Yu G, Gai W, Li Y, Chen X. DCDB 2.0: a major update of the drug combination database. Database (Oxford). 2014;2014:bau124.
105. Bansal M, Yang J, Karan C, et al. A community computational challenge to predict the activity of pairs of compounds. Nat Biotechnol. 2014;32(12):1213–22.
106. Barretina J, Caponigro G, Stransky N, et al. The Cancer Cell Line Encyclopedia enables predictive modelling of anticancer drug sensitivity. Nature. 2012;483(7391):603–7.
107. Zhao J, Zhang XS, Zhang S. Predicting cooperative drug effects through the quantitative cellular profiling of response to individual drugs. CPT Pharmacometrics Syst Pharmacol. 2014;3(2):e102.

Chapter 7
Drug-Based Network Pharmacology Practice Process

Xiaobo Sun, Xiaoyan Xing, and Min Wang

7.1 Guide to this Chapter

TCM has a long history and notable therapeutic effect in China [1, 2]. Starting from the holistic and systematic of drug–target–disease interactions, network pharmacology employs complex network models to enunciate and scrutinize drug–target–disease network relationships [3]. The holistic and methodical characteristics of network pharmacology coincide with the holistic view of TCM theory and the principle of syndrome differentiation and treatment, which provides new ideas and perspectives for the systematic research of TCM [4].

Considering the classic and reputed Guanxin Danshen Formulation and the commonly used Chinese medicines Ginseng Radix et Rhizoma, Notoginseng Radix et Rhizoma, and Salviae miltiorrhizae Radix et Rhizoma as examples, this chapter introduces the practice process of network pharmacology based on drugs from six aspects: active ingredients identification, mechanism analysis, compatibility theory of TCM, interaction between Chinese and Western medicines, drug repurposing, and multi-targets drug development, and attempts to provide clues with reference value for the application of network pharmacology in TCM research.

X. Sun (✉) · X. Xing · M. Wang
Institute of Medicinal Plant Development, Chinese Academy of Medical Sciences and Peking Union Medical College, Beijing, China

S. Li (ed.), *Network Pharmacology*, https://doi.org/10.1007/978-981-16-0753-0_7

7.2 Finding the Active Ingredients of a Single Chinese Medicine or Prescription

Indefinite material basis and indefinite mechanism of action are the salient hurdles to the wider acceptance of TCM in the international community. Therefore, the identification of active ingredients in TCM is a crucial challenge to be decoded in the modernization of traditional Chinese medicine. The typical measures for network pharmacology to identify the effective ingredients of TCM are as follows: Primarily, the information related to chemical components, chemical component targets, and disease targets of TCM are collated based on database retrieval and computer simulation technology. Subsequently, these data are taken as nodes in the network, and the "TCM–component" network, the "component–target" network, and the "disease–gene" network are constructed based on the interconnection between the nodes. Finally, the overall "TCM–component–target–disease" network is fabricated by a network composite. The interconnection between the elements is scrutinized based on the overall network, in order to detect the potential effective component group of TCM for the treatment of specific diseases.

Guanxin Danshen Formulation (GXDSF) is a classic prescription commonly used in clinical practice. It consists of three Chinese herbs: Salvia miltiorrhiza, Panax notoginseng, and Dalbergia odorifera oil. It is effective in improving blood circulation and disperse stasis, regulating qi and relieving pain. It is predominantly used in the treatment of coronary heart disease with qi stagnation and blood stasis. Modern compound preparations developed on the basis of GXDSF, such as Guanxin Danshen tablet, Guanxin Danshen capsule, and Guanxin Danshen dripping pills, have significant clinical efficacy and are widely used in the prevention and treatment of coronary heart disease [5]. Expounding the active ingredient basis of GXDSF can provide expedient clues for the R&D of new drugs in the treatment of cardiovascular disease (CVD). Therefore, case in point of GXDSF, identifying the effective component groups of TCM prescriptions based on network pharmacology is introduced exhaustively below. The research flow is as demonstrated in Fig. 7.1.

7.2.1 Data Acquisition and Processing

7.2.1.1 Chemical Component Collection of Complete GXDSF Prescription

The chemical components of the complete GXDSF prescription were assembled based on two classic Chinese herbal medicine databases—ETCM and TCM-MESH. The "Herbs" option was selected under the MENU option of the ETCM database menu bar, and "Salvia miltiorrhiza" was entered in the search box to obtain the chemical composition list 1 of radix Salviae Miltiorrhizae. "Herb" was selected under the Search Type option of TCM-MESH database, "Pinyin name" was selected

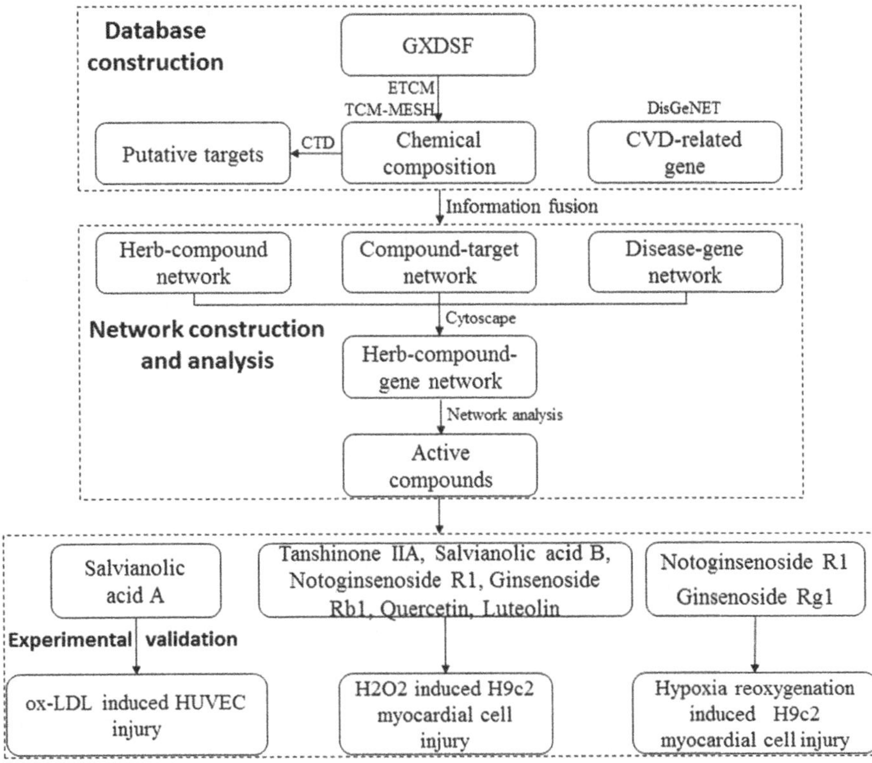

Fig. 7.1 Research ideas and processes

under Herb Name Type option, and "Dan Shen" entered in the search box to obtain the chemical composition list two of radix Salviae Miltiorrhizae. The two chemical component lists of Danshen assembled based on the ETCM and TCM-MESH databases were integrated and deduplication processing was performed to obtain a complete chemical component list of Salvia miltiorrhiza medicinal materials. The chemical components of the two medicinal materials of Panax notoginseng and Dalbergia odorifera were assembled using the same method. The corresponding relationship between each Chinese medicine and its chemical composition was saved in the form of a two-dimensional table.

7.2.1.2 Collection of Chemical Component Targets

The "Chemicals" option was selected under the Keyword Search option of the CTD database, the appropriate English name of each chemical component was entered in the search box, and the target data of each chemical component was assembled. The corresponding relationship between each chemical component and its target was saved in the form of a two-dimensional table. The mass search function provided by the CTD database can also be used to retrieve the target data of each chemical component.

7.2.1.3 Collection of CVD-Related Disease Genes

The "Search" option was selected in the menu bar of the DisGeNET database, the search type was set to "diseases," and cardiovascular disease was entered in the search box, to assemble the CVD-related target gene data. The corresponding relationship between the disease and its related genes was saved in the form of a two-dimensional table.

7.2.2 *Network Construction and Visualization*

The "TCM–ingredient" list, "ingredient–target" list, and "disease–gene" list obtained in the data source were entered into Cytoscape 3.5.0 network analysis and visualization software. The merge function under the "Tools" option in the menu bar was used to superimpose networks to construct a "TCM–ingredient–disease–target" network. To increase the self-evidence of the network, different attributes (shape, size, color, font, etc.) can be set for different nodes in the network. At the same time, the visualization effect of the network can be adjusted through the network layout function under the "Layout" option in the menu bar.

The Network Analyzer function under the "Tools" option in the Cytoscape 3.5.0 menu bar was used to analyze the topological attributes (connectivity) of each node in the network.

7.2.3 *Network Analysis and Prediction*

7.2.3.1 Chemical Components of Complete GXDSF Prescription and Its Targets

Based on the ETCM and TCM-MESH database, there are a total of 115 chemical components of Salvia miltiorrhiza, 121 chemical components of Panax notoginseng, and 35 chemical components of Dalbergia odorifera assembled in this study. By means of chemical component deduplication treatment, a total of 267 chemical components of Complete GXDSF Prescription are collected. The number of chemical component targets corresponding to Salvia miltiorrhiza, Panax notoginseng, Dalbergia odorifera, and GXDSF is 241, 215, 101, and 398, respectively (as shown in Table 7.1). The Venn diagram distribution shows that there are pronounced differences in the chemical composition of the three medicinal materials of salvia miltiorrhiza, Panax notoginseng, and Dalbergia odorifera (As shown in Fig. 7.2).

Table 7.1 Chemical components of complete GXDSF prescription and its targets

Data type	Traditional Chinese medicine			Total
	Salvia miltiorrhiza	Panax notoginseng	Dalbergia odorifera	
Chemical composition	115	121	35	267
Targets	241	215	101	398

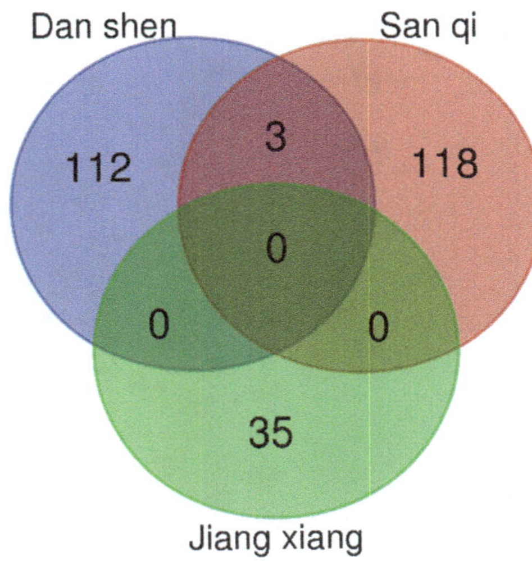

Fig. 7.2 Venn diagram—chemical composition of GXDSF

7.2.3.2 Analysis of TCM–Ingredient–Disease Target Network

Figure 7.3 shows the TCM–component–disease target network of GXDSF for CVD treatment. As demonstrated in Fig. 7.3, the three traditional Chinese medicines Salvia miltiorrhiza, Panax notoginseng, and Dalbergia odorifera have certain regulatory effects on CVD-related genes. A total of 37 ingredients in GXDSF are associated in the regulation of CVD. Among them, 21 ingredients are from Salvia miltiorrhiza, 2 ingredients are from Dalbergia odorifera, and 16 ingredients are from Panax notoginseng. The results confirm that Salvia miltiorrhiza, Dalbergia odorifera, and Panax notoginseng execute a synergistic role in the treatment of CVD by means of distinct active components.

Yellow, green, and red round nodes represent TCM, TCM chemical components, and disease targets, respectively. The size of each node is adjusted according to the topology parameter—connectivity of nodes in the network. The larger the node, the greater the connectivity of the node in the network, and vice versa. The size of the node reflects the importance of the node in the network to a certain extent. The gray edge represents the inclusive or regulating relationship between the two nodes.

By and large, kaempferol, luteolin, palmitic acid, tanshinone IIB, tanshinone IIA, tanshinone I, and other ingredients, together totaling 37 ingredients, constitute the effective ingredient group of GXDSF that plays a synergistic role in the treatment of CVD. Table 7.2 shows the source, English name, Chinese name, CAS number, and

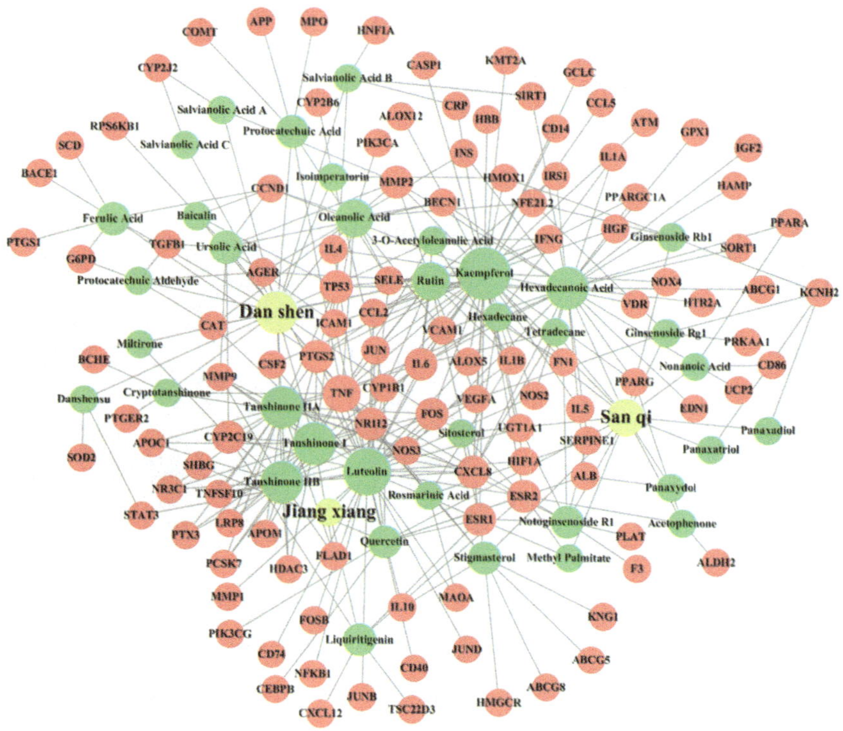

Fig. 7.3 TCM–component–disease target network

topological parameter information of each component in the GXDSF effective ingredient group.

7.2.4 *Verification and Summary*

Integrating the content of each chemical component in the medicinal components and its topological parameter—connectivity in the network, we hand-picked nine components (Kaempferol, luteolin, tanshinone IIA, quercetin, Notoginsenoside R1, salvianolic acid B, Ginsenoside Rg1, ginsenoside Rb1, and salvianolic acid A) from the above 37 to verify the activity of cardiovascular protection.

Through experiments, we verified that (1) Protective effects of tanshinone IIA, salvianolic acid B, Notoginsenoside R1, ginsenoside Rb_1, quercetin, and luteolin on H_2O_2 induced H9c2 myocardial cell injury; (2) Protective effects of Notoginsenoside R1 and ginsenoside Rg1 on H9c2 cardiomyocytes injury were induced by hypoxia reoxygenation; (3) Protective effects of salvianolic acid A on oxidative low-density lipoprotein (ox-LDL) induced injury of human umbilical vein endothelial cells; (4) Protective effects of kaempferol on doxorubicin-induced H9c2

Table 7.2 Effective component group of GXDSF

Serial No.	Source of medicinal materials	Chemical compound	Chinese name	CAS	Connectivity
1	Panax notoginseng	Kaempferol	Kaempferol	520-18-3	44
2	Dalbergia odorifera	Luteolin	Luteolin	491-70-3	36
3	Panax notoginseng	Hexadecanoic acid	Palmitic acid	1957-10-3	26
4	Salvia miltiorrhiza	Tanshinone IIb	Tanshinone IIB	17397-93-2	19
5	Salvia miltiorrhiza	Tanshinone IIa	Tanshinone IIA	568-72-9	19
6	Salvia miltiorrhiza	Tanshinone I	Tanshinone I	568-73-0	19
7	Salvia miltiorrhiza	Rutin	Rutin	153-18-4	15
8	Salvia miltiorrhiza	Oleanolic acid	Oleanolic acid	508-02-1	12
9	Panax notoginseng	Quercetin	Quercetin	117-39-5	8
10	Salvia miltiorrhiza	Ursolic acid	Ursolic acid	77-52-1	8
11	Panax notoginseng	Notoginsenoside R1	Notoginsenoside R1	80418-24-2	8
12	Salvia miltiorrhiza, Panax notoginseng	Stigmasterol	Stigmasterol	83-48-7	7
13	Salvia miltiorrhiza	Ferulic acid	Ferulic acid	1135-24-6	6
14	Salvia miltiorrhiza	Protocatechuic acid	Protocatechuic acid	99-50-3	5
15	Dalbergia odorifera	Liquiritigenin	Liquiritigenin	578-86-9	5
16	Salvia miltiorrhiza	Salvianolic acid B	Salvianolic acid B	115939-25-8	4
17	Salvia miltiorrhiza	Protocatechuic aldehyde	Protocatechuic aldehyde	139-85-5	4
18	Panax notoginseng	Ginsenoside Rg1	Ginsenoside Rg1	22427-39-0	4
19	Salvia miltiorrhiza	Cryptotanshinone	Cryptotanshinone	35825-57-1	4
20	Salvia miltiorrhiza	3-O-Acetyloleanolic acid	Oleanolic acid 3-acetate	4339-72-4	4
21	Salvia miltiorrhiza	Rosmarinic acid	Rosmarinic acid	537-15-5	4
22	Panax notoginseng	Hexadecane	N-hexadecane	544-76-3	3
23	Panax notoginseng	Tetradecane	N-tetradecane	629-59-4	3
24	Panax notoginseng	Acetophenone	Acetophenone	98-86-2	3

(continued)

Table 7.2 (continued)

Serial No.	Source of medicinal materials	Chemical compound	Chinese name	CAS	Connectivity
25	Panax notoginseng	Ginsenoside Rb1	Ginsenoside Rb1	41753-43-9	3
26	Salvia miltiorrhiza	Isoimperatorin	Isoimperatorin	482-45-1	3
27	Panax notoginseng	Nonanoic acid	Nonanoic acid	112-05-0	2
28	Panax notoginseng	Methyl palmitate	Methyl palmitate	112-39-0	2
29	Salvia miltiorrhiza	Baicalin	Baicalin	21967-41-9	2
30	Salvia miltiorrhiza	Danshensu	Tanshinol	23028-17-3	2
31	Salvia miltiorrhiza	Salvianolic acid A	Salvianolic acid A	96574-01-5	2
32	Salvia miltiorrhiza, Panax notoginseng	Sitosterol	β-sitosterol	83-46-5	2
33	Panax notoginseng	Panaxadiol	Panaxadiol	19666-76-3	1
34	Salvia miltiorrhiza	Miltirone	Miltirone	27210-57-7	1
35	Panax notoginseng	Panaxatriol	Panaxatriol	32791-84-7	1
36	Panax notoginseng	Panaxydol	Panaxydol	72800-72-7	1
37	Salvia miltiorrhiza	Salvianolic acid C	Salvianolic acid C	115841-09-3	1

cardiomyocyte injury. By and large, the effective component group of GXDSF was identified by using the network pharmacology method, and the cardiovascular protective effects of some components were verified by different in vitro cell models. The results of network analysis are highly consistent with the experimental results, which signify that network pharmacology is an effective means to identify the material basis of traditional Chinese medicines/TCM compound prescriptions.

7.2.4.1 Effects of Tanshinone IIA, Salvianolic Acid B, Notoginsenoside R1, Ginsenoside Rb_1, Quercetin, and Luteolin on H_2O_2 Induced H9c2 Myocardial Cell Injury; Protective Effect of H_2O_2 on H9c2 Myocardial Cell Injury

After pre-incubating different concentrations of tanshinone IIA, salvianolic acid B, notoginsenoside R1, ginsenoside Rb1, and luteolin for a corresponding time, 150 μM H_2O_2 was allowed to react for 6 h. The MTT method was employed to detect the consequences of each active ingredient on H9c2 myocardial cell activity.

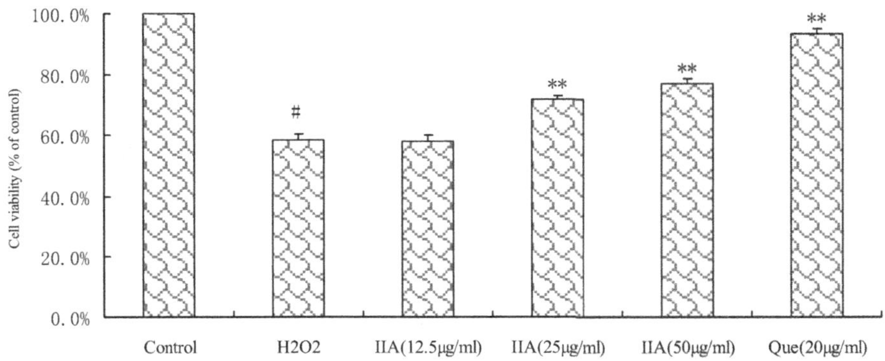

Fig. 7.4 Effect of tanshinone IIA on H_2O_2-induced H9c2 myocardial cell injury. *IIA* tanshinone IIA, *Que* quercetin, $^{\#}P < 0.01$ (model group vs control group), $^{**}P < 0.01$ (processing group vs model group)

The results demonstrate that: Tanshinone IIA, a fat-soluble component of Salvia miltiorrhiza, exhibits significant myocardial cell protective effect at 50 μg/ml and 25 μg/ml (as shown in Fig. 7.4). Salvianolic acid B, a water-soluble component, has protective effects on myocardial cells at 12.5 μg/ml and 6.25 μg/ml (as shown in Fig. 7.5). Ginsenoside Rb1 in Panax notoginseng has a significant inhibitory effect on H_2O_2-induced decline in myocardial cell activity at 50 μg/ml and 25 μg/ml (as shown in Fig. 7.6). However, notoginsenoside R1 has no significant effect on H_2O_2-induced H9c2 cell damage within the detection concentration range (3.125–200 μg/ml) (as shown in Fig. 7.7). Luteolin, a flavonoid from Dalbergia odorifera, has significant protective effects on myocardial cells. The cardiomyocyte activity in the model group is 52.7%±1.1% of that in the normal group, while that in the luteolin 12.5 μg/ml and 25 μg/ml pre-incubation groups are 81.9%±1.4% and 89.2%±1.4%, respectively. The cardiomyocyte activity in the luteolin group is significantly higher than that in the model group (as shown in Fig. 7.8). Quercetin shows significant protective effects on myocardial cells at concentrations of 20 μg/ml and 40 μg/ml. In the same dose, its protective effect on myocardial cells is significantly higher than that of tanshinone IIA, ginsenoside Rb1, and notoginsenoside R1 (as shown in Figs. 7.4, 7.6, and 7.7).

7.2.4.2 Protective Effects of Notoginsenoside R1 and Ginsenoside Rg1 on H9c2 Myocardial Cell Injury Induced by Hypoxia Reoxygenation

After pre-incubation with different concentrations of notoginsenoside R1 and ginsenoside Rg1 for a corresponding time, hypoxia reoxygenation damage occurred on myocardial cells. The CCK-8 method was employed to detect the activity of myocardial cells. Compared to the control group, the survival rate of H9c2 cells was significantly reduced due to 6 h of hypoxia and 12 h of reoxygenation. After

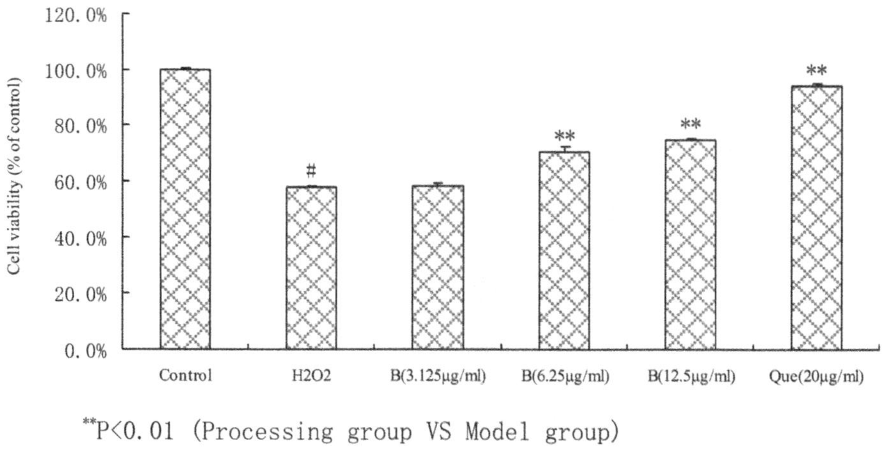

Fig. 7.5 Effect of salvianolic acid B on H_2O_2-induced H9c2 myocardial cell injury. *B* salvianolic acid B, *Que* quercetin, $^{\#}P < 0.01$ (model group vs control group), $^{**}P < 0.01$ (processing group vs model group)

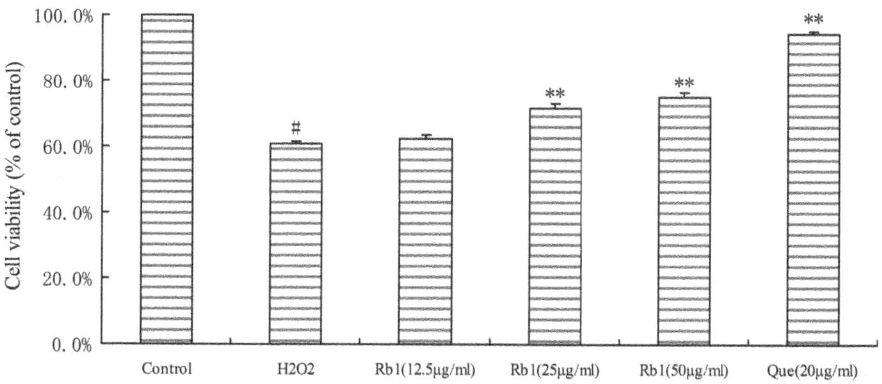

Fig. 7.6 Effects of ginsenoside Rb1 on H_2O_2-induced H9c2 myocardial cell injury. *Rb1* ginsenoside Rb1, *Que* quercetin, $^{\#}P < 0.01$ (model group vs control group), $^{**}P < 0.01$ (processing group vs model group)

pre-incubation with different concentrations of notoginsenoside R1 and ginsenoside Rg1 (2.5, 5, 10, 20, 40, 80 μmol/L) for 24 h, they all demonstrated sublime cell protective effects, and significantly enhanced the cell survival rate, demonstrating a dose-dependent trend (as shown in Fig. 7.9).

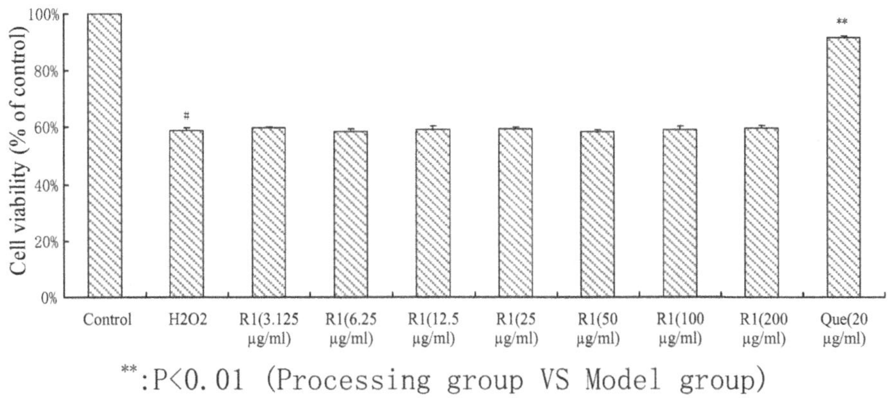

Fig. 7.7 Effects of notoginsenoside R1 on H_2O_2-induced H9c2 myocardial cell injury. *R1* notoginsenoside R1, *Que* quercetin, $^{\#}P < 0.01$ (model group vs control group), $^{**}P < 0.01$ (processing group vs model group)

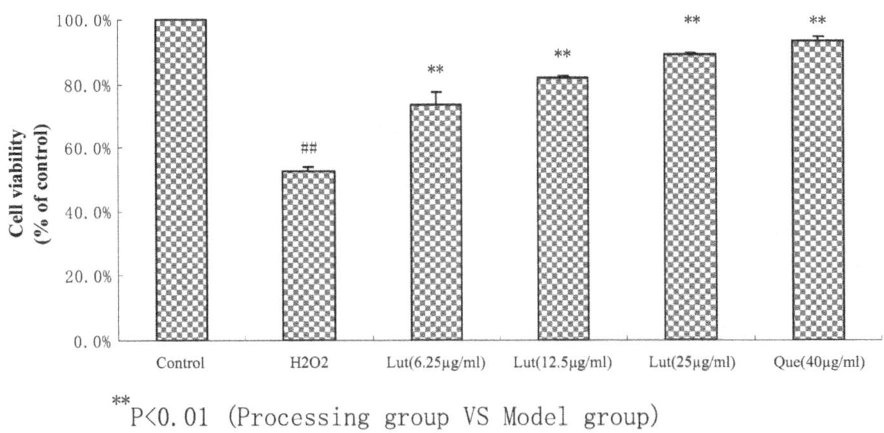

Fig. 7.8 Effects of luteolin on H_2O_2-induced H9c2 myocardial cell injury. *Lut* luteolin, *Que* quercetin, $^{\#\#}P < 0.01$ (model group vs control group), $^{**}P < 0.01$ (Processing group vs model group)

7.2.4.3 Protective Effects of Salvianolic Acid A on ox-LDL-Induced Injury of Human Umbilical Vein Endothelial Cells

After 12 h pre-incubation with different concentrations of salvianolic acid A, 70 μg/ml ox-LDL was allowed to react for 24 h. The CCK-8 method was employed to detect the activity of cells. The results demonstrate that salvianolic acid A protects ox-LDL-induced injury to human umbilical vein endothelial cells, in acceptable doses. At the outset, the effective concentration of salvianolic acid A is low, and it significantly reduce the ox-LDL-induced injury to human umbilical vein endothelial

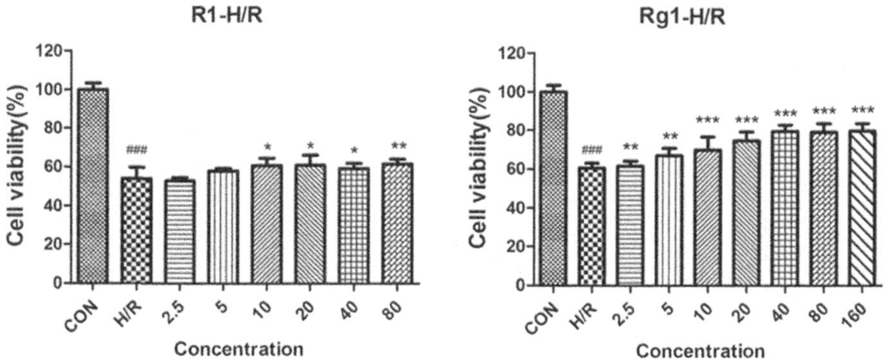

Fig. 7.9 Effects of notoginsenoside R1 and ginsenoside Rg1 on H9c2 myocardial cell injury induced by hypoxia reoxygenation. *R1* notoginsenoside R1, *Rg1* ginsenoside Rg1. ###$P < 0.001$ (model group vs control group), *$P < 0.05$ (processing group vs model group), **$P < 0.01$ (processing group vs model group), ***$P < 0.001$ (processing group vs model group)

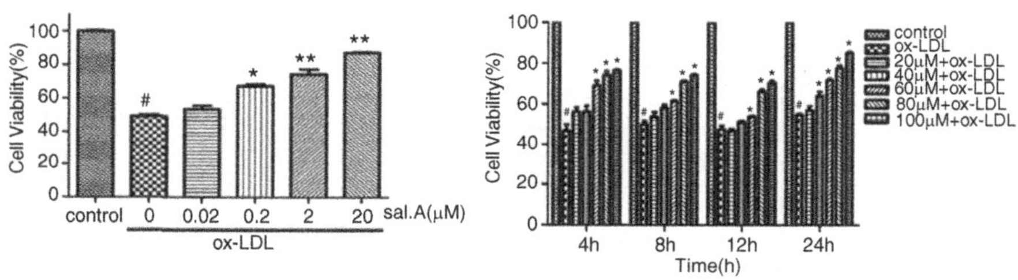

Fig. 7.10 Effect of salvianolic acid A on ox-LDL-induced injury of human umbilical vein endothelial cells. *Sal.A* salvianolic acid A, #$P < 0.001$ (model group vs control group), *$P < 0.05$ (processing group vs model group), **$P < 0.01$ (processing group vs model group)

cell at a concentration of 0.2 μm. However, salvianolic acid A shows obvious cytotoxic effects at concentrations above 25 μmol (as shown in Fig. 7.10).

7.2.4.4 Protective Effects of Kaempferol on h9c2 Cardiomyocyte Injury Induced by Doxorubicin

After 24 h pre-incubation with different concentrations of kaempferol, 1 μM doxorubicin was allowed to react for 4 h. The MTT method was employed to detect the effects of different concentrations of kaempferol on H9c2 myocardial cell activity. The results demonstrate that kaempferol at different concentrations significantly reduced the doxorubicin-induced H9c2 cardiomyocyte injury (as shown in Fig. 7.11).

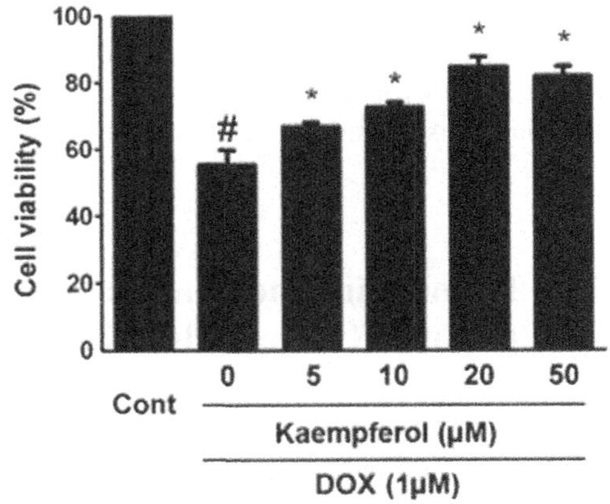

Fig. 7.11 Effect of kaempferol on doxorubicin-induced H9c2 cardiomyocyte injury. $^{\#}P < 0.05$ (model group vs control group), $^{**}P < 0.05$ (processing group vs model group)

7.2.4.5 Summary

Taking Guanxin Danshen Formulation (GXDSF), a classic and famous prescription as an example, this section exhaustively introduces the experimental reasoning and measures of identifying the effective component groups of TCM/TCM compound prescriptions based on the network pharmacology method, in an attempt to provide reference for the application of network pharmacology in the research of the component basis of TCM/TCM compound prescriptions. Contingent on ETCM, TCM-MESH, CTD, and DisGeNET databases, this section constructs a TCM–ingredient–disease target network of GXDSF in the treatment of CVD diseases based on the network pharmacology method. By means of network analysis, we identified 37 monomer chemical components, which collectively constitute the active component group of GXDSF. Based on the component of each chemical component in the medicinal ingredients and its topological parameter—connectivity in the network, we hand-picked 9 components (kaempferol, luteolin, tanshinone IIA, quercetin, Notoginsenoside R1, salvianolic acid B, Ginsenoside Rg1, ginsenoside Rb1, and salvianolic acid A) from the above 37 to verify the activity of cardiovascular protection. The results demonstrate that tanshinone IIA, salvianolic acid B, ginsenoside Rb1, quercetin, and luteolin have protective effects on H_2O_2-induced H9c2 myocardial cell injury. Ginsenoside Rg1 has protective effect on H9c2 myocardial cell injury induced by anoxic reoxygenation. Albeit notoginsenoside R1 has no significant consequence on H_2O_2-induced H9c2 cell injury, it could significantly enhance H9c2 myocardial cell injury induced by hypoxia reoxygenation. Different concentrations of kaempferol can significantly enhance doxorubicin-induced H9c2 myocardial cell injury. Based on the ox-LDL-induced injury model of human umbilical vein endothelial cells, we verified the effect of salvianolic acid A pretreatment on cell activity. The results demonstrate that salvianolic acid A can protect ox-LDL-induced human umbilical vein endothelial cells from damage in a dose-dependent manner. By and large, we detected the effective component group of GXDSF based on the network pharmacology method, and the cardiovascular protective effects of some components were verified by different in vitro cell models. The results of network analysis have high consistency with the experimental results, which signifies that network pharmacology is an effective means to identify the material basis of traditional Chinese medicines/TCM compound prescriptions.

7.3 Expounding the Pharmacodynamic Mechanism of Single Chinese Medicine or Prescription

Traditional Chinese medicine and TCM prescriptions have multi-component, multi-target, and multi-pathway functional characteristics, and have significant advantages in the treatment of complex diseases. Traditional research procedures predominantly employ phytochemical separation, extraction, identification, and other technologies to explore the primary effective components in TCM or compound prescriptions, and subsequently employ modern pharmacological means to investigate the primary action target and signaling pathway, as a means to explore its mechanism of action. However, this "single target–single component" chemical drug development model is inconsistent with the application of synergistic compatibility of TCM and their compounds, and cannot comprehensively explain the clinical effect of TCM and its compound prescription. The emergence of network pharmacology promotes the discovery, research, and development of drugs and the elucidation of therapeutic mechanism [6], providing a new research idea and method for TCM and its compounds [7–9].

Guanxin Danshen Formulation is a classic compound prescription composed of Salvia miltiorrhiza, Panax notoginseng, and Dalbergia odorifera oil. In the preceding research of its protective effect on Ischemia-Reperfusion Injury-Induced Left Myocardial Ventricular Remodeling (MIRI-LVR), the author discovered that Guanxin Danshen Formulation can enhance the cardiac systolic function of MIRI-LVR model rats in acceptable doses, and demonstrates a significant inhibitory effect on MIRI-LVR, however, its mechanism of action is not comprehensible. Although the pharmacological action and mechanism of action of certain chemical components in Guanxin Danshen Formulation have been researched and documented, the joint action mechanism of several complex components in the compound cannot be validated. In this section, we employ the network pharmacology method to predict the possible action targets and mechanism of action of Guanxin Danshen Formulation on MIRI-LVR, providing research ideas for elucidating the complex mechanism of action of TCM compounds.

7.3.1 Data Acquisition and Processing

The research ideas and processes are shown in Fig. 7.12.

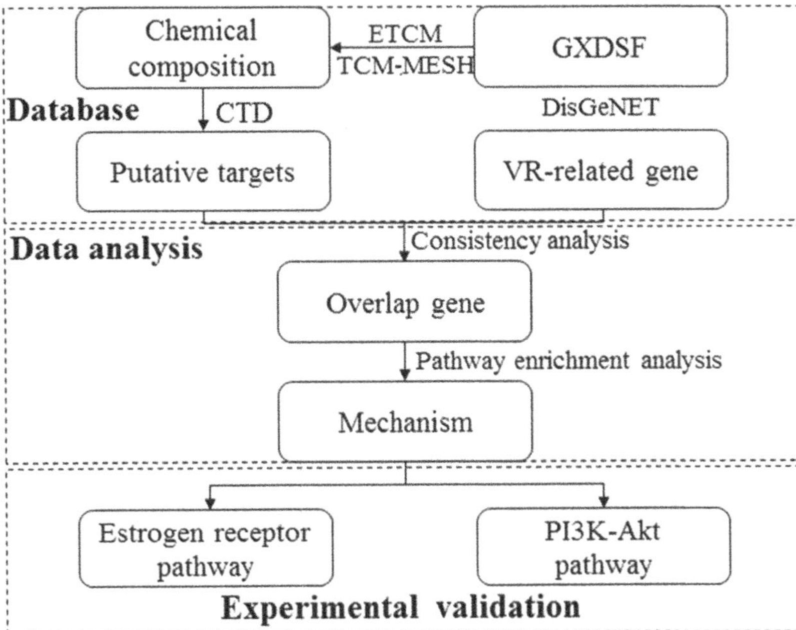

Fig. 7.12 Research ideas and processes

7.3.1.1 Chemical Component Collection of GXDSF Prescription

Based on two classic Chinese herbal medicine databases, ETCM and TCM-MESH, the chemical ingredients of GXDSF prescription were assembled. (1) The "Herbs" option is selected under the MENU option in the ETCM database menu bar, and "danshen" is entered in the search box, to obtain chemical composition list 1 of Radix Salviae Miltiorrhizae. (2) "Herb" is selected under the Search Type option in the TCM-MESH database, the "Pinyin Name" option is selected under Herb Name Type option, and "Dan Shen" is entered in the search box to get the chemical composition list 2 of Radix Salviae Miltiorrhizae. (3) The two chemical composition lists of Salviae Miltiorrhizae collected based on ETCM and TCM-MESH databases are integrated and de-duplicated, creating the complete chemical composition list of Radix Salviae Miltiorrhizae. (4) The chemical components of panax notoginseng and dalbergia odorifera are assembled employing the same method. The corresponding relationship between each traditional Chinese medicine and its chemical components are saved in the form of a two-dimensional list.

7.3.1.2 Collection of Chemical Component Targets

The "Chemicals" option was selected under Keyword Search in the CTD database and the English name of each chemical component was entered in the search box, to assemble the target data of each chemical component. The corresponding relationship between each chemical component and its target was saved in the form of a two-dimensional list. The mass search function provided by the CTD database can also be employed to retrieve the target data of each chemical component.

7.3.1.3 Collection of VR-Related Disease Genes

The "Search" option was selected under the menu bar in the CTD database, the search type was set to "diseases," and Ventricular remodeling was entered in the search box to assemble the top 100 VR-related genes in the Inference Score. The corresponding relationship between the disease and its related genes was saved in the form of a two-dimensional list.

7.3.2 Network Construction and Visualization

7.3.2.1 Pathway Enrichment Analysis

The "set analyzer" option was selected under the "analyze" option in the CTD database, Genes was selected as the input type, and the abbreviation of the target gene entered in the input box. "Enriched pathways" was selected as the analysis type, and the corrected P-value threshold value was set to 0.001.

7.3.2.2 TCM–Target Network

The corresponding relationships between various TCM and VR-related genes in GXDSF were saved in the form of a two-dimensional list. Cytoscape 3.5.0 software was used to realize the visualization of the TCM–target network.

The NetworkAnalyzer function under the "Tools" option under the menu bar in Cytoscape 3.5.0 was employed to analyze the topology attributes (connectivity) of each node in the network.

7.3.3 Network Analysis and Prediction

7.3.3.1 Coincidence Degree Between GXDSF Component Target Proteins and VR-Related Genes

By implementing the consistency analysis of the chemical composition target proteins of the complete GXDSF prescription and VR-related genes, it was established that a total of 56 target proteins in GXDSF appear in the list of VR-related genes,

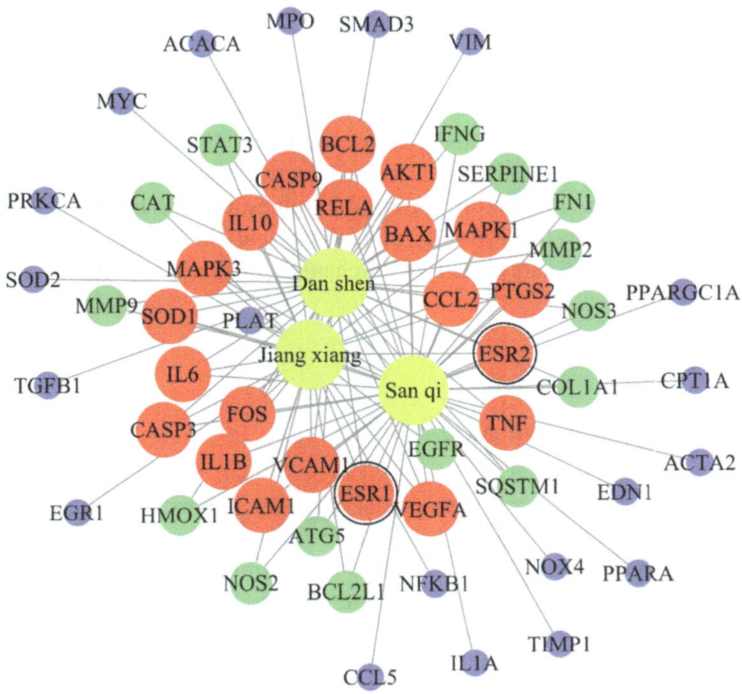

Fig. 7.13 TCM–target network of GXDSF in the treatment of VR. The yellow square nodes represent TCM. The red, green, and blue circular nodes represent VR-related genes with connectivity degrees 1, 2, and 3, respectively. The size of connectivity represents the number of Chinese medicines involved in the regulation of this gene in GXDSF. The genes in black circles are ESR1 and ESR2

accounting for 56% (56/100) of all VR-related genes. GXDSF may achieve direct regulation of VR by means of these target proteins.

7.3.3.2 TCM–Target Network of GXDSF in the Treatment of VR

By means of the connectivity analysis of the TCM–target network, it was established that among the 56 genes involved in regulation by GXDSF, the number of genes with connectivity degrees 1, 2, and 3 are 20, 15, and 21, respectively (as shown in Fig. 7.13). This implies that in GXDSF, there are 21 VR-related genes that 3 Chinese herbs act on concurrently, 15 VR-related genes that at least two kinds of Chinese herbs act on concurrently, and 20 VR-related genes that only 1 kind of Chinese herb acts upon.

7.3.3.3 Discovery of the Potential Pathway of GXDSF in the Treatment of VR

The KEGG pathway enrichment analysis was implemented using GXDSF target protein overlapped with VR-related genes as the input. The results demonstrate that there are 75 VR-related pathways involved in the regulation through GXDSF. Table 7.3 provides the names, the corrected P-values, and the involved VR-related genes of each pathway. The results of pathway enrichment analysis reflect the characteristics of multi-target and multi-channel treatment of TCM compound prescriptions.

7.3.4 Verification and Summary

Through experimental research in the initial stage, the authors found that a variety of main active ingredients in Guanxin Danshen Formulation can combine with estrogen receptor to produce an estrogen like effect, and exhibit anti-inflammatory, antioxidant, anti-apoptotic [4], and neuroprotective effects [10] by regulating ERs-PI3K/Akt signaling pathway. Based on the results of pathway enrichment and its topological parameter—connectivity in the network, and combined with previous studies, we hand-picked ERs-PI3K/Akt signaling pathway from the above 75 pathways to verify the pharmacodynamic mechanism of action of ERs-PI3K/Akt signaling pathway in the Guanxin Danshen Formulation against MIRI-LVR.

7.3.4.1 Expression of ERs-PI3K/Akt Signaling Pathway-Related Proteins of Guanxin Danshen Formulation Against MirI-LVR Rat Myocardial Tissue

Western Blot results demonstrate that compared to the sham-operated group, the expression quantity of estrogen receptor α and β in the MIRI-LVR model group increased, but there was no significant difference. Simvastatin also had no significant effect on the expression of estrogen receptors. Upon being treated with Guanxin Danshen Formulation, the expression of ERα in myocardial tissue was not significantly affected either, however, the expression quantity of Erβ increased in acceptable doses. Correspondingly, with the increase of ERβ expression quantity, the phosphorylation level of PI3K/Akt in the downstream signaling pathway protein PI3K/Akt in myocardial tissue increased significantly. The results are shown in Fig. 7.14.

The effect of Guanxin Danshen Formulation on the distribution of ERβ/α-SMA in myocardial tissue of MIRI-LVR model rats was investigated by immunofluorescence double staining. The results demonstrate that the expression of ERβ in the MIRI-LVR model group did not significantly increase compared to the

Table 7.3 Potential Pathway of GXDSF in the Treatment of VR

Serial No.	Pathway	Corrected P-value	Related genes
1	AGE-RAGE signaling pathway in diabetic complications	5.72×10^{-55}	AKT1|BAX|BCL2|CASP3|CCL2|COL1A1|EDN1|EGR1|FN1|ICAM1|IL1A|IL1B|IL6|MAPK1|MAPK3|MMP2|NFKB1|NOS3|PRKCA|RELA|SERPINE1|SMAD3|STAT3|TGFB1|TNF|VCAM1|VEGFA
2	Fluid shear stress and atherosclerosis	2.82×10^{-33}	AKT1|BCL2|CCL2|EDN1|FOS|HMOX1|ICAM1|IFNG|IL1A|IL1B|MMP2|MMP9|NFKB1|NOS3|PLAT|RELA|SQSTM1|TNF|VCAM1|VEGFA
3	HIF-1 signaling pathway	1.27×10^{-31}	AKT1|BCL2|EDN1|EGFR|HMOX1|IFNG|IL6|MAPK1|MAPK3|NFKB1|NOS2|NOS3|PRKCA|RELA|SERPINE1|STAT3|TIMP1|VEGFA
4	TNF signaling pathway	1.03×10^{-28}	AKT1|CASP3|CCL2|CCL5|EDN1|FOS|ICAM1|IL1B|IL6|MAPK1|MAPK3|MMP9|NFKB1|PTGS2|RELA|TNF|VCAM1
5	IL-17 signaling pathway	1.12×10^{-20}	CASP3|CCL2|FOS|IFNG|IL1B|IL6|MAPK1|MAPK3|MMP9|NFKB1|PTGS2|RELA|TNF
6	Colorectal cancer	1.42×10^{-18}	AKT1|BAX|BCL2|CASP3|CASP9|FOS|MAPK1|MAPK3|MYC|SMAD3|TGFB1
7	PI3K-Akt signaling pathway	3.64×10^{-18}	AKT1|BCL2|BCL2L1|CASP9|COL1A1|EGFR|FN1|IL6|MAPK1|MAPK3|MYC|NFKB1|NOS3|PRKCA|RELA|VEGFA
8	Inflammatory bowel disease (IBD)	3.70×10^{-18}	IFNG|IL10|IL1A|IL1B|IL6|NFKB1|RELA|SMAD3|STAT3|TGFB1|TNF
9	EGFR tyrosine kinase inhibitor resistance	3.6×10^{-17}	AKT1|BAX|BCL2|BCL2L1|EGFR|IL6|MAPK1|MAPK3|PRKCA|STAT3|VEGFA
10	MAPK signaling pathway	1.46×10^{-16}	AKT1|CASP3|EGFR|FOS|IL1A|IL1B|MAPK1|MAPK3|MYC|NFKB1|PRKCA|RELA|TGFB1|TNF
11	Apoptosis	2.46×10^{-16}	AKT1|BAX|BCL2|BCL2L1|CASP3|CASP9|FOS|MAPK1|MAPK3|NFKB1|RELA|TNF
12	Prion diseases	2.56×10^{-16}	BAX|CCL5|EGR1|IL1A|IL1B|IL6|MAPK1|MAPK3|SOD1
13	Endocrine resistance	3.13×10^{-16}	AKT1|BAX|BCL2|EGFR|ESR1|ESR2|FOS|MAPK1|MAPK3|MMP2|MMP9
14	Th17 cell differentiation	1.23×10^{-15}	FOS|IFNG|IL1B|IL6|MAPK1|MAPK3|NFKB1|RELA|SMAD3|STAT3|TGFB1
15	NOD-like receptor signaling pathway	3.20×10^{-15}	ATG5|BCL2|BCL2L1|CCL2|CCL5|IL1B|IL6|MAPK1|MAPK3|NFKB1|RELA|TNF
16	Small cell lung cancer	1.05×10^{-14}	AKT1|BCL2|BCL2L1|CASP9|FN1|MYC|NFKB1|NOS2|PTGS2|RELA
17	FoxO signaling pathway	1.34×10^{-14}	AKT1|CAT|EGFR|IL10|IL6|MAPK1|MAPK3|SMAD3|SOD2|STAT3|TGFB1

(continued)

Table 7.3 (continued)

Serial No.	Pathway	Corrected P-value	Related genes
18	Apelin signaling pathway	2.22×10^{-14}	ACTA2|AKT1|EGR1|MAPK1|MAPK3|NOS2|NOS3|PLAT|PPARGC1A|SERPINE1|SMAD3
19	Estrogen signaling pathway	5.23×10^{-14}	AKT1|EGFR|ESR1|ESR2|FOS|MAPK1|MAPK3|MMP2|MMP9|NOS3
20	Non-alcoholic fatty liver disease (NAFLD)	5.26×10^{-14}	AKT1|BAX|CASP3|IL1A|IL1B|IL6|NFKB1|PPARA|RELA|TGFB1|TNF

sham-operated group, but the expression distribution of α-SMA in the myocardial infarction area and the infarction boundary area significantly increased. Compared to the model group, the expression distribution of α-SMA in the infarct zone and the infarct border zone of the simvastatin group decreased; the expression of ERβ in myocardial tissue in the border zone of infarction increased with the increase of dose in low, medium, and high dose groups of Guanxin Danshen Formulation. Concurrently, the expression of α-SMA in the infarct area and infarct border area decreased with the increase of dose. The results are demonstrated in Fig. 7.15.

The results advocate that the Guanxin Danshen Formulation can promote the expression of ERβ in myocardial tissue in acceptable doses, and in the interim, increase the phosphorylation of PI3K/Akt in its downstream signaling pathway. It indicates that the myocardial protective effect of Guanxin Danshen Formulation may be related to the selective activation of ERβ/PI3K/Akt signaling pathway.

7.3.4.2 Verification of the Pharmacodynamic Mechanism of Action of ERs-PI3K/Akt Signaling Pathway in Guanxin Danshen Formulation Against MIRI-LVR

Effect of Inhibiting ERβ on the Therapeutic Effect of Guanxin Danshen Prescription Against MIRI-LVR

The test results of myocardial three enzymes show that the levels of myocardial three enzymes do not change significantly after MIRI-LVR model rats are treated with PHTPP alone. Compared with the Guanxin Danshen Formulation treatment group, the LDH ($P < 0.001$) and CK-MB ($P < 0.05$) increased significantly in the +PHTPP Guanxin Danshen Formulation treatment group. The results are shown in Fig. 7.16.

The results of Masson staining demonstrate that there is no significant change in the area of myocardial fibrosis in MIRI-LVR model rats after being treated with PHTPP. Compared to the Guanxin Danshen Formulation treatment group, the area of myocardial fibrosis increased significantly in the +PHTPP Guanxin Danshen Formulation treatment group ($P < 0.01$). Western Blot testing of α-SMA expression level in myocardial tissue exhibits no significant change in the expression level of α-SMA in MIRI-LVR model rats treated with PHTPP. Compared to the Guanxin

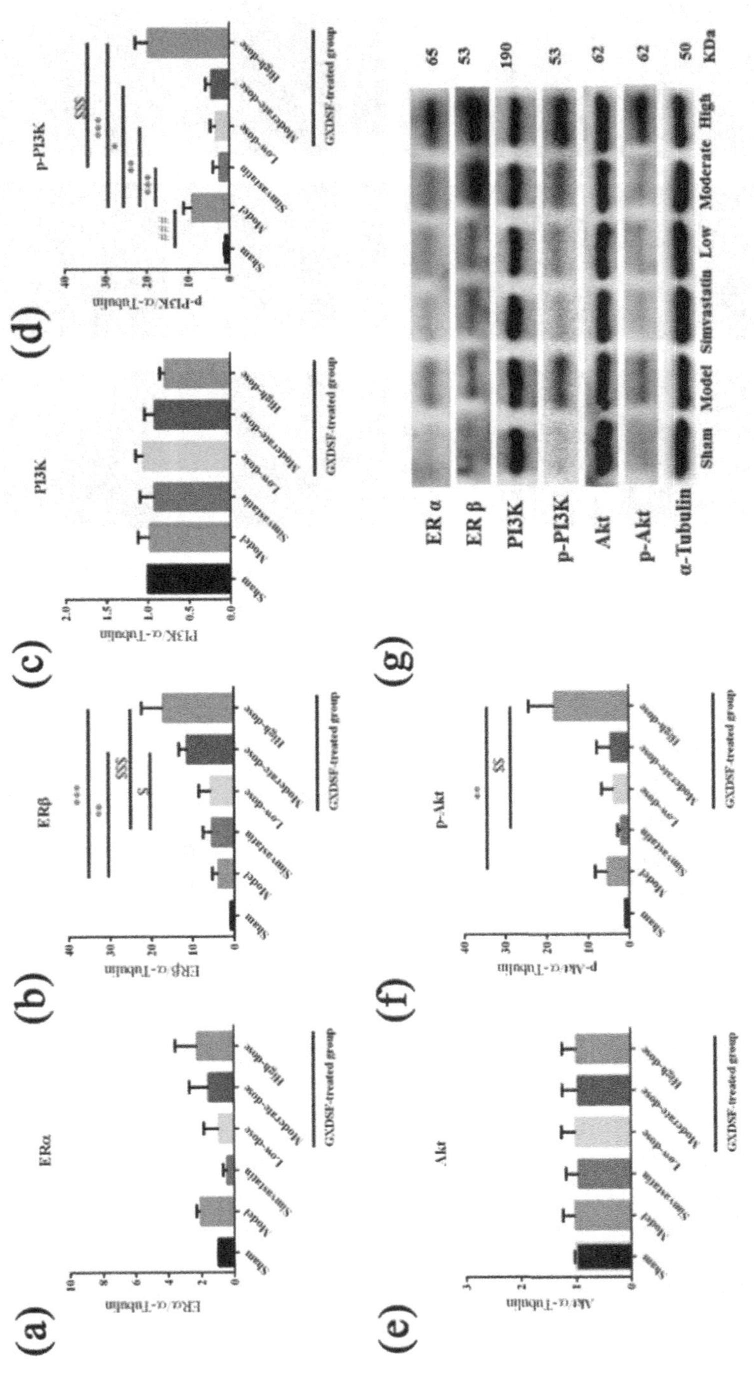

Fig. 7.14 Effect of Guanxin Danshen formulation on protein expression in estrogen receptor and its downstream signaling pathway

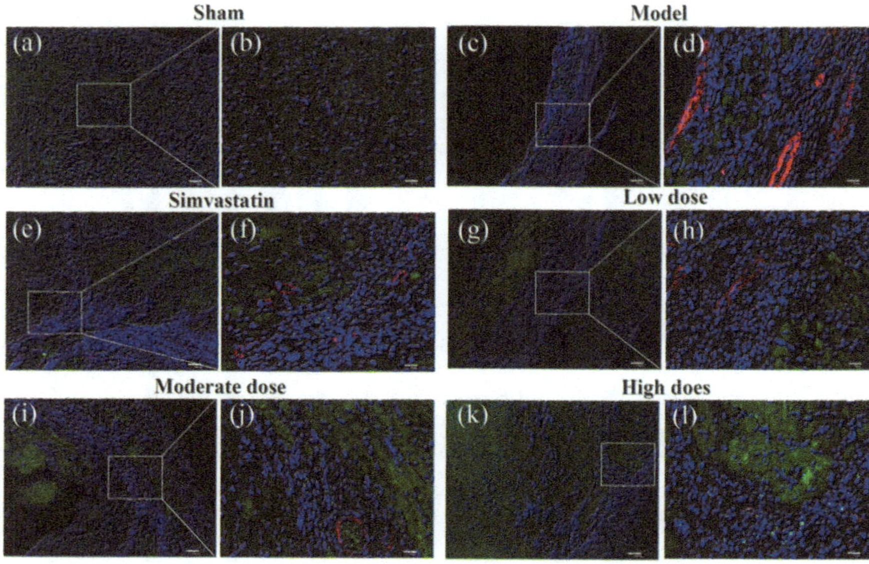

Fig. 7.15 Effect of Guanxin Danshen formulation on expression and distribution of ERβ/α-SMA in myocardial tissues (the bar value of (**a**, **c**, **e**, **g**, **i**, and **k**) is 100 μm, and that of (**b**, **d**, **f**, **h**, **j**, and **i**) is 25 μm)

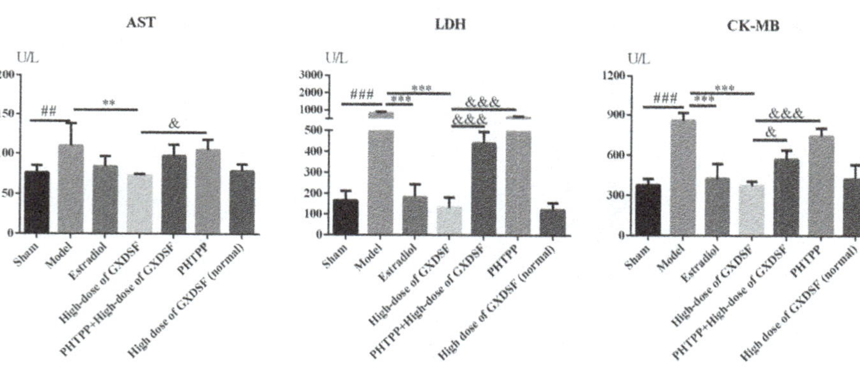

Fig. 7.16 Effect of ERβ inhibitor PHTPP on the expression of three enzymes in myocardium of Guanxin Danshen formulation

Danshen Formulation treatment group, the expression level of α-SMA increased significantly in the +PHTPP Guanxin Danshen Formulation treatment group ($P < 0.001$). The results are shown in Fig. 7.17.

The shown heart function test results of Hemodynamics (as shown in Fig. 7.18) and echocardiography (as shown in Fig. 7.19) indicate that there are no significant changes in the LVSP, +DP/DT, LVEF, and LVFS of MIRI-LVR model rats after being treated with PHTPP. Compared to the Guanxin Danshen Formulation treatment group, the LVSP ($P < 0.05$), +dp/dt ($P < 0.05$), LVEF ($P < 0.01$), and LVFS

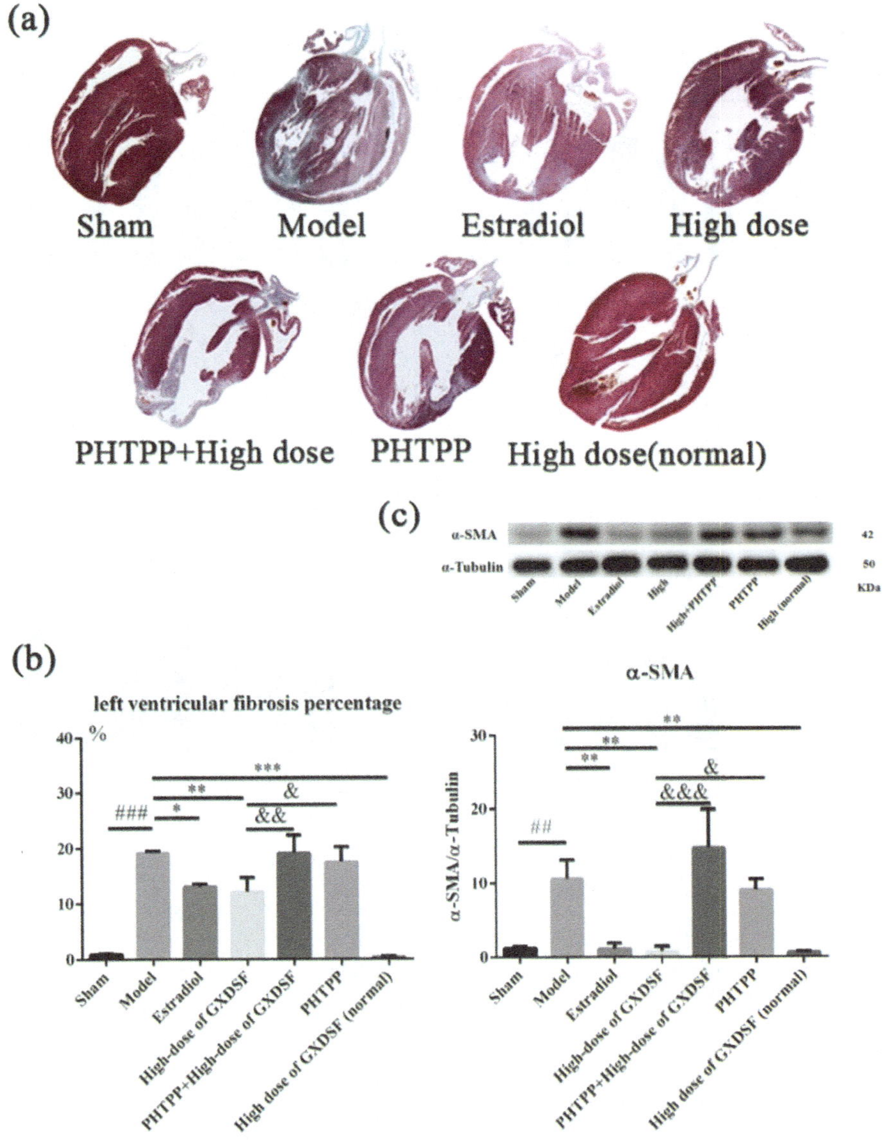

Fig. 7.17 Effect of ERβ Inhibitor PHTPP on reversing myocardial fibrosis of Guanxin Danshen formulation. (**a**) Results of Masson staining in myocardial tissue sections; (**b**) Statistical results of fibrotic area in Masson staining sections; (**c**) Western blot detection of α-SMA expression quantity results in myocardial tissue

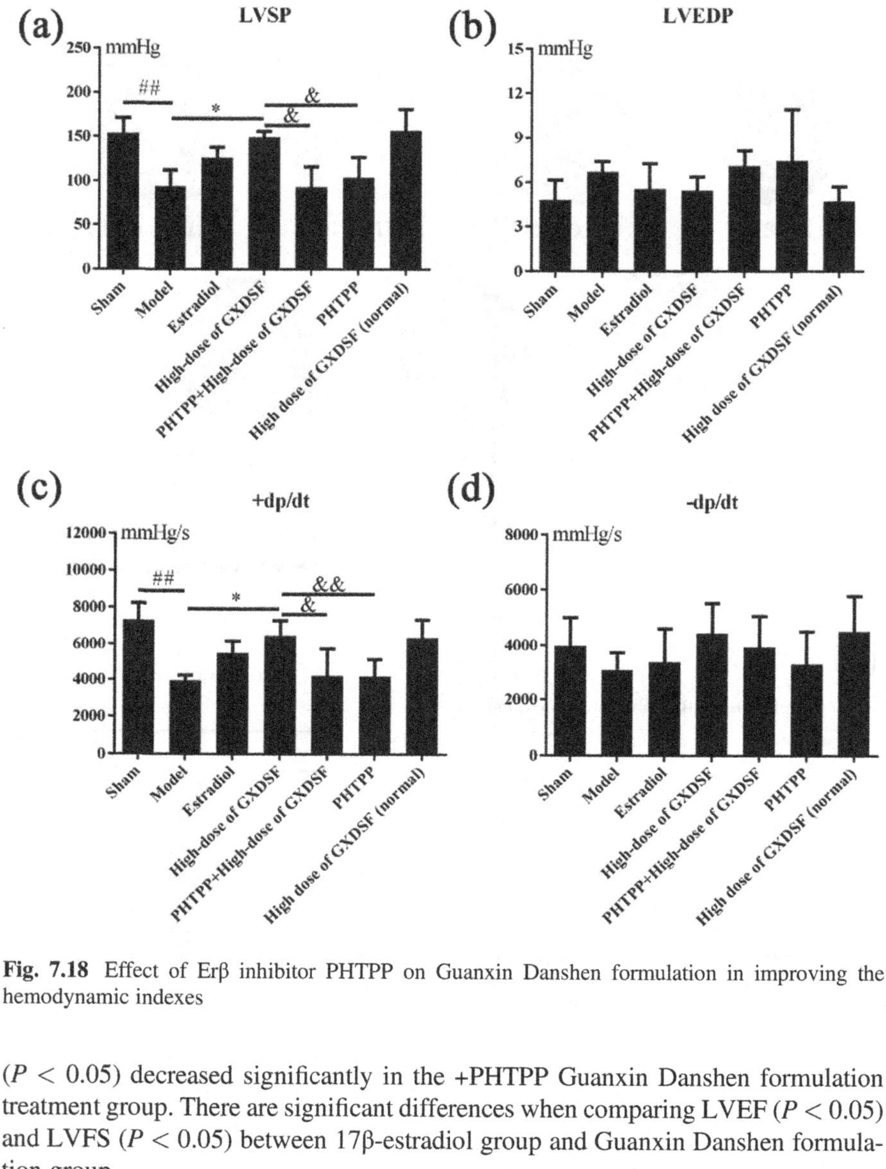

Fig. 7.18 Effect of Erβ inhibitor PHTPP on Guanxin Danshen formulation in improving the hemodynamic indexes

($P < 0.05$) decreased significantly in the +PHTPP Guanxin Danshen formulation treatment group. There are significant differences when comparing LVEF ($P < 0.05$) and LVFS ($P < 0.05$) between 17β-estradiol group and Guanxin Danshen formulation group.

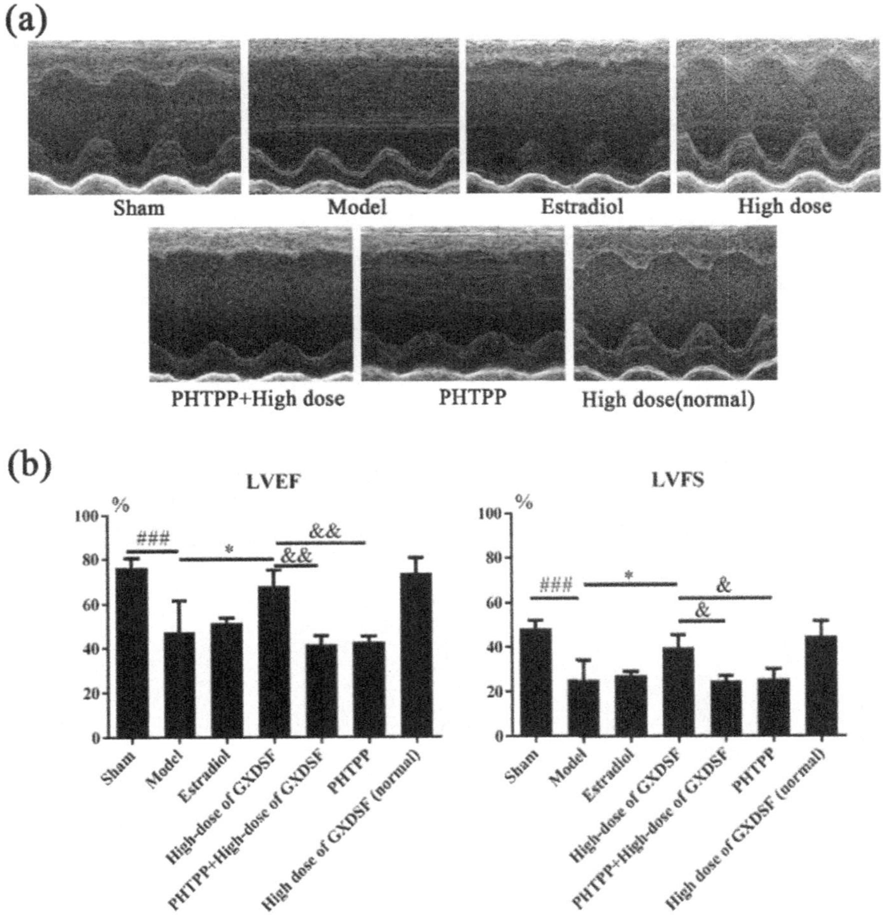

Fig. 7.19 Effect of Erβ inhibitor PHTPP on Guanxin Danshen formulation in improving the echocardiographic indexes

Effects of Inhibiting ERβ on the Protein and Signaling Pathway that Guanxin Danshen Formulation Acts Upon

The results of expression of estrogen receptor β and its downstream signaling pathway PI3K/Akt detected by Western Blot indicate that, compared to the sham-operated group, Guanxin Danshen Formulation has no significant effect on the expression of estrogen receptor β and its downstream signaling pathway PI3K/Akt in normal rat myocardial tissue. Upon PHTPP treatment, compared to the Guanxin Danshen Formulation treatment group, the expression of estrogen receptor β in the +PHTPP group of Guanxin Danshen Formulation significantly decreased ($P < 0.001$), and its phosphorylation level of PI3K/Akt in downstream signaling pathway also significantly decreased ($P < 0.001$). The results are shown in Fig. 7.20.

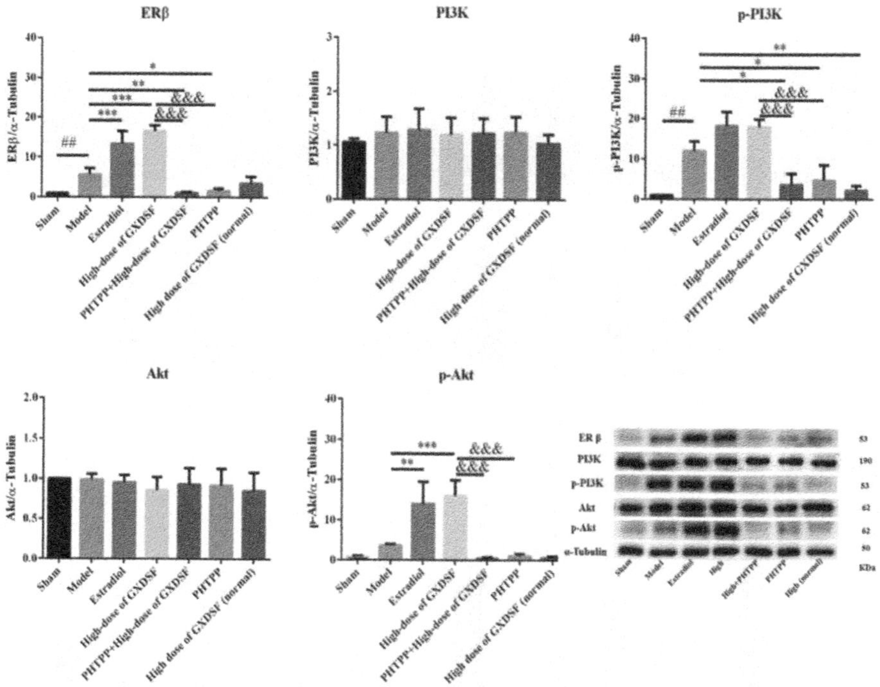

Fig. 7.20 Effect of ERβ Inhibitor PHTPP on the protein and signaling pathway that Guanxin Danshen formulation acts upon

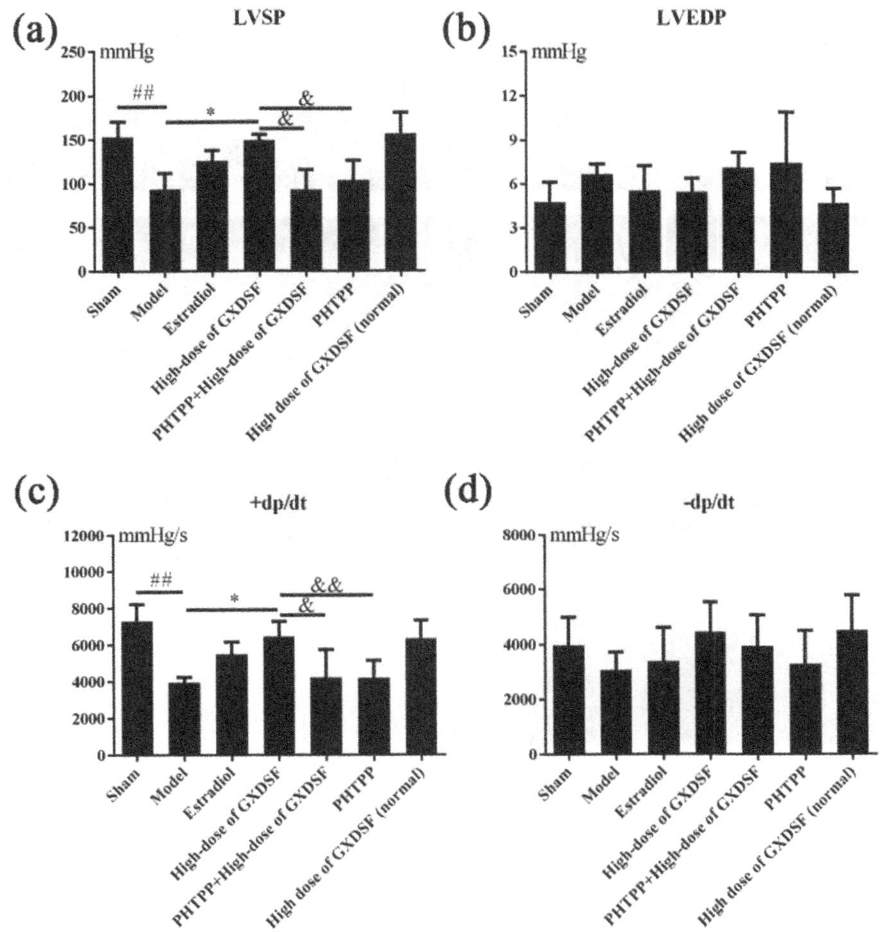

The effects of PHTPP on the expression distribution of ERβ/α-SMA tested by immunofluorescence double staining indicate that, after treatment with PHTPP, the expression of estrogen receptor β in the infarct area and the infarct border area of MIRI-LVR rats significantly decreased, and the expression of α-SMA in the infarct area and the infarct border area significantly increased. Compared to the Guanxin Danshen Formulation treatment group, the expression of ERβ in the myocardial tissue of infarction area and infarct boundary area was significantly inhibited in the +PHTPP Guanxin Danshen Formulation treatment group, and in the interim, a large number of expression and distribution of α-SMA can be observed. The results are shown in Fig. 7.21.

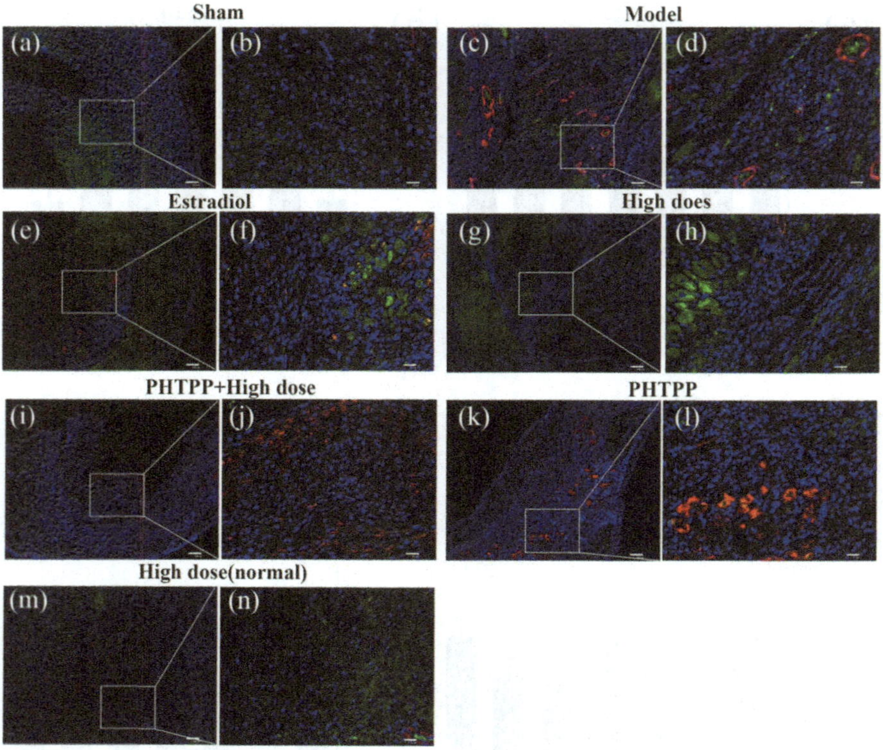

Fig. 7.21 Effect of ERβ Inhibitor PHTPP on the Expression Distribution of ERβ/α-SMA (the bar value of (**a**, **c**, **e**, **g**, **i**, **k**, and **m**) is 100 μm, and that of (**b**, **d**, **f**, **h**, **j**, **i**, and **n**) is 25 μm)

7.3.4.3 Summary

This section cites the classic and famous GXDSF Formulation as an example to exhaustively introduce the experimental reasoning and measures of investigating the efficacy mechanism of Chinese herbal compound prescriptions based on the network pharmacology method, with a view to provide research reasoning and reference for the investigation of the mechanism of action of TCM/TCM compound prescriptions. Contingent on ETCM, TCM-MESH, CTD database, and Cytoscape analysis software, this section constructs a TCM–target–disease network of GXDSF against MIRI-LVR based on the network pharmacology method. Using network analysis, we identified 75 signaling pathways, which collectively constitute the pharmacodynamic network of GXDSF. The pathway enrichment results and topological parameters—connectivity in the network, were integrated and combined with the basis of previous research, and we hand-picked the ERs-PI3K/Akt signaling pathway from the above 75 pathways to verify the pharmacodynamic mechanism of GXDSF against MIRI-LVR through experiments. The verification results demonstrated that Guanxin Danshen Formulation could significantly promote the expression of ERβ and its downstream signaling pathway protein PI3K/Akt in the myocardial tissue of MIRI-LVR model rats in acceptable doses. PHTPP, a specific inhibitor of ERβ in rats, was rendered to verify the role of ERβ in the myocardial protection capabilities of Guanxin Danshen Formulation. The results demonstrated that PHTPP could significantly aggravate the improvement of three myocardial enzymes and the improvement of cardiac structure and function by Guanxin Danshen Formulation. It indicates that the myocardial protective effect of Guanxin Danshen Formulation is closely related to the activation of ERβ/PI3K/Akt signaling pathway. In summation, we discovered the pharmacodynamic mechanism network of GXDSF by employing the analysis method of network pharmacology, and verified the significant function of ERβ/PI3K/Akt signaling pathway in the pharmacodynamics of GXDSF by means of animal model experiments [11]. The results of network analysis are highly consistent with the experimental results, which indicate that network pharmacology is an effective means to investigate the pharmacodynamic mechanism of TCM/TCM compound prescriptions.

7.4 Explanation of the Interaction Between TCM and Western Medicine: Combined Use of Chinese and Western Medicines Enhances Efficacy and Reduces Toxicity

Ischemic stroke is a global health problem, accounting for more than 77% of all strokes, and is the leading cause of disability and the second leading cause of mortality globally, with a growing mortality rate [12]. Although great progress has been made in the pathophysiological mechanism of ischemic stroke in China and overseas in recent years, there are still very limited clinical drugs for the treatment of ischemic stroke. So far, the only drug approved for the treatment of acute ischemic stroke is recombinant tissue plasminogen activator (rt-PA). However, the application of rt-PA is limited due to the short treatment time window (3 h) and potential side effects (intracranial hemorrhage) [13]. Thrombolytic therapy is only suitable for acute stage of ischemic stroke. At present, aspirin, which is commonly used in clinical treatment and prevention of cerebrovascular disease, is only effective for patients with mild stroke, and the therapeutic effect is not satisfactory. The CHANCE study conducted by Professor Wang Yong-jun found that, for patients with mild stroke and TIA within 24 h of onset, giving them a combination of aspirin and clopidogrel for 21 consecutive days (grade B evidence, grade IIb recommendation) was effective in reducing stroke recurrence within 90 days, confirming that the combined use of aspirin and clopidogrel is more effective than using aspirin alone. Although the efficacy of combined antiplatelet therapy is better than that of aspirin alone, combined antiplatelet therapy also has limitations related to the appropriate population, bleeding risk, and gastrointestinal mucosal injury. As existing clinical drugs have not yet met the clinical needs, there is an urgent need for new treatment strategies for acute ischemic stroke. The activating blood and removing blood stasis agent, clearing heat and resuscitating agent, replenishing qi and promoting blood circulation agent among Chinese patent medicines, such as Panax notoginseng, Salvia miltiorrhiza, Ligusticum chuanxiong, and Ginkgo biloba preparations with clinically definite curative effects, have received increasing attention recently due to their unique effects. Therefore, finding more effective treatment methods and drugs for stroke has become a key topic of discussion in the field of pharmaceutical research.

Panax notoginseng is a traditional and precious traditional Chinese medicine in China, enjoying the reputation of "Jinbuchang," "Magic medicine from Nan'guo," "King of Ginseng," and "surgical elixir." [14] The *Supplement to Compendium of Materia Medica* records that: "Ginseng supplements qi first, panax notoginseng supplements blood first, having the same taste but different functions, thus it is called panax notoginseng, the most precious of Traditional Chinese medicine." [15] Panax notoginseng is the root of the perennial herbaceous plant Araliaceae. It is sweet and slightly bitter in taste, wet in nature, and attributive to liver, and stomach channels. Raw Panax notoginseng reduces blood stasis and stops bleeding, and can be used for hemoptysis, vomiting blood, bruises, swelling and pain, and traumatic bleeding; cooked Panax notoginseng replenishes blood and promotes blood circulation, and is used for blood loss and anemia [16]. By constructing an integrated pharmacology based on the integration of network pharmacology, genomics, systematic pharmacology, and other technologies, this research group analyzed the multi-level research technology of the mechanism of action of panax notoginseng, promoted the clinical positioning and re-evaluation of original new drugs, and clarified panax notoginseng's pharmacodynamic material basis. Xuesaitong is developed from the effective active ingredients in Panax notoginseng. In vivo and in vitro studies in China and overseas have proved that it has definite cardioprotective effect, such as inhibiting platelet aggregation, reducing blood viscosity, antithrombotic effect, improving microcirculation, inhibiting inflammatory reaction, activating estrogen receptor in playing an anti-apoptosis role, etc. [17] The Xuesaitong Soft Capsule has the effect of promoting blood circulation and removing blood stasis, dredging blood vessels, and activating collaterals. It is mainly used during the recovery period of the meridian in stroke for the blood stasis and closed channels and collaterals syndrome. Symptoms include hemiplegia, askew tongue, hard tongue, tough pronunciation of words, or inability to speak. Symptoms include hemiplegic paralysis, hemiparalysis, deviation of the eye and mouth, stiff tongue. In vitro and in vivo studies in China and overseas have proved that it has anti-oxidative stress and anti-inflammatory effects, and has definite neuroprotective effects.

According to the big data analysis of clinical data, at present, the traditional Chinese patent medicines for the treatment of acute ischemic stroke are mainly drugs for promoting blood circulation and removing blood stasis. To achieve symptomatic treatment, it is supplemented by Huatan Xingnao Kaiqiao medicine, while the use of Western medicine is recommended according to the guidelines for diagnosis and treatment of acute ischemic stroke. The combination of Chinese patent medicine and

Western medicine is mostly blood activating and stasis removing drugs + antiplatelet drugs [18]. Clinical findings show that the efficacy of using aspirin alone and the combined use of aspirin and clopidogrel could not meet the clinical needs. Moreover, due to the side effects of long-term use of aspirin, such as gastrointestinal mucosal injury and the risk of bleeding, antiplatelet drugs are not used alone in clinical use. Although it was found that the effect of combined use of Chinese patent medicine and antiplatelet drug is better than that of single use, there is a lack of quantitative data support for combined applications, and its action link, efficacy target, use dosage, multi-target synergistic effect enhancement, and toxicity reduction mechanism are as yet unclear. Therefore, we chose to adopt MCAO/R model rats.

7.4.1 Data Acquisition and Processing

The research idea and process are shown in Fig. 7.22.

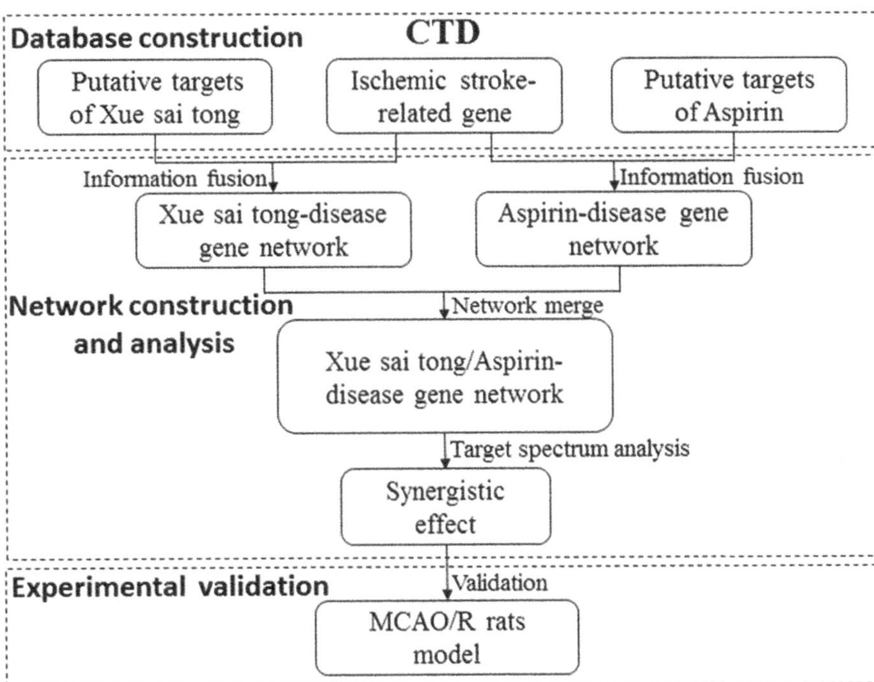

Fig. 7.22 Research ideas and processes

7.4.1.1 Selection of Target Components

Based on references and our previous experimental results, five main effective ingredients—notoginsenoside R1, ginsenoside Rg1, ginsenoside Rb1, ginsenoside Rd, and ginsenoside Re (as shown in Table 7.4) were selected as the representative ingredients of Xuesaitong for carrying out the subsequent study.

7.4.1.2 Collection of Chemical Composition Targets

"Chemicals" was selected under the Keyword Search option of the CTD database, the English name of each chemical component was entered in the search box, and the target data of each chemical component collected. The corresponding relationship between each chemical component and its targets was saved in the form of a two-dimensional list.

7.4.1.3 Gene Collection of Ischemic Stroke-Related Diseases

"Diseases" was selected under the Keyword Search option of the CTD database, and "Cerebral infarction/Brain infarction" was entered in the search box to collect the gene data related to ischemic stroke. The corresponding relationship between each gene and ischemic stroke was saved in the form of a two-dimensional list.

Table 7.4 Main effective ingredients of Xuesaitong

Serial No.	Compound	Chinese name	CAS	Molecular formula	Molecular weight
1	Notoginsenoside R1	三七皂苷 R1	80418-24-2	$C_{47}H_{80}O_{18}$	933.139
2	Ginsenoside Rg1	人参皂苷 Rg1	22427-39-0	$C_{42}H_{72}O_{14}$	801.024
3	Ginsenoside Rb1	人参皂苷 Rb1	41753-43-9	$C_{54}H_{92}O_{23}$	1109.307
4	Ginsenoside Rd	人参皂苷 Rd	52705-93-8	C48H82O18	947.15
5	Ginsenoside Re	人参皂苷 Re	52286-59-6	C48H82O18	947.15

7.4.2 Network Construction and Visualization

7.4.2.1 Network Construction and Visualization

The "component–target" list and "disease–gene" list obtained from the data source were entered into the Cytoscape 3.5.0 network analysis and visualization software. The merge function under the "Tools" in the menu bar was used to superimpose the network, and construct "Xuesaitong-ischemic stroke target network," "Aspirin-ischemic stroke target network," and "Xuesaitong and Aspirin-Ischemic Stroke target network." Based on the drug–target network, the target profiles and the interaction between Xuesaitong and Aspirin were analyzed.

7.4.2.2 Analysis Index and Algorithm

The NetworkAnalyzer function under the "Tools" option in the Cytoscape 3.5.0 menu bar was used to analyze the topological attributes (connectivity) of each node in the network.

7.4.3 Network Analysis and Prediction

7.4.3.1 Target Network of Xuesaitong in the Treatment of Ischemic Stroke

Figure 7.23 shows the target network of Xuesaitong in the treatment of ischemic stroke. Notoginsenoside R1, Ginsenoside Rg1, ginsenoside Rb1, ginsenoside Rd, and ginsenoside Re regulate ischemic stroke by regulating 29, 18, 8, 9, and 23 genes related to ischemic stroke, respectively. There is a certain degree of crossover between the genes related to ischemic stroke regulated by each component. At the same time, each component has its specific regulatory target, reflecting the multi-component and multi-target characteristics of TCM. The genes with connectivity greater than 3 in the network are CASP3, CAT, TNF, BAX, BCL2, MAPK3, IL6, and MAPK1. These genes may be the key targets of Xuesaitong in the treatment of ischemic stroke.

7.4.3.2 Target Network of Aspirin in the Treatment of Ischemic Stroke

In treating ischemic stroke, aspirin regulates 62 genes related to ischemic stroke (as shown in Fig. 7.24). CASP3, CAT, TNF, BAX, BCL2, MAPK3, IL6, and MAPK1, which are regulated by Xuesaitong, are all reflected in the aspirin-ischemic stroke-related gene network, which further demonstrates the important role of these genes in the treatment process of ischemic stroke.

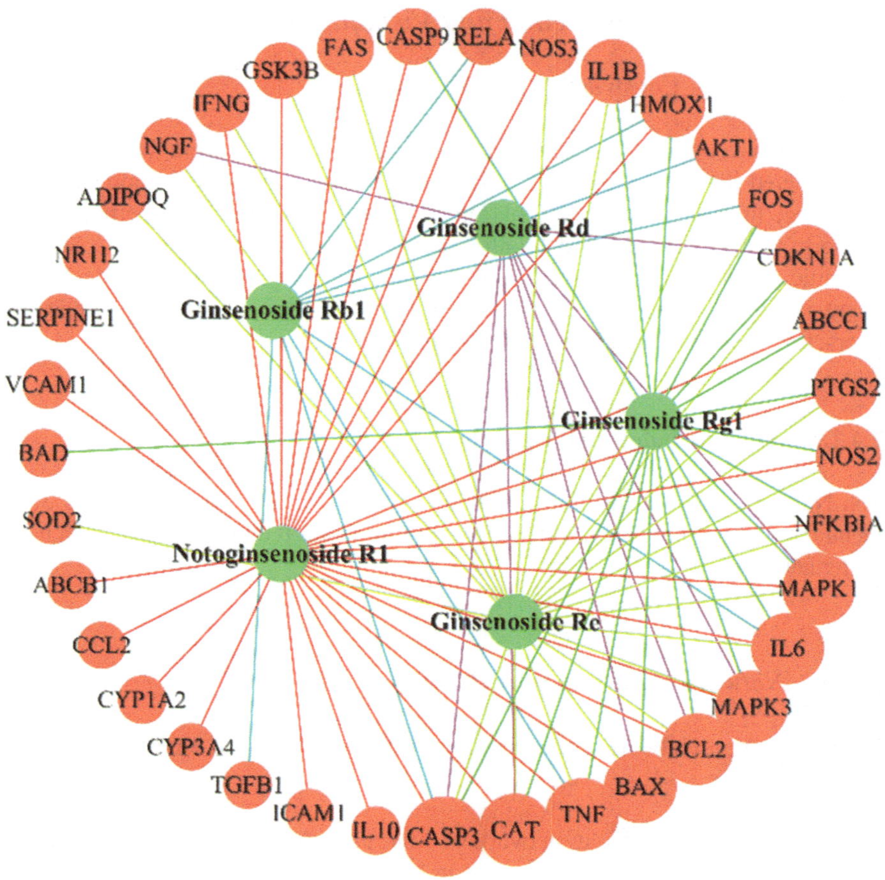

Fig. 7.23 Xuesaitong-ischemic stroke-related gene network. The green and red round nodes represent the main components of Xuesaitong and genes related to ischemic stroke, respectively

7.4.3.3 The Combined Use of Xuesaitong and Aspirin Enhances the Effect of Aspirin in Treating Ischemic Stroke

Figure 7.25 shows the molecular target network of combined use of aspirin and Xuesaitong. There is a high degree of overlap between aspirin and ischemic stroke-related genes regulated by Xuesaitong. Among the 37 genes regulated by Xuesaitong, 31 genes are overlapped with those regulated by aspirin, suggesting that the combined use of Xuesaitong and aspirin may have the potential to enhance the effect of aspirin in the treatment of ischemic stroke (as shown in Fig. 7.26). Compared with using aspirin alone, ischemic stroke-related genes regulated by the combined use of aspirin and Xuesaitong increased by 6 genes (CYP3A4, NRI12, NGF, CYP1A2, SERP1NE1, and ADIPOQ). However, the specific role of these genes in the combined use of aspirin and Xuesaitong still needs further research.

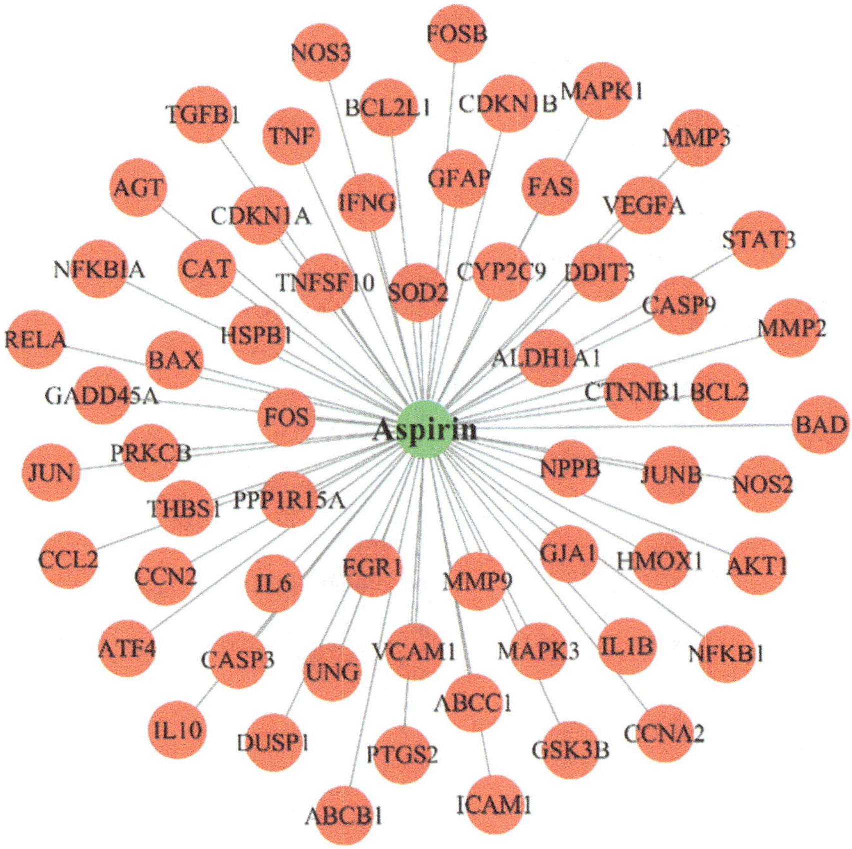

Fig. 7.24 Aspirin-ischemic stroke-related gene network. Green and red round nodes represent aspirin and ischemic stroke-related genes, respectively

7.4.4 Verification and Summary

7.4.4.1 Clinical Therapeutic Effect

A total of 120 patients with cerebral infarction treated from August 2015 to October 2017 were taken as research subjects and randomly divided into the treatment group and the control group with 60 cases each [19]. The treatment group was treated with the combined use of panax notoginseng saponins and aspirin, while the control group was treated with aspirin only. The therapeutic effect, platelet aggregation rate, recurrence rate, and complication rate of the two groups were compared. The total effective rate of 86.67% (52/60) in the treatment group was significantly higher than that of 71.67% (43/60) in the control group ($P < 0.05$). After treatment, the NIHSS score of the treatment group was significantly lower than that of the control group, the platelet aggregation rate was significantly lower than that of the control group,

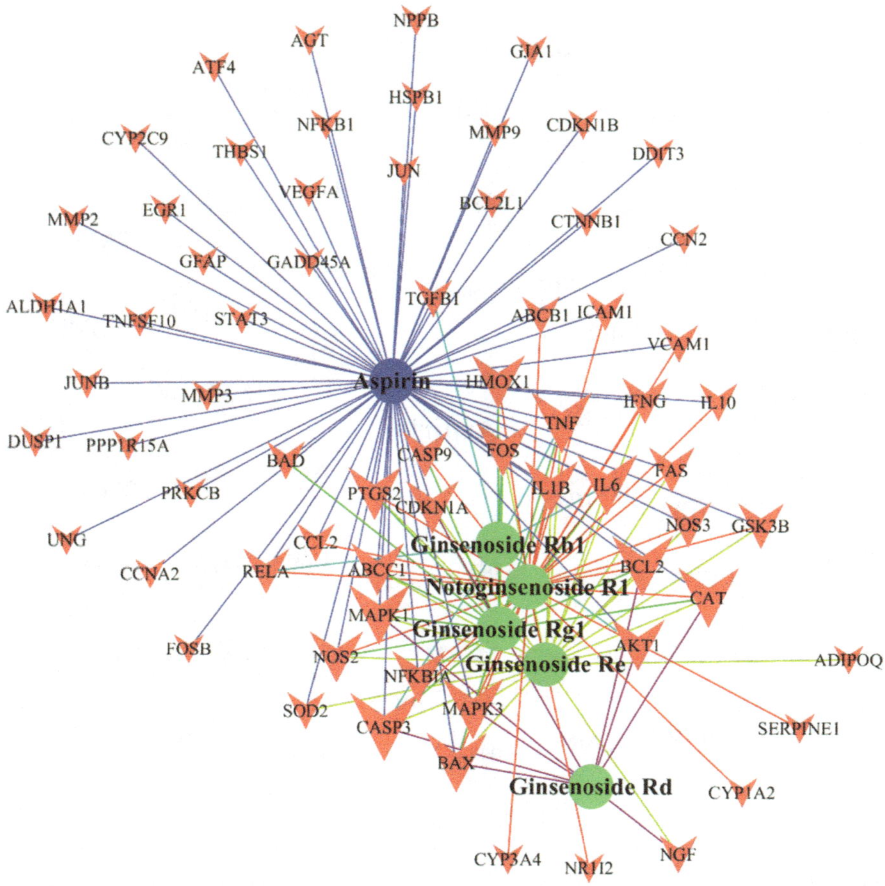

Fig. 7.25 Aspirin and Xuesaitong-ischemic stroke-related gene network. The green round nodes represent the main components of Xuesaitong, and the blue round nodes represent aspirin; the red V-shaped nodes represent genes associated with ischemic stroke. The blue, red, purple, yellow, green, and blue edges connect to the ischemic stroke-related genes associated with aspirin, notoginsenoside R1, ginsenoside Rd, ginsenoside Re, ginsenoside Rg1, and ginsenoside Rb1, respectively

the recurrence rate was significantly lower than that of the control group, and the incidence of complications was also significantly lower than that of the control group ($P < 0.05$). The combined use of panax notoginseng saponins and aspirin can achieve a certain preventive effect, which is safe and has a remarkable therapeutic effect on cerebral infarction.

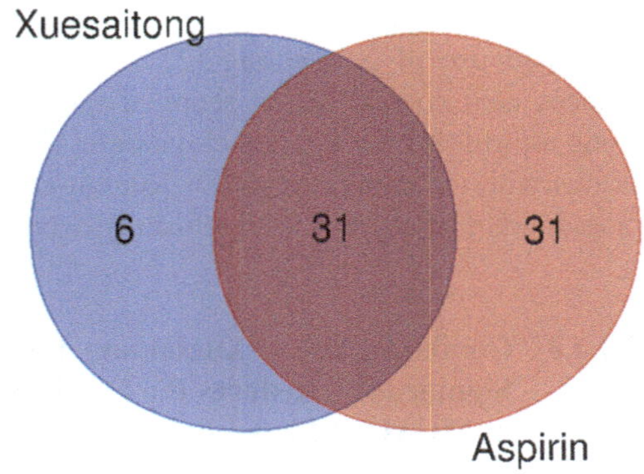

Fig. 7.26 Venn diagram—aspirin vs Xuesaitong (genes associated with ischemic stroke)

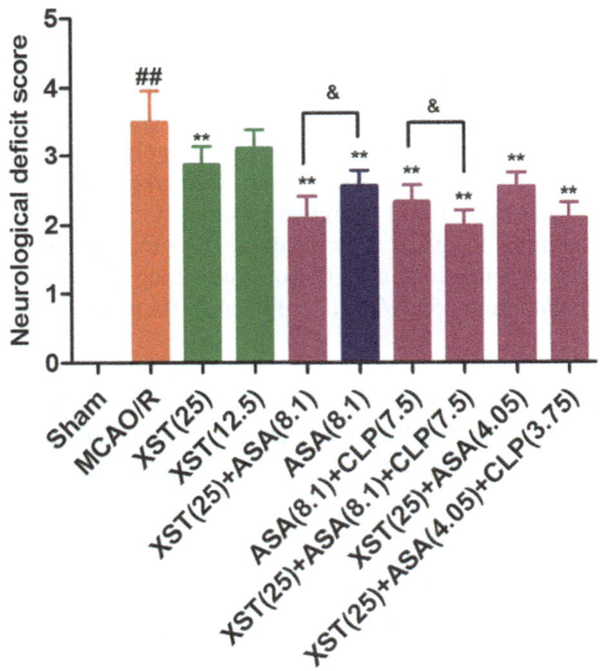

Fig. 7.27 Combined use of Xuesaitong and antiplatelet drugs significantly reduces the neurological deficit score of MCAO/R model rats. Note: ##, $P < 0.01$ vs sham-operated group; *, $P < 0.05$ vs MCAO/R Model group; △, $P < 0.05$ vs ASA group; &, $P < 0.05$ vs ASA+CLP group

7.4.4.2 Combined Use of Xuesaitong and Antiplatelet Drugs can Significantly Reduce the Neurological Deficit Score of MCAO/R Model Rats

As shown in Fig. 7.27, compared with the sham-operated group, the neurological deficit score of rats in the MCAO/R model group is increased significantly ($P < 0.05$); compared with the MCAO/R model group, Xuesaitong, aspirin, combined use of Xuesaitong and aspirin, combined use of clopidogrel and aspirin, combined use of Xuesaitong, aspirin, and clopidogrel, all significantly reduced the neurological deficit score of rats ($P < 0.05$). Compared with aspirin (8.1 mg/kg) group, the combined use of Xuesaitong (25 mg/kg) and aspirin (8.1 mg/kg) significantly reduces neurological deficit score of rats ($P < 0.05$). Compared with the group using aspirin (8.1 mg/kg) and clopidogrel (7.5 mg/kg), the neurological deficit score of rats with the combined use of Xuesaitong (25 mg/kg), aspirin (8.1 mg/kg), and clopidogrel (7.5 mg/kg) is significantly decreased ($P < 0.05$).

7.4.4.3 Combined Use of Xuesaitong and Antiplatelet Drugs Significantly Reduces the Cerebral Infarction Volume in MCAO/R Model Rats

As shown in Fig. 7.28, compared with the sham-operated group, the cerebral infarction volume of rats in the MCAO/R model group is significantly increased ($P < 0.05$); compared with the MCAO/R model group, Xuesaitong, aspirin, combined use of Xuesaitong and aspirin, combined use of clopidogrel and aspirin, and combined use of Xuesaitong, aspirin, and clopidogrel, all significantly reduce the cerebral infarction volume ($P < 0.05$). Compared with the aspirin (8.1 mg/kg) group, the combined use of Xuesaitong (25 mg/kg) and aspirin (8.1 mg/kg) significantly reduces the cerebral infarction volume ($P < 0.05$). Compared with the group using aspirin (8.1 mg/kg) and clopidogrel (7.5 mg/kg), the cerebral infarction volume of rats with the combined use of Xuesaitong (25 mg/kg), aspirin (8.1 mg/kg), and clopidogrel (7.5 mg/kg) is significantly decreased ($P < 0.05$).

7.4.4.4 Combined Use of Xuesaitong and Antiplatelet Drugs Improves the Inhibitory Effect of Aspirin or Penicillin-Streptomycin on Platelets

As shown in Fig. 7.29, compared with the sham-operated group, the maximum platelet aggregation rate of the MCAO/R model group is significantly increased. Compared with the MCAO/R model group, use of aspirin, or combined use of clopidogrel and aspirin significantly reduces the maximum platelet aggregation rate. Combined use of Xuesaitong and aspirin, and combined use of Xuesaitong, aspirin, and clopidogrel significantly improve the inhibition of aspirin on platelets.

7.4.4.5 Xuesaitong Significantly Reduces Aspirin-Induced Gastric Mucosal Damage in Rats

As shown in Fig. 7.30, compared with the control group, gastric mucosal epithelial cells of rats are necrotic and inflammatory cells are infiltrated in the aspirin group. Compared with the aspirin group, Xuesaitong significantly reduces gastric mucosal epithelial cell necrosis and inflammatory cell infiltration induced by aspirin. Using Xuesaitong alone has no significant effect on the gastric mucosa of rats.

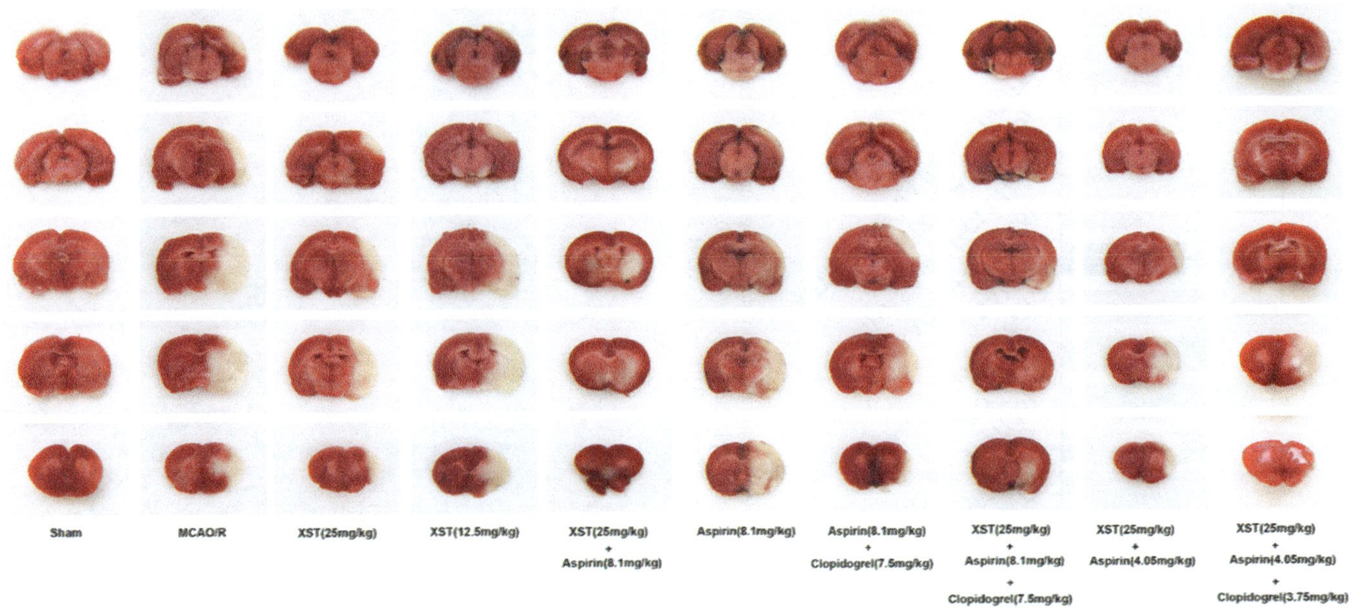

Fig. 7.28 Combined use of Xuesaitong and antiplatelet drugs significantly reduces the cerebral infarction volume in MCAO/R model rats. Note: ##, $P < 0.01$ vs sham-operated group *, $P < 0.05$ vs MCAO/R Model group; △, $P < 0.05$ vs ASA group; &, $P < 0.05$ vs ASA+CLP group

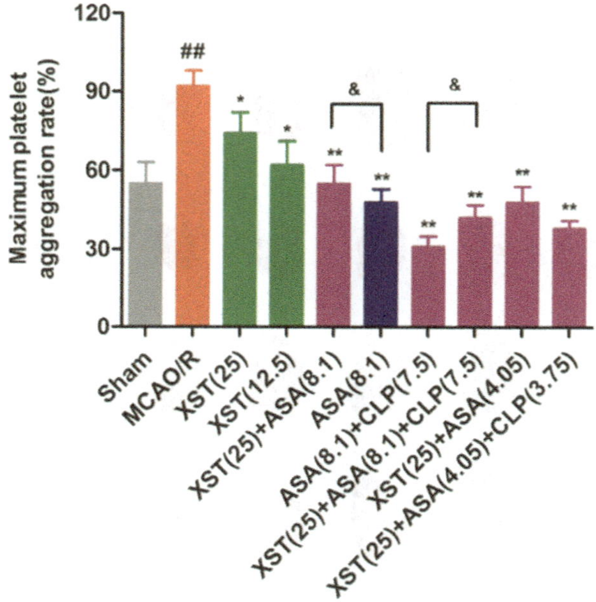

Fig. 7.29 Combined use of Xuesaitong and antiplatelet drugs improves the inhibitory effect of aspirin or penicillin-streptomycin on platelets. Note: ##, $P < 0.01$ vs sham-operated group; *, $P < 0.05$ vs MCAO/R Model group; **, $P < 0.01$ vs MCAO/R Model group; △, $P < 0.05$ vs ASA group; &, $P < 0.05$ vs ASA+CLP group

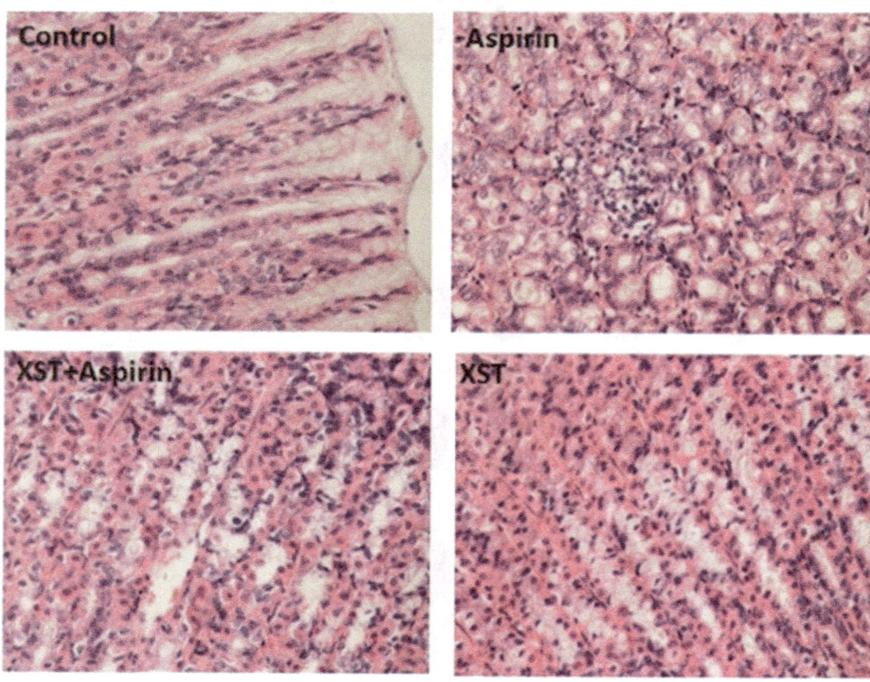

Fig. 7.30 Xuesaitong significantly reduces aspirin-induced gastric mucosal damage in rats

7.4.4.6 Xuesaitong Significantly Reduces Aspirin-Induced Duodenal Microvilli Injury in Rats

As shown in Fig. 7.31, compared with the control group, the number of microvilli on the surface of rat duodenum in the aspirin group significantly reduces. Compared with the aspirin group, Xuesaitong significantly reduces the decrease in microvilli on the duodenum surface induced by aspirin, however, using Xuesaitong alone has no significant effect on microvilli on the surface of rat duodenum.

7.4.4.7 Combined Use of Xuesaitong and Aspirin has Synergistic Effect on the Influence of Gene Expression of MCAO Model Rats

As shown in Fig. 7.32, aspirin has little influence on gene expression of MCAO model rats, while Xuesaitong has significant influence on gene expression of MCAO model rats. The combined use of Xuesaitong and aspirin has synergistic effect on the influence of gene expression of MCAO model rats.

7.4.4.8 Combined Use of Xuesaitong and Aspirin Significantly Affects the Gene Expression of MCAO Model Rats

As shown in Fig. 7.33, compared with the MCAO model group, aspirin causes 58 differential gene expressions, PNS (Panax notoginseng saponins) administration causes 267 differential gene expressions, and ALI Therapy causes 677 differential

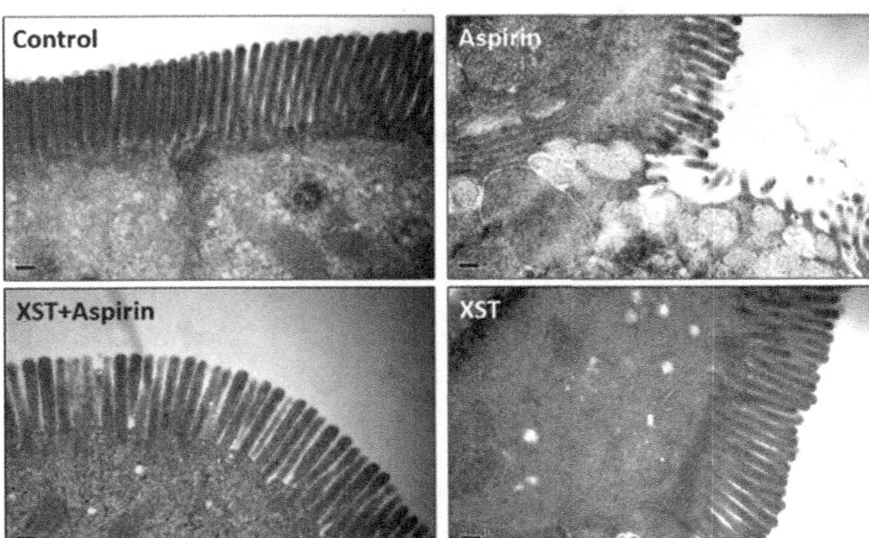

Fig. 7.31 Xuesaitong significantly reduces aspirin-induced duodenal microvilli injury in rats

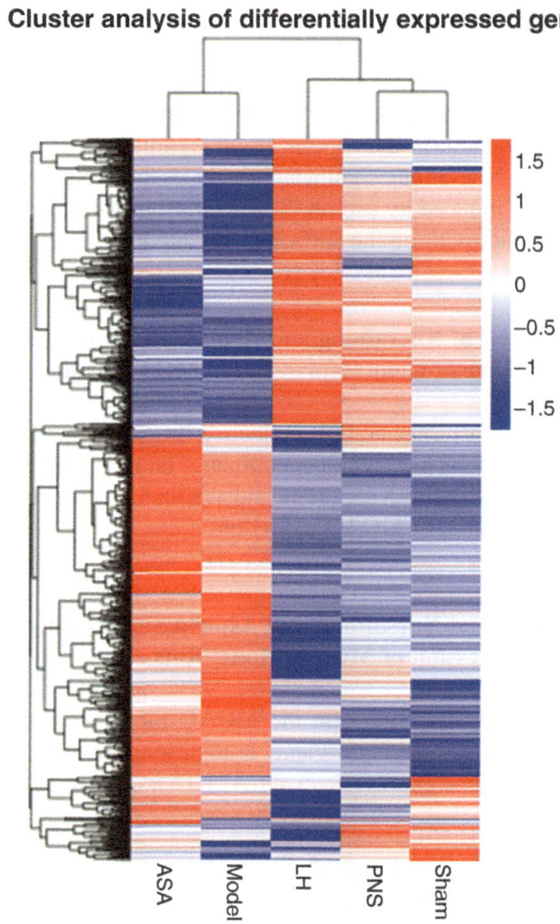

Fig. 7.32 Differential gene cluster diagram of ALI therapy

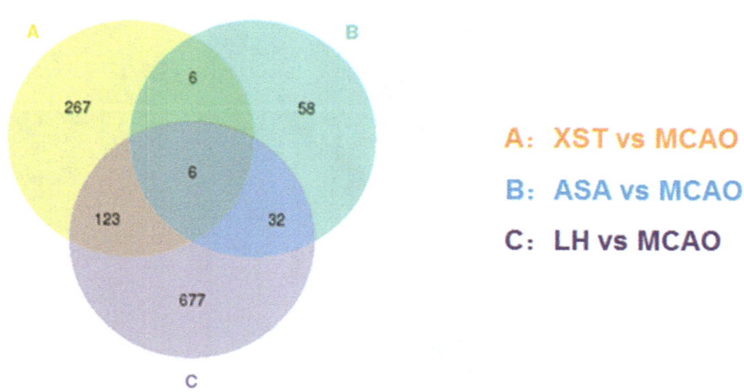

Fig. 7.33 Differential gene venn diagram of ALI therapy

gene expressions; Compared with aspirin, ALI Therapy causes 32 differential gene expressions; Compared with Panax notoginseng saponins, ALI Therapy causes 132 differential gene expressions.

7.4.4.9 Summary

Taking the combined use of Xuesaitong and aspirin as an example, this section comprehensively introduces the experimental ideas and processes of the interaction between TCM and Western medicine based on network pharmacology, and tries to provide reference for the application of network pharmacology in the study of interaction between Chinese and Western medicine. Based on the results of the CTD database and literature research, this section constructs the molecular target networks of Xuesaitong and aspirin in regulating ischemic stroke using network pharmacology. The consistency analysis of the target spectrum of Xuesaitong and aspirin is carried out through the network superposition technology. It was found that there is a high degree of overlap in the ischemic stroke-related genes regulated by aspirin and Xuesaitong. Among the 37 genes regulated by Xuesaitong, 31 genes are completely consistent with those regulated by aspirin, suggesting that the combined use of the two has the potential to enhance the effect of aspirin in the treatment of ischemic stroke. Based on the MCAO/R model of SD rats, we tested the effects of Xuesaitong, aspirin, and Xuesaitong + aspirin on the neurological deficit score and cerebral infarction volume. The results showed that the effect of the combined use of aspirin and Xuesetong is better than using aspirin or Xuesetong alone. In addition, Xuesaitong has a certain alleviating effect on gastrointestinal mucosal damage caused by aspirin or penicillin-streptomycin. In general, based on network pharmacology, this section infers from the drug–target level that the combined use of Xuesaitong and aspirin has the potential to enhance the effect of aspirin in the treatment of ischemic stroke; the network analysis results were verified from the overall level based on the MCAO/R rat model. The experimental results are highly consistent with the network analysis results, indicating that network pharmacology has broad application prospects in explaining the interaction between Chinese and Western medicines.

7.5 Repositioning of Clinical Application of Drugs: New Uses of TCM Ingredients in Protecting Cerebral Ischemia-Reperfusion Injury

Thrombolytic therapy is still the main treatment methodology for acute ischemic stroke. However, cerebral ischemia-reperfusion injury that is a side effect of thrombolytic therapy hinders the successful treatment of acute ischemic stroke. Although reperfusion is the key to the recovery of brain function, reperfusion leads to excessive production of reactive oxygen species (free radicals), which leads to oxidative stress and further deterioration of brain injury [20]. Elimination of the produced free radicals seems to be a therapeutic strategy for treating acute ischemic stroke. Although pre-clinical experiments proved effective antioxidants that remove active oxygen, the results of clinical trials did not support the same. Nevertheless, the disappointing clinical trial results cannot deny the important role of oxidative stress in cerebral ischemia-reperfusion injury. Targeting the source of free radicals may be a new therapeutic strategy. Although the source of free radicals has not been completely determined, many studies show that NADPH oxidase and mitochondria are the main sources of free radicals in the pathological process of cerebral ischemia-reperfusion [21, 22].

There is increasing evidence that phytoestrogens and notoginseng have protective effects on neurodegenerative diseases including on acute ischemic stroke. Phytoestrogens ginsenoside Rg1 and Rb1 isolated from notoginseng have significant neuroprotective effects on cerebral ischemia-reperfusion injury [23, 24]. Our recent study found that notoginsenoside R1 activates the Akt/Nrf2/HO-1 signaling pathway through an estrogen receptor-dependent pathway and inhibits oxidative stress in PC12 cells [10]. Moreover, HO-1 inhibits the activity of NADPH oxidase and mitochondrial dysfunction [25]. Based on the above research results, we speculate that notoginsenoside R1 may inhibit NADPH oxidase activity and mitochondrial dysfunction by inducing the expression of HO-1, thus playing a neuroprotective role in cerebral ischemia-reperfusion injury.

We used both in vivo and in vitro cerebral ischemia-reperfusion injury models, namely the rat middle cerebral artery occlusion reperfusion model and oxygen glucose deprivation in primary cortical neuronal cells, to evaluate the neuroprotective effects of notoginsenoside R1. In addition, we elucidated the neuroprotective mechanism of Notoginsenoside R1, that is, Notoginsenoside R1 activates Akt/Nrf2 signaling pathway through estrogen receptor-dependent pathway, thus inhibiting NADPH oxidase activity and mitochondrial dysfunction. The research idea and process are shown in Fig. 7.34.

7.5.1 Data Acquisition and Processing

7.5.1.1 Collection of Chemical Component Targets

"Chemicals" was selected under the Keyword Search option of the CTD database, and Notoginsenoside R1 entered in the search box to collect target data of Notoginsenoside R1. "Chemicals" was selected under the Menu option in the ETCM Database menu bar and "Notoginsenoside R1" was entered in the search box, to collect the target data of Notoginsenoside R1. The target data of Notoginsenoside R1 collected from the CTD and ETCM databases were integrated for deduplication processing. The correspondence between Notoginsenoside R1 and its targets was saved in the form of a two-dimensional list.

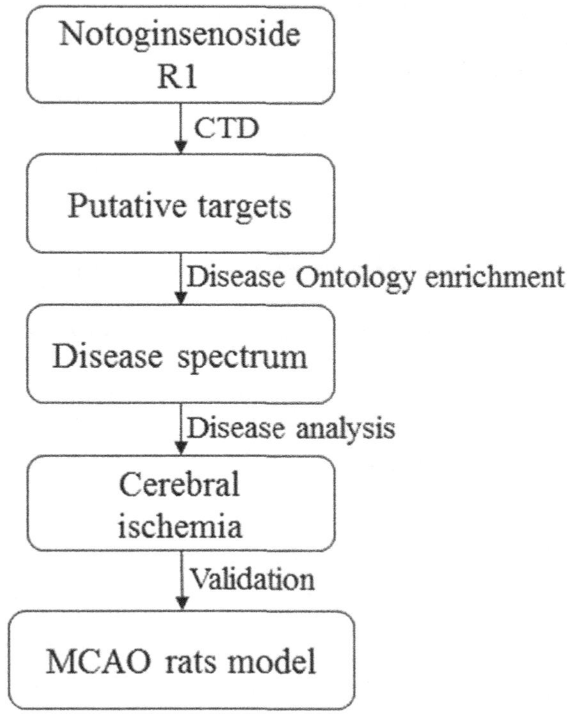

Fig. 7.34 Research ideas and process

7.5.1.2 Disease Ontology Enrichment Analysis

"Set Analyzer" was selected under the Analyze option of the CTD database, "Genes" was selected as the input type, and the abbreviation of the target gene was entered in the input box. "Enriched diseases" was selected as the analysis type, and the corrected P-value threshold was set to 0.01.

7.5.2 Network Construction and Visualization

7.5.2.1 Network Construction and Visualization

The disease spectrum of notoginsenoside R1 obtained through the enrichment analysis of the disease ontology was entered into Cytoscape 3.5.0, to visualize the disease spectrum of notoginsenoside R1. The nervous system diseases and disease-related genes related to notoginsenoside R1 were imported into Cytoscape 3.5.0 to construct a molecular network of "notoginsenoside R1–target–nervous system disease."

7.5.2.2 Analysis Index and Algorithm

The diseases with significant differences were screened and selected according to the corrected p-value (Corrected P-value < 0.01) of each disease in the disease ontology enrichment analysis results.

7.5.3 Network Analysis and Prediction

7.5.3.1 Disease Spectrum Analysis of Notoginsenoside R1

The disease spectrum (as shown in Fig. 7.35) of Notoginsenoside R1 was drawn by selecting the top 60 diseases in the results of disease ontology enrichment analysis, involving 19 disease types (as shown in Fig. 7.36). The top five disease types are cancer, cardiovascular disease, digestive system disease, urogenital disease (male and female), and nervous system disease. In recent years, researchers in China and overseas have reported on the neuroprotective effects of Panax notoginseng,

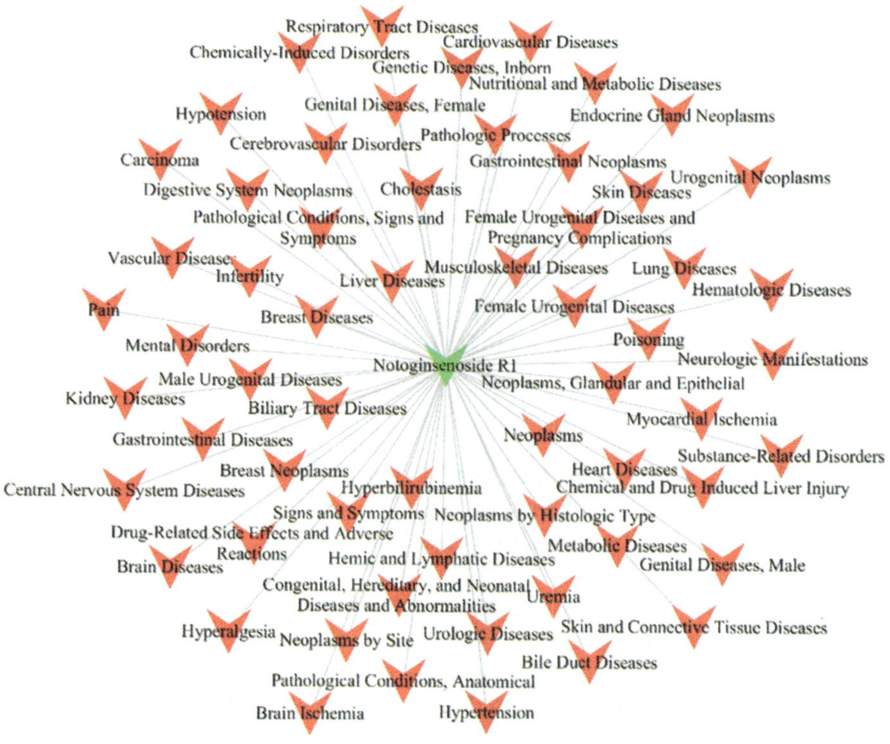

Fig. 7.35 Disease spectrum of notoginsenoside R1. Green and red V-shaped nodes represent Notoginsenoside R1 and diseases related to Notoginsenoside R1, respectively

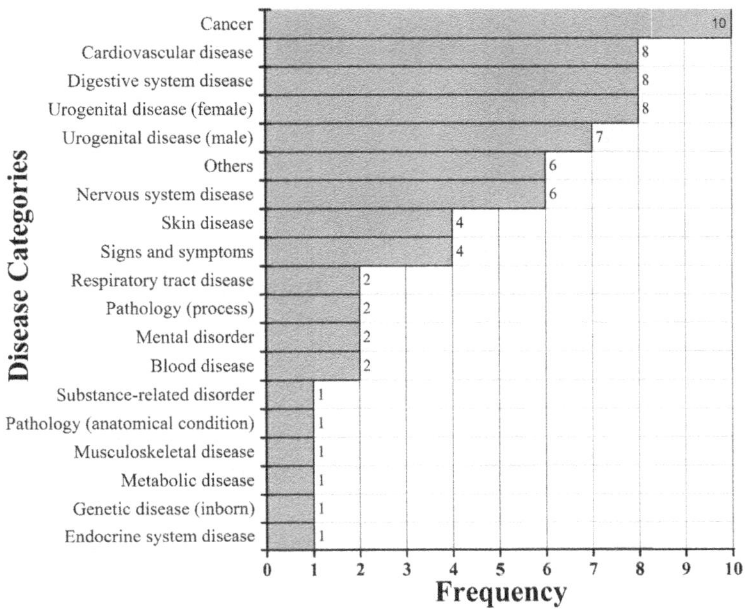

Fig. 7.36 Statistical analysis of panax notoginsenoside R1-related disease types (TOP60). Frequency represents the kinds of diseases involved in each disease type

however, the material basis of neuroprotective activity of Panax notoginseng has not been systematically studied, let alone its mechanism of action. The results of disease spectrum analysis show that Notoginsenoside R1 may play an important role in the neuroprotective effect of Panax notoginseng.

7.5.3.2 Discovery of New Uses of Notoginsenoside R1 in Protecting Cerebral Ischemia-Reperfusion Injury

Figure 7.37 shows the molecular network of Notoginsenoside R1 regulating neurological diseases, the involved disease kinds include cerebral ischemia, cerebrovascular diseases, brain diseases, nervous system manifestations, central nervous system diseases, and hyperalgesia. In addition to cerebral ischemia, the other five disease types (cerebrovascular disease, brain disease, nervous system performance, central nervous system disease, and hyperalgesia) are collectively referred to as a class of diseases. Considering the feasibility and rationality of experimental verification, we next verified the protective effect of Notoginsenoside R1 on cerebral ischemia.

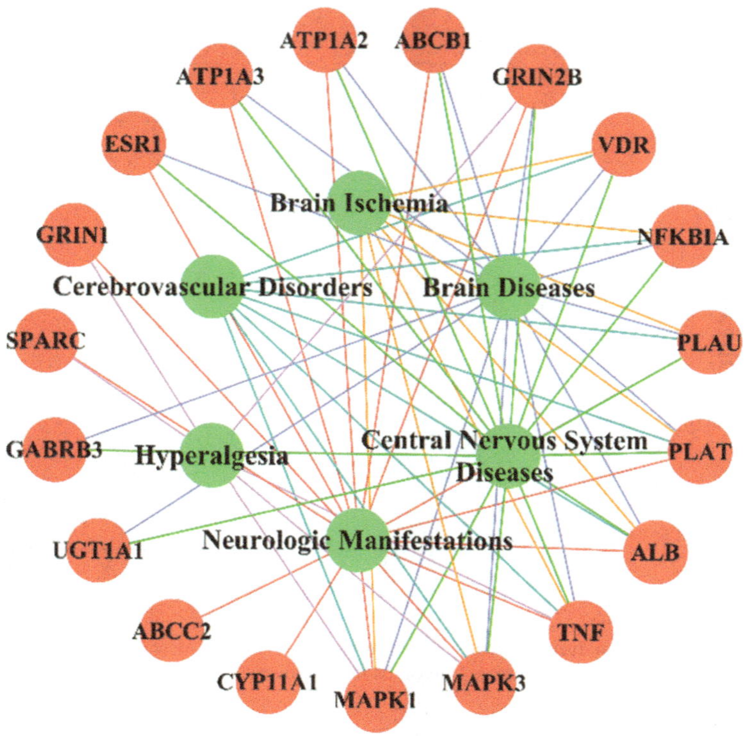

Fig. 7.37 Notoginsenoside R1–target–neural system disease molecular network. The green and red round nodes represent the nervous system diseases related to Notoginsenoside R1 and the nervous system disease-related genes regulated by Notoginsenoside R1, respectively. The orange, blue, red, green, blue, and purple edges are connected to disease genes associated with cerebral ischemia, brain diseases, nervous system manifestations, central nervous system diseases, cerebrovascular disease, and hyperalgesia, respectively

7.5.4 *Verification and Summary*

7.5.4.1 Notoginsenoside R1 Reduces Neurological Impairment and Cerebral Infarction Volume Caused by Cerebral Ischemia-Reperfusion

It has been reported that Notoginsenoside R1 can reduce the neurological impairment and cerebral infarction volume caused by cerebral ischemia-reperfusion [26]. As shown in Fig. 7.38, the rats in the sham and the NGR1-treated group presented no neurologic deficits and infarction volumes. After 48-h reperfusion, the rats that received I/R treatment displayed a marked increase in neurologic deficit score (Fig. 7.38c, $n = 10$, $P < 0.01$), and a well-defined infarct involving both ischemic core and penumbra (Fig. 7.38a, b, $n = 10$, $P < 0.01$). However, NGR1

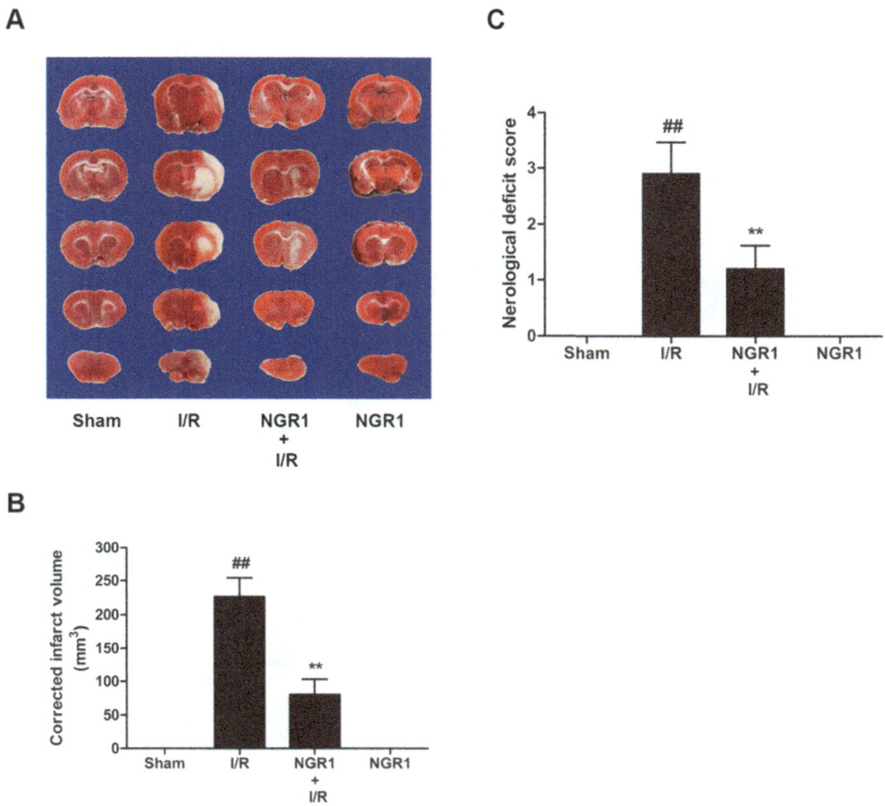

Fig. 7.38 Notoginsenoside R1 reduces neurological impairment and cerebral infarction volume caused by cerebral ischemia-reperfusion. (**a**) TTC staining method to detect cerebral infarction volume. (**b**) Statistical results of cerebral infarction volume. (**c**) Neurological function score

pretreatment provided a significant improvement in neurologic deficit score and remarkably reduced infarct volumes (Fig. 7.38a–c, $n = 10$, $P < 0.01$).

7.5.4.2 Notoginsenoside R1 Increases the Expression of HO-1 in Rat Cerebral Cortex

HO-1 is an antioxidant enzyme with neuroprotective effect. As shown in Fig. 7.39a, b, both histo-cytometer analysis and Western blot analysis show that there are few HO-1 positive cells in the cortex of rats in the sham-operated group, while the expression of HO-1 around the lesions in the I/R model group increases, however, most of them are weak positive cells. Compared with the I/R model group, higher HO-1 level was noted in the NGR1+ I/R group. Interestingly, administration of Notoginsenoside R1 alone significantly increases HO-1 immunoreactivity. We further detected the activity of HO-1. The results show that the HO-1 activity was also

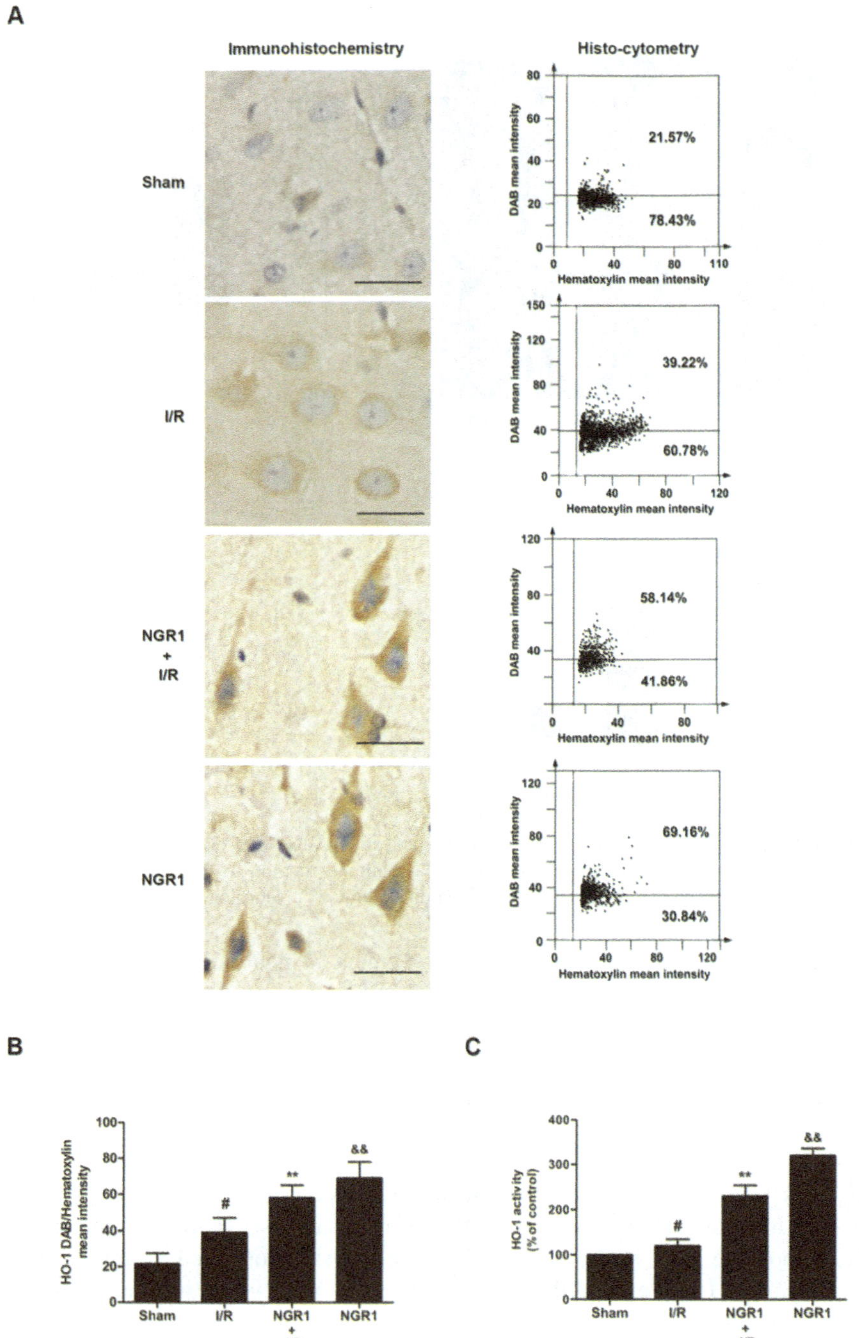

Fig. 7.39 Notoginsenoside R1 increases the expression of HO-1 in rat cerebral cortex. (**a**) Detect the expression of HO-1 in cerebral cortex tissue of rats by immunohistochemistry (left) and analyze the expression level of HO-1 by flow-like analysis (right). (**b**) Statistical map of HO-1 expression

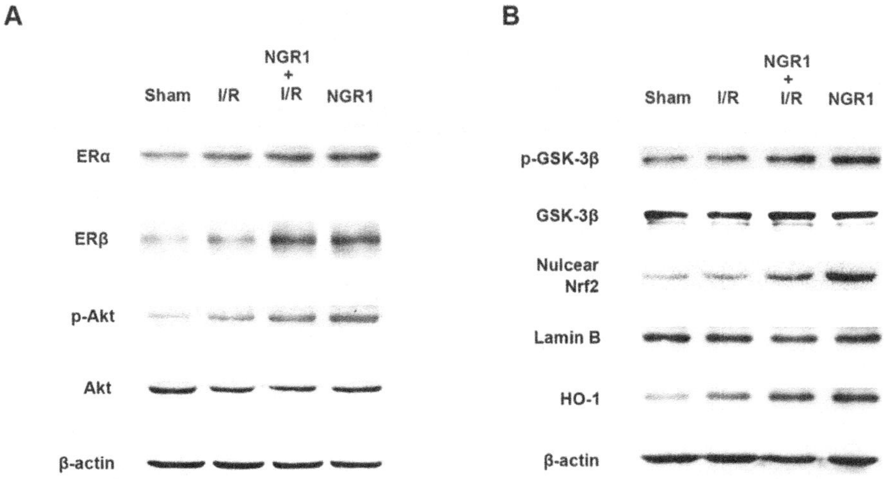

Fig. 7.40 Notoginsenoside R1 activates estrogen receptor-dependent Akt/Nrf2 signaling pathway. (**a**) Notoginsenoside R1 increases the protein expression of ERα and ERβ and the phosphorylation of Akt in the cerebral cortex tissues of rats. (**b**) Notoginsenoside R1 increases the phosphorylation of GSK-3β, accumulation of Nrf2 in nucleus, and protein expression of HO-1 in the cerebral cortex tissues of rats

increased in the I/R, NGR1+ I/R, and NGR1-treated groups (as shown in Fig. 7.39c, $n = 6$, $P < 0.01$).

7.5.4.3 Notoginsenoside R1 Activates Estrogen Receptor-Dependent Akt/Nrf2 Signaling Pathway

Western blot results show that in the I/R model group, the protein expression of HO-1 is significantly up-regulated in the NGR1+ I/R and the NGR1-treated groups, respectively (as shown in Fig. 7.40b, $n = 6$, $P < 0.01$). Moreover, Notoginsenoside R1 significantly increases nuclear accumulation of Nrf2 (as shown in Fig. 7.40b, $n = 6$, $P < 0.01$). We investigated the estrogen receptor and Akt/GSK-3β signaling pathway to clarify the mechanism of Nrf2 activation. As shown in Fig. 7.40a, Notoginsenoside R1 significantly increases the expression of ERα and ERβ proteins and the phosphorylation of Akt and GSK-3β ($n = 6$, $P < 0.01$).

Notosaponin R1 up-regulates HO-1 protein expression and activity by activating the estrogen-receptor-dependent Akt/Nrf2 signaling pathway both in vitro and in vivo, and inhibits NADPH oxidase activity and mitochondrial dysfunction,

Fig. 7.39 (continued) level in cerebral cortex tissue of rats. (**c**) Notoginsenoside R1 increases the activity of HO-1 in cerebral cortex tissue of rats

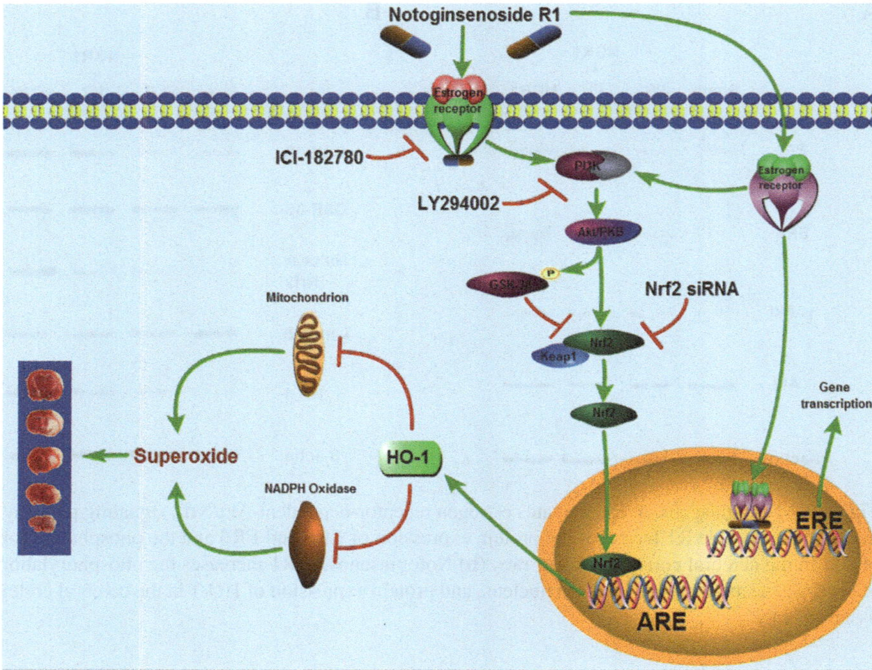

Fig. 7.41 Molecular mechanism illustration of notoginsenoside R1 against cerebral ischemia

thereby inhibiting cerebral ischemia-reperfusion injury and oxygen glucose deprivation reperfusion injury (as shown in Fig. 7.41).

7.5.4.4 Study on Other Mechanisms of the Neuroprotective Effect of Notoginsenoside R1

In-depth studies have been conducted on the neuroprotective mechanism of action of Notoginsenoside R1 in China and overseas. Notoginsenoside R1 activates estrogen receptors, causing crosstalk between Akt and ERK1/2 signaling pathways, thereby activating Nrf2/ARE signaling pathway [10]. Through the estrogen receptor-mediated endoplasmic reticulum, panax Notoginseng saponin R1 stress plays an anti-neonatal cerebral ischemia and hypoxia injury role [27], and the release of stress calcium plays a neuroprotective role by inhibiting the endoplasmic reticulum through PLC [28].

7.5.4.5 Summary

Taking Notoginsenoside R1 as an example, this section comprehensively introduces the experimental ideas and processes of drug repositioning based on network pharmacology, with the aim to provide reference for the application of network pharmacology in drug repositioning research. Based on the CTD database, we collected the target data of Notoginsenoside R1 and predicted the disease spectrum of Notoginsenoside R1 through disease ontology enrichment. The results of disease ontology enrichment indicate that Notoginsenoside R1 has protective effect on nervous system diseases such as cerebral ischemia. To investigate the reliability of the prediction results, we tested the protective effect of Notoginsenoside R1 on cerebral ischemia based on the MCAO model. The results show that: Notoginsenoside R1 activates the Akt/Nrf2/HO-1 pathway in an estrogen receptor-dependent manner, and inhibits NADPH oxidase activity and mitochondrial dysfunction, thereby inhibiting the production of peroxides, and finally plays a neuroprotective role in cerebral ischemia-reperfusion injury. In general, based on network pharmacology, this section predicts the disease spectrum of Notoginsenoside R1, and discovers a new use of Notoginsenoside R1 in protecting against cerebral ischemia. This use of Notoginsenoside R1 has been verified on the MCAO model, indicating that network pharmacology is an effective method and strategy for drug relocation research.

7.6 Development of Multi-target Drugs: Low-Density Lipoprotein-Induced Endothelial Cell Injury Protected by Synergistic Compatibility of TCM Ingredients

As a complex disease, the occurrence and development of atherosclerosis involves multiple targets, and the commercially available single-target drugs have limited therapeutic effects [29]. The traditional drug development concept of "one gene, one disease, one drug" is facing great challenges in the prevention and treatment of atherosclerosis. In recent years, the rise of the "multi-gene, multi-target" drug development model has pointed the way for new drug development in atherosclerosis. TCM has rich practical experience in the treatment of complex diseases, and has been widely recognized for its multi-channel, multi-target, and low toxicity treatment features. However, due to the complex ingredients, slow onset of action, difficulty in quality control, and lack of systematic toxicological studies, it is difficult to determine the material basis of its efficacy. Both, the unclear mechanism of action, and unclear target of action, limit the promotion and application of TCM in the international community. Therefore, developing innovative TCM prescriptions with definite curative effect, controllable quality, and clear mechanism of action has become a critical requirement in the treatment of atherosclerosis.

Network pharmacology is a novel method developed on the basis of systems biology and multidirectional pharmacology [30]. By integrating the drug–target protein interaction network and the biological network, it analyzes the interaction between drugs and other nodes in the network, and then analyzes the effectiveness and toxicity of drugs. Guanxin Danshen Formulation is an effective prescription for the treatment of coronary cardiovascular diseases developed by our research group. It is mainly composed of three herbs: Salvia miltiorrhiza, Panax notoginseng, and Dalbergia odorifera. Clinically, it is effective in treating coronary cardiovascular disease caused by qi stagnation and blood stasis, but there have been few studies on its efficacy in treating atherosclerosis. In recent years, relevant experimental studies have shown that salvianolic acid B, the main water-soluble component of Salvia miltiorrhiza, can effectively reduce blood lipids, reduce lipid content in plaque, reduce plaque area, increase fiber thickness, and reduce plaque erosion and angiogenesis in plaque [31], thus effectively preventing the occurrence of atherosclerosis and stabilizing atherosclerotic plaque. Although ginsenoside Re in Panax notoginseng has not been reported directly in the prevention and treatment of atherosclerosis, it can effectively reduce the content of malondialdehyde (MDA), enhance the activities of superoxide dismutase (SOD) and glutathione (GSH-Px), reduce the release of lactate dehydrogenase (LDH), and enhance the scavenging of DPPH free radicals, thereby reducing oxidative damage. In addition, ginsenoside Re effectively reduces the secretion of IL-6, TNF-α, IL-10, and other related inflammatory factors in serum, and inhibit inflammation [32]. The role of ginsenoside Re in regulating apoptosis-related proteins has also been reported. [33] Previous studies suggest that ginsenoside Re can exert anti-atherosclerotic effects through its anti-inflammatory, antioxidant, and anti-apoptotic effects.

Based on network pharmacology, this section investigates the overall protective effect of salvianolic acid B (Sal B) and ginsenoside Re (Re) on oxidative low-density lipoprotein (Ox-LDL)-induced injury of human umbilical vein endothelial cells (HUVECs) through multiple targets and pathways.

7.6.1 Data Acquisition and Processing

First, the pathological database of atherosclerosis, the Ox-LDL-induced HAEC cell damage expression profile database, and the Ox-LDL-induced HUVECs damage protein chip database were constructed. Then, using the molecular docking technology combined with literature statistics, the direct-action targets of salvianolic acid B and ginsenoside Re were determined. The targets of salvianolic acid B (Sal B) and ginsenoside Re (RE) were imported into the constructed disease pathology database, to find overlapping targets. Finally, through relevant GO function annotation, KEGG pathway analysis, and protein interaction analysis the mechanism of action of the two compounds' cooperative protection of Ox-LDL-induced HUVECs damage was explored, to provide research ideas and technical support for the in-depth development of Guanxin Danshen Formulation (as shown in Fig. 7.42).

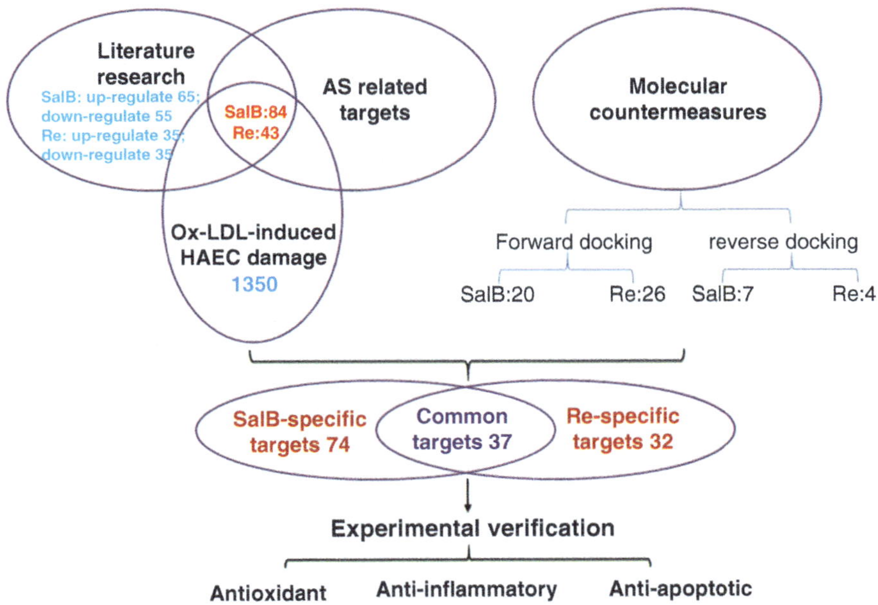

Fig. 7.42 Research ideas and processes

7.6.1.1 Collection of Chemical Component Targets

Using salvianolic acid B and ginsenoside Re as keywords, we searched the CNKI, Pubmed, SCI, ScienceDirect, and Springer databases to obtain related literature on salvianolic acid B and ginsenoside Re. The end date for the literature search was 2016-6-17. We extracted the relevant targets of salvianolic acid B and ginsenoside Re by reading the full text. We used PharmMapper and idTarget to predict the potential action targets of salvianolic acid B and ginsenoside Re, and all the docking parameters were set according to the default values on the website. Finally, we integrated the literature search results with the molecular docking prediction results.

7.6.1.2 Atherosclerosis-Related Genes

We searched genes related to atherosclerosis diseases based on the GeneCards database, the end date was 2016-6-30.

7.6.1.3 Differential Gene Analysis Based on Gene Expression Profile

We downloaded GSE13139 gene expression profile data based on NCBI's GEO database. This group of data contains five groups of data: inducing HAEC cell damage without adding Ox-LDL, and inducing HAEC cells for 2 h, 6 h, 12 h, and

24 h with Ox-LDL. The data was normalized based on the R language bioconductor toolkit, and differentially expressed genes were determined.

7.6.1.4 Analysis of Apoptosis Targets and Inflammatory Factors in Ox-LDL-Induced HUVECs Damage

This part mainly includes the data on apoptosis and inflammatory factors: inducing HUVECs cell damage without adding Ox-LDL and inducing HUVECs cells for 12 h with Ox-LDL. Human apoptotic protein chip (RayBiotech, USA) and human inflammatory factor protein chip (RayBiotech, USA) were used to detect apoptotic proteins and inflammatory factors.

7.6.2 Network Construction and Visualization

Each network involved in this study was drawn by using Cytoscape 3.5.0.

7.6.2.1 GO Function Enrichment Analysis

The online enrichment analysis tool DAVID was used to perform Gene Ontology (GO) enrichment analysis. GO enrichment analysis mainly includes three parts: Molecular Function (MF), Cellular Component (CC), and Biological Process (BP).

7.6.2.2 KEGG Pathway Analysis

In this experiment, the Cluster Profiler package and Kobas2.0 were used to analyze the KEGG pathway of target genes, and the obtained data were imported into Cytoscape, to construct the compound–target gene–pathway–disease network diagram.

7.6.2.3 Analysis Index and Algorithm

Differential gene expression analysis, KEGG analysis, and GO function analysis all use false discovery rate (FDR) test. When FDR$<$ 0.05 or $P < 0.05$, the difference is considered significant and statistically significant.

7.6.3 Network Analysis and Prediction

7.6.3.1 Statistics of Potential Target Genes on the Protective Effects of SalB and Re on Ox-LDL-Induced Endothelial Cell Damage

After standardizing the targets of salvianolic acid B and ginsenoside Re retrieved from CNKI, Pubmed, SCI, ScienceDirect, and Springer databases by NCBI gene data and correlated with protein chip data, 120 target genes related to salvianolic acid B and 70 target genes related to ginsenoside Re were finally obtained. The obtained target genes were correlated with the atherosclerotic disease gene library and the differential genes of Ox-LDL-induced HAEC cell damage; the overlapping target genes were removed, and finally there are 84 target genes related to salvianolic acid B and 43 target genes related to ginsenoside Re [32].

According to the pharmacophore simulation docking and reverse docking, two molecular docking databases of both salvianolic acid B and ginsenoside Re were obtained. According to the scoring and ranking rules of their respective websites, the top 100 proteins with the docking scores were taken, and their protein names were converted into gene names, and finally associated with the atherosclerosis disease gene library, to find the overlapping parts. Finally, 27 target genes related to salvianolic acid B and 30 target genes of ginsenoside Re were obtained.

By integrating the target genes and molecular docking results of database three, a total of 111 target genes related to salvianolic acid B and 69 target genes of ginsenoside Re were obtained. Further analysis shows that salvianolic acid B and ginsenoside Re have a common target gene 37. Therefore, the specific target of salvianolic acid B is 74, and the specific target gene of ginsenoside Re is 32.

7.6.3.2 Go Enrichment Analysis of Potential Target Genes on the Protective Effects of SalB and Re on Ox-LDL-Induced Endothelial Cell Damage

First, the GO function enrichment analysis on the common target genes between salvianolic acid B and ginsenoside Re was performed, and the common 37 target genes between them were imported into the DAVID web database. A total of 376 annotations were obtained with respect to cell components, molecular functions, and biological processes. With FDR < 0.05 as the screening condition, 69 annotations were finally obtained. As shown in Fig. 7.43, the common target genes mainly play an antioxidant role in the cell fluid and extracellular sites. The biological process mainly involves antioxidant, anti-apoptotic, and maintenance of cell ion balance; the key genes are GPX and SOD.

Next, the GO function enrichment analysis was performed on the specific target genes of salvianolic acid B, and its specific 74 target genes were imported into the DAVID web database. A total of 684 annotations were obtained with respect to cell components, molecular functions, and biological processes. With FDR < 0.05 as the

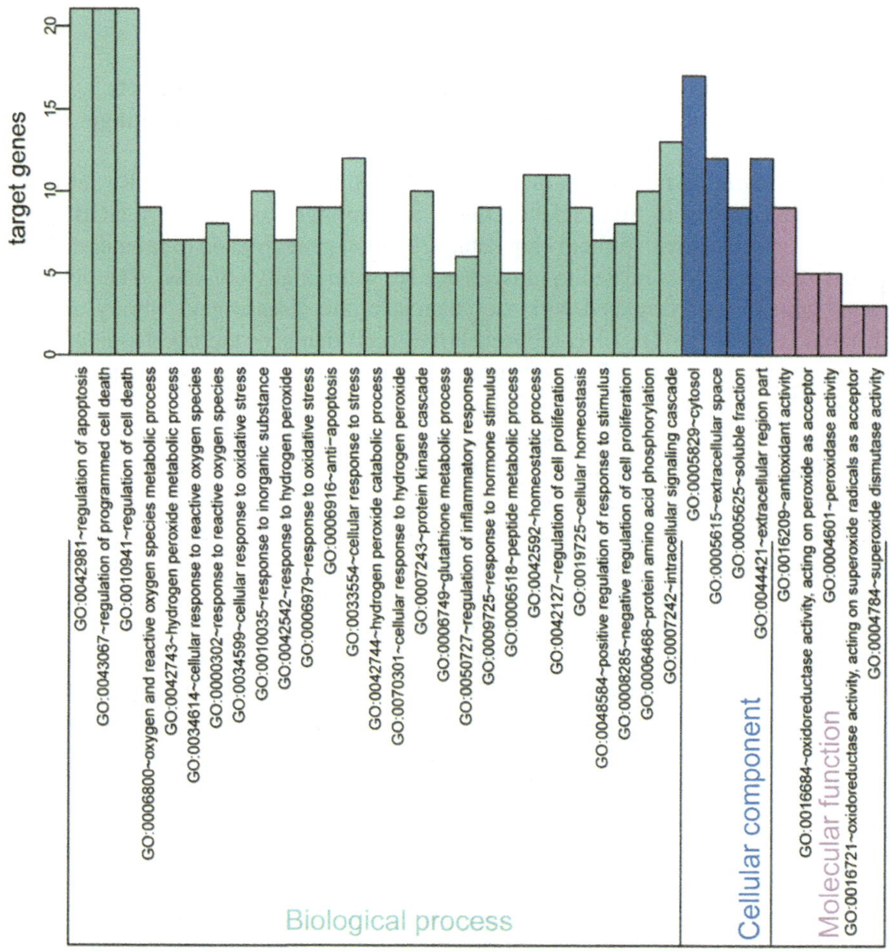

Fig. 7.43 GO function enrichment analysis on the common target genes between salvianolic acid B and Ginsenoside Re

screening condition, 113 annotations were finally obtained. As shown in Fig. 7.44, the common target genes mainly play antioxidant and electron transport functions in the cytoplasmic membrane and extracellular sites, and biological processes mainly involve antioxidant, cell proliferation, cell migration, anti-inflammatory, and other functions; the key genes are GSR, NOX5, NOX1, and NOS3.

Lastly, the GO function enrichment analysis was performed on the specific target genes of ginsenoside Re, and the specific 32 target genes were imported into the DAVID web database. A total of 282 annotations were obtained with respect to cell components, molecular functions, and biological processes. With FDR < 0.05 as the screening condition, 16 annotations were finally obtained. As shown in Fig. 7.45, the common target genes mainly play the role of steroid hormone in cell processes, and

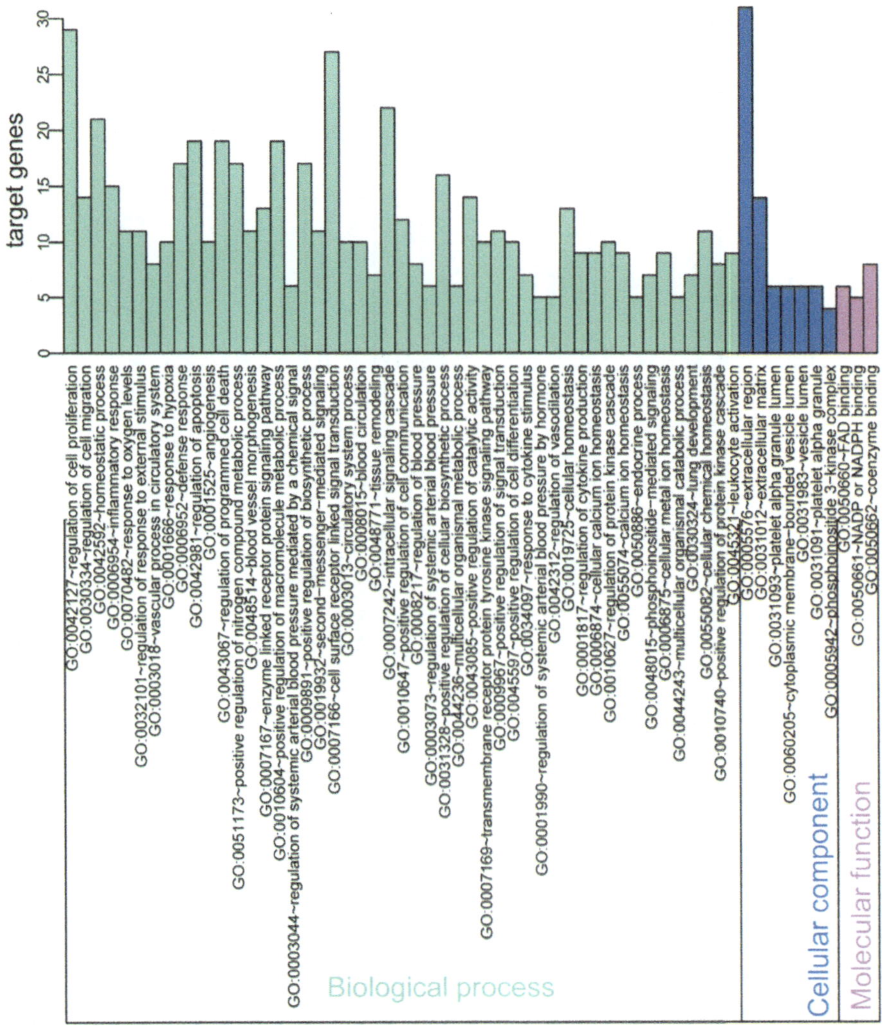

Fig. 7.44 GO function enrichment analysis on the specific target genes of salvianolic acid B

the main biological processes mainly involve hormone stimulation, cell proliferation, insulin stimulation, etc.; the key genes are AR, RXRB, RXRA, ESR1, and ESR2.

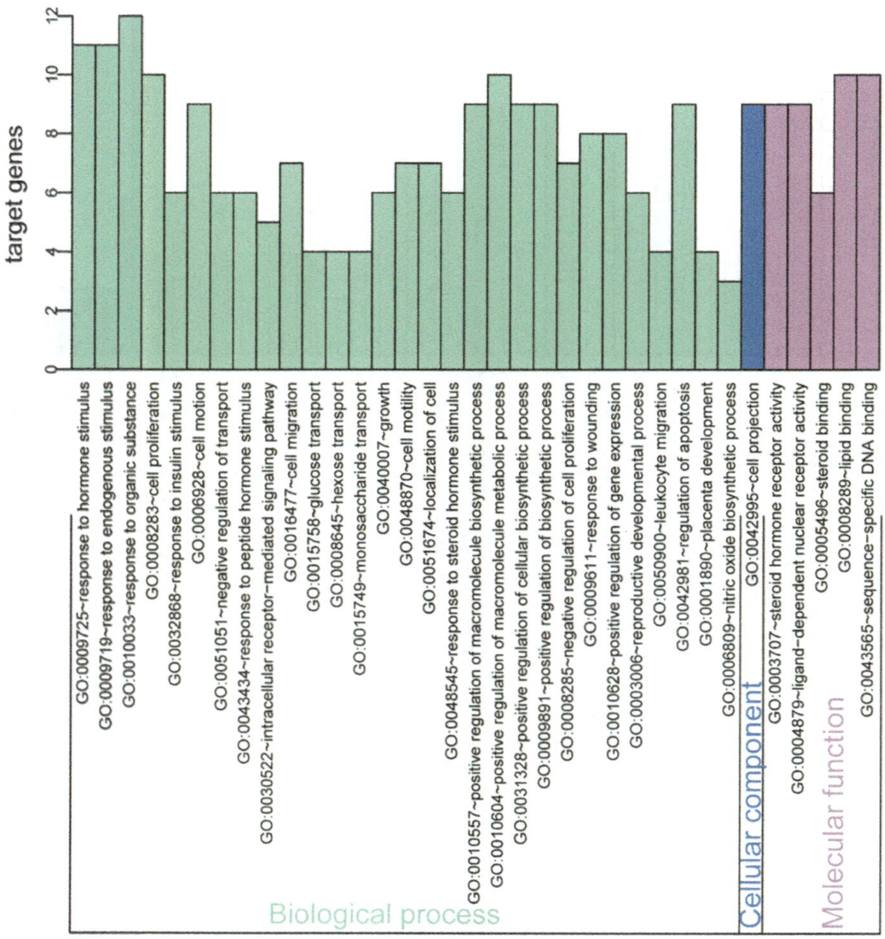

Fig. 7.45 GO function enrichment analysis on the specific target genes of ginsenoside Re

7.6.3.3 KEGG Pathway Analysis of Potential Target Genes on the Protective Effects of SalB and Re on Ox-LDL-Induced Endothelial Cell Damage

First, KEGG Pathway analysis was performed on the common target genes between salvianolic acid B and ginsenoside Re, and the common 37 target genes between them were imported into the Cluster Profiler package and Kobas 2.0, using FDR < 0.05 or $P < 0.05$ as the screening condition. The results are shown in Fig. 7.46. These target genes are mainly enriched in Toll-like receptor pathway, NF-κB pathway, MAPK signaling pathway, viral and bacterial disease-related pathway, and energy metabolism. The 37 target genes are involved in a total of 71 pathways, and many genes are involved in multiple signaling pathways concurrently. For

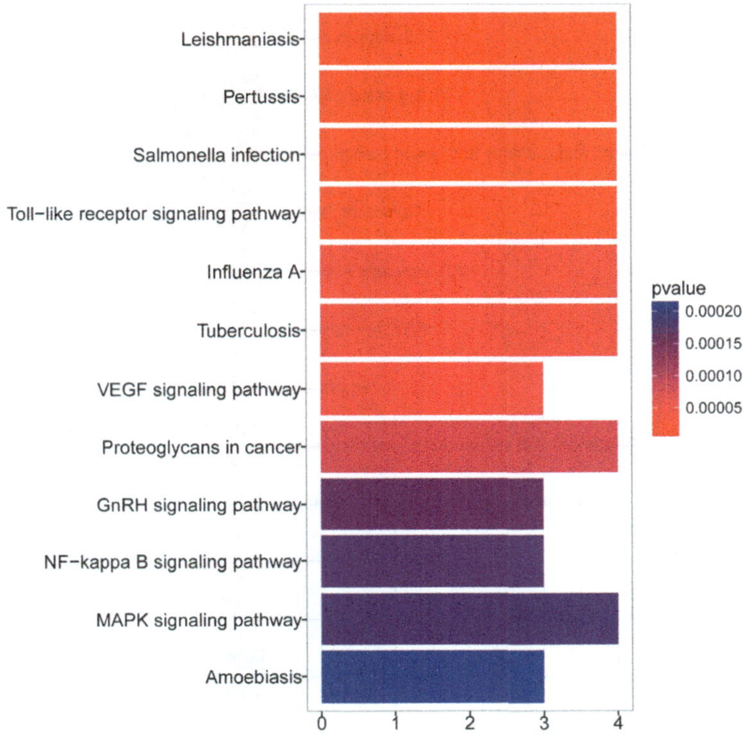

Fig. 7.46 KEGG pathway analysis of the common target genes between salvianolic acid B and Ginsenoside Re

example, CD14 gene plays a role in Toll-like receptor pathway, NF-κB pathway, and MAPK signaling pathway.

Next, the KEGG Pathway analysis was performed on the specific target genes of salvianolic acid B, and the specific 74 target genes were imported into the Cluster Profiler package and Kobas 2.0, using FDR < 0.05 or $P < 0.05$ as the screening condition. The results are shown in Fig. 7.47. These target genes are mainly enriched in TNF signaling pathway, AGE-RAGE signaling pathway, Ras signaling pathway, monocyte migration, and local adhesion signaling pathways. The 74 target genes are involved in a total of 34 pathways, and many genes are involved in multiple signaling pathways concurrently. For example, PIK3CD gene plays a role in Toll-like receptor pathway, TNF signaling pathway, and AGE-RAGE signaling pathway.

Last, the KEGG Pathway analysis was performed on the specific target genes of ginsenoside Re, and the specific 32 target genes were imported into the Cluster Profiler package and Kobas 2.0, using FDR < 0.05 or $P < 0.05$ as the screening condition. The results are shown in Fig. 7.48. These target genes are mainly enriched in adipocytokine signaling pathway, hormone signaling pathway, insulin resistance signaling pathway, and PPAR signaling pathway. The 32 target genes are involved in a total of 21 pathways, and many genes are involved in multiple signaling

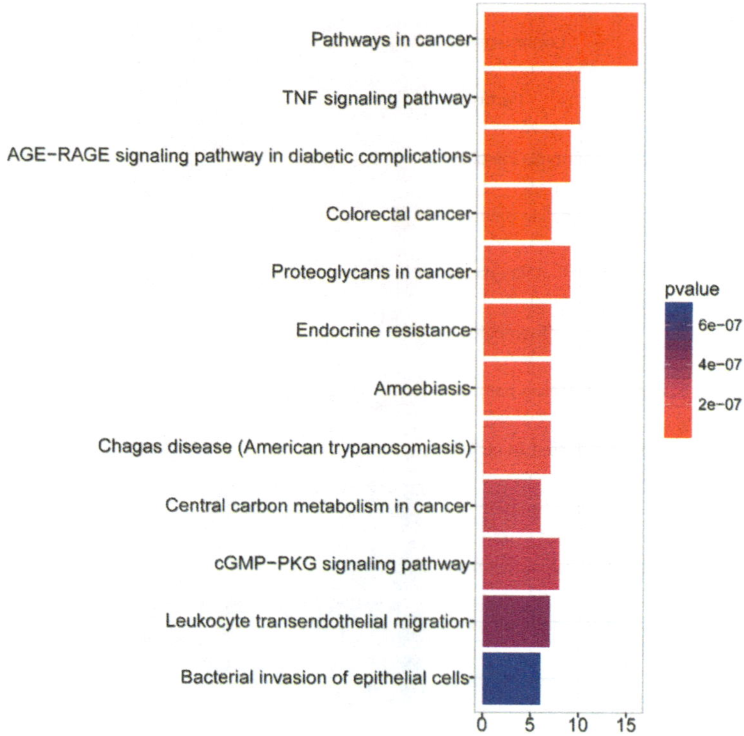

Fig. 7.47 KEGG pathway analysis of the specific target genes of salvianolic acid B

pathways concurrently. For example, RXRB gene plays a role in adipocytokine signaling pathway, hormone signaling pathway, insulin resistance signaling pathway, and PPAR.

7.6.3.4 Related Network Construction and Analysis of Potential Target Genes on the Protective Effects of SalB and Re on Ox-LDL-Induced Endothelial Cell Damage

Drug targets are the active sites of direct action of drugs in organisms, including gene sites, nucleic acids, various enzymes, ion channels, membrane proteins, and other biological macromolecules. Strictly speaking, drug targets refer to biomacromolecules with specific drugs in the market. The key to new drug research and development is to determine potential drug targets and lead compounds, which is also the key to researching drug molecules that can play a role in the treatment of diseases. In this experiment, Cytoscape 3.4.0 was used to construct and analyze the "compound–target–pathway–disease" network by analyzing the common and specific target gene pathway annotations and corresponding diseases of salvianolic acid B and ginsenoside Re. The network map of specific target genes shows that there are

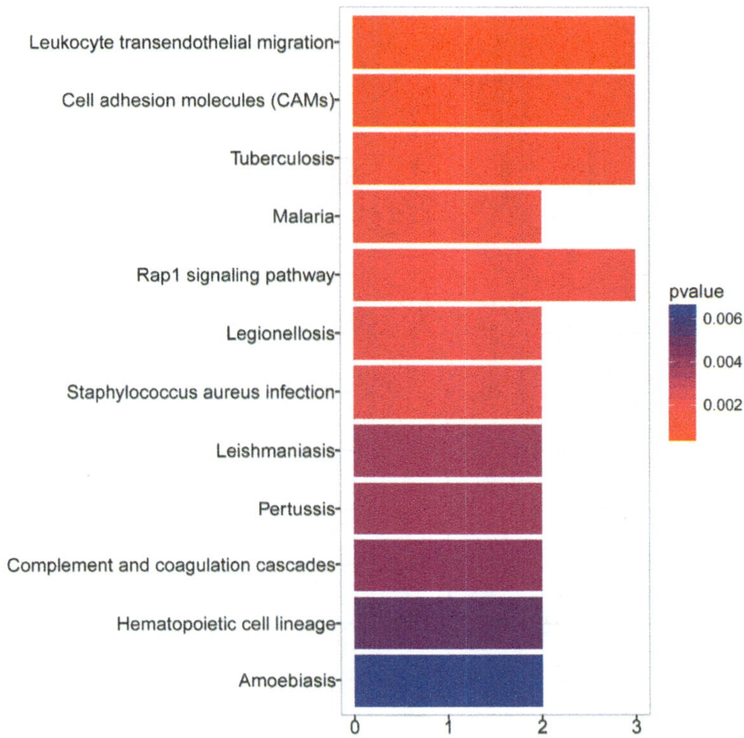

Fig. 7.48 KEGG pathway analysis of the specific target genes of Ginsenoside Re

five target genes that are only involved in the regulation of pathways, but not that of cardiovascular-related diseases; 23 genes are only involved in regulating cardiovascular diseases, without specific pathway positioning; and there are 9 genes involved in both regulation of cardiovascular disease and that of related pathways (as shown in Fig. 7.49) [32].

Next, the "compound–target–pathway–disease" network of each specific target gene of salvianolic acid B and ginsenoside Re was analyzed. The results are shown in Fig. 7.50 [32]. The regulation pathways of specific target genes of salvianolic acid B and ginsenoside Re and diseases have both commonness and specificity. They both regulate insulin resistance and monocyte migration-related pathways and immune-related diseases. The difference is that the regulation pathway of salvianolic acid B is mainly related to the inflammation and energy metabolism, while ginsenoside Re focuses on regulating the signal pathway related to fat metabolism. In terms of disease regulation, salvianolic acid B mainly regulates cardiovascular diseases, but ginsenoside Re mainly regulates vascular inflammation diseases.

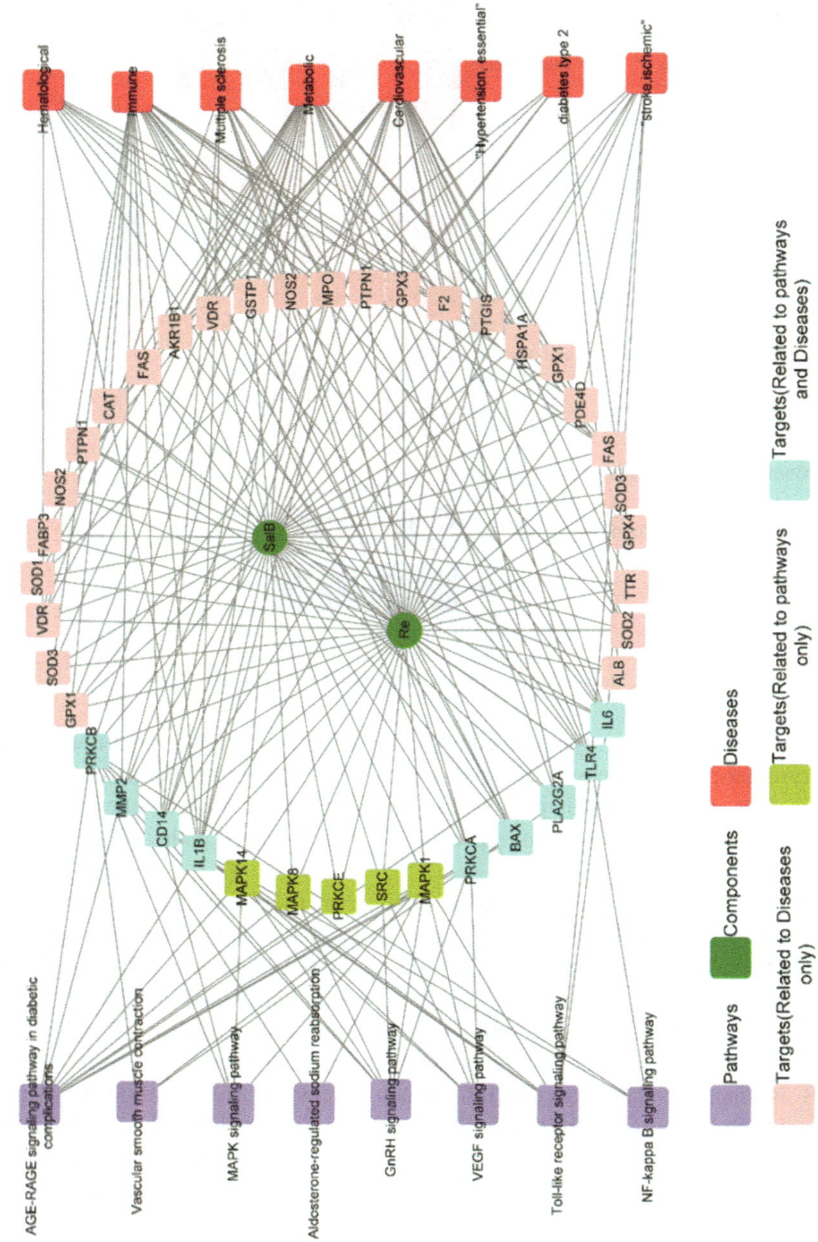

Fig. 7.49 “Compound–target–pathway–disease” network regulation diagram of common target genes of salvianolic acid B and ginsenoside Re [32]

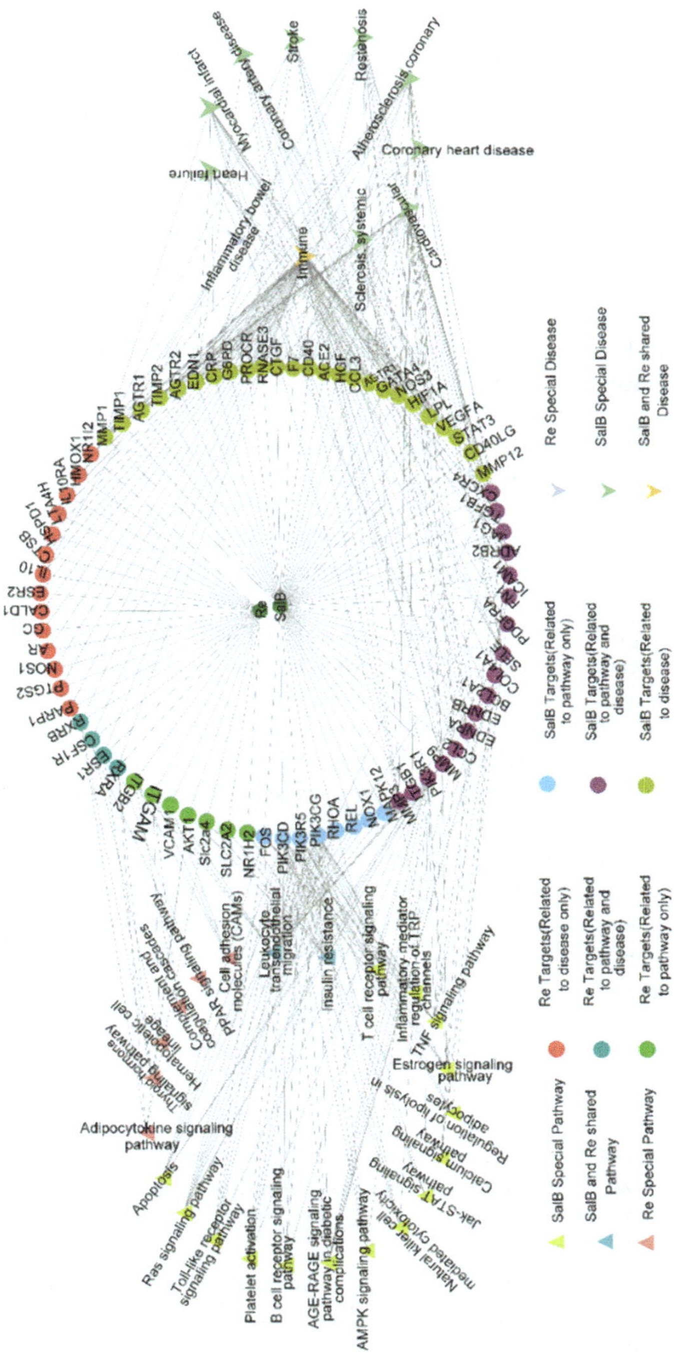

Fig. 7.50 "Compound–target–pathway–disease" network regulation diagram of specific target genes of salvianolic acid B and ginsenoside Re [32]

7.6.4 Verification and Summary

Network pharmacology was used to mine the action target information of salvianolic acid B and ginsenoside Re. The results revealed the mode of action between salvianolic acid B and ginsenoside Re synergy anti-Ox-LDL-induced HUVECs injury through multi-targets and multi-pathways, at the molecular network level. The molecular mechanism of salvianolic acid B and ginsenoside Re in synergistic protection of ox-LDL-induced HUVECs injury through multi-targets and multi-pathways was verified in vitro.

7.6.4.1 SalB, Re, and SR Inhibited Ox-LDL-Induced HUVECs Oxidative Stress Injury

In this study, flow cytometry was used to analyze the effects of Ox-LDL-induced intracellular ROS levels in HUVECs. The experimental results show that after Ox-LDL treatment, intracellular ROS levels increase significantly, which is manifested by increased fluorescence of carboxy-H2DCF (Fig. 7.51a) [32]. The statistical results (Fig. 7.51b) show that compared with the control group, Ox-LDL treatment can cause significant increase in the intracellular ROS level. Compared with the model group, the intracellular ROS levels of SalB, Re, and SR pretreatment decrease significantly. However, the SR group has the strongest inhibitory effect on ROS production in Ox-LDL-induced HUVECs, which is more statistically significant compared with the two monomers. Between the two monomers, the inhibitory effect of SalB on ROS in HUVECs is stronger than that of Re (Fig. 7.51b) [32].

Intracellular antioxidant enzyme activity detection showed that compared with the control group, the Ox-LDL treatment caused a significant decrease in intracellular CAT, SOD, and GSH-Px enzyme activities; compared with the model group, the activities of CAT, SOD, and GSH-Px increase after pretreatment with SalB, Re, and SR. The enhanced enzyme activities of CAT, SOD, and GSH-px in the SR group are stronger than those of the two monomers, between the two monomers, the enhancing effect of SalB on CAT, SOD, and GSH-Px-enhanced enzyme activities is stronger than that of Re (Fig. 7.51c–e) [32]. The results of intracellular antioxidant enzyme activities are consistent with the results of intracellular ROS level detection.

7.6.4.2 Effects of SalB, Re, and SR on the Expression of Cytoinflammatory Factors and Adhesion Molecules in HUVECs Damage Induced by Ox-LDL

In this study, the ELISA method was used to analyze the expression of inflammatory factors in HUVECs cells induced by Ox-LDL. The research results show that the secretion of inflammatory factors IL-6 and TNF-α in the cells increases significantly after Ox-LDL treatment. Compared with the model group, the secretion of

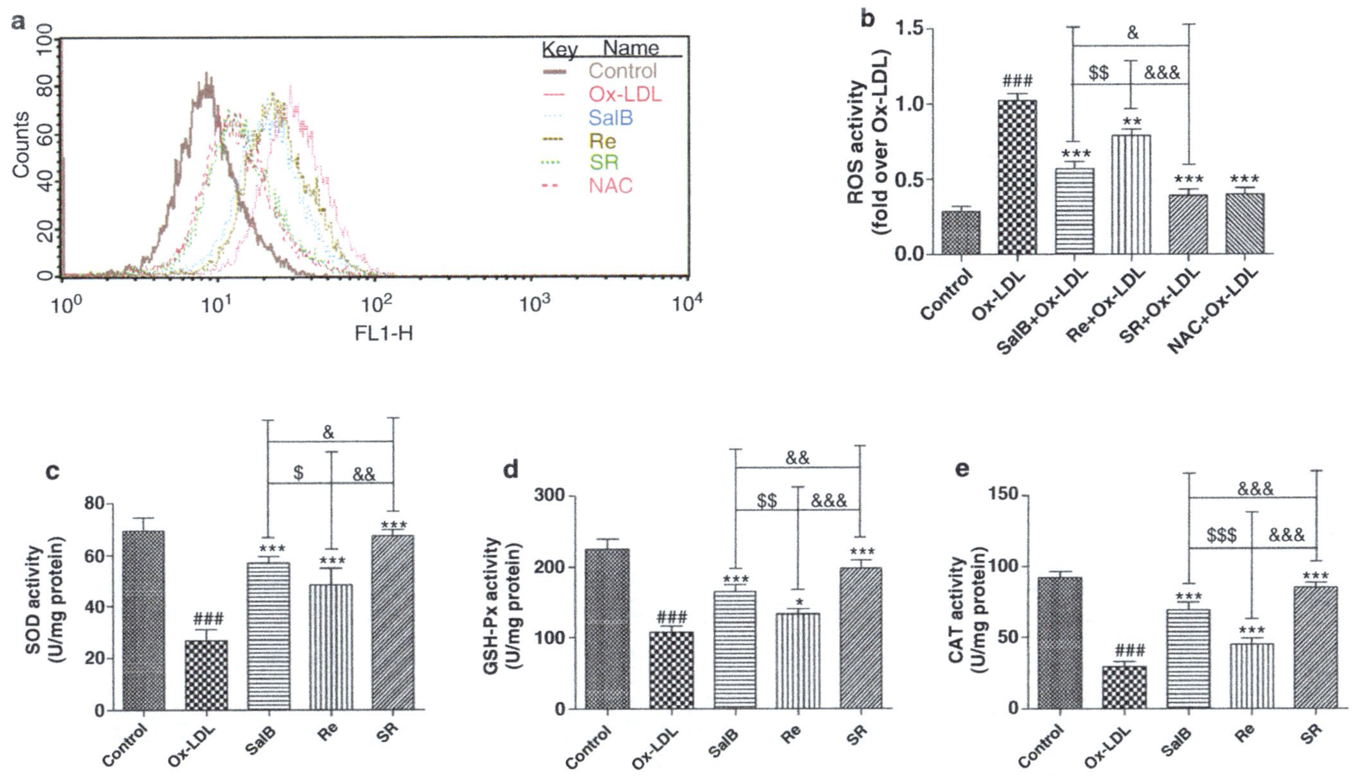

Fig. 7.51 Protective effects of SalB, Re, and SR on Ox-LDL-induced oxidative stress in HUVECs [32]. (**a**) Protective effect of SalB, Re, and SR pre-incubation for 12 h on Ox-LDL-induced over-production in HUVECs cell ROS; (**b**) Statistical diagram of ROS over-production in HUVECs cells induced by Ox-LDL; (**c**) Protective effect of SalB, Re, and SR pre-incubation for 12 h on Ox-LDL-induced production in HUVECs cell SOD; (**d**) Protective effect of SalB, Re, and SR pre-incubation for 12 h on Ox-LDL-induced production in HUVECs cell GSH-Px; (**e**) Protective effect of SalB, Re, and SR pre-incubation for 12 h on Ox-LDL induced production in HUVECs cell CAT. $^{***}P < 0.001$, $^{**}P < 0.01$, $^{*}P < 0.05$ compared with Ox-LDL; $^{\#\#\#}P < 0.001$ compared with Control; $^{\$\$\$}P < 0.001$, $^{\$\$}P < 0.01$, $^{\$}P < 0.05$ and SalB; $^{\&\&\&}P < 0.001$, $^{\&\&}P < 0.01$, $^{\&}P < 0.05$ compared with SR

intracellular inflammatory factors significantly reduces after SalB, Re, and SR pretreatment. However, the SR group has the strongest reducing effect on the secretion of inflammatory factors, followed by SalB, and Re, which is the weakest. The comparison between every neighboring two groups is statistically significant (as shown in Fig. 7.52a–c) [32].

Western blot is used to study the effects of SalB, Re, and SR on the expression of adhesion molecules (as shown in Fig. 7.52d–f). Compared with the control group, Ox-LDL significantly up-regulates the expression of adhesion molecules ICAM-1 and VCAM-1, while SalB and SR pretreatment can reverse the expression of ICAM-1 and VCAM-1. When adding p38MAPK agonist and PI3K inhibitor, it can block the protective effects of SalB and SR. Studies have shown that Re has no effect on the expression of adhesion molecules ICAM-1 and VCAM-1 [32]. At the same time, the results of MCP-1 secretion analysis using the ELISA method show that after Ox-LDL treatment, intracellular MCP-1 secretion increases significantly. Compared with the model group, the secretion of intracellular MCP-1 reduces significantly after SalB, Re, and SR pretreatment. However, the SR group has the strongest reducing effect on the secretion of MCP-1, followed by SalB, and Re, which is the weakest. Re has a significant effect on the secretion of McP-1, and the comparison between every neighboring two groups is statistically significant.

7.6.4.3 SalB, Re, and SR Regulate the Expression of Apoptosis-Related Proteins in the Damage Process of Ox-LDL-Induced HUVECs Through PI3K/Akt Pathway and p38MAPK/NF-κB Pathway

Western blot is used to study the effects of SalB, Re, and SR on apoptosis-related protein expression (as shown in Fig. 7.53a–d) [32]. Compared with the blank control group, Ox-LDL significantly inhibits the expression of anti-apoptotic proteins Bcl-2 and cIAP2. While up-regulating the expression of pro-apoptotic protein Bax and Smac and down-regulating the ratio of Bcl-2/Bax, the pretreatment with SalB, Re, and SR significantly inhibits the effect of Ox-LDL on Bcl-2 family proteins. Increasing the ratio of Bcl-2/Bax and reversing the expression of cIAP2 and Smac, the SR group has strongest regulatory effect, followed by SalB group, and the Re group being the weakest, however, they all have significant differences. After adding PI3K-specific inhibitor LY294002 or p38MAPK agonist, the regulatory effect of SR on apoptosis protein expression in HUVECs significantly reduces, thus suggesting that the regulation of SR on apoptotic proteins in HUVECs' injury induced by OX-LDL is regulated by the PI3K/Akt pathway and the p38MAPK/NF-κB pathway. At the same time, SalB, Re, and SR can inhibit the increased activity of the pro-apoptotic protein cleaved Caspase3 caused by Ox-LDL (as shown in Fig. 7.53e, f) [32].

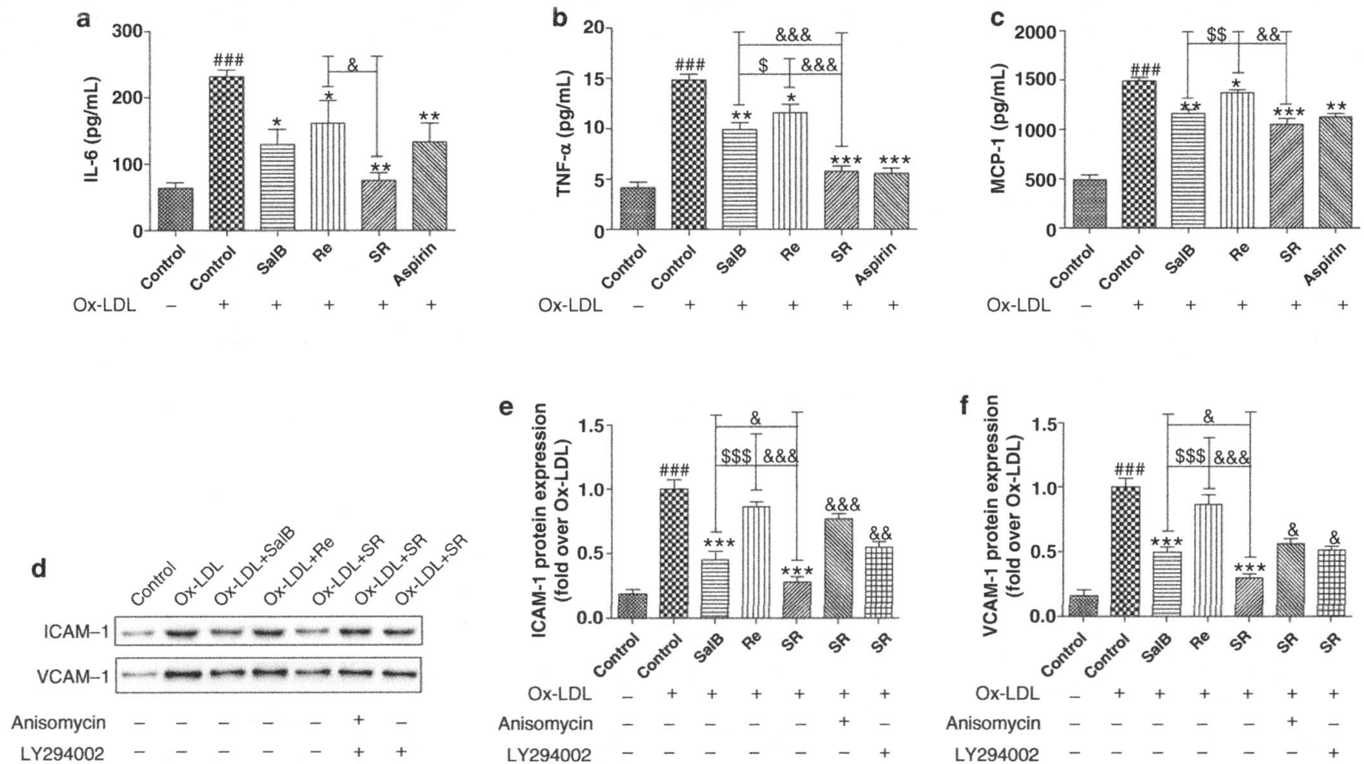

Fig. 7.52 SalB, Re, and SR inhibit the secretion of inflammatory factors in HUVECs induced by Ox-LDL [32]. (**a**) Protective effect of SalB, Re, and SR pre-incubation for 12 h on Ox-LDL-induced over-production in HUVECs IL-6; (**b**) Protective effect of SalB, Re, and SR pre-incubation for 12 h on Ox-LDL-induced over-production in HUVECs TNF-α; (**c**) Protective effect of SalB, Re, and SR pre-incubation for 12 h on Ox-LDL-induced over-production in HUVECs MCP-1; (**d**) effects of pre-incubation with SalB, Re, and SR for 12 h on the expression of ICAM-1 and VCAM-1 in HUVECs induced by Ox-LDL; (**e**) statistical diagram of ICAM-1 expression in HUVECs induced by OX-LDL after pre-incubation with SalB, Re, and SR for 12 h; (*f*) Statistical diagram of VCAM-1 expression in HUVECs induced by OX-LDL after pre-incubation with SalB, Re, and SR for 12 h. $^{***}P < 0.001$, $^{**}P < 0.01$, $^{*}P < 0.05$ compared with Ox-LDL; $^{\#\#\#}P < 0.001$ compared with control; $^{\$\$\$}P < 0.001$, $^{\$\$}P < 0.01$, $^{\$}P < 0.05$ and SalB; $^{\&\&\&}P < 0.001$, $^{\&\&}P < 0.01$, $^{\&}P < 0.05$ compared with SR

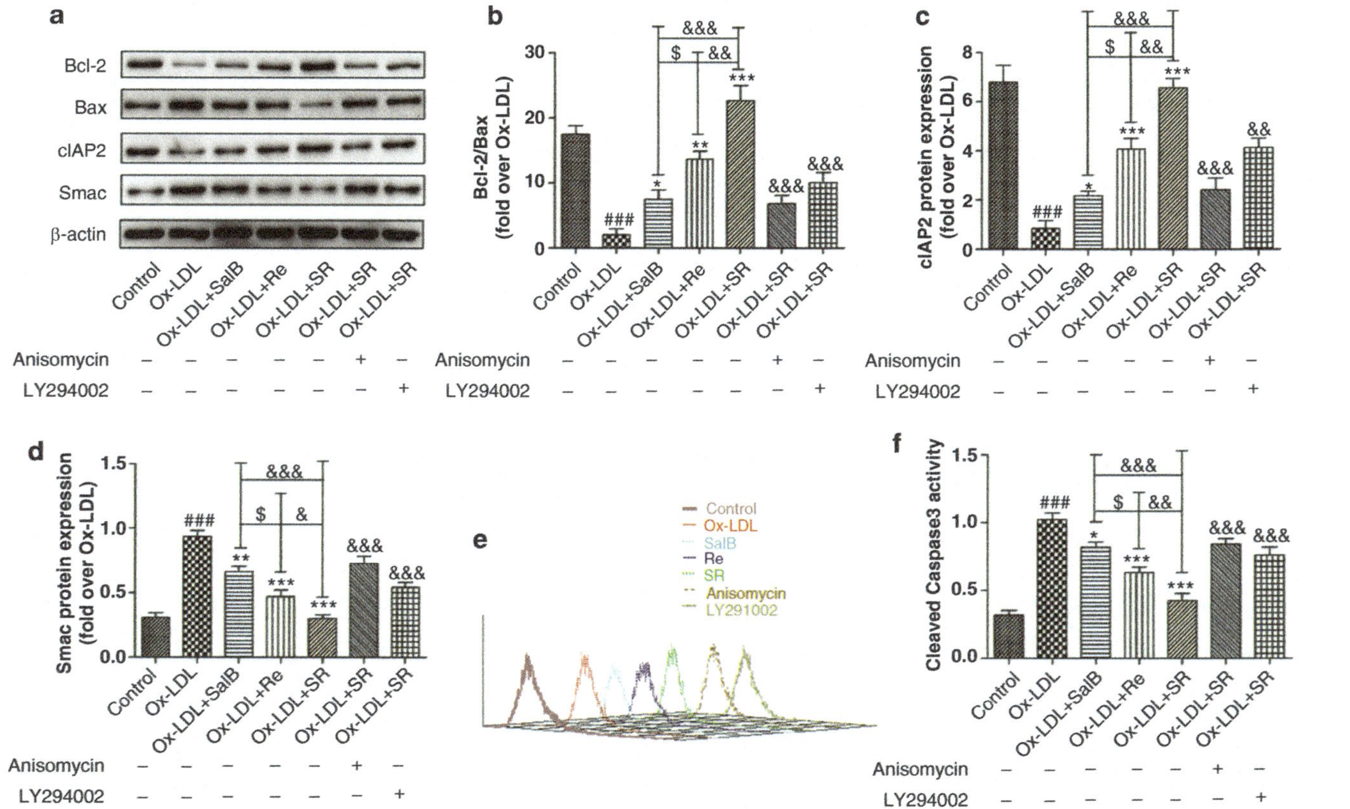

Fig. 7.53 SalB, Re, and SR regulate the expression of apoptosis-related proteins in the damage process of Ox-LDL-induced HUVECs through PI3K/Akt/NF-κB pathway and p38MAPK/NF-κB pathway [32]. (**a**) Regulatory effect of SalB, Re, and SR pre-incubation for 12 h, on the expression of Bcl-2, Bax, cIAP2, and Smac induced by Ox-LDL in HUVECs; (**b**) Statistical diagram of SalB, Re, and SR pre-incubation for 12 h, on the expression of Bcl-2 and Bax induced by

Ox-LDL in HUVECs; (**c**) Statistical diagram of SalB, Re, and SR pre-incubation for 12 h, on the expression of cIAP2 induced by Ox-LDL in HUVECs; (**d**) Statistical diagram of SalB, Re, and SR pre-incubation for 12 h, on the expression of Smac induced by Ox-LDL in HUVECs; (**e**) 3D model diagram of cleaved Caspase3 activity detected by flow cytometry when SalB, Re, and SR are pre-incubated for 12 h, on Ox-LDL-induced HUVECs' injury; (**f**) Statistical diagram of cleaved Caspase3 activity detected by flow cytometry when SalB, Re, and SR are pre-incubated for 12 h, on Ox-LDL-induced HUVECs' injury. $^{***}P < 0.001$, $^{**}P < 0.01$, $^{*}P < 0.05$ compared with Ox-LDL; $^{\#\#\#}P < 0.001$ compared with Control; $^{\$}P < 0.05$ and SalB; $^{\&\&\&}P < 0.001$, $^{\&\&}P < 0.01$, $^{\&}P < 0.05$ compared with SR

7.6.4.4 Summary

This section takes the combined use of salvianolic acid B and ginsenoside Re as an example, to introduce in detail the experimental ideas and procedures for the development of multi-target drugs based on the network pharmacology method, and provides reference for the application of network pharmacology in multi-target drug research. Relying on literature and database retrieval technologies, this section constructs a molecular target network based on the network pharmacology method to protect endothelial cell damage induced by low-density lipoprotein by combining salvianolic acid B and ginsenoside Re, and analyzes the rationality of multi-target drug development based on the combined use of drugs from three different levels, i.e. target, gene ontology, and KEGG pathway. Finally, using oxidative low-density lipoprotein-induced human umbilical cord vein endothelial cell injury as a model, and by adopting relevant effect indicators such as oxidative stress, inflammatory response, and endothelial cell apoptosis, this section verifies the protective effects of salvianolic acid B, ginsenoside Re monomer, and their compatibility on oxidized low-density lipoprotein-induced human umbilical cord vein endothelial cell injury. The results show that salvianolic acid B, ginsenoside Re monomer, and their compatibility play a role in protecting endothelial cells by interfering with the oxidative stress, inflammation, and apoptosis in the process of oxidized low-density lipoprotein-induced human umbilical cord vein endothelial cell injury.

References

1. Zeng K. Modernization research strategy and thinking of complex system of traditional Chinese medicine. Beijing: Science Press; 2016.
2. Guo W. Brief discussion on old and new technology of traditional Chinese medicine extraction process. Chem Pharm Eng. 2005;26(1):41–7.
3. Hopkins AL. Network pharmacology: the next paradigm in drug discovery. Nat Chem Biol. 2008;4(11):682–90.
4. Han B, Huang W, Xie X, et al. Thought and methodology of toxicity-efficacy network integrated analysis of toxic aconitum. World Chin Med. 2017;12(11):2585–97.
5. Tang S, Xing X, Deng X, et al. Research progress of Guanxin Danshen formula and its effective components in treating coronary artery heart disease. J Chin Mater Med. 2016;41(20):3721–6.
6. Xie L, Draizen E, Bourne P. Harnessing big data for systems pharmacology. Annu Rev Pharmacol Toxicol. 2017;57:245–62.
7. Wang J, Liu R, Liu B, et al. Systems pharmacology-based strategy to screen new adjuvant for hepatitis B vaccine from traditional Chinese medicine ophiocordyceps sinensis. Sci Rep. 2017;7:44788.
8. Li Y, Wang J, Xiao Y, et al. A systems pharmacology approach to investigate the mechanisms of action of Semen Strychni and Tripterygium wilfordii Hook F for treatment of rheumatoid arthritis. J Ethnopharmacol. 2015;175(2015):301–14.
9. Sun B, Xiao J, Sun X, et al. Notoginsenoside R1 attenuates cardiac dysfunction in endotoxemic mice: an insight into oestrogen receptor activation and PI3K/Akt signalling. Br J Pharmacol. 2013;168(7):1758–70.

10. Meng X, Sun G, Ye J, et al. Notoginsenoside R1-mediated neuroprotection involves estrogen receptor-dependent crosstalk between Akt and ERK1/2 pathways: a novel mechanism of Nrf2/ ARE signaling activation. Free Radic Res. 2014;48(4):445–60.
11. Deng X, Xing X, Sun G, et al. Guanxin Danshen formulation protects against myocardial ischemia reperfusion injury-induced left ventricular remodeling by upregulating estrogen receptor β. Front Pharmacol. 2017;8(2017):777.
12. Goldstein L, Adams R, Alberts M, et al. Primary prevention of ischemic stroke: a guideline from the American Heart Association/American Stroke Association Stroke Council: cosponsored by the Atherosclerotic Peripheral Vascular Disease Interdisciplinary Working Group; Cardiovascular Nursing Council; Clinical Cardiology Council; Nutrition, Physical Activity, and Metabolism Council; and the Quality of Care and Outcomes Research Interdisciplinary Working Group. Stroke. 2006;37(6):1583–633.
13. Donnan G-A, Fisher M, MacLeod M, et al. Stroke. Lancet. 2008;371(9624):1612–23.
14. Lin J, Zhang Y, Cui J, et al. Development status and prospects of the panax notoginseng industry in our country. Chin Pharm. 2005;14(2):18.
15. Yu N. Pharmacological effects of panax notoginseng saponins on cardiovascular system. Zhejiang J Integr Trad Chin West Med. 2000;10(4):66–7.
16. Sun F, Sun M, Lv X. Research progress on the effect of Chinese medicine panax notoginseng on hemostasis and promoting blood circulation. J Med Res. 2013;42(9):24–6.
17. Xie W, Meng X, Zhai Y, et al. Panax notoginseng saponins: a review of its mechanisms of antidepressant or anxiolytic effects and network analysis on phytochemistry and pharmacology. Molecules. 2018;23(4):940.
18. Yang W, Li Y, Sun L, et al. Complex network analysis on dynamic change regularity of combining use of Chinese and western medicine in 27678 cases with ischemic stroke in acute phase. J Chin Mater Med. 2015;40(24):4783–90.
19. Chen L, Chen S, Yang M, et al. Analysis on the clinical value of notoginseng total saponin combined with aspirin in the treatment of cerebral infarction for 120 cases. Chin Med Mod Distance Educ China. 2018;16(10):54–6.
20. Rodrigo R, Fernandez-Gajardo R, Gutierrez R, et al. Oxidative stress and pathophysiology of ischemic stroke: novel therapeutic opportunities. CNS Neurol Disord Drug Targets. 2013;12 (5):698–714.
21. Radermacher K, Wingler K, Kleikers P, et al. The 1027th target candidate in stroke: will NADPH oxidase hold up? Exp Transl Stroke Med. 2012;4(1):11.
22. Moskowitz M, Lo E, Iadecola C. The science of stroke: mechanisms in search of treatments. Neuron. 2010;67(2):181–98.
23. Serrano-Pozo A, Frosch M, Masliah E, et al. Neuropathological alterations in Alzheimer disease. Cold Spring Harb Perspect Med. 2011;1(1):6189.
24. Zhou Y, Li HQ, Lu L, et al. Ginsenoside Rg1 provides neuroprotection against blood brain barrier disruption and neurological injury in a rat model of cerebral ischemia/reperfusion through downregulation of aquaporin 4 expression. Phytomedicine. 2014;21(7):998–1003.
25. Taille C, El-Benna J, Lanone S, et al. Induction of heme oxygenase-1 inhibits NAD(P)H oxidase activity by down-regulating cytochrome b558 expression via the reduction of heme availability. J Biol Chem. 2004;279(27):28681–8.
26. Liu WJ, Tang HT, Jia YT, et al. Notoginsenoside r1 attenuates renal ischemia-reperfusion injury in rats. Shock. 2010;34(3):314–20.
27. Wang Y, Tu L, Li Y, et al. Notoginsenoside R1 protects against neonatal cerebral hypoxic-ischemic injury through estrogen receptor-dependent activation of endoplasmic reticulum stress pathways. J Pharmacol Exp Ther. 2016;2016:230359.
28. Wang Y, Tu L, Li Y, et al. Notoginsenoside R1 alleviates oxygen–glucose deprivation/ reoxygenation injury by suppressing endoplasmic reticulum calcium release via PLC. Sci Rep. 2017;7(1):16226.
29. Norata GD, Tibolla G, Catapano AL. Statins and skeletal muscles toxicity: from clinical trials to everyday practice. Pharmacol Res. 2014;88:107–13.

30. Hopkins AL. Network pharmacology. Nat Biotechnol. 2007;25(10):1110–1.
31. Zheng F, Guo M, Gu L, et al. Effects of salvianolic acid B on stability of atherosclerotic plaque in apolipoprotein E gene knock-out mice treated with STZ and high fat diet. Chin J Arterioscler. 2011;19(11):885–90.
32. Ke Y, Yun L, Shan L, et al. Salvianolic acid B and ginsenoside Re synergistically protect against Ox-LDL-induced endothelial apoptosis through the antioxidative and antiinflammatory mechanisms. Front Pharmacol. 2018;9:662.
33. Fang F, Qiu L, Miao J, et al. Anti-inflammatory and antioxidant effect of ginsenoside Re on the lung injury induced by intestinal ischemia reperfusion in rats. Central South Pharm. 2014;12 (06):521–4.

Chapter 8
Disease-Based Network Pharmacology Practice Process

Xiaohui Fan and Xiang Li

Guide to This Chapter

Network pharmacology is a new research strategy [1] to understand the molecular and drug mechanisms of complex diseases based on the structure and function of the "molecular biological network." The network-based method is a powerful tool for studying complex diseases and the nonlinear modes of drug-disease interactions [2]. The WHO drafted guidelines for traditional medicine from 2014 to 2023. Traditional Chinese Medicine (TCM), as important inheritance of the Chinese nation and the critical constituent of China's existing medical and health care system, play great role in the field of healthcare of Chinese people [3]. Currently, researches on modernization of traditional medicine, including TCM, have attracted increasing attention both at home and abroad. Based on network visions and methods, it can facilitate the systematically understanding of the mechanism of disease pathology from biological network equilibrium view, promoting study of the relationships among different diseases and also the study of drug repositioning. What's more, network visions and methods could also promote the systematic deciphering of complex interactions between TCM and disease biomolecular network, and enhance the R&D on combinatorial drugs.

Fan's research group from Zhejiang University focus on key scientific issues such as network regulation of TCM Formulae's components compatibility. With application of omics technologies including transcriptomics, several research strategies for TCM network pharmacology with disease network as core have been established, which contributed to the formation of the concept of network formulaology [4, 5]. A series of significant progresses have made, including establishment of several basic

X. Fan (✉)
Zhejiang University, Hangzhou, China
e-mail: fanxh@zju.edu.cn

X. Li
Hangzhou Medical College, Hangzhou, China

S. Li (ed.), *Network Pharmacology*, https://doi.org/10.1007/978-981-16-0753-0_8

databases, such as TCM-PTD, which is a database of potential TCM targets. Based on the characteristics of integrated regulation of TCM, Fan's research group proposed a TCM Formulae's components compatibility optimization strategy according to their network balance construction algorithm, after which a series of experimental studies were conducted to establish a comprehensive evaluation method for TCM efficacy analysis. They also created a multi-component/multi-target/multi-pathway network construction method for TCM, and the method was successfully applied for the study of integrated regulation mechanism of TCM, such as Shengmai and Qishen Yiqi Formulae [6–27]. This chapter took ischemic heart disease as an example, together with several research examples [12, 13, 15, 18, 19] to introduce disease-based network pharmacology research, which can provide references for the development and application of network pharmacology associated research works.

8.1 Disease Network Construction and Analysis of Coronary Heart Disease

Coronary heart disease (CHD), as a chronic and complex disease, its occurrence and development involves multi-genes, multi-signaling pathways, and multi-links. The construction of disease network could fully integrate the disease-related gene–gene interactions, and the interactions were abstractly presented as network in the way of network visualization. Meanwhile, network analysis technology helps study of disease-associated gene groups and biological pathways at a holistic level. Therefore, disease networks provide a platform for systematically study interactions among molecules, which shows important scientific research and application value for understanding the pathogenesis of CHD and drug development.

8.1.1 Data Acquisition and Processing

8.1.1.1 Text Mining of CHD-Related Genes

The keywords "Coronary heart disease" were applied to searched in the PubMed database with year limited from 2000/1/1 to 2013/1/23. The search retrieved about 110,000 literatures. In the PubMed retrieved panel, select "Send to" → "Choose Destination" → "File" → "Format" → "Abstract (text)" → "Create File" from pull-down menu to save the .txt file containing abstracts. The abstracts information can be extracted using text mining technology.

Words were extracted from abstracts and the ArrayTrack (V 3.5.0) gene database was queried to get the potentially related genes, and these genes were retrieved in the obtained abstracts to attain genes with literatures support. Three researchers then independently carried out manual confirmations work. Genes associated with CHD were determined by reading relevant abstracts, full text, and other related references to acquire CHD-related genes. The researchers retained 660 CHD-related genes for further research.

8.1.1.2 Extraction of CHD-Related Genes by Manually Reading of Literatures

Compared to text mining technology, manual literature mining is time-consuming and labor-consuming, but it has a high accuracy rate. According to JCR Science Edition report published by Thomson Reuters, *Circulation* is the most authoritative professional journal in the field of cardiac & cardiovascular systems. Therefore, *Circulation* was selected as the literature source, with the year set from 2006 to 2011. By reading literature abstracts, gene and protein information were extracted from 151 abstracts and inconsistent formats were standardized. Official names of genes (Official Symbol) and gene numbers Entrez ID in NCBI were applied to normalization of gene names. Standard protein names adopted were "UniProt ID" and "UniProt Consortium Protein Name." Finally, 252 related genes were obtained.

8.1.1.3 Mining CHD-Related Genes from Public Databases

Public databases, containing information on cardiovascular disease-related genes and proteins, are important resources to study the pathogenesis of cardiovascular diseases and the mechanism of drug action. Cardiovascular disease-related genes were selected from the rat genome research database (RGD) [28] by February 11th, 2014. 161 genes related to the cardiovascular disease portal and myocardial ischemia were selected. These genes were extracted and removed duplications for the construction of CHD@ZJU research platform.

8.1.1.4 Integration of CHD-Related Genes from Different Sources

CHD-related genes were normalized through the three methods by application of their official names (official symbol) and gene Entrez ID in NCBI, after integration and removal of duplicated genes, 1073 genes were finally identified. Compared with the CHD@ZJU version 1.0, 413 new genes were added. Further gene-related information was annotated, including gene name, gene Entrez Gene ID, and gene description, literature evidence of the genes, other literature information related to CHD, PPI relationship information related with the genes, and FDA drug information of the genes, etc., new genes in version 2.0 were especially highlighted in red.

8.1.2 Network Construction and Visualization

CHD@ZJU V2.0 integrates PPI-related information from databases HPRD and BioGRID. We optimized the internal data structure of the CHD@ZJU database and the computation and access speed of the website was improved.

Pairwise relationships of 1073 genes were extracted from the integrated PPI relationships to generate a gene–gene interaction relationship table, including 4030 pairs. Cytoscape Web [29] was used to construct a CHD disease network. The network model includes 1073 nodes and 4030 edges, with the largest sub-network containing 819 nodes and 3988 edges.

In disease network, gene groups with similar biological functions (corresponding to the sub-network or sub-cluster in the network), also known as biological function modules, can concurrently involve in certain phase of disease biogenesis. Thus, further analysis of biological functional modules is expected to reveal the pathogenesis of complex diseases and to provide support for the design and R&D of therapeutic drugs.

8.1.3 Network Analysis and Prediction

Network analysis was conducted using network topological attribute analysis, cluster analysis of sub-network/sub-cluster, and biological function gene ontology (GO) analysis.

8.1.3.1 Network Topological Attribute Analysis

The topological properties of the disease network were evaluated, and results showed that the distribution of node connectivity of the constructed disease network conformed to the power-law distribution ($R^2 = 0.890$), that is, the CHD network indicated scale-free properties and obtain the general characteristics of biological network.

The network analyzer plug-in in Cytoscape software was applied to calculate the node degree (Degree) and betweenness (Betweenness Centrality) of disease network. In biological networks, nodes with large degrees are usually considered as "Hubs" of the network, while nodes with high betweenness are called "bottleneck" (Bottleneck Node). These topological properties represent the importance of nodes in the network [30]. In addition, some studies showed that important genes related to diseases usually tend to form hub nodes in biological networks [31–34].

The degree and betweenness of nodes in disease network can be calculated and two strategies were adopted for node ranking analysis:

Betweenness as the Screening Criteria

23 network nodes were obtained with betweenness greater than 0.02 and sorted from large to small according to betweenness values from the CHD-related gene network topology parameters (betweenness > 0.02).

23 genes were imported into ArrayTrack 3.5, "Pathway Enrichment Analysis" was performed to retrieve 32 signaling pathways. Pathways were divided into six categories according to their biological functions: cell adhesion and connection, apoptosis, myocardial and smooth muscle contraction, energy metabolism, immune inflammation, and cell signal transduction-related pathways.

If the threshold value of betweenness is set at 0.01, 65 nodes can be obtained. The signaling pathway enrichment analysis revealed 32 pathways in 7 types. These pathways were basically the same as those obtained when the betweenness threshold was set at 0.02. Three new signaling pathways were different, i.e., Cytosolic DNA-sensing pathway ($p = 0.025$) related to immune inflammation and RIG-I-like receptor signaling pathway ($p = 0.046$); Signal molecular related pathways of extracellular matrix: ECM-receptor interaction ($p = 0.002$).

Degree as the Screening Standard

Nodes with degrees greater than 10 were sorted in descending order of degree value. Simultaneously, the betweenness was greater than 0.02, and 22 nodes were obtained for the topological parameters of CHD-related gene network (degree > 10, betweenness > 0.02).

The signaling pathway enrichment analysis of these 22 genes indicated that there were mainly 32 signaling pathways in 6 categories.

If the degree is set as greater than 10, it returned 221 nodes meeting the criteria. Signaling pathway enrichment analysis of these genes can be performed to get 35 signaling pathways in 7 categories with 5 newly-added signaling pathways, i.e., PPAR signaling pathway related to energy metabolism ($P = 0.019$); Immune inflammation-related signaling pathway RIG-I-like receptor signaling pathway ($p = 0.000$), Cytosolic DNA-sensing pathway ($p = 0.006$); Extracellular signal molecule related signaling pathway ECM-receptor interaction ($p = 0.002$), Cytokine-cytokine receptor interaction ($p = 0.002$).

The pathways enriched using the key genes can reflect the biological functions of the gene group and can provide support for explanation of CHD pathogenesis. Our network analysis results indicated that the abnormal function of one or several signaling pathways in the biological pathways, such as cell adhesion and connection, apoptosis, contraction of myocardium and smooth muscle, energy metabolism, immune inflammation, cell signal transduction, and so on, may be related to the pathogenesis of CHD.

8.1.3.2 Cluster Analysis of Sub-Network/Sub-Cluster

Network medicine investigates human diseases in the view of network. Its theories and methods are based on the associations between human diseases occurrence and the disturbance of the disease module. The tacit hypothesis is that "Topological Modules," "Functional Modules," and "Disease Modules" could overlap in the network. Therefore, functional modules are equivalent to topological modules, and disease can be regarded as disturbance and disruption of functional modules [35].

The topological module can be obtained by applying a network clustering algorithm. MCODE plug-in in Cytoscape was adopted to analyze the network topological properties to discover highly interactive areas, namely clusters [36]. The MCODE sub-cluster analysis was carried out for the entire CHD disease network, and a total of 38 sub-clusters were returned. These sub-clusters were further analyzed for their biological functions (GO_Biological_Process, GO_BP).

8.1.3.3 GO Analysis of Biological Functions

BiNGO, another plug-in in Cytoscape, can integrate the molecular interaction networks, visualize and analyze the GO categories of genes in biological networks to discover functional modules of the network [37].

GO_BP analysis was performed on the top 15 sub-clusters obtained from the extraction and analysis of the MCODE sub-clusters. Homo sapiens was selected as the species with other parameters in BiNGO settings dialog box setting to the default, i.e., the statistical significance level is set as 0.05, the whole annotation is taken as the reference set for analysis. Finally, a total of 13 sub-cluster GO analysis results were returned, however, results for sub-cluster 9 were not returned, and sub-cluster 15 had only 2 nodes, hence GO analysis was not performed.

This chapter set sub-clusters 1, 2, and 3 as examples to conduct GO_BP analysis. The analysis results and discussion are listed as follows:

1. Sub-cluster 1, cluster genes included E2F1, IRS2, RELA, SOCS1, ESR1, RB1, SIRT1, IRS1, STAT3, BRCA1, STAT6, HIF1A, HDAC1, JAK1, PARP1, PIK3R1, and GHR. GO_BP analysis found that the functions of these genes were involved in three aspects: intracellular and extracellular stimulation signals, synthesis and metabolism of biological molecules in the body, regulation of cell proliferation and apoptosis.
   (a) The responses to intracellular and extracellular stimulation signals may be mainly due to the organisms response to various biomolecules (hormones, cytokines, etc.) during the occurrence and developmental stages of CHD.
   (b) The synthesis and metabolic regulation of biomolecules, including glycolipid metabolism and other processes related to body energy metabolism. For example, insulin-related signaling pathways in sub-cluster 1 were involved in regulating the transport and metabolism of glucose, β-oxidation of fatty

acids, etc., which show important role in the pathogenesis of CHD. The related GO_BP categories included: GO-ID 10907, positive regulation of glucose metabolic process; GO-ID 45913, positive regulation of carbohydrate metabolic process; GO-ID 10828, positive regulation of glucose transport; GO-ID 19216, regulation of lipid metabolic process; GO-ID 32000, positive regulation of fatty acid beta-oxidation; GO-ID 43550, regulation of lipid kinase activity; GO-ID46321, positive regulation of fatty acid oxidation, etc.

(c) Cell proliferation and apoptosis are involved in the pathological process of myocardial infarction. The main related GO_BP categories included: GO-ID 42127, regulation of cell proliferation; GO-ID 8284, positive regulation of cell proliferation; GO-ID 42981, regulation of apoptosis; GO-ID 43067, regulation of programmed cell death; GO-ID 10,941, regulation of cell death, etc.

2. Sub-cluster 2, cluster genes included PPARA, CAV1, TNF, IL6ST, GRB2, PPARG, NFKBIA, FOXO1, NR3C1, CTNNB1, RPA1, FOS, GATA2, CD44, RAC1, RUNX1, MYC, CCNA2, CHUK, HSPA8, AKT2, NFATC1, IRAK1, MAP 2K1, RXRA, SMAD5, TP53, SMAD3, SMAD1, CDK4, PRKCD, KDR, HDAC4, HDAC3, CDKN1A, ETS1, MAPK3, MAPK8, and MDM4. GO_BP analysis found that the functions of these genes were mainly involved in the responses to intracellular and extracellular stimulation signals, regulation of cell proliferation, differentiation, and apoptosis, and the regulation of immune inflammatory related processes:

   (a) The responses to intracellular and extracellular stimulation signals may be produced by the corresponding response of the body caused by myocardial infarction, for example: GO-ID 9611 response to wounding.
   (b) Cell proliferation, differentiation, and apoptosis are involved in the pathological process of myocardial ischemia and infarction. The corresponding GO_BP categories are: GO-ID 42127, regulation of cell proliferation; GO-ID 8285, negative regulation of cell proliferation; GO-ID 45595, regulation of cell differentiation; GO-ID 43069, negative regulation of programmed cell death; GO-ID 42981, regulation of apoptosis; GO-ID 43067, regulation of programmed cell death; GO-ID 10941, regulation of cell death; GO-ID 45767, regulation of anti-apoptosis; GO-ID 51726, regulation of cell cycle, etc.
   (c) Immune inflammatory reaction occurs throughout the development of CHD, the main GO_BP categories include: GO-ID 2376, immune system process; GO-ID 2682, regulation of immune system process; GO-ID 2520, immune system development; GO-ID 6954, inflammatory response; GO-ID 2673, regulation of acute inflammatory response; GO-ID 50727, regulation of inflammatory response, etc.

3. Sub-cluster 3, cluster genes included: BID, TRAF1, THRA, ERBB2, NFKB1, BCL2L1, FOXO3, SRC, ATF2, IGF1R, VDR, CSNK2A1, CXCR4, RHOA, FAS, APEX1, AR, SOCS3, SMAD2, PTPN11, CCND1, TNFRSF10B, EP300,

HDAC2, JUN, MDM2, JAK2, PTPN1, and TNFAIP3. GO_BP analysis found that the main functions of these genes are regulation of cell proliferation, differentiation and apoptosis, and regulation of hypoxic and oxidative stress.

(a) In myocardial infarction, cell proliferation, differentiation, and apoptosis involve myocardial cells, endothelial cells, smooth muscle cells, immune inflammatory cells, etc. The main GO_BP categories include: GO-ID 42981, regulation of apoptosis; GO-ID 43067, regulation of programmed cell death; GO-ID 10941, regulation of cell death; GO-ID 45595, regulation of cell differentiation; GO-ID 8219, cell death; GO-ID 6915, apoptosis; GO-ID 12501, programmed cell death; GO-ID 6916, anti-apoptosis; GO-ID 42127, regulation of cell proliferation; GO-ID 8633, activation of pro-apoptotic gene products; GO-ID 51726, regulation of cell cycle; GO-ID 6917, induction of apoptosis; GO-ID 12502, induction of programmed cell death, etc.

(b) Hypoxia and oxidative stress play an important role in the occurrence and development of systolic heart disease. The GO_BP categories include: GO-ID 51341, regulation of oxidoreductase activity; GO-ID 1666, response to hypoxia; GO-ID 70482, response to oxygen levels; GO-ID 42542, response to hydrogen peroxide; GO-ID 6979, response to oxidative stress; GO-ID 302, response to reactive oxygen species, etc.

Similarly, this chapter also conducted GO_BP analysis of the other 10 sub-clusters, results mainly involving angiogenesis, leukocyte chemotactic migration, and cell apoptosis; oxidative stress injury, damage repair; cell proliferation, migration and apoptosis, fatty acid oxidative metabolism; immune inflammation-related biological processes; calcium ion channel regulation; Cell-extracellular matrix interaction regulation; coagulation function cascade reaction, and other biological pathways.

8.1.4 Validation and Summary

8.1.4.1 Enrichment Results Discussion

Functions of signaling pathways enriched through disease network analysis and their association relationships with diseases are discussed and analyzed as follows:

1. The role of apoptosis and necrosis in CHD: In acute myocardial infarction (AMI), cardiomyocyte apoptosis and necrosis occur rapidly, and the related signaling pathways like cell cycle, apoptosis, and p53 signaling pathway play a key role in the pathological process of cardiomyocyte apoptosis and necrosis [38–40].
2. The immune inflammatory response involves throughout the entire occurrence and development process of atherosclerosis (AS), and is the key biological process of CHD [41–44]. Inflammatory response involves throughout the entire process of AMI. Hypoxia is one of the causes of inflammation. Inflammation

involves all stages of ischemic injury [45]. Of all the 37 enriched signaling pathways, 11 are associated with immune inflammation, including: T cell receptor signaling pathway, Chemokine signaling pathway, B cell receptor signaling pathway, Fc epsilon RI signaling pathway, Fc gamma R-mediated phagocytosis, natural killer cell mediated cytotoxicity, toll-like receptor signaling pathway, leukocyte transendothelial migration, NOD-like receptor signaling pathway, cytosolic DNA-sensing pathway, RIG-I-like receptor signaling pathway. Studies indicate that MAPK signaling pathway, with regulatory effects on cell proliferation, differentiation, and apoptosis, plays an important role in inflammatory response, and is a potential target of anti-inflammatory therapy [46].

3. Energy metabolism plays an essential role in the occurrence and development of CHD. Myocardial energy metabolism includes the metabolism and utilization of fatty acids and glucose. Cardiac insulin promotes cardiomyocytes to utilize fatty acids and glucose for ATP synthesis, while myocardial ischemia inhibits normal conduction of insulin signaling pathway [47], with subsequent inducing of the occurrence of adverse left ventricular remodeling after myocardial infarction. This process is related to the decreased function of mitochondrial fatty acid oxidation in cardiomyocytes [48]. For PPAR signaling pathway, it can inhibit myocardial ischemia by promoting glucose utilization and anti-inflammatory effects [49], in which adiponectin is a key adipocytokine that can promote fatty acids β-oxidation and increase the utilization of glucose [50].
4. The role of angiogenesis in CHD: VEGF signaling pathway regulates the proliferation, migration or cell viability of vascular endothelial cells, promotes vasodilation, and improves blood supply post-myocardial infarction [51–53]. The mTOR signaling pathway has a regulatory effect on hypoxia induced angiogenesis, and can promote the recovery of blood flow supply to ischemic myocardium post-myocardial infarction [54, 55].
5. The role of cell adhesion and junction in CHD: Focal adhesion is the medium for cells to connect with the ECM through the cytoskeleton, while AS is the internal pathological basis of CHD. The disturbance of blood "Fluid Shear Stress" at the bifurcation point of arteries is transmitted through focal adhesion and causes morphological and functional changes of endothelial cells, which promotes the occurrence and development of AS [56]. At the same time, focal adhesion also mediates endothelial injury due to lipoproteins and promotes the progress of AS [57]. The integrity of the structure and function of endothelial cells is an vital basis for maintaining the normal functions of the cardiovascular system. Adherens junction, Gap junction, and Tight junction are three critical connections between endothelial cells. Abnormal connection between these cells changes the morphology and function of the endothelium, increases the permeability of the endothelium, and promotes the occurrence and development of AS [58]. In addition, injury to endothelial cells causes pro-inflammatory cells to adhere to the surface of damaged endothelial cells, and to migrate and invade farther into the blood vessel wall in the endothelium, participating in the formation of atherosclerotic plaques together with the involving of actin cytoskeleton [59]. Endothelial tissue is a continuous monolayer structure of endothelial cells

in the inner wall of blood vessels, which plays the role of a functional barrier between blood and vascular smooth muscle. The changes in endothelial structure and function directly affect the contraction function of blood vessels. On one hand, the functional barrier of endothelial tissue is changed with increased permeability, which induces some vasoactive substances in blood circulation to invade into the vascular wall. On the other hand, the injured endothelium synthesizes and secretes vasoactive substances (such as endothelin), or metabolizes the precursor substances in the blood circulation into vasoactive substances (such as AngI transforming to AngII), which cause vasoconstriction and affect the blood and oxygen supply to the myocardium [60].

6. The role of ventricular remodeling and myocardial injury repair in CHD: The TGF-beta signaling pathway is activated in the repair process post-myocardial infarction, which has a pleiotropic and multifunctional regulatory effect on different types of cells involved in the repair [61]. Myocardial infarction triggers inflammation, which eventually forms scar tissue. In the early stage of infarction repair, TGF-β inhibits the activity of macrophages with subsequent inhibition of synthesis of chemokines and cytokines by endothelial cells to show anti-inflammatory effects. In the followed process, TGF-β causes ECM deposition, activates the fibrosis signaling pathway, and induces fibrosis and hypertrophy of non-infarcted myocardium, which all contribute to left ventricular remodeling [62]. The notch signaling pathway plays a key role in mammalian heart development [63] as well as in the myocardial repair [64] and regeneration process after infarction. The hedgehog signaling pathway, another signaling pathway regulating the development and formation of tissues and organs, plays an important role in cardiac repair post-myocardial infarction. Erythropoietin (EPO) can promote angiogenesis through the hedgehog signaling pathway and plays a protective role [65] in the heart after infarction. Another mechanism of the hedgehog signaling pathway on cardiac function recovery post-myocardial infarction is to upregulate the expression of angiogenic genes and to enhance the migration of bone marrow progenitor cells to the infarcted myocardium [66].
7. The role of other biological processes in CHD: ErbB and Wnt signaling pathways have multiple roles in regulating biological processes, including cardiac development, cardiomyocyte proliferation, myocardial cell viability, etc. ErbB signaling pathway is especially vital for cardiac development and can regulate the balance of both sympathetic vagus nerve and hemodynamics. The activation of ErbB signaling pathway can reverse the declining cardiac function post-myocardial infarction [67]. Wnt signaling pathway plays an significant role in stem cell biological activity, cardiac development and differentiation, angiogenesis, etc. [68–70] What's more, the Jak-STAT signaling pathway has a versatile biological functions, involving cell proliferation, differentiation, migration, and apoptosis, and is an essential signaling cascade for organisms [71]. Studies have found that under pathological conditions, the renin-angiotensin system (RAS) is activated, and Ang II binds to its receptor to further activate Jak-STAT signaling pathway, participating in cardiac dysfunction caused by myocardial ischemia-reperfusion [72]; In addition, the Jak-STAT signaling pathway plays an important

role in the occurrence of myocardial infarction and post-myocardial infarction ventricular remodeling, which may be related to the activation of the pro-inflammatory signaling pathway of Jak-STAT signaling pathway [73].

The abovementioned analysis indicates that the pathogenesis of CHD involves immune inflammatory reaction, apoptosis and necrosis, energy metabolism of cells, cell adhesion and connection, angiogenesis, myocardial injury repair, ventricular remodeling, and other related biological processes.

8.1.4.2 Conclusion

1. The disease network of CHD was improved and the CHD@ZJU2.0 disease network research platform was established through application of the integrated text knowledge mining, manually literature validation and public database knowledge methods. With the guidance of network biology, network pharmacology and network medicine concepts and methods, network analysis was applied to identify key genes and biological pathways of the CHD disease network. CHD@ZJU, the disease network research platform, has currently been updated to version 3.0.
2. The results of network analysis preliminarily show that CHD is a polygenic, multi-biological pathways associated disease. Pathogenesis related biological processes mainly include: Immune inflammatory response, cell proliferation, differentiation and apoptosis-related processes, angiogenesis, hypoxia and oxidative stress response, glucose and fatty acid related energy metabolism, myocardial injury repair, and ventricular remodeling. The construction and improvement of the CHD disease network research model can facilitate the subsequent experimental research works.

8.2 Research Practice of the Application of Disease Network in TCM Prescriptions

8.2.1 Integrated Mechanism Study of TCM Prescriptions Modes of Action

The Qishen Yiqi formulae mainly contain water-soluble components from Radix Astragali, Salvia Miltiorrhiza, and Panax Notoginseng, together with volatile oil components from Dalbergia Odorifera. Our previous research results [74, 75] show that the pharmacodynamic material basis for Qishen Yiqi formulae are mainly saponins from Radix Astragali, phenolic acids from Salvia Miltiorrhiza, saponins from Panax Notoginseng, and volatile oil components from Dalbergia Odorifera. Shi Pei-ying [75] studied the non-volatile and volatile chemical constituents of Qishen Yiqi formulae by application of liquid chromatography mass spectrometry (LC/TOF/MS), liquid chromatography ion trap mass spectrometry (LC/IT/MS), and gas chromatography mass spectrometry (GC/MS). A total of 35 non-volatile components were identified, and the compounds with highest contents were of danshensu, salvianolic acid B, salvianolic acid A, isosalvianolic acid C, ginsenoside Rb_1, and ginsenoside Rd. 24 volatile components were identified in the Qishen Yiqi extract. By comparing the total ion flow diagram of Qishen Yiqi and Dalbergia Odorifera extracts, 5 volatile components with high content amount were obtained, notably *cis*-α-santalol, nerolidol, E-nerolidol (ENL), (3S,6R,7R)-3,7,11-trimethyl-3,6-epoxy-1,10-dodecadien-7-ol (RDL), and (3S,6S,7R)-3,7,11-trimethyl-3,6-epoxy-1,10-dodecadien-7-ol (SDL), respectively. Analysis of plasma samples of SD rats after intragastric administration of Qishen Yiqi extract (6 g/kg) revealed that the constituents absorbed into the blood were four phenolic acid compounds and seven saponins compounds.

In addition, our research group's Li et al. [76, 77] used HPLC-UV-ELSD and HPLC-DAD-ESI-MS^n methods to study the content of related components in Qishen Yiqi dropping pills. Combined with results of this study, Shi Pei-ying suggested that astragaloside IV (Ast), Danshensu (DSS), Ginsenoside Rg_1 (Rg_1), and ginsenoside Rb_1 (Rb_1) in the Qishen Yiqi formulae may be its representative effective components in blood corresponding to drugs in Qishen Yiqi. Other domestic research groups have also conducted research on the pharmacodynamic material basis of Qishen Yiqi formulae [78].

Based on the research results of the chemical composition of TCM prescription and in vivo pharmacokinetics, effective components of the Qishen Yiqi formulae are the saponins of Radix Astragali, phenolic acids of Salvia Miltiorrhiza, saponins of Panax Notoginseng, and volatile oil of Dalbergia Odorifera. Representative compounds were selected from corresponding TCM fractions, i.e., Ast, DSS, Rg_1, and ENL were identified as the four main active compounds. Study was designed to investigate the effects of single compound administration and combined compounds administration on rat AMI models. Gene chip technology and network pharmacology methods were used, together with CHD@ZJU V2.0 ischemic heart disease network, and the synergistic mechanism of four main active components of the Qishen Yiqi formulae against the rat AMI at the transcriptional level.

8.2.1.1 Data Acquisition and Processing

Left Anterior Descending Coronary Artery (LAD) ligation was done under anesthesia in rats. Myocardial infarction model rats were randomly divided into groups with intragastric administration (i.g) on every morning for 7 consecutive days (i.g volume 10 ml/kg). The sham operation group (1% sodium carboxymethyl cellulose solution, 1% CMCNa), model group (1% CMCNa), Ast group (80 mg/kg), DSS group (44 mg/kg), Rg_1 group (8 mg/kg), ENL (53.3 mg/kg), 4H group, Qishen Yiqi decoction group (QSYQ). Five rats in each group were used for gene chip research, i.e., sham, model, Ast, DSS, Rg1, ENL, and 4H.

Extraction of rat myocardial tissue for gene chip detection required surgical instruments with DEPC RNase-free water treatment, autoclaved, and dried.

Ophthalmic scissors and ophthalmic tweezers were used to obtain about 300 mg of myocardial tissue at the junction between the infarcted and normal myocardium below the site of ligation. The Affymetrix Rat Genome 230 2.0 chip was selected and entrusted to the chip company for testing. The company used Affymetrix GeneChip Command Console software (version 4.0, Affymetrix) to process and extracts the original data from the scanned original images.

The original data document was downloaded from the Arraytrack server, and Excel was used to standardize with median set as 1000 for all data. The standardized calculation is as follows:

$$\begin{aligned}&\text{Probe expression value after standardization}\\&\quad = \text{original expression value in the chip}/\text{median} \times 1000.\end{aligned}$$

The average value of probe expression was calculated. The expression value obtained after normalization was further calculated through a logarithm of base 2 ($\text{Log}2^{\text{expression value}}$) to attain the average log2 value of each probe. 1073 ischemic heart disease-related genes were downloaded from the CHD disease network platform CHD@ZJUV2.0, constructed in Sect. 8.1, and 902 ischemic heart disease-related genes were extracted and returned from the 26,430 genes on the chip. Reverse Rate (RR) of each gene was calculated, and finally the signaling pathway enrichment analysis was done in Arraytrack.

The formula for calculating the gene callback rate is as follows:

$$\text{RR} = (D - M)/(S - M)$$

where RR stands for the callback rate, that is, the ability of drug to regulate gene expression in the opposite direction of the model's change against the sham operation group, so it can return to the sham operation level. *D* stands for component or component combination, *M* stands for model, and *S* stands for sham operation.

Where a gene is up-regulated relative to the sham operation after LAD ligation, i.e., $M > S$, the effective callback condition is $M > D \geq S$, then the callback rate is $0 < \text{RR} \leq 1$. If the gene is down-regulated relative to the sham operation after LAD ligation, i.e., $S > M$, the effective callback condition is $S \geq D > M$, then the callback rate is $0 < \text{RR} \leq 1$, that is, the closer the RR value getting to 1, the stronger the callback effect shows.

However, callback rate $\text{RR} > 1$ indicates the over-callback effect, that is, the gene continues to be regulated in the direction of sham surgery after the gene was recalled to the level of sham surgery due to drug intervention, and the callback rate $\text{RR} \leq 0$ indicates no callback effect.

8.2.1.2 Network Analysis and Prediction

ArrayTrack software was used to conduct signaling pathway enrichment analysis of those effective callback genes. There were 466 effective callback genes for Ast, 365 effective callback genes for DSS, 495 effective callback genes for Rg_1, 425 effective callback genes for ENL, and 444 effective callback genes for the 4H group. The respective groups of regulated signaling pathways and signaling pathway network were constructed and referred to as the drug-signaling pathway network. The network attributes included 49 nodes, 179 edges, and 44 signaling pathways. There were 26 signaling pathways with significant regulation of single administration of the four components and combined administration of the four components, accounting for 59.1% of the total enriched signaling pathways. These signaling pathways mainly involved biological processes such as immune inflammation, cell adhesion and connection, angiogenesis, ventricular remodeling and myocardial repair, and energy metabolism. There were 34 signaling pathways that are significantly regulated by Ast ($p < 0.05$), 35 by Rg_1 ($p < 0.05$), 39 by DSS ($p < 0.05$), 36 by ENL ($p < 0.05$), and 35 by 4H ($p < 0.05$).

The results of network analysis show that each component can regulate multiple ischemic heart disease-related signaling pathways. Some signaling pathways are regulated by only one component, while others are regulated by two to four components simultaneously.

Glycerolipid metabolism signaling pathway is only regulated by Ast, while the three signaling pathways of nicotinate and nicotinamide metabolism, steroid biosynthesis, and cell cycle are only modulated by DSS. And methane metabolism signaling pathway is only regulated by ENL.

Ast and Rg_1 can significantly regulate PPAR signaling pathway and pyruvate metabolism. DSS and ENL can both significantly regulate p53 signaling pathway, tight junction, and RIG-I-like receptor signaling pathway.

The three components of Ast, DSS, and Rg_1 can significantly regulate cardiac muscle contraction and Fc gamma R-mediated phagocytosis. Ast, DSS, and ENL can significantly regulate ABC transporters; Ast, Rg_1, and ENL can significantly regulate ECM-receptor interaction; DSS, Rg_1, and ENL can significantly regulate Leukocyte transendothelial migration, Hematopoietic cell lineage, and natural killer cell mediated cytotoxicity.

The four components of Ast, DSS, Rg_1, and ENL can significantly regulate arachidonic acid metabolism.

There are 26 signaling pathways with significant regulation of single and combined administration of the four components, including: adherens junction, adipocytokine signaling pathway, apoptosis, B cell receptor signaling pathway, calcium signaling pathway, chemokine signaling pathway, complement and coagulation cascades, cytokine-cytokine receptor interaction, ErbB signaling pathway, Fc epsilon RI signaling pathway, focal adhesion, gap junction, GnRH signaling pathway, insulin signaling pathway, Jak-STAT signaling pathway, MAPK signaling pathway, mTOR signaling pathway, NOD-like receptor signaling pathway, regulation of actin cytoskeleton, renin-angiotensin system, T cell receptor signaling pathway, TGF-beta signaling pathway, toll-like receptor signaling pathway, vascular smooth muscle contraction, VEGF signaling pathway, and Wnt signaling pathway.

8.2.1.3 Validation and Summary

Experimental Validation

Lipopolysaccharide (LPS)-induced inflammatory cellular model in RAW264.7 mouse mononuclear macrophages was applied to study the anti-inflammatory effect and mechanism of ENL (the main component of the volatile oil of Dalbergia Odorifera) and the two components SDL and RDL (isolated from the oil of Dalbergia Odorifera for the first time). Meanwhile, the synergistic anti-inflammatory effects of the four main components of QSYQ, i.e., Ast, DSS, Rg_1, and ENL, were studied.

The effects of ENL, SDL, and RDL were investigated in order to identify their safety concentration ranges which would have no affections to the viability of RAW264.7 cells, and the inhibitory effect of these compounds against the production of NO in RAW264.7 cells induced by LPS was evaluated. The synergistic inhibitory effects of sodium danshensu and ginsenoside Rg_1 against LPS-induced secretion of NO in RAW264.7 were also investigated. The inhibitory effects of the combined treatment of the four components against LPS induced NO secretion in RAW264.7 were detected by the Griess method. Further, the effects of small molecule (Tool Compound), i.e., U0126, T0070907, Pioglitazone hydrochloride (Pio), ZnPPIX on the NO secretion in LPS stimulated RAW264.7 were investigated. Among them, U0126 is a selective ERK1/2 phosphorylation inhibitor, T0070907 is an inhibitor of PPARγ phosphorylation, Pio is a PPARγ agonist, and ZnPPIX is a specific inhibitor of HO-1. Western blot method was selected to detect the protein expression levels of ERK1/2, phospho-ERK1/2, PPARγ, and HO-1.

Main Conclusions

1. Gene chip technology and network pharmacology method were applied, the synergetic mechanisms of the four main components of the QSYQ against AMI in rats were studied at the transcriptome level, and the four main components have regulatory effects on multiple genes related to ischemic heart disease. Among the genes with effective callbacks from the combination of the four components, more than 50% of genes are involved in effective callbacks by at least two components, reflecting the synergistic effects of all four active components on the regulation of related genes. In the component combination administration group, there were 40 genes that are up-regulated and the four components had synergistic effects against LAD ligation. 36 genes that were down-regulated indicated synergistic effects by the four components after modeling. Biological

function and signaling pathway enrichment analysis of these genes revealed several pathways, including immune inflammation, angiogenesis, ventricular remodeling and myocardial repair, energy metabolism, etc., which may be the key biological pathways for the four components of the QSYQ to play a multi-target and multi-pathway integrated synergy against rat AMI.

2. Experimental verification studies revealed that ENL, SDL, and RDL inhibit the secretion of NO in LPS-induced RAW264.7 monocytes macrophages. The mechanism of action of the three components (especially ENL and SDL) may be partly through inhibition of ERK1/2 and PPARγ phosphorylation, and increase of PPARγ and HO-1 expression involving NF-κB, ROS, iNOS, and so on, which all contributed to inhibition of LPS-induced NO production in RAW264.7 macrophages. The combined co-culture of DSS and Rg_1 with RAW264.7 could synergistically enhance the inhibition effects of LPS induced NO secretion in a dose-effect relationship. This effect of DSS and Rg_1 could be attenuated or even abolished by ZnPPIX, an HO-1-specific inhibitor. Thus, DSS and Rg_1 may play an anti-inflammatory role by partially promoting the expression of HO-1. Meanwhile, compared to the single component administration group, the combined administration of Ast, DSS, Rg_1, and ENL of the four components could synergistically enhance the inhibition effects on the LPS-induced NO secretion and exhibited a good dose-response relationship.
3. The component-target-pathway network of the main pharmacodynamic substance of the QSYQ was constructed, and experimental data revealed that the regulation network of Qishen Yiqi dropping pills consist of 12 effective components and 55 targets acting on 17 pathways, involving both AMI stage (Vasodilation, anti-myocardial apoptosis, anti-inflammatory protection of the endothelium, and improved energy metabolism) and ventricular remodeling stage (promoting angiogenesis, improving cardiac function, anti-myocardial fibrosis, and anti-platelet aggregation). This indicated the integrative regulation effects of QSYQ as multi-components, multi-targets, and multi-pathways modes of action.

8.2.2 Compatibility Law: "Sovereign-Minister-Assistant-Courier" in TCM Formulae

Network pharmacology technology provides a new perspective for the systematic exploration of integrated regulation modes of TCM formulae. Qishen Yiqi formulae were set as an example to explain the scientific connotation of its compatibility law in combating AMI. This section proposes a new research model of integrated regulation of TCM based on biological network equilibrium analysis. Firstly, the Organism Disturbed Network (ODN) model was constructed by integrating disease-related gene information, transcriptome expression, and interaction related information. We also analyze the ability of the Qishen Yiqi formulae and its components of Radix Astragali, Salvia Miltiorrhiza, Panax Notoginseng, and Dalbergia Odorifera on recovering and regulating of the ODN. The network recovery ability algorithm was improved and applied to quantitatively evaluate the efficacy of Qishen Yiqi formulae. Results indicated that the Qishen Yiqi formulae was significantly better than the four TCM drugs of QSYQ administered alone against AMI, and had a synergistic mode of effect. As for the ability of network recovery, the sovereign drug and minister drug (Radix Astragali and Salvia Miltiorrhiza) is significantly better than that of the assistant drug and courier drug (Panax Notoginseng and Dalbergia Odorifera), which complies with the compatibility law of "sovereign-minister-assistant-courier or Jun-Chen-Zuo-Shi rules." Pathway enrichment analysis sheds light on the compatibility rules of the Qishen Yiqi formulae and its components at the pathway level.

8.2.2.1 Data Acquisition and Processing

Preparation of Myocardial Tissue Samples from AMI Rats

The AMI rat myocardial tissue samples were provided by the Institute of Pharmacoinformatics, Zhejiang University. A total of seven groups of samples were involved in this study, including normal group (Ctrl), model group (MI), Qishen Yiqi Decoction group (QSYQ), Salvia Miltiorrhiza group (DS), Radix Astragali group (HQ), Panax Notoginseng group (SQ), and Dalbergia Odorifera group (JX). Three biological replicate samples were included in each group.

Chip Experiment and Data Preprocessing

RNA extraction, purification, sample quality inspection, chip experiment, and data acquisition were completed by chip company. The Affymetrix Rat 230 2.0 chip was used, and the final chip data was saved in the .CEL format files. ArrayTrack software was applied to read the .CEL files and the chip data was exported to Excel in .txt format files for normalization processing. Data from 21 chips was processed for data standardization. The median expression value for each chip was set to 1.000 (Median = 1000) by multiplying with the weight coefficient.

8.2.2.2 Network Construction and Visualization

Construction of Organism Disturbed Network (ODN)

The whole process can be divided into four parts: data collection, data arrangement, network construction and visualization, and network analysis.

In the data collection process, the AMI-related gene information, correlation, and expression profile information were collected through knowledge mining techniques and transcriptomics experiments. In the data management process, genes related to CHD and myocardial ischemia in CHD@ZJU and RGD databases were integrated. Protein–protein interaction (PPI) relationship information in both HPRD and BioGRID databases was also integrated. Gene expression information was attained through chip expression data processing using data normalization. AMI disease biological network was constructed by using integrated genetic information and PPI relationship as nodes and edges, respectively. Each node in the network represents a gene, and each edge represents the interaction relationship between the corresponding proteins of two genes. Then, the gene expression profile information of AMI was obtained by transcriptomics technology, and it was combined with the disease biological network in the form of network annotation (including node annotation and edge annotation) to form ODN. Cytoscape software was applied to conduct visualization research of the ODN.

Calculation of Network Recovery Index (NRI) of ODN Model

NRI-ODN, which is oriented to the Organism Disturbed Network model, enables to integrate node topology attributes and callback efficiency, to comprehensively evaluate the ability of network recovery regulation of drugs. In this study, node topology attributes are defined by the degree of nodes. The node callback efficiency is evaluated by "Efficiency of Recovery regulation" (EoR).

EoR is an index describing the callback efficiency of a node based on a quantitative callback state (RL′). RL′ is a continuous variable form of the callback state index RL, and the calculation is shown in Formula 8.1. The EoR calculation is shown in Formula 8.2, and its maximum value is 100%, that is, the drug can eliminate the expression change caused by the AMI modeling. For example, if the mean Log2 value of expression intensity in the normal control group is 5, and that in the model group is 10. EoR = 50% indicates that the expression intensity of this gene was regulated in recovery by 50% (value = 7.5) or over-regulated by 50% (value = 12.5) after drug administration. While EoR = 100% indicates that the gene expression intensity returned to the normal control state after administration (value = 10). If EoR < 0, it means that the drug does not have a callback effect (value < 5) or produces an excessive over-callback effect (>15) on the gene, and this type of gene does not contribute to the efficacy of the drug.

$$\mathrm{RL}' = \frac{\mathrm{Log}E_{\mathrm{drug}} - \mathrm{Log}E_{\mathrm{disease}}}{\mathrm{Log}E_{\mathrm{control}} - \mathrm{Log}E_{\mathrm{disease}}}, \tag{8.1}$$

$$\mathrm{EoR} = 100\% - |100\% - \mathrm{RL}'|, \tag{8.2}$$

$\mathrm{NRI}_{\mathrm{ODN}}$ was calculated by Formula 8.4. The callback level (Recovery Regulation-ODN, RRODN) comprehensively considers the influence of node topology and callback efficiency on the callback level, as shown in Formula 8.3. Where W_{topo} represents the degree of the node and $EoR_{positive}$ indicates that only those nodes with positive EoR (value > 0) are used in the RRODN calculation. Finally, NRI_{ODN} was obtained by calculating the overall network, the sum of the RRODN of significantly up-regulated genes and significantly down-regulated genes.

$$\mathrm{RRODN} = \sum W_{\mathrm{topo}} \times \mathrm{EoR}_{\mathrm{positive}}, \tag{8.3}$$

$$\mathrm{NRI}_{\mathrm{ODN}} = \mathrm{RRODN}_{\mathrm{all}} + \mathrm{RRODN}_{\mathrm{up}} + \mathrm{RRODN}_{\mathrm{down}}, \tag{8.4}$$

8.2.2.3 Network Analysis and Prediction

The study applied the NRI-ODN to evaluate the efficacy of the Qishen Yiqi formulae against AMI, and analyzed the impact of the node's Fold Change (FC) on the callback level RRODN and NRI_{ODN}. The callback efficiency of Qishen Yiqi and its single drugs to the nodes of the ODN were calculated through EoR. The genes with effective callback ability were defined with EoR $> 50\%$ as the threshold, and the effective callback genes lists of Qishen Yiqi and its four drugs were obtained.

Pathway enrichment analysis methods were used to analyze the biological signaling pathways involved in each gene list. ArrayTrack (version 3.5.0) software was cited to analyze the pathway of the effective callback gene list. The KEGG pathway database was selected as the pathway information source, and fisher p value < 0.05 was set as the standard to identify the significant pathways. The KEGG pathway database contains cellular processes, environmental information processes, metabolism, human diseases, etc. Considering the relevance with PPI, only cellular and environmental information processes were studied in this research.

8.2.2.4 Validation and Summary

Network Construction and EoR Calculation Results

The AMI-related disease biological network based on the Qishen Yiqi data involves a total of 324 genes and 623 pairs of interaction relationships. The largest sub-network is the ODN, involving 281 genes and 616 interaction relationships. Each node represents a gene, and each edge represents an interaction relationship between the corresponding proteins of the genes. The color of the nodes represents the changed state of expression in the modeling group, where red represents the up-regulated expression of the modeling group as compared to the normal group; and green represents the down-regulated expression of the modeling group versus the normal group (as shown in Fig. 8.1a).

The EoR index was used to annotate the callback ability of the Qishen Yiqi decoction after administration (as shown in Fig. 8.1b). A blue node indicated that the

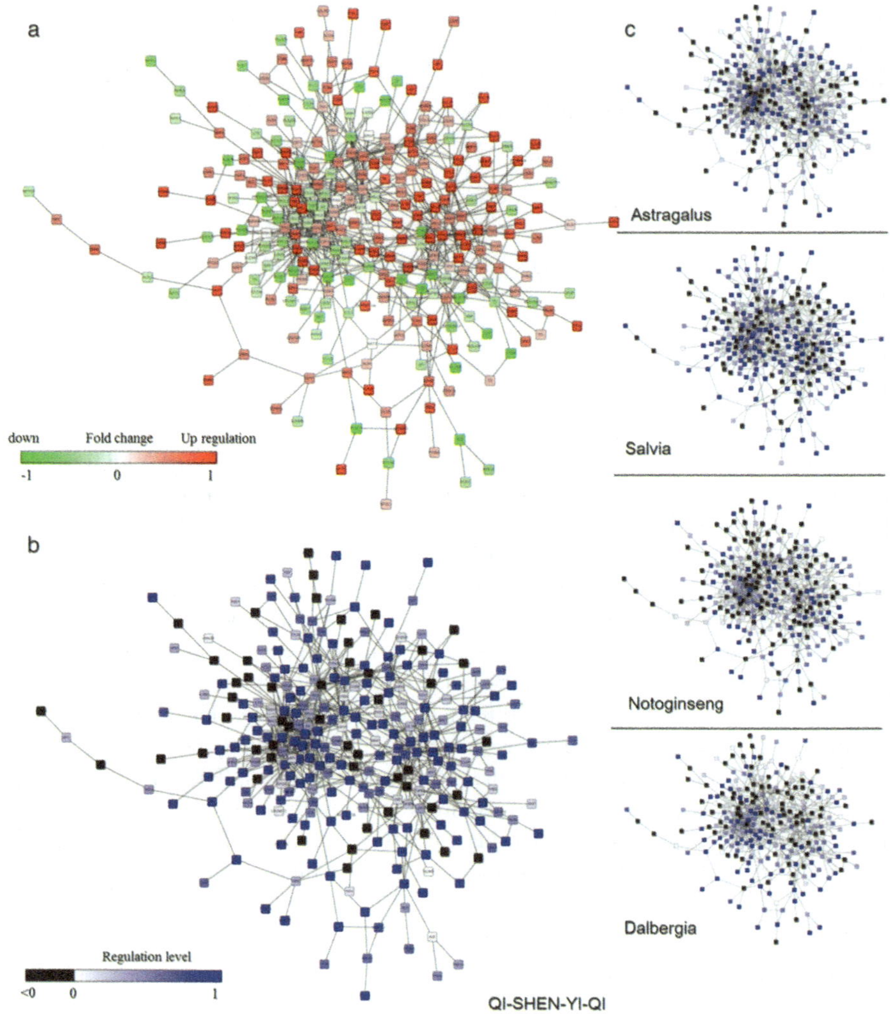

Fig. 8.1 Graph of the AMI-related Organism Disturbed Network (ODN) (Qishen Yiqi network) based on the Qishen Yiqi gene chip expression data

Qishen Yiqi formulae could callback the expression imbalance caused by AMI after its administration, while a gray node indicated that there was no callback effect. The four drugs of Qishen Yiqi formulae—Salvia Miltiorrhiza (Salvia), Radix Astragali (Astragalus), Panax Notoginseng (Notoginseng), and Dalbergia Odorifera (Dalbergia), are shown in Fig. 8.1c.

Calculation Results of RRODN and NRI_{ODN} of Qishen Yiqi Formulae

Among the four drugs, the NRI_{ODN} index of Salvia Miltiorrhiza and Radix Astragali was higher than that of Panax Notoginseng and Dalbergia Odorifera. The Qishen Yiqi formulae, Radix Astragali, and Salvia Miltiorrhiza had a very significant callback effect on the ODN ($p < 0.01$). Dalbergia Odorifera had a significant callback effect ($p < 0.05$), and the Panax Notoginseng alone showed an insignificant callback effect on the ODN ($p > 0.1$).

Results of Network Recovery Regulation Ability

In this study, the absolute value of FC > 0.5 was used as the screening criterion for significantly up-regulated and down-regulated genes, and the influence of this screening criterion on the calculation results of RRODN was investigated. The RR value of Qishen Yiqi formulae is always higher than those of its four drugs alone. When the FC threshold is greater than 1, the RRODN levels of Salvia Miltiorrhiza and Radix Astragali are higher than those of Panax Notoginseng and Dalbergia Odorifera. When the FC is greater than 1, the significant RRODN value of Qishen Yiqi formulae shows little difference with that of Salvia Miltiorrhiza, while the significant RRODN values corresponding to Radix Astragali, Panax Notoginseng, and Dalbergia Odorifera are similar.

Compatibility Rules of Qishen Yiqi at the Pathway Level

EoR > 50% was used as the threshold value to define the effective callback genes of the Qishen Yiqi formulae and its four drugs against ODN, and the biological pathway enrichment of the genes with EoR > 50% were counted and analyzed. The results indicated that Radix Astragali could affect more pathways, while the other three drugs had similar number of signaling pathways. The 14 pathways regulated by the Qishen Yiqi formulae can be also regulated by at least one of its drugs. Radix Astragali and Salvia Miltiorrhiza could both regulate 10 pathways of the 14 pathways, Panax Notoginseng could regulate 8 pathways, while Dalbergia Odorifera could only regulate 5 pathways, which all indicates that Radix Astragali and Salvia Miltiorrhiza may play a major role in the regulation effects of Qishen Yiqi formulae at the pathway level.

8.2.3 *Study of "Tonifying Qi and Activating Blood" Efficacy in TCM Formulae*

The Qishen Yiqi formulae is composed of Salvia Miltiorrhiza, Radix Astragali, Panax Notoginseng, and Dalbergia Odorifera, and it is prescribed for treatment of ischemic heart disease [79]. The Qishen Yiqi dripping pills manufactured according to Qishen Yiqi formulae [80] are clinically used for the treatment of CHD due to Qi deficiency and blood stasis with definite curative effects. The four herbs are formulated in accordance with the prescription of "sovereign-minister-assistant-courier," however, their mechanism of the treatment of ischemic heart disease and related complications needs to be further studied [81]. The preparation was originally called Huangqi Danshen Dropping Pills [82–84], and then renamed as Qishen Yiqi dropping pills. TCM theory indicates that Qi deficiency and blood stasis lead to the pathogenesis of ischemic heart disease. Tonifying Qi and activating blood circulation is the basic treatment regimen for ischemic heart disease. Therefore, research on the efficacy of Qi tonifying and blood activating could conducted from the view of the Qi tonifying and blood activating of Radix Astragali and Salvia Miltiorrhiza. Based on the ischemic heart disease network, with the regulation of Salvia Miltiorrhiza and Radix Astragali and network regulation analysis method, it is feasible to carry out research of efficacy of Qi tonifying and blood activating on the disease molecular network view. What's more, further cellular and molecular biology experiments are warranted to verify related molecular mechanisms.

8.2.3.1 Data Acquisition and Processing

Construction of Ischemic Heart Disease Network

The disease network was constructed with application of CHD@ZJU cardiovascular disease network pharmacology research platform, which was used to investigate the efficacy of the Qishen Yiqi formulae of its Qi tonifying and blood circulation promoting.

Construction of Molecular Network of Radix Astragali and Salvia Miltiorrhiza for Regulating of Ischemic Heart Disease

The myocardial tissue samples of AMI rats were provided by the Institute of Pharmacoinformatics, Zhejiang University. A total of seven groups of samples were involved in this study, including normal group (Ctrl), model group (MI), Qishen Yiqi Decoction group (QSYQ), Salvia Miltiorrhiza group (DS), Radix Astragali group (HQ), Panax Notoginseng group (SQ), and Dalbergia Odorifera group (JX). Three biological replicate samples were included in each group.

RNA extraction, purification, sample quality inspection, chip experiment, and data acquisition were completed by chip company. The Affymetrix Rat 230 2.0 chip was used, and the final chip data was saved in the. CEL format files. ArrayTrack software was applied to read the. CEL files and the chip data was exported to Excel in .txt format files for normalization processing. Data from 21 chips was processed for data standardization. The median expression value for each chip was set to 1.000 (Median = 1000) by multiplying with the weight coefficient.

8.2.3.2 Network Construction and Visualization

In the network modeling process, the PPI relationships were obtained with integration of HPRD and BioGRID databases. As for disease-associated genes collection, CHD@ZJU was applied, together with CHD and myocardial ischemia related genes from RGD database were also used. The chip expression data was processed with normalization to attain gene expression information. Gene expression profile information of AMI was obtained through transcriptomics technology, then Cytoscape software (version 3.0.1) was used to conduct the research on visualization of the ODN.

8.2.3.3 Network Analysis and Prediction

Efficacy exploration of Radix Astragali and Salvia Miltiorrhiza in "tonifying Qi and promoting blood circulation" in ischemic heart disease at molecular network level.

In Sect. 8.2.2, the NRI_{ODN} was used to study the compatibility rules of the Qishen Yiqi formulae with "sovereign-minister-assistant-courier." At the molecular network level, the network recovery regulation ability of the sovereign and minister drugs (Radix Astragali and Salvia Miltiorrhiza) is significantly better than that of assistant and courier drugs (Panax Notoginseng and Dalbergia Odorifera), which is accord with the compatibility rules "sovereign-minister-assistant-courier" of these drugs. In our previous pharmacodynamic and proteomics research, results showed that Radix Astragali and Salvia Miltiorrhiza, the sovereign and minister drugs in Qishen Yiqi formulae, targeted on the energy metabolism and blood circulation pathways of the imbalance network, respectively, which was consistent with the traditional efficacy of "replenishing Qi and promoting blood circulation."

In this section, NRI-ODN algorithm was cited to calculate the callback ability of the drug to the organisms network balance, and the drug efficacy was evaluated systematically. The NRI-ODN algorithm further considered the influence of network topology and node callback efficiency on the overall recovery regulation ability, so it could reflect the influence of TCM drugs on the network more reasonably.

Further pathway enrichment analysis was carried out. Effective callback genes with a threshold value (EoR > 50%) were defined and obtained for Qishen Yiqi formulae and its constituent drugs. ArrayTrack (version 3.5.0) software was cited to analyze the pathway of the effective callback gene list. The KEGG pathway database was selected as the pathway information source, and fisher p value < 0.05 was set as the standard to identify the significant pathways. The KEGG pathway database contains cellular processes, environmental information processes, metabolism, human diseases, etc. Considering the relevance with PPI, only cellular and environmental information processes were studied in this research.

8.2.3.4 Validation and Summary

"Tonifying Qi" Effects of Radix Astragali: Detecting Energy Metabolism-Related Indicators

The rats LAD ligation model was used on under anesthesia. Myocardial infarction Rats were divided randomly into different groups with intragastric administration of TCM every morning for 7 consecutive days. The rats were administered 10 ml/kg in the Sham operation group (1% CMCNa), model group model (1% CMCNa), high-dose Radix Astragali group (200 mg/kg/day, ARE-H), and Radix Astragali low-dose group (100 mg/kg/day, ARE-L). Radix Astragali extract was provided by Tianjin Tasly Pharmaceutical Co., Ltd.

After 7 days of administration, the rats were anesthetized by intraperitoneal injection of 360 mg/kg chloral hydrate. Blood was collected from the abdominal aorta and allowed to stand for 30 min at room temperature, then was centrifuged at 4000 rpm for 15 min. The supernatant was collected and stored in the refrigerator at −80 °C. Then the heart was perfused with 20 ml of precooled normal saline, and was cut off and washed in precooled normal saline. The connective tissue and right ventricle were removed. Myocardium below the ligation site were placed in a precooled 2 ml cryopreservation tube and stored at −80 °C.

The test kit was used to measure biochemical indicators in the serum and myocardial tissue, HPLC chromatography method was used to detect the content of high-energy phosphate compounds in myocardial tissue, and Western Blot was used to detect the expression of proteins related to energy metabolism in the myocardial tissue.

Serum and myocardial tissue homogenate: detecting of content or activity of lactate dehydrogenase (LDH), pyruvate (PA), lactic acid (LD), creatine kinase (CK), and free fatty acid (FFA).

Effects of Representative Ingredients of Radix Astragali on Energy Metabolism of Hypoxic Cardiomyocytes

The effects of the three representative compounds, i.e. Astragaloside IV, calycosin, and formononetin, against ATPase activity in H9c2 cardiomyocytes were detected respectively. The hypoxic device consists of a hypoxic culture chamber (Modular Incubator Chamber, Billups-Rothenberg). Hypoxic conditions were created by using mixed air to replace the air in the hypoxic culture chamber (ventilate mixed air for about 15 min). The culture chamber was placed in a 37 °C, 5% CO_2 incubator for 12 h. The ATP content of cardiomyocytes was detected using the CellTiter-Glo™ reagent, and the luminescence intensity was measured with a fluorescence chemiluminescence analyzer (Tecan F200, USA).

At the same time, the effects of the three representative compounds against ATPase activity in cardiomyocytes were detected, using a reference ultra-trace ATPase test kit according to kit instructions.

Finally, Western Blot was conducted to detect the effects of the three active compounds on the expression of the PGC-1 and PPAR-α, two proteins which are associated with energy metabolism in hypoxic cardiomyocytes.

Main Conclusions

1. Based on the ischemic heart disease network and transcriptomics information, NRI-ODN algorithm application can reflect the recovery regulation ability of Radix Astragali and Salvia Miltiorrhiza on the organisms network balance and is able to evaluate TCM drug efficacy systematically. Pathway level studies indicated that the "Qi tonifying and blood circulation activating" of Radix Astragali and Salvia Miltiorrhiza may be associated with the regulation of myocardial energy metabolism and blood circulation.
2. Radix Astragali extract showed effects on LDH activity and CK, FFA, PA, and LA levels in the serum and myocardial tissue of AMI rats. Compared to the sham operation group, the LDH activity and CK level in the serum and ischemic myocardial tissue were significantly increased. After administration of Radix Astragali extract (200 mg/kg/day, 100 mg/kg/day), the LDH activity and CK level in the serum and ischemic myocardium significantly decreased compared to those of the model group. The serum LDH activity and CK levels of ischemic myocardial tissue in the high-dose group were significantly different from those in the model group ($P < 0.05$). These results show that the Radix Astragali extract could effectively alleviate ischemic injury of AMI rats. Compared with the sham operation group, the levels of FFA, PA, and LA in serum and ischemic myocardial tissue were significantly increased. After intragastric administration of the Radix Astragali extract (200 mg/kg/day, 100 mg/kg/day), the levels of FFA, PA, and LA in serum and ischemic myocardial tissue decreased compared to those in the model group. The levels of FFA, PA, and LA in serum and ischemic myocardium of the high-dose group (200 mg/kg/day) significantly decreased ($P < 0.01$, $P < 0.05$), while the FFA level in ischemic myocardium with the low-dose administration (100 mg/kg/day) showed significantly decreased ($P < 0.05$). The results showed that the Radix Astragali extract could effectively regulate the energy metabolism-related metabolites in serum and myocardial tissue of AMI rats.
3. Effects of Radix Astragali extract on high-energy phosphate compounds in ischemic myocardial tissues of rats with myocardial ischemia. The HPLC detection showed that after LAD ligation, the levels of ATP, ADP, AMP, and TAN in

myocardial tissue decreased. Compared to the model group, the concentrations of ATP, ADP, AMP, and TAN increased with treatment of Radix Astragali extract of high and low dosages.

4. Effects of active compounds of Radix Astragali on ATP level of hypoxic cardiomyocytes. Ast can promote the production of ATP in H9c2 cardiomyocytes under hypoxic conditions in a dose-dependent manner. Compounds Cal and For can also increase the production of ATP, showing a good dose-effect relationship.
5. Effects of Radix Astragali active compounds on ATPase activity of hypoxic cardiomyocytes. Compounds Ast, Cal, and For can enhance the activities of Na^{+}-K^{+}-ATPase and Ca^{2+}-Mg^{2+}-ATPase of H9c2 under hypoxic conditions with a good dose-effect relationship.
6. Effects of active compounds of Radix Astragali on PGC-1 and PPAR-α in hypoxic cardiomyocytes. Compared with the normal group, the protein expression of PPAR-α decreased significantly while protein expression of PGC-1 decreased a little. Ast, Cal, and For can significantly promote the expression of PGC-1, but the expression of PPAR-α increases slightly.

In summary, Radix Astragali can improve the energy metabolism of ischemic myocardium, and PPAR pathway activation may be the involved mode of action.

8.3 Practice of Disease Network Application for Holistic Efficacy Evaluation of TCM Drug

The rational application of network pharmacology techniques in the field of TCM research and the development of TCM network pharmacology are currently hotspots of TCM drug research. Currently, the applications of network pharmacology in TCM research mainly involve the construction of TCM information database, construction of TCM network model, study of the TCM components-target relationships, analysis of TCM biological network, and so on. Establishing a scientific and systematic evaluation system to conduct activity evaluation of TCM is a key technical link [85] in the creation and optimal design of modern new TCM drugs, which is also a difficult point in the current research. With the discovery of drug multi-target effects, drug optimization design strategy based on multiple targets is able to more reasonably reflect drug efficacy, side effects, in vivo processes, and other characteristics [86]. Network pharmacology research has further developed the concept of multi-objective optimization. The effects of a drug on the overall network as a comprehensive evaluation index to replace the traditional single-indicator or multi-objective evaluation system, in which pharmacodynamic evaluation based on system biology data has made remarkable progresses [87, 88] in the field of the drug repositioning. By constructing the system network model, drug actions were represented as the characteristics of the holistic network, which makes breakthrough against the bottleneck that single target could not fully represent the overall effects of drugs against the biological system, while it also solves the faced problem of multi-objective optimization when using multi-efficacy indicators for evaluation. What's more, the network model also reflects changes in the biological system responding to diseases and drugs at the molecular level. This allows for further research on the mode of action and reveals the biological pathways and molecular mechanisms involved during the drug treatment process. This type of research does not rely on the drug structural characteristics, nor does it aim to a specific disease target, which reduces the research limitations. Therefore, compared to the structure-dependent traditional chemical medicine research, it is more suitable for the development of holistic Chinese medicine research.

Holistic biological network analysis is different from the study of drug-target network, which adopts homogeneous network or a hybrid network model integrating both homogeneous and heterogeneous networks to replace the heterogeneous drug-target network. More emphasis is placed on the relationship within the biological system together with the impact of drugs on the whole biological network, rather than only focusing on the direct effect and impact of drugs on the target.

Considering Shenmai injection as an example, the Network Recovery Index (NRI) was used to quantitatively to evaluate the callback effect of Shenmai Injection on acute myocardial ischemia imbalance network.

8.3.1 Data Acquisition and Processing

8.3.1.1 Research on Acute Myocardial Ischemia in Rats

Male SD rats were subjected to LAD ligation, and divided into three groups, sham, model, and drug. The dosage of Shenmai injection was 10 ml/kg, and the rats were intraperitoneally injected for 7 consecutive days ($n = 8$ in each group). After 7 days of administration, rat cardiac function was evaluated by echocardiography. The ischemic penumbra area between the necrotic area and normal tissue in the myocardium were sampled and used for mRNA extraction and chip analysis research. The animal experiment was conducted by the department of pharmacology, the second military medical university, and the echocardiography measurement results were processed by Zhongshan Hospital affiliated to Fudan University.

8.3.1.2 Chip Experiments and Data Preprocessing

The chip used in this study was the Affymetrix Rat 230 2.0 chip based on rat genome-wide chip, including 31,099 probes. There were 24 samples, $n = 4$ for red ginseng group, and $n = 5$ for the Ophiopogon japonicus group, Shenmai injection group, normal group, and model group. Affymetrix expression profiling chip matching kit—GeneChip 3′IVT Express Kit (Cat#901229, Affymetrix, Santa Clara, CA, US) and standard operating procedures (SOPs) were applied to amplify, label, and purify mRNA in the total RNA of the samples to obtain Biotin-labeled cRNAs.

According to the hybrid standard procedure and matching kit provided by the Affymetrix expression profile chip—GeneChip® Hybridization, Wash and Stain Kit (Cat#900720, Affymetrix, Santa Clara, CA, US), rolling hybridization was carried out for 16 h in a 45 °C Hybridization Oven 645 (Cat#00-0331-220V, Affymetrix, Santa Clara, CA, US). After the hybridization was completed, the chip was then washed in a Fluidics Station 450 (Cat#00-0079, Affymetrix, Santa Clara, CA, US) according to the SOPs provided by Affymetrix.

The chip results were scanned by GeneChip® Scanner 3000 (Cat#00-00212, Affymetrix, Santa Clara, CA, US). The original data were read by Command Console Software 3.1 (Affymetrix, Santa Clara, CA, US). Qualified data was normalized using Gene Spring Software 11.0 (Agilent technologies, Santa Clara, CA, US) with application of MAS 5.0 as the algorithm.

The chip experiments were completed by the Shanghai Biotechnology Corporation.

8.3.2 Network Construction and Visualization

The network model, used to evaluate the effects of Shenmai injection against AMI, is referred to the enriched pathway network model, and was mainly based on the significantly enriched signaling pathways and related gene-association information in AMI. The specific construction process is as follows: (1) P value < 0.01 and Fold change > 1.5 were selected as the threshold, the genes were extracted and pathway enrichment analysis was conducted to obtain the corresponding information. (2) KEGG database was used to retrieve all of the genes contained in these pathways. (3) The HPRD database was used to acquire the correlation relationships between these genes, and network model was constructed.

With p value < 0.01 and fold change > 1.5 as the threshold, a total of 1957 probes, with differential expressions produced with comparing of the model and control groups, were obtained and involved a total of 1376 related genes. Pathway enrichment analysis was performed on these genes, and 27 enriched KEGG signaling pathways (Fisher P value < 0.05) were obtained, including 10 metabolism pathways and 10 cellular process pathways, 2 environmental signal transduction pathways, 4 disease pathways, and DNA replication pathway. These pathways involve a total of 1478 related genes. By searching the HPRD database, 905 genes were found to have at least one PPI association with other genes (or themselves), involving a total of 2618 PPIs. 700 genes were found to form the largest sub-network. The enriched pathway network diagram was generated, in which nodes of different colors represented that they belong to different signaling pathways. Network parameter analysis showed that the connectivity distribution is in accordance with the characteristics of scale-free network ($R^2 = 0.868$), indicating that it has the properties of general biological network.

8.3.3 Network Analysis and Prediction

Analysis of the alleviation effects of Shenmai injection against network imbalance induced by AMI.

Changes of gene expression levels were used to create networks to reflect the status of the network before and post-modeling and Shenmai injection administration, as well as the recovery regulation trend post-Shenmai injection administration. In the drug regulation network, the red node represents the up-regulated expression level, while the green node represents the down-regulated node. By conducting network comparing, i.e., Model vs sham, Shenmai vs sham, Shenmai vs Model, holistic network expression changes were analyzed both for post-AMI and post-Shenmai injection administration treatments. Information on regulation of the overall network expression on MI was obtained, and efficacy associated mechanism post-Shenmai administration was found.

Shenmai injection shows the ability to make recovery regulation effects against the network imbalance caused by ischemic modeling. What's more, NRI index was applied to evaluate the network recovery capability. For NRI calculation, refer to Sect. 8.2.2.

8.3.4 Main Conclusions

1. Echocardiography evaluation of left ventricular function in the rats was done 7 days after AMI as the apparent pharmacodynamic index of Shenmai injection, to calculate the evaluation indexes of left ventricular function, including Ejection Fraction (EF) and Fractional Shortening (FS). The EF and FS values of rats in the modeling group decreased significantly after 7 days of AMI and increased significantly after Shenmai injection administration ($P < 0.05$), showing myocardial repair effects. However, the changes of EF and FS values after administration of red ginseng and Ophiopogon japonicus alone, respectively, were not statistically significant ($p > 0.05$).
2. The administration of Shenmai injection alleviates network disorders caused by AMI. It was found that the holistic network expression change-related trend is similar to that of after the administration of the Shenmai injection, that is, the injection does not produce excessively strong regulatory effects that affect the balance of the organisms. Compared to the regulatory trend of MI modeling, the change in expression levels of the Shenmai injection is almost opposite, that is, the Shenmai injection could alleviate the imbalance of the enrichment pathway network caused by AMI and regulate it back to a normal status.
3. By analyzing the expression levels of the top 10 genes with the most significant expression imbalance after MI modeling, it was found that the expression levels of all nodes that were significantly regulated were recalled after the administration of the Shenmai injection, which further confirms the conclusion that the

Shenmai injection has a callback to the network imbalance caused by ischemic modeling.

4. Shenmai injection has over 90% recovery regulation ability for genes that are significantly dysregulated after AMI, and the overall network callback ability was 77.9%. In contrast, the network callback ability of red ginseng and Ophiopogon japonicus is relatively weak. Red ginseng can only callback about 50% of the ODN, while the effect of Ophiopogon japonicus is even lower, with only about 16.4–35.4%. Finally, the NRI score of Shenmai injection was 0.876, much higher than the NRI scores of red ginseng and Ophiopogon japonicus (0.498 and 0.269, respectively), indicating that red ginseng and Ophiopogon japonicus have a significant synergistic enhancing effect when administered concurrently in Shenmai injection. They also produce a stronger callback effect on the expression imbalance that occurs in the enriched pathway network.

Human disease spectrum has changed from communicable diseases to non-communicable diseases (NCDs). The mortality and disability rate of NCDs has brought severe challenges to the human medical and health system. The occurrence and development of diseases are often not limited to a single gene, but a manifestation of the interactions among internally associated multi-molecular processes. Humans have made new progress in understanding complex diseases. From the view of structure and function of the "molecular biological network" to systematically reveal the molecular mechanisms of complex diseases, the internal relationships between disease and disease, and the modes of action of drugs is a new research strategy.

Humanity's understanding of the role of drugs has changed from the traditional "one drug, one target" model to the "network target, multi-component treatment" pattern. As a historical heritage and treasure of China, TCM plays an important role in China's medical and health care system, and thus makes positive contributions to the world's medical and health system. TCM is the most important way for preventing and treating diseases in China. As a complex system with multiple ingredients, TCM has a nonlinear interaction relationship with complex diseases. Therefore, the understanding and analysis of this mode of action need to break through the traditional pharmacological research methods. With the rapid development of bioinformatics, systems biology, and polypharmacology, web-based methods have become a powerful tool for the study of complex diseases and nonlinear drug-disease complex modes of action.

In summary, this chapter studies cardiovascular disease, which is rank first in the diseases to cause human deaths, and analyzes the occurrence and development of ischemic heart disease through disease network construction and analysis. Based on the disease network, we conducted the research on the integrated mechanisms of TCM, the law of compatibility, the efficacy of "supplementing Qi and promoting blood circulation," and the regulation of ODN. In the research process, pharmacodynamics, pharmacokinetics, transcriptomics, proteomics, metabolomics, bioinformatics, network pharmacology, and other methods and technologies were integrated to design experimental studies at the organism, cellular, molecular, and other levels.

Examples of several famous TCM products mentioned in this chapter, namely Qishen Yiqi dropping pills, Xuesaitong injection, and Shenmai injection, have obvious clinical efficacy and social benefits. They play integrated regulation roles, including multi-components, multi-targets, and multi-pathways in the prevention and treatment of ischemic heart disease. Therefore, the research in this chapter was also designed and carried out based on a systematic and integrated perspective. The research concepts and methods in this chapter can provide references for the study of other diseases and the effects of other drugs.

Certainly, for disease-based network pharmacology study there will be more extended applications, including deciphering of disease–disease associations (DDAs), drug repositioning research, drug-target prediction, and research on network toxicology of TCM. Future research also needs to integrate multi-dimensional "-omics" information, including genes, RNA, proteins, endogenous metabolites, etc., which could facilitate the network-based research to play a key role in the modernization and internationalization of TCM.

References

1. Li S. Exploring traditional Chinese medicine by a novel therapeutic concept of network target. Chinese J Integr Med. 2016;22(9):647–52.
2. Zhang C, Zhou W, Guan DG, et al. Network intervention, a method to address complex therapeutic strategies. Front Pharmacol. 2018;9:754.
3. World Health Organization. Who traditional medicine strategy 2014–2023. 2013. https://www.who.int/publications/list/traditional_medicine_strategy/zh/ (in Chinese) [世界卫生组织. 世卫组织2014-2023年传统医学战略. 2013. https://www.who.int/publications/list/traditional_medicine_strategy/zh/].
4. Fan X, Xiao S, Ai Ni, et al. Study on the effective substance group of Xiaoqinglong Decoction based on network prescription science. Chinese J Traditional Chinese Med. 2015;40(13):2634–2638 (in Chinese) [范骁辉, 肖舜, 艾妮, 等. 基于网络方剂学的小青龙汤类方功效物质组研究. 中国中药杂志, 2015, 40(13):2634–2638].
5. Fan X, Cheng Y, Zhang B. Network pharmacology: a new strategy for modern research of prescriptions. Chinese J Traditional Chinese Med. 2015;40(1):1–6 (in Chinese) [范骁辉, 程翼宇, 张伯礼. 网络方剂学: 方剂现代研究的新策略. 中国中药杂志, 2015, 40(1):1–6].
6. Fan X, Zhao X, Jin Y, et al. On the establishment of network toxicology and traditional Chinese medicine network toxicology research ideas. Chinese J Traditional Chinese Med. 2011;36(21):2920–2 (in Chinese) [范骁辉, 赵筱萍, 金烨成, 等. 论建立网络毒理学及中药网络毒理学研究思路. 中国中药杂志, 2011, 36(21):2920–2922].
7. Wu L, Wang Y, Fan X. Internet pharmacology technology tools: network visualization and network analysis. Chinese J Traditional Chinese Med. 2011;36(21):2923–5 (in Chinese) [吴磊宏, 王毅, 范骁辉. 网络药理学技术工具: 网络可视化及网络分析. 中国中药杂志, 2011, 36(21):2923–2925].
8. Wu L, Gao X, Cheng Y, et al. Research on network pharmacology of decoction pieces of traditional Chinese medicine based on correlation between indications and indications of traditional Chinese medicine. Chinese J Traditional Chinese Med. 2011;36(21):2907–10 (in Chinese) [吴磊宏, 高秀梅, 程翼宇, 等. 基于中医主治关联的中药饮片网络药理学研究. 中国中药杂志, 2011, 36(21):2907–2910].
9. Wu L, Gao X, Wang L, et al. Prediction of multi-component action target and network pharmacology of Aconitum carmichaeli. Chinese Herbal Med. 2011;36(21):2916–9

(in Chinese) [吴磊宏, 高秀梅, 王林丽, 等. 附子多成分作用靶点预测及网络药理学研究. 中国中药杂, 2011, 36(21):2916–2919].
10. Li X, Wu L, Fan X, et al. Study on network pharmacology of main active components of Compound Danshen Prescription. Chinese J Traditional Chinese Med. 2011;36(21):2911–5 (in Chinese) [李翔, 吴磊宏, 范骁辉, 等. 复方丹参方主要活性成分网络药理学研究. 中国中药杂志, 2011, 36(21):2911–2915].
11. Wang Y, Fan XH, Qu HB, et al. Strategies and techniques for multi-component drug design from medicinal herbs and traditional Chinese medicine. Curr Top Med Chem. 2012;12 (12):1356–62.
12. Wu LH, Wang Y, Nie J, et al. A network pharmacology approach to evaluating the efficacy of Chinese medicine using genome-wide transcriptional expression data. Evid Based Complement Alternat Med. 2013;2013:915343.
13. Wu LH, Li X, Yang JH, et al. CHD@ZJU: a knowledgebase providing network-based research platform on coronary heart disease. Database. 2013;2013:bat047.
14. Yang ZZ, Yang JH, Liu W, et al. T2D@ZJU: a knowledgebase integrating heterogeneous connections associated with type 2 diabetes mellitus. Database. 2013;2013:bat052.
15. Wang LL, Li Z, Zhao XP, et al. A network study of Chinese medicine Xuesaitong injection to elucidate a complex mode-of-action with multi-compound, multi-target and multi-pathway. Evid Based Complement Alternat Med. 2013;2013:652373.
16. Yang JH, Li Z, Fan XH, et al. A three step network based approach (TSNBA) to finding disease molecular signature and key regulators: a case study of IL-1 and TNF-alpha stimulated inflammation. PLoS One. 2014;9(4):e94360.
17. Wang LL, Li Z, Shao Q, et al. Dissecting active ingredients of Chinese medicine by content-weighted ingredient-target network. Mol BioSyst. 2014;10:1905–11.
18. Li X, Wu LH, Liu W, et al. A network pharmacology study of Chinese medicine QiShenYiQi to reveal its underlying multi-compound, multi-target, multi-pathway mode of action. PLoS One. 2014;9(5):e95004.
19. Wu LH, Wang Y, Li Z, et al. Identifying roles of "Jun-Chen-Zuo-Shi" component herbs of QiShenYiQi formula in treating acute myocardial ischemia by network pharmacology. Chinese Med. 2014;9:24.
20. Yang JH, Li Z, Fan XH, et al. Drug-disease association and drug-repositioning predictions in complex diseases using causal inference-probabilistic matrix factorization. J Chem Inf Model. 2014;54(9):2562–9.
21. Liu YF, Ai N, Keys A, et al. Network pharmacology for traditional Chinese medicine research: methodologies and applications. Chinese Herbal Med. 2015;7(1):18–26.
22. Ai N, Fan XH, Ekins S. In silico methods for predicting drug-drug interactions with cytochrome P-450s, transporters and beyond. Adv Drug Deliv Rev. 2015;86:46–60.
23. Liu YF, Ai N, Liao J, et al. Transcriptomics: a sword to cut the Gordian knot of traditional Chinese medicine. Biomark Med. 2015;9(11):1201–13.
24. Chen Q, Zheng J, Shao Y, et al. Network-based assessment on chemical-induced cholestatic liver injury. Curr Top Med Chem. 2016;16(30):3668–77.
25. Chen Q, Ai N, Liao J, et al. Revealing topics and their evolution in biomedical literature using bio-DTM: a case study of ginseng. Chinese Med. 2017;12:27.
26. Wang Y, Zhao Y, Jiang W, et al. iTRAQ-based proteomic analysis reveals recovery of impaired mitochondrial function in ischemic myocardium by Shenmai formula. J Proteome Res. 2018;17 (2):794–803.
27. Liao J, Hao C, Huang WH, et al. Network pharmacology study reveals energy metabolism and apoptosis pathways-mediated cardioprotective effects of SHENQI FUZHENG. J Ethnopharmacol. 2018;227:155–65.
28. Dwinell MR, Worthey EA, Shimoyama M, et al. The rat genome database 2009: variation, ontologies and pathways. Nucleic Acids Res. 2009;37(suppl 1):D744–9.
29. Lopes CT, Franz M, Kazi F, et al. Cytoscape web: an interactive web-based network browser. Bioinformatics. 2010;26(18):2347–8.

30. Yang M, Chen J-L, Xu L-W, et al. Navigating traditional chinese medicine network pharmacology and computational tools. Evid Based Complement Alternat Med. 2013;2013:731969.
31. Gandhi T, Zhong J, Mathivanan S, et al. Analysis of the human protein interactome and comparison with yeast, worm and fly interaction datasets. Nat Genet. 2006;38(3):285–93.
32. Xu J, Li Y. Discovering disease-genes by topological features in human protein–protein interaction network. Bioinformatics. 2006;22(22):2800–5.
33. Goh K-I, Cusick ME, Valle D, et al. The human disease network. Proc Natl Acad Sci. 2007;104 (21):8685–90.
34. Feldman I, Rzhetsky A, Vitkup D. Network properties of genes harboring inherited disease mutations. Proc Natl Acad Sci. 2008;105(11):4323–8.
35. Barabási A-L, Gulbahce N, Loscalzo J. Network medicine: a network-based approach to human disease. Nat Rev Genet. 2011;12(1):56–68.
36. Bader GD, Hogue CW. An automated method for finding molecular complexes in large protein interaction networks. BMC Bioinformatics. 2003;4(1):2.
37. Maere S, Heymans K, Kuiper M. BiNGO: a cytoscape plugin to assess overrepresentation of gene ontology categories in biological networks. Bioinformatics. 2005;21(16):3448–9.
38. Yaoita H, Ogawa K, Maehara K, et al. Apoptosis in relevant clinical situations contribution of apoptosis in myocardial infarction. Cardiovasc Res. 2000;45(3):630–41.
39. Palojoki E, Saraste A, Eriksson A, et al. Cardiomyocyte apoptosis and ventricular remodeling after myocardial infarction in rats. Am J Physiol Heart Circ Physiol. 2001;280(6):H2726–31.
40. Crow MT, Mani K, Nam Y-J, et al. The mitochondrial death pathway and cardiac myocyte apoptosis. Circ Res. 2004;95(10):957–70.
41. Weber C, Noels H. Atherosclerosis: current pathogenesis and therapeutic options. Nat Med. 2011;17(11):1410–22.
42. Hansson GK, Hermansson A. The immune system in atherosclerosis. Nat Immunol. 2011;12 (3):204–12.
43. Hansson GK, Robertson A-KL, Söderberg-Nauclér C. Inflammation and atherosclerosis. Annu Rev Pathol. 2006;1:297–329.
44. Hansson GK. Inflammation, atherosclerosis, and coronary artery disease. N Engl J Med. 2005;352(16):1685–95.
45. Schwartz RS, Eltzschig HK, Carmeliet P. Hypoxia and inflammation. N Engl J Med. 2011;364 (7):656–65.
46. Kaminska B. MAPK signalling pathways as molecular targets for anti-inflammatory therapy—from molecular mechanisms to therapeutic benefits. Biochim Biophys Acta. 2005;1754 (1):253–62.
47. Bertrand L, Horman S, Beauloye C, et al. Insulin signalling in the heart. Cardiovasc Res. 2008;79(2):238–48.
48. Sena S, Hu P, Zhang D, et al. Impaired insulin signaling accelerates cardiac mitochondrial dysfunction after myocardial infarction. J Mol Cell Cardiol. 2009;46(6):910–8.
49. Finck BN. The PPAR regulatory system in cardiac physiology and disease. Cardiovasc Res. 2007;73(2):269–77.
50. Yamauchi T, Kamon J, Minokoshi YA, et al. Adiponectin stimulates glucose utilization and fatty-acid oxidation by activating AMP-activated protein kinase. Nat Med. 2002;8 (11):1288–95.
51. Robinson ES, Khankin EV, Karumanchi SA, et al. Hypertension induced by vascular endothelial growth factor signaling pathway inhibition: mechanisms and potential use as a biomarker. Proceedings of the seminars in nephrology. Elsevier; 2010:591–601.
52. Aramoto H, Breslin JW, Pappas PJ, et al. Vascular endothelial growth factor stimulates differential signaling pathways in in vivo microcirculation. Am J Physiol Heart Circ Physiol. 2004;287(4):H1590–8.
53. Olsson A-K, Dimberg A, Kreuger J, et al. VEGF receptor signalling? In control of vascular function. Nat Rev Mol Cell Biol. 2006;7(5):359–71.

54. Kiefer FN, Berns H, Resink TJ, et al. Hypoxia enhances vascular cell proliferation and angiogenesis in vitro via rapamycin (mTOR)-dependent signaling. FASEB J. 2002;16 (8):771–80.
55. Laplante M, Sabatini DM. mTOR signaling at a glance. J Cell Sci. 2009;122(20):3589–94.
56. Katoh K, Kano Y, Ookawara S. Role of stress fibers and focal adhesions as a mediator for mechano-signal transduction in endothelial cells in situ. Vasc Health Risk Manag. 2008;4 (6):1273.
57. Pellegrino M, Furmaniak-Kazmierczak E, Leblanc JC, et al. The apolipoprotein (a) component of lipoprotein (a) stimulates actin stress fiber formation and loss of cell-cell contact in cultured endothelial cells. J Biol Chem. 2004;279(8):6526–33.
58. De Caterina R, Libby P. Endothelial dysfunctions and vascular disease. Wiley; 2008.
59. Thomas T, Advani A. Inflammation in cardiovascular disease and regulation of the actin cytoskeleton in inflammatory cells: the actin cytoskeleton as a target. Cardiovasc Hematol Agents Med Chem. 2006;4(2):165–82.
60. Vanhoutte PM, Rubanyi GM, Miller VM, et al. Modulation of vascular smooth muscle contraction by the endothelium. Annu Rev Physiol. 1986;48(1):307–20.
61. Dobaczewski M, Chen W, Frangogiannis NG. Transforming growth factor (TGF)-β signaling in cardiac remodeling. J Mol Cell Cardiol. 2011;51(4):600–6.
62. Bujak M, Frangogiannis NG. The role of TGF-β signaling in myocardial infarction and cardiac remodeling. Cardiovasc Res. 2007;74(2):184–95.
63. Niessen K, Karsan A. Notch signaling in cardiac development. Circ Res. 2008;102 (10):1169–81.
64. Li Y, Hiroi Y, Liao JK. Notch signaling as an important mediator of cardiac repair and regeneration after myocardial infarction. Trends Cardiovasc Med. 2010;20(7):228–31.
65. Ueda K, Takano H, Niitsuma Y, et al. Sonic hedgehog is a critical mediator of erythropoietin-induced cardiac protection in mice. J Clin Invest. 2010;120(6):2016.
66. Roncalli J, Renault M-A, Tongers J, et al. Sonic hedgehog-induced functional recovery after myocardial infarction is enhanced by AMD3100-mediated progenitor-cell mobilization. J Am Coll Cardiol. 2011;57(24):2444–52.
67. Lemmens K, Doggen K, De Keulenaer GW. Role of neuregulin-1/ErbB signaling in cardiovascular physiology and disease implications for therapy of heart failure. Circulation. 2007;116 (8):954–60.
68. Rao TP, Kühl M. An updated overview on Wnt signaling pathways a prelude for more. Circ Res. 2010;106(12):1798–806.
69. Goodwin A, D'Amore P. Wnt signaling in the vasculature. Angiogenesis. 2002;5(1–2):1–9.
70. Cohen ED, Tian Y, Morrisey EE. Wnt signaling: an essential regulator of cardiovascular differentiation, morphogenesis and progenitor self-renewal. Development. 2008;135 (5):789–98.
71. Rawlings JS, Rosler KM, Harrison DA. The JAK/STAT signaling pathway. J Cell Sci. 2004;117(8):1281–3.
72. Mascareno E, El-Shafei M, Maulik N, et al. JAK/STAT signaling is associated with cardiac dysfunction during ischemia and reperfusion. Circulation. 2001;104(3):325–9.
73. Zhang S, Liu X, Goldstein S, et al. Role of the JAK/STAT signaling pathway in the pathogenesis of acute myocardial infarction in rats and its effect on NF-κB expression. Mol Med Rep. 2013;7(1):93–8.
74. Hong C. Comparative proteomics study on compatibility mechanism of effective components of Qishen Yiqi formula. Hangzhou: Zhejiang University; 2010. (in Chinese) [洪诚韬. 比较蛋白质组学研究芪参益气方有效组分的配伍机制. 杭州:浙江大学, 2010].
75. Shi P. Fragmentation of four components of traditional Chinese medicine by mass spectrometry and pharmacokinetics of Qishen Yiqi formula. Hangzhou: Zhejiang University; 2010. (in Chinese) [史培颖. 中药四类成分质谱裂解规律及芪参益气方药代动力学研究. 杭州:浙江大学, 2010].

76. Li YF, Qu HB, Cheng YY. Identification of major constituents in the traditional Chinese medicine "QI-SHEN-YI-QI" dropping pill by high-performance liquid chromatography coupled with diode array detection-electrospray ionization tandem mass spectrometry. J Pharm Biomed Anal. 2008;47(2):407–12.
77. Li Y, Wang Y, Qu H, et al. Simultaneous determination of seven bioactive compounds in Chinese medicine "QI-SHEN-YI-QI" dropping pill by LC-UV and LC-ELSD. Chromatographia. 2008;67(3–4):293–7.
78. Wang J. Chemical basis and mechanism of Qishen Yiqi dropping pills. Tianjin: Nankai University; 2011. (in Chinese) [王静. 复方中药芪参益气滴丸化学物质基础与作用机理研究. 天津:南开大学, 2011].
79. Hong C, Wang Y, Lou J, et al. The effect of Qi Shen Yiqi prescription on myocardial proteome in rats with acute myocardial infarction. Chinese J Traditional Chinese Med. 2009;34 (8):1018–21 (in Chinese) [洪诚韬, 王毅, 楼剑洲, 等. 芪参益气方对急性心肌梗死大鼠心肌蛋白质组的影响. 中国中药杂志, 2009, 34(8): 1018–1021].
80. Yan X, Wu N, Guo Z, et al. Traditional Chinese medicine preparation for treating angina pectoris of coronary heart disease and its preparation method. China. 2005 (in Chinese) [闫希军, 吴迺峰, 郭治昕, 等. 治疗冠心病心绞痛的中药制剂及其制备方法. 中国. 2005].
81. Wei C, Zhu M, Du W, et al. Research progress on clinical application of Qishen Yiqi dropping pills. Western Chinese Med. 2011;24(10):102–6 (in Chinese) [魏聪聪, 朱明丹, 杜武勋, 等. 芪参益气滴丸临床应用研究进展. 西部中医药, 2011, 24(10): 102–106].
82. Zhu X. Clinical observation of Huangqi Danshen dripping pills in treating angina pectoris of coronary heart disease. Beijing: Beijing University of Traditional Chinese Medicine; 2002. (in Chinese) [朱晓泉. 黄芪丹参滴丸治疗冠心病心绞痛临床观察. 北京:北京中医药大学, 2002].
83. Li Y. Clinical study on Huangqi Danshen dripping pill in treating angina pectoris of coronary heart disease with qi deficiency and blood stasis syndrome. Beijing: Beijing University of Traditional Chinese Medicine; 2003. (in Chinese) [李玉峰. 黄芪丹参滴丸治疗冠心病心绞痛气虚血瘀证的临床研究. 北京:北京中医药大学, 2003].
84. Wang Y, Gao X. Experimental study on the anti-acute myocardial ischemia induced by pituitrin with Huangqi Danshen drop pills. New Chinese Med Clin Pharmacol. 2003;14(2): 91–3 (in Chinese) [王怡, 高秀梅. 黄芪丹参滴丸抗垂体后叶素致大鼠急性心肌缺血的实验研究. 中药新药与临床药理, 2003, 14(2): 91–93].
85. Zhang B, Wang Y. Basic research on key scientific problems of prescriptions--development of modern Chinese medicine based on component compatibility. Chinese Nat Med. 2005;3(5): 258–61 (in Chinese) [张伯礼,王永炎. 方剂关键科学问题的基础研究--以组分配伍研制现代中药. 中国天然药物, 2005, 3(5):258–261].
86. Nicolaou CA, Brown N. Multi-objective optimization methods in drug design. Drug Discov Today Technol. 2013;10(3):e315–450.
87. Sirota M, Dudley JT, Kim J, et al. Discovery and preclinical validation of drug indications using compendia of public gene expression data. Sci Transl Med. 2011;3(96):96ra77.
88. Dudley JT, Sirota M, Shenoy M, et al. Computational repositioning of the anticonvulsant topiramate for inflammatory bowel disease. Sci Transl Med. 2011;3(96):96ra76.

Chapter 9
Drug-Disease-Based Network Pharmacology Practice Process

Weiwei Su and Panlin Li

Abstract The chemical composition of traditional Chinese medicine (TCM) is inordinately complex; therefore, it is a daunting task to reflect on its integrity and methodology by means of adopting the reductionist philosophy of western medicine. It cannot quintessentially manifest the scientific nature of TCM. The augmentation of modern scientific research and the introduction of network pharmacology have gradually transformed the research idea of single component and single target to the overall regulation of a complex system. Network pharmacology studies problems from the perspective of interrelation, which coincides with the core holistic view of Chinese medicine. Therefore, the application of network pharmacology in the study of TCM has unique advantages, and is conducive to a thorough understanding of the value and significance of the overall view of TCM. Several related studies have also emerged. In this chapter, single medicinal components and compound preparations are taken as examples to demonstrate the commonly used drug-disease-based network pharmacology analysis methods from two research examples.

9.1 Study on Network Pharmacology of Exocarpium Citri Grandis in the Treatment of Respiratory Diseases

Exocarpium Citri Grandis is an authentic medicinal materials in Lingnan. It has a significant effect on relieving cough and reducing phlegm and has a history of thousands of years of clinical application. Studies have validated that Exocarpium Citri Grandis not only has antitussive and expectorant effects, but also has an obvious inhibitory effect on acute and chronic respiratory inflammation, and can also promote the regression of inflammation [1–3]. However, due to the complexity of the ingredients and mechanism of action of TCM, it is difficult to carry out in-depth research on the pharmacodynamic mechanism of Exocarpium Citri Grandis, and such research conducted so far has lacked pertinence. Network

W. Su (✉) · P. Li
Sun Yat-sen University, Guangzhou, China

S. Li (ed.), *Network Pharmacology*, https://doi.org/10.1007/978-981-16-0753-0_9

pharmacology provides new research ideas and technical channels to resolve this issue. The overall research idea is first, clarify the chemical component basis of TCM by means of HPLC-MS and construct a library of chemical ingredients. At the same time, use data mining methodology to collect disease-related protein targets and construct a protein target library. Subsequently, calculate the correlation between ingredients and targets by means of molecular docking, and construct the component-target network. Furthermore, employ proteomics, transcriptomics, and disease-related biochemical indicators to verify the prediction results, and establish a regulatory network linking ingredients, targets, pathways, and efficacy of TCM, to explore the complex mechanism of TCM from the holistic perspective.

9.1.1 Prediction of Action Target of Exocarpium Citri Grandis in the Treatment of Respiratory Diseases

9.1.1.1 Analysis of Chemical Ingredients in Exocarpium Citri Grandis Based on UFLC-Triple TOF-MS/MS

We implemented a systematic online separation and identification of chemical components in medicinal components of Exocarpium Citri Grandis by employing UFLC-Triple TOF-MS/MS technology. By comparing with reference substances, accurate molecular weight, and analysis of mass spectrometry cracking behavior, a total of 48 compounds were confirmed and indicated, including 19 flavonoids, 16 coumarins, eight limonoids, and five organic acid compounds (as shown in Fig. 9.1). In addition, the flavonoid components in Exocarpium Citri Grandis mostly exist in the form of glycosides. After oral administration, flavonoid glycosides rapidly remove the glycosylates and turn into corresponding glycosides [4] under the action of intestinal flora β-glucosidase. Therefore, when the molecules are docked, the corresponding aglycones can be used for calculation. The chemical structure of each compound (shown in Table 9.1) was saved in the MOL file format, and used as the ligand for molecular docking calculation.

9.1.1.2 Construction of Target Database for Respiratory Diseases

Protein target information related to respiratory diseases were mined and sorted from multiple public databases such as ChEMBL, DrugBank, ClinicalTrials, BindingDB, Scifinder, SuperTarget, Protein Data Bank, KEGG, and other literature. At present, there are 426 protein targets included in the database, which are divided into the following categories: (1) 153 enzymes, such as 6-phosphate glucose dehydrogenase, histone deacetylase, and arachidonic acid-5-lipoxygenase, phosphodiesterase, etc.; (2) 105 membrane receptors, such as adenosine receptors, adrenergic receptors, chemokine receptors, etc.; (3) 73 unclassified proteins, such as calmodulin protein,

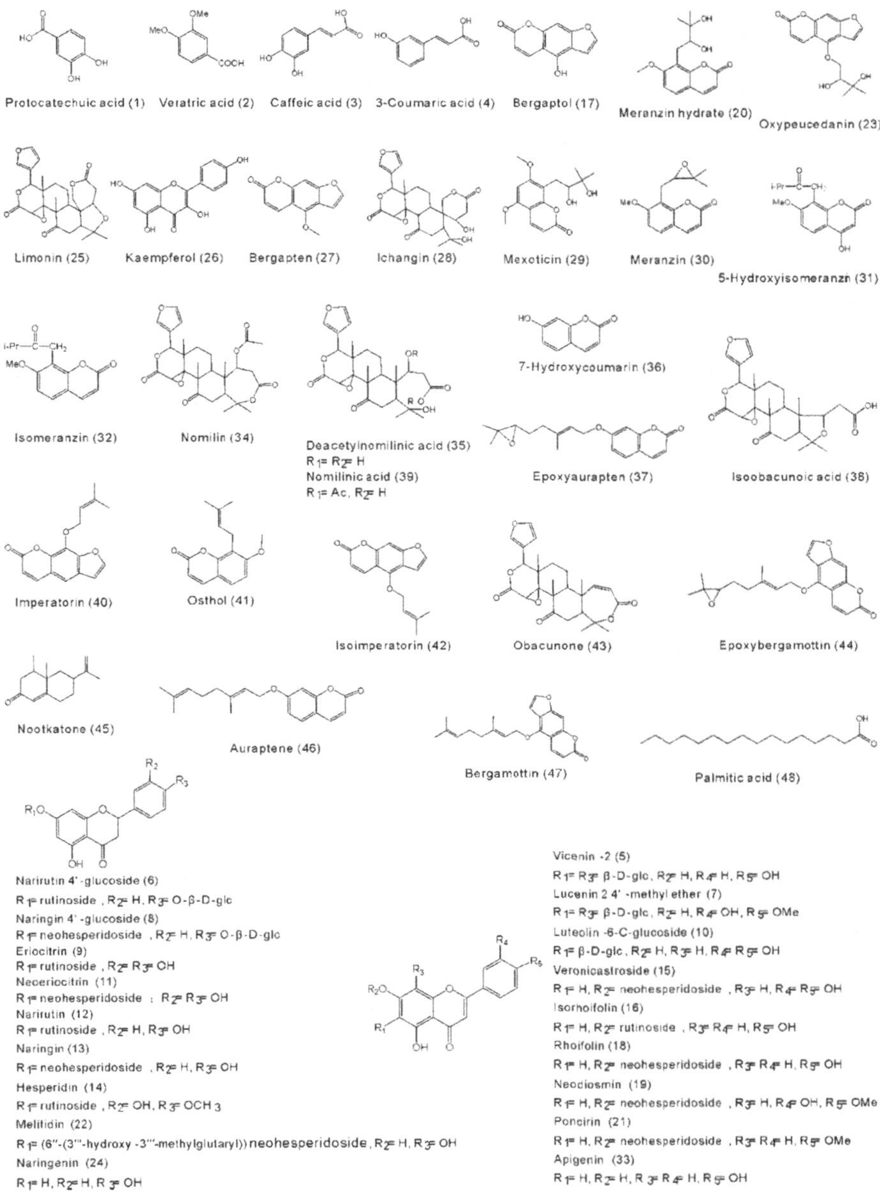

Fig. 9.1 Chemical components of Exocarpium Citri Grandis

integrin protein, heat shock protein, etc.; (4) 37 ion channel proteins, such as voltage-dependent potassium channel, calcium-activated potassium ion channel, sodium channel proteins, etc.; (5) 19 transcription factors, such as peroxisome proliferator activated receptor, glucocorticoid receptor, etc.; (6) 15 secretory

Table 9.1 Compounds used for molecular docking calculation

No.	Compounds	No.	Compounds
F01	Naringenin (Naringin, Narirutin, Melitidin)	C11	Imperatorin
F02	Apigenin (Rhoifolin, Isorhoifolin)	C12	Osthole
F03	Eriodictyol (Eriocitrin, Neoeriocitrin)	C13	Isoimperatorin
F04	Luteolin (Isoorientin, Lonicerin)	C14	Epoxybergamottin
F05	Diosmetin (Neodiosmin)	C15	Auraptene
F06	Hesperetin (Hesperidin)	C16	Bergamottin
F07	Isosakuranetin (Poncirin)	L01	Limonin
F08	Kaempferol	L02	Ichangin
F09	Lucenin-2 4′-methyl ether	L03	Nomilin
F10	Vicenin-2	L04	Deacetylnomilin acid
C01	Bergaptol	L05	Isoobacunoic acid
C02	Meranzin hydrate	L06	Nomilinic acid
C03	Oxypeucedanin	L07	Obacunone
C04	Bergaptene	L08	Nootkatone
C05	Mexoticin	O01	Protocatechuic acid
C06	Meranzin	O02	Veratric acid
C07	Hydroxyisohesperidin	O03	Caffeic acid
C08	Isomeranzin	O04	Coumaric acid
C09	Hydroxycoumarin	O04	Palmitic acid
C10	Epoxyaurapten		

Note: *F* flavone, *C* coumarin, *L* limonin, *O* organic acid. The flavone glycosides represented by aglycones are in brackets

proteins, such as tumor necrosis factor, interleukin, chemokine, etc.; (7) 14 transporter proteins, such as solute transporter, ATP binding cassette, etc.; (8) seven adhesion proteins, such as intercellular adhesion molecules, selectins, etc.; (9) three surface antigen proteins, such as T cell wall glycoprotein, T lymphocyte activation antibody, etc. The three-dimensional structure of each protein was downloaded from the Protein Data Bank as a receptor for the molecular docking calculations.

9.1.1.3 Target Prediction and Network Analysis

AutoDock Vina software was employed in molecular docking calculation. The docking score was evaluated and ranked based on the interaction between the compound molecule and the target protein structure, as in the case of hydrogen bonding, van der Waals force, hydrophobic interaction, etc. The docking score represents the predicted value of $-\log_{10}(K_d)$ between the compound and the target protein. The target with the docking score >6, that is, the protein dissociation constant K_d value $<10^{-6}$, was selected as the potential action target of the target compound. Cytoscape software was employed to visualize the results of molecular docking. Nodes represent chemical components, action targets, and signaling pathways, and the connecting lines represent the connections between components,

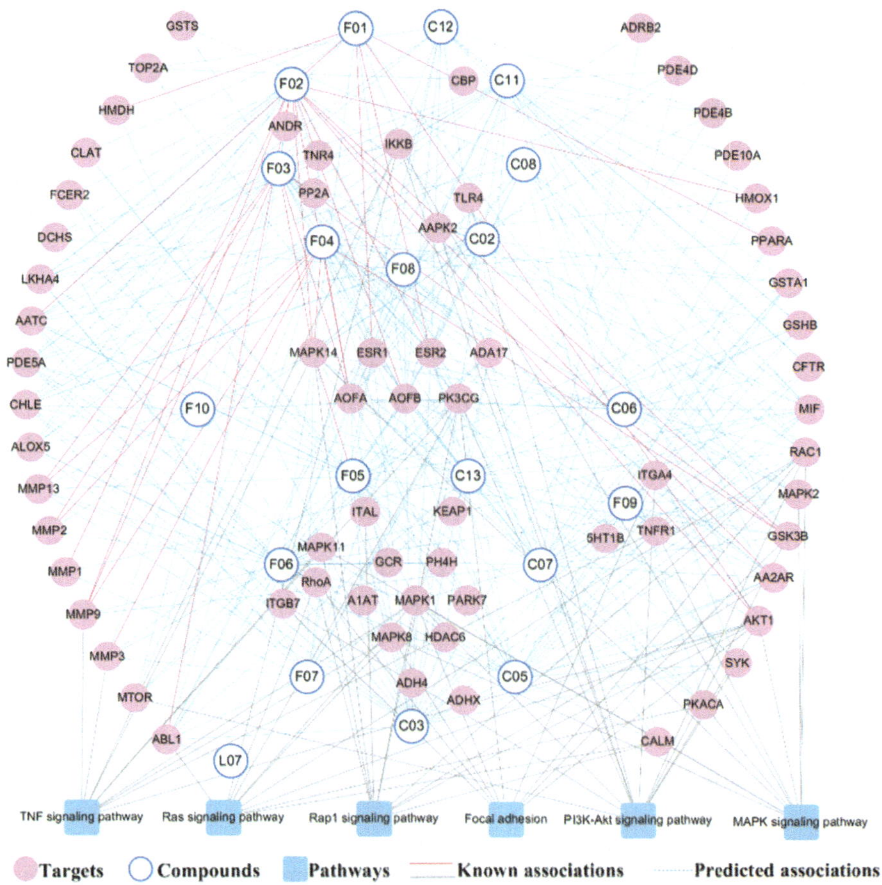

Fig. 9.2 Component-target-pathway network diagram of Exocarpium Citri Grandis

targets, and pathways to construct a network diagram (as shown in Fig. 9.2). The signaling pathway information was obtained using DAVID analysis tools [5, 6], and all the targets in the respiratory disease target library were used as the background; the calculated potential targets of the compounds were subjected to KEGG signaling pathway enrichment analysis.

The results demonstrate that most flavonoids and coumarins have more targets that associate with each other, with all the organic acids, and with most of the limonin and individual coumarin components. A total of 19 compounds were excluded due to fewer related targets (<5). Hence, flavonoids and coumarins are the main active components of Exocarpium Citri Grandis in the treatment of respiratory diseases. The chemical components with the largest number of related targets are diosmetin (F05), imperatorin (C11), luteolin (F04), oxypeucedanin (C03), and eriodictyol (F03). The targets with the largest number of related compounds include MAPK14, AOFB, ESR1, ESR2, AOFA, and PK3CG. The interactions between a handful of ingredients and targets have been confirmed in literature and are shown in pink lines in Fig. 9.2. The potential targets of Exocarpium Citri Grandis are closely related to many signaling pathways, including key inflammatory signal transduction pathways such as TNF signaling pathway, PI3K-Akt signaling pathway, and MAPK signaling pathway; and cell connection-related pathways such as Ras signaling pathway, Rap1 signaling pathway, and Focal adhesion. The calculation results were combined with the experimental verification data for a comprehensive analysis.

9.1.2 Verification of the Action Targets of Exocarpium Citri Grandis in the Treatment of Respiratory Diseases

Due to the complexity of target prediction results, high-throughput iTRAQ quantitative proteomics technology was employed for experimental verification. Employing a mouse model of acute lung inflammation caused by cigarette smoke, iTRAQ was used to investigate the regulatory effect of Exocarpium Citri Grandis on the overall protein expression level, and to comprehensively analyze the mechanism of action of Exocarpium Citri Grandis in the treatment of respiratory diseases by combining with the target prediction results.

9.1.2.1 Animal Model

The stimulation of cigarette smoke can initiate various pathological changes in the respiratory system, such as increasing parasympathetic excitability, bronchoconstriction and spasms, mucosal hyperemia, edema and increased secretion, inflammation, etc. Therefore, the mouse model of acute pulmonary inflammation caused by cigarette smoke was selected for the experiments. The Balb/c mice were divided into six groups randomly, each with ten mice, namely: normal group, model group, positive drug dexamethasone (DEX) group (5 mg/kg), and Exocarpium Citri Grandis extract (CGE) group (80 mg/kg). Intragastric administration was given 1 h before the first cigarette smoking event every day. The intragastric administration volume was 0.1 mL/10 g body weight. The normal group and the model group were given an identical amount of normal saline.

The animals were first adapted to the new environment and raised for 7 days before initiating the smoking events and modeling. The smoking events were conducted twice a day, with an interval of 4 h. During each smoking event, eight cigarettes were smoked for 1 h, for five consecutive days. The mice were sacrificed by removing the cervical vertebrae 16 h after the last smoking event; the thorax was incised, and the left and right lung tissues were removed, quickly placed on ice, and washed with PBS buffer solution. The right lung was fixed with 4%

paraformaldehyde after cleaning and used to make hematoxylin-eosin-stained tissue sections. The left lung was cut into pieces with small scissors, the residual blood was fully washed, and it was then stored in a sealed bag in at refrigerator at −80 °C, for proteomics analysis.

9.1.2.2 Histopathological Examination

First, the pathological changes in the lung tissue of the mouse caused by the cigarette smoke were observed in the pathological sections. As shown in Fig. 9.3, the results of hematoxylin-eosin-stained lung tissue slices of mice after the acute smoking model demonstrate that compared to the normal group, the alveolar cavity of the model group was reduced, and the alveolar wall and alveolar compartment were thickened. There was proliferation of fibrous tissue and normal alveolar tissue had changed. At the same time, thickening of bronchiole wall, inflammatory cell infiltration, and exudation of inflammatory cells in the lumen were also observed (as shown by the arrow). After administration of positive drug and Exocarpium Citri Grandis, the thickening of alveolar wall and bronchial wall was reduced to various degrees and the degree of pulmonary edema and lesion level alleviated.

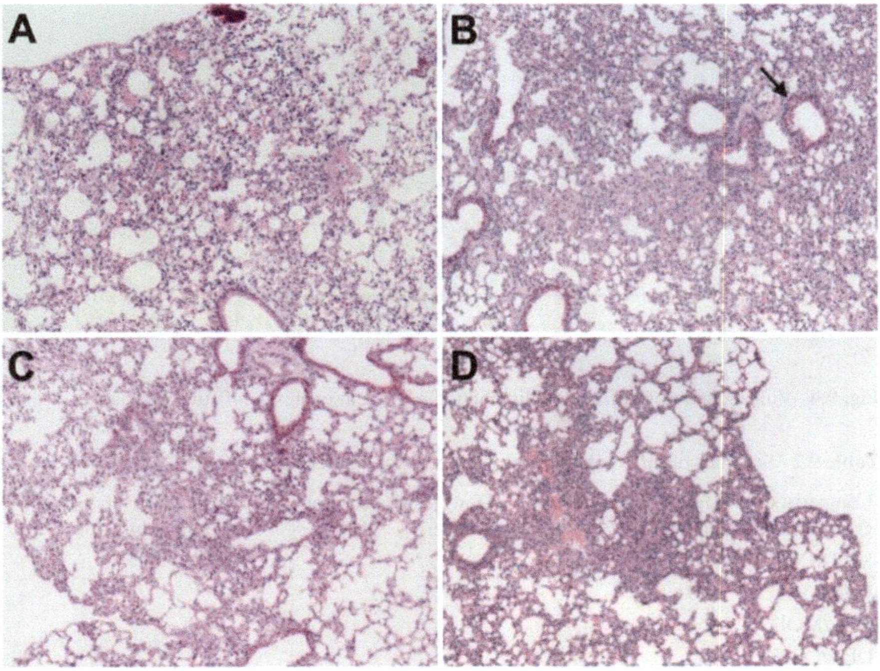

Fig. 9.3 Hematoxylin-eosin staining results of mouse lung tissue. (**a**) Normal group; (**b**) Model group; (**c**) Dexamethasone group; (**d**) Exocarpium Citri Grandis group

9.1.2.3 Proteomic Analysis of iTRAQ

Protein Identification and Differential Protein Expression Analysis

The iTRAQ kit (AB Sciex) was employed for proteomics detection. There are four groups of samples, namely the normal group (CON), the model group (MOD), the dexamethasone group (DEX), and the Exocarpium Citri Grandis extract group (CGE), and each set has one technical replicate. A total of 12,232 peptides and 3528 proteins were identified. IQuant (BGI) software was used for quantitative analysis. The results of each pair of neighboring samples of the four groups of samples were compared. According to the volcanogram of protein expression differential distribution (as shown in Fig. 9.4), proteins with differential expression Q value <0.05 were selected as differential proteins (as shown in Table 9.2).

Bioinformatics Analysis of Differentially Expressed Proteins

Cluster analysis: Cluster analysis was performed on differential proteins, and maps were employed for visualization processing (as shown in Fig. 9.5) to investigate the

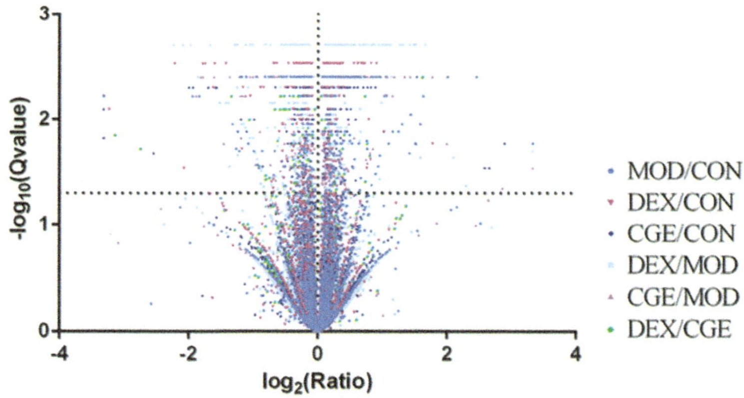

Fig. 9.4 Volcanogram of differential distribution of protein expression between groups

Table 9.2 Statistics of differentially expressed proteins between groups

Comparison group	Up-regulated protein number	Down-regulated protein number	Total number of differential proteins
MOD/CON	57	60	117
DEX/MOD	119	113	232
CGE/MOD	63	58	121
DEX/CON	94	86	180
CGE/CON	46	41	87
DEX/CGE	79	57	136

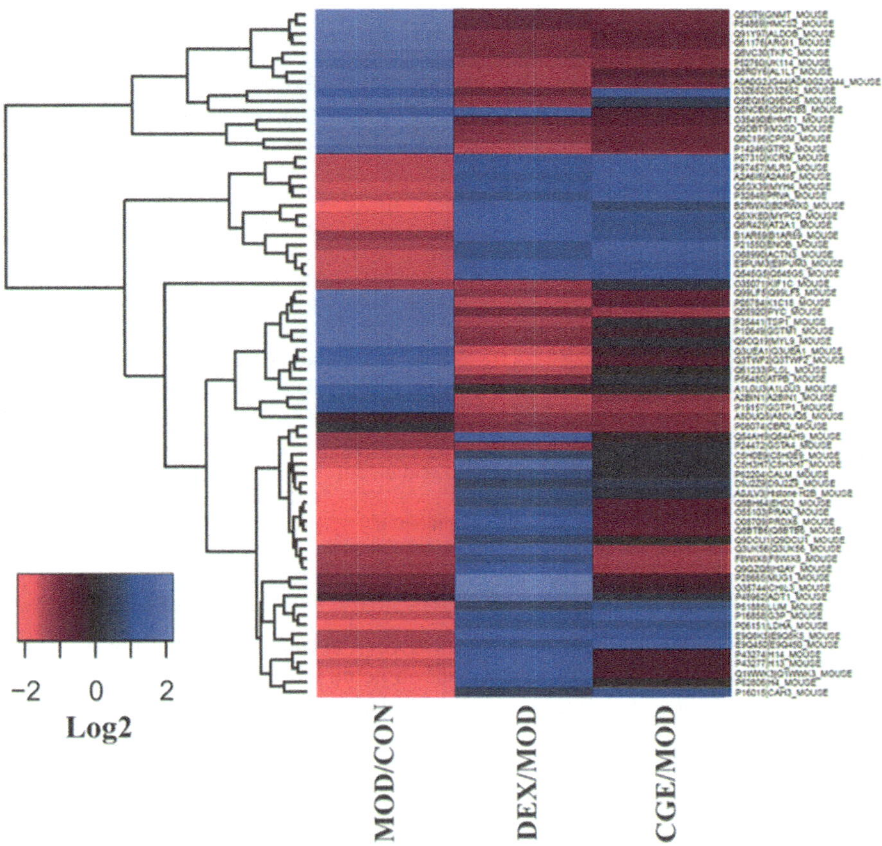

Fig. 9.5 Cluster analysis of differentially expressed proteins

correlation and difference of differential proteins between different groups. The results demonstrate that the positive drug dexamethasone (DEX) has distinct degrees of callback to the differential expression protein (MOD/CON) caused by modeling, which indicates that dexamethasone had a wide, rapid, and powerful therapeutic effect on acute inflammation. Exocarpium Citri Grandis (CGE) has similar regulation effect to dexamethasone on differential proteins related to cell junction and metabolism but has no effect on mitochondrial function and histone-related differential proteins.

Gene Ontology (GO) enrichment analysis: The enrichment results are demonstrated in Table 9.3. The enrichment results of different proteins between the model group and the normal group in terms of biological processes show the presence of stimulation of the mouse lung tissue by the cigarette smoke and activation of the metabolism process of exogenous small molecules. At the same time, the smoke stimulation also affects the process of actin, which may be related to the morphological changes of pulmonary vascular smooth muscle cells. In terms of molecular

Table 9.3 Enrichment analysis results of differentially expressed protein GO

Group	Cellular component	Molecular function	Biological process
MOD/CON	Actin cytoskeleton Myosin complex Filamentous actin	Calcium ion binding	Generation of precursor metabolites and energy Small molecule metabolic process Response to chemical stimulus Muscle system process
DEX/MOD	Extracellular region part Myosin complex Extracellular space	Oxygen binding	Response to lipid Response to extracellular stimulus Response to purine-containing compound Response to nutrient levels Response to glucocorticoid stimulus Response to endogenous stimulus
CGE/MOD	Contractile fiber Actin cytoskeleton Myosin complex	Modified amino acid binding Structural constituent of cytoskeleton	Muscle system process Cellular amino acid metabolic process

functions, differential proteins are mainly enriched in calcium ion binding activities. On the one hand, calcium ions directly act on actin, and are also important second messengers, participating in various signal regulation processes including the release of inflammatory factors. In terms of cellular components, the differentially expressed proteins are mainly enriched in the actin cytoskeleton and myosin structure, which indicates that the smoking modeling may also affect the proliferation and migration of pulmonary vascular smooth muscle cells and the integrity of epithelial cells. The differentially expressed proteins affected by dexamethasone are involved in the response to glucocorticoids in biological processes, including regulating the synthesis and metabolism of nutrients such as lipids and purine compounds, and regulating the immune response induced by endogenous and extracellular response. In terms of cellular components, there is enrichment of extracellular components and compartments and the myosin complex, which may be related to the pharmacological effects in regulating vascular permeability and inhibiting the directional migration of inflammatory cells. The enrichment results of Exocarpium Citri Grandis show that its effect is mainly reflected in the regulation of cytoskeleton and amino acid modification binding activity.

Enrichment analysis of KEGG signaling pathway: Proteins usually perform certain biological functions through mutual connection. Based on the KEGG database, differentially expressed proteins were analyzed for signaling pathway enrichment. The enrichment results are shown in Table 9.4. The signaling pathways closely related to the differential proteins between the model group and the normal group include: Metabolism of xenobiotics by cytochrome P450 related to the metabolism of exogenous substances, tight junction pathways associated with cellular connectivity and barrier function, focal adhesion pathways, leukocyte

Table 9.4 Enrichment analysis results of KEGG signaling pathway of differentially expressed proteins

Group	Pathway	DEPs with pathway annotation	*P* value
MOD/CON	Carbon metabolism	10	1.41E-04
	Biosynthesis of amino acids	9	1.90E-04
	Focal adhesion	9	1.29E-03
	Tight junction	8	1.45E-02
	Metabolism of xenobiotics by cytochrome P450	7	1.48E-03
	Glycolysis/gluconeogenesis	5	4.74E-03
	Leukocyte transendothelial migration	5	3.65E-02
DEX/MOD	Carbon metabolism	14	6.86E-05
	Focal adhesion	14	7.54E-03
	Biosynthesis of amino acids	11	2.36E-04
	Glycolysis/gluconeogenesis	8	9.04E-03
	ECM-receptor interaction	8	2.79E-02
	Leukocyte transendothelial migration	8	9.39E-03
	Metabolism of xenobiotics by cytochrome P450	7	3.54E-02
	Small cell lung cancer	6	2.40E-02
CGE/MOD	Carbon metabolism	14	1.20E-10
	Biosynthesis of amino acids	11	5.00E-09
	Glycolysis/gluconeogenesis	10	1.80E-08
	Tight junction	8	5.20E-04
	Focal adhesion	8	5.10E-03
	Adrenergic signaling in cardiomyocytes	6	1.80E-02
	Metabolism of xenobiotics by cytochrome P450	6	1.20E-02
	Glutathione metabolism	5	2.30E-03
	Leukocyte transendothelial migration	5	3.50E-02
	Dilated cardiomyopathy	5	1.00E-02
	Cardiac muscle contraction	4	4.40E-02

transendothelial migration, material and energy metabolism related pathways, carbon metabolism, biosynthesis of amino acids, and glycolysis/gluconeogenesis. The enrichment results of dexamethasone show that its effect is related to maintaining the stability of actin filament, which is the specific protective effect of the glucocorticoid [7]. At the same time, it may also play a role in reducing vascular permeability, reducing tissue congestion and leucocyte exudation, and recruitment of white blood cells through adhesion plaques, extracellular matrix receptors, and leukocyte migration signaling pathways across the endothelium, in order to reduce tissue inflammation reaction, which is consistent with its known mechanism of action. There are many signaling pathways enriched by the differentially expressed proteins caused by

Exocarpium Citri Grandis, which reflects the complexity of the regulation methods of multi-component drugs. The role of Exocarpium Citri Grandis is related to pathways such as tight junctions, focal adhesion, and actin cytoskeleton regulation. In addition, it is also involved in the process of muscle excitation and contraction.

9.1.3 Analysis of the Regulatory Network of Exocarpium Citri Grandis in the Treatment of Respiratory Diseases

The overall regulatory network of Exocarpium Citri Grandis in the treatment of respiratory diseases is discussed combining the results of molecular docking, iTRAQ proteomics testing, and reported pharmacological experiment results (as shown in Fig. 9.6). In terms of antitussive effect, the mechanism may be related to airway smooth muscle relaxation related to cGMP level, wherein the PDE5 is the key target. At the same time, it may also act on PP2A and CALM in the tight junction pathway to maintain the stability of the airway barrier function, thereby reducing the exposure of peripheral RARs receptors, inhibiting the release of substance P, and reducing cough. In addition, the predicted major potential targets of Exocarpium Citri Grandis are the upstream regulatory molecules of PI3K-Akt and Mapk14 pathway. There have been several studies that demonstrate that Exocarpium Citri Grandis has an agreeable anti-inflammatory effect on respiratory inflammation [1–3], and can affect the gene expression of inflammatory cytokines such as TNF-α. Therefore, based on comprehensive analysis it is speculated that the regulatory network is associated with anti-respiratory inflammation in Exocarpium Citri Grandis. Adhesion spot pathway and other cell connection-related pathways can mediate cell adhesion and migration and are closely related to promoting the release of inflammatory factors and the development of tissue inflammation. They may also be a key link in the anti-inflammatory mechanism of Exocarpium Citri Grandis. Inflammation also has a vast impact on the secretion of mucin in sputum. Our previous research demonstrated that naringin, the main active ingredient of Exocarpium Citri Grandis, can inhibit the increase of MUC5AC content and goblet cell proliferation by inhibiting MAPKs-AP-1 and IKKs-IkB-NF-κB B pathways [1–3], which is consistent with the speculated regulatory network of Exocarpium Citri Grandis, and can also explain the mechanism of Exocarpium Citri Grandis in relieving of cough and phlegm.

The association between the binding ingredients and the target was analyzed. The key proteins ITGB, RhoA, and PP2A in the adhesion junction regulation pathway have flavonoids acting on their own, suggesting that flavonoids may play a major role in maintaining the airway barrier function. At the same time, CALM, the target of coumarins acting on their own may affect actin synthesis through calcium ion signals, and on the other hand, affect barrier function. Most of the targets in inflammation-related signaling pathways are common targets of flavonoids and coumarins. This also reflects several possible mechanisms of multi-component

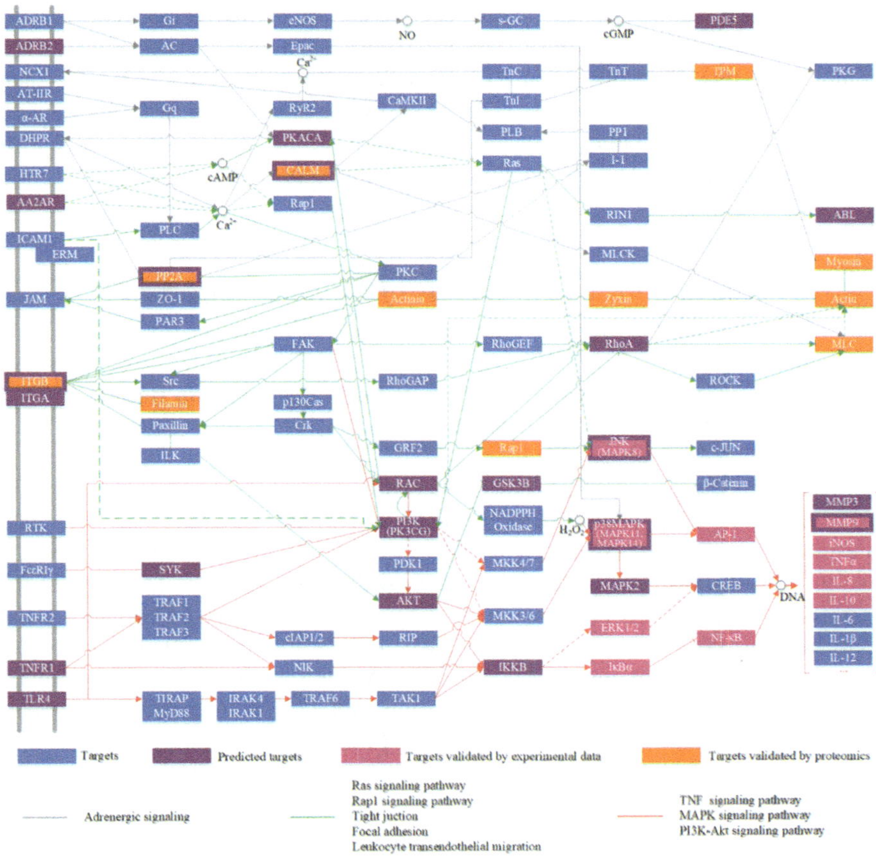

Fig. 9.6 Regulatory network of Exocarpium Citri Grandis in the treatment of respiratory diseases

synergistic action of TCM, including different components acting on the same target, acting on different targets of the same signaling pathway, or interrelated different signaling pathway targets. The results of this study provide an important basis for further exploration of the mechanism of action of Exocarpium Citri Grandis and its active ingredients and guide the clinical application of Exocarpium Citri Grandis.

9.2 Network Pharmacological Study on the Treatment of Cardiovascular Diseases with Danhong Injection

Danhong injection is a TCM preparation composed of Salvia miltiorrhiza and safflower. It is widely used clinically in the treatment of coronary heart disease, angina pectoris, myocardial infarction, and other cardiovascular diseases. The pathogenesis of cardiovascular disease is complex, involving coagulation, inflammation, oxidative stress, and other systems; at the same time, Danhong injection is a complex mixture. Network pharmacology provides a new method to resolve such complex problems. This section employs network pharmacology technology to study the overall regulatory mechanism of Danhong injection in the treatment of cardiovascular disease and the scientific compatibility of its prescription.

9.2.1 Prediction of Action Targets of Danhong Injection in the Treatment of Cardiovascular Diseases

9.2.1.1 Chemical Composition Analysis of Danhong Injection Based on UFLC-Triple ToF-MS/MS

The chemical components of Danhong injection were detected online and sorted using UFLC-DAD-Q-TOF-MS/MS technology. Through comparison of reference substances, precise molecular weight search, and secondary lysis pattern analysis, a total of 82 chemical components were confirmed and identified in Danhong injection, including two alkaloids, three nucleosides, six amino acids, five organic acids, four iridoid glycosides, seven flavonoids, five quinone chalcones, 39 phenolic acids, eight tanshinone, and three other compounds. At the same time, the attribution of each component was determined by comparing with a single medicinal component. There are 17 components in both salvia and Carthamus tinctorius, mainly amino acids and nucleosides; there are 32 components only attributable to Salvia, mainly including phenolic acids and tanshinones; and there are 22 components only attributable to Carthamus tinctorius, mainly flavonoids, quinone chalcones, and iridoid glycosides. In addition, 11 kinds of phenolic acids were not detected in the two medicinal components, and were newly generated during the production process. The molecular structure of each compound is stored in MOL format as a ligand for molecular docking.

9.2.1.2 Action Target Prediction and Network Construction Analysis of Danhong Injection

The existing cardiovascular and cerebrovascular disease target database was employed for molecular docking calculation. The database includes 984 candidate protein targets and involves multiple pathophysiological processes such as thrombosis, endothelial function, energy metabolism, inflammation reaction, oxidative stress, etc. [8] The 82 chemical components of Danhong injection were molecularly docked with 984 protein targets, and a total of 64 active chemical components and 470 potential action targets were screened. The higher the number of components associated with the target, the stronger the influence of the components of Danhong, therefore it may be the main target of Danhong. The targets ranked high in the

Table 9.5 Potential action targets of chemical components of Danhong Injection (number of associated compounds ≥34)

No.	Target	Target name	Number of associated compounds
1	RENI	Renin	45
2	PDE5A	cGMP-specific 3′,5′-cyclic phosphodiesterase	45
3	HMDH	3-hydroxy-3-methylglutaryl-coenzyme A reductase	43
4	GDN	Glia-derived nexin	43
5	PDE4D	cAMP-specific 3′,5′-cyclic phosphodiesterase 4D	41
6	FOLH1	Glutamate carboxypeptidase 2	41
7	ACE	Angiotensin-converting enzyme	37
8	DPP4	Dipeptidyl peptidase 4	35
9	ANT3	Antithrombin-III	35
10	MK14	Mitogen-activated protein kinase 14	34

number of associated compounds are shown in Table 9.5, and mainly include: PDE5A, PDE4D, and MK14 that are associated with inflammatory response; ACE related to renin angiotensin system (angiotensin-converting enzyme); Reni (renin), FA10 (coagulation factor X), ANT3 (SERPINC1, antithrombin), PAFA, and PROC (protein C—coagulation factor VA and VIIIA inhibitors) associated with fibrinolysis system; HMDH associated with lipid metabolism; NOS3 (endothelial nitric oxide synthase) associated with endothelial function; and HMOX1 (heme oxygenase gene 1) associated with blood oxygen metabolism. Similarly, the more targets the compound is associated with, the stronger the regulatory activity of the component, thus it may be the main active component of Danhong. As shown in Table 9.6, the components with a large number of related targets are mainly salvianolic acid H, salvianolic acid I, and salvianolic acid A, followed by flavonoids such as Kaempferol-O-rutinoside, Kaempferol-di-O-glucoside, etc., as well as quinone chalcone such as Cartormin and Isocarthamin.

The correlation between the calculated components and targets was visualized by employing Cytoscape software. At the same time, the ClueGO plug-in was used to analyze the KEGG signal pathway of the targets in the network, to interpret the biological significance of the calculation results and the correlation between the targets, and to construct a component-target-signal pathway network. The results demonstrate that the potential action targets of Danhong injection are mainly enriched in antigen processing and presentation, B cell receptor signaling pathway and other pathways related to inflammation and immunity, complement and coagulation cascades signaling pathway related to the coagulation process, fluid shear stress and atherosclerosis pathway associated with cardiovascular disease, focal adhesion and other pathways related to endothelial function, and the key signal transduction pathways, namely PI3K Akt signaling pathway, MAPK signaling pathway, TNF signaling pathway, and Rap1 signaling pathway.

Table 9.6 Potential active ingredients of Danhong Injection (number of associated targets ≥100)

Compound serial no.	Compound name	Number of associated targets
SR-52	Salvianolic acid H	203
SR-53	Salvianolic acid I	199
SR-70	Salvianolic acid A	196
SR-65	Salvianolic acid E	174
SR-66	Salvianolic acid B	160
SR-56	Salvianolic acid D	157
SR-50	Salvianolic acid K	152
SR-59	Monomethyl lithospermate	152
SR-58	Salvianolic acid G	145
SR-62	Lithospermic acid	142
SR-61	Rosmarinic acid	109
SR-76	Salvianolic acid C	105
SR-67	Ethyl lithospermate	101

Furthermore, the associations between Danhong injection components and signaling pathways were explored by analyzing the number of targets associated with components in each signaling pathway. The results are shown in Fig. 9.7. The key signal transduction pathways, namely PI3K Akt signaling pathway, MAPK signaling pathway, TNF signaling pathway, Rap1 signaling pathway, and HIF-1 signaling pathway are strongly related to phenolic acids, flavonoids, and other ingredients. In addition, phenolic acids are also closely related to inflammation and immune-related pathways, such as antigen processing and presentation, B cell receptor signaling pathway, etc.; flavonoids are closely related to complement and coagulation cascades. The amino acids, nucleosides, organic acids, tanshinones, and other components in Danhong injection are associated with fewer targets, suggesting that the drug efficacy is also weak.

In summary, through molecular docking and network pharmacology analysis, the main active ingredients of Danhong injection in the treatment of cardiovascular diseases may be salvianolic acid H, salvianolic acid I, salvianolic acid A, and other salvianolic acids, as well as flavonoids such as Kaempferol-O-rutinoside and Kaempferol-di-O-glucoside, and quinoid chalcones such as Cartormin and Isocarthamin. The targets of these ingredients are enriched in the key signal transduction pathways PI3K-Akt and the MAPK signal pathway. In addition, the action target of Danhong injection is firmly correlated with inflammation, immunity, coagulation, endothelial function, and other related pathways. The phenolic acids derived from salvia focus more on inflammation and immune-related pathways, while the flavonoids derived from Carthamus tinctorius focus more on blood coagulation-related pathways, suggesting a mutual collaboration between the two herbs.

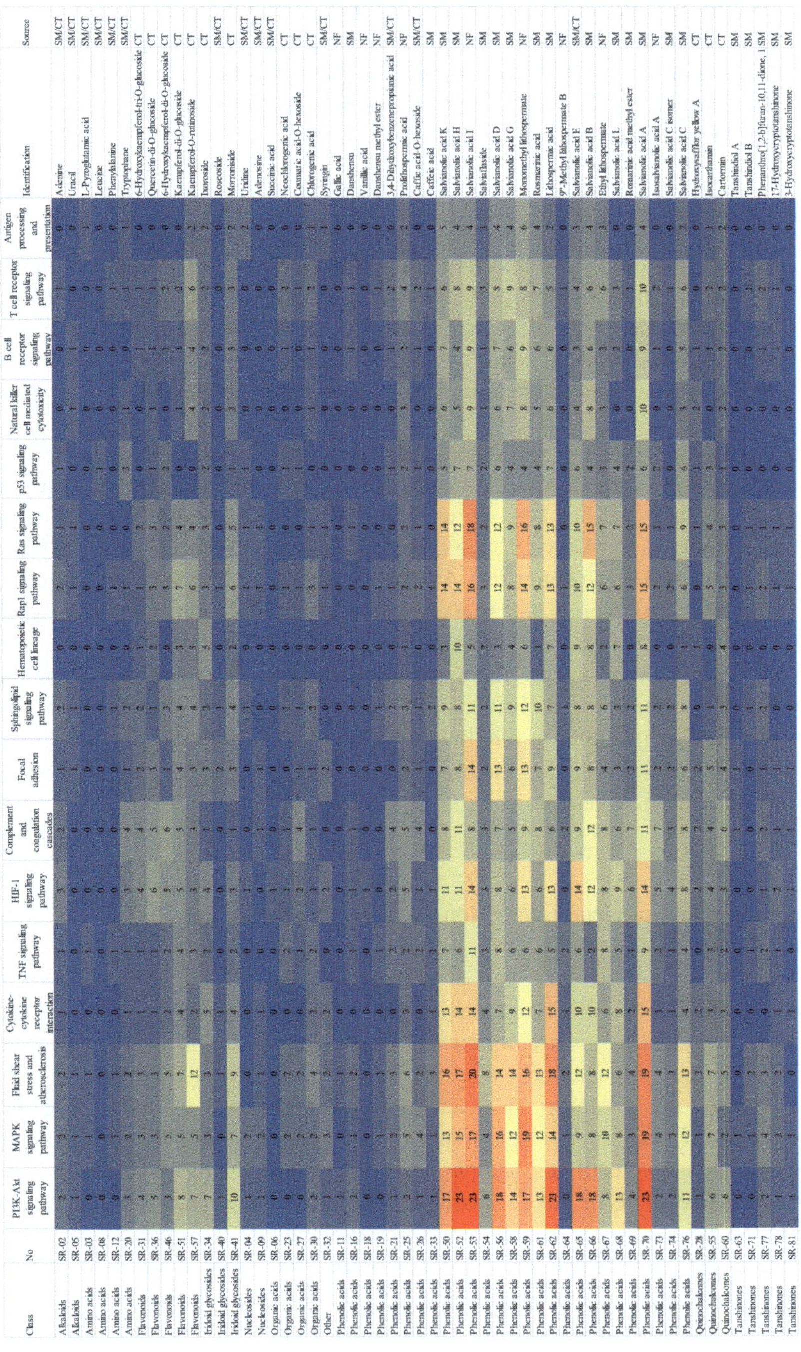

Fig. 9.7 Distribution of target points of active ingredients of Danhong injection in signal pathways of cardiovascular diseases (the numbers in the table refer to the number of targets)

9.2.2 Verification of Action Targets of Danhong Injection in the Treatment of Cardiovascular Diseases

9.2.2.1 Investigation of the Effect of Danhong Injection on Gene Expression in Rats with Acute Blood Stasis Based on Transcriptome

Animal Model

The SD rats were randomly divided into three groups: blank group (control), acute blood stasis model group (model), and Danhong injection group (3 mL/kg/d) (DHI), respectively, with three rats in each group. The Danhong injection group was administered intramuscular injection; and the blank control group and model group were injected with the same volume of normal saline, once a day for a period of ten consecutive days.

Thirty minutes after the last administration, except in the blank control group, rats in the other groups were injected subcutaneously with adrenaline hydrochloride 0.8 mg/kg, and rats in the blank group were injected subcutaneously with the same amount of normal saline. After 2 h, the rats in each group except the blank control group were immersed in ice water at 0–4 °C for 5 min. After 2 h, they were injected with adrenaline hydrochloride 0.8 mg/kg again [9]. After treatment, rats in each group were kept on fasting for 12 h and then administered with DHI or normal saline, respectively. And 15 min later, the rats were anesthetized by intraperitoneal injection of 10% chloral hydrate 0.35 mL/100 g, and blood was taken from the heart and they were sacrificed. One milliliter of whole blood was taken from each rat; three times the amount of trizol was added to the blood and it stored in a refrigerator at −80 °C for transcriptome detection.

Analysis of Amount of Gene Expression and Detection of Differentially Expressed Genes

Employing the BGISEQ-500RS sequencing platform, quantitative gene analysis and differential gene screening were conducted on the samples. The genes with Fold Change $\geq$4.00 and Adjusted *P* value $\leq$0.001 were employed as differentially expressed genes, and bioinformatics analysis was performed on them. The test results demonstrate that the average output of each sample is 23.70 M of data, the average comparison rate of the sample comparison genome is 96.24%, and the average comparison rate of the comparison gene set is 94.08%; a total of 13,416 genes were detected. The percentage of bases after filtering low-quality data was >90%, indicating that the sequencing quality is good. Compared to the model group, a total of 176 up-regulated genes and 145 down-regulated genes were detected in the blank group; compared to the Danhong group, a total of 1671 up-regulated genes and 14 down-regulated genes were detected in the model group.

Accuracy Verification of Transcriptome Sequencing

RT-qPCR method was employed to detect and calculate the relative expression amount of 15 genes, namely FN1, TLR4, PIK3cb, iNOS, IL-1R1, ITGB3, AP-1, JNK, NFκB, MHCII, IL-6R, Hif-1α, Ctsb, Xop7, and Retn, and the difference multiple of relative expression amount between the Danhong group and model group (as shown in Fig. 9.8), where Log_2 Fold Change (DHI/model) = Log_2 (Relative expression amount of Danhong group/relative expression amount of model group). The results demonstrate that the relative expression trend of each gene in qPCR results is consistent with that of transcriptome, signifying the accuracy and reliability of the transcriptome results.

Bioinformatics Analysis of Differentially Expressed Genes

Gene Ontology (GO) enrichment analysis: Go function enrichment analysis was conducted for the differentially expressed genes with respect to three aspects—molecular function, cell composition, and biological process. When comparing the model group and Danhong group (Model-VS-DHI) (as shown in Fig. 9.9), in terms of molecular functions, the differentially expressed genes were significantly enriched in adenyl ribonucleotide binding, kinase binding, transcription factor binding, and cation binding; in terms of cell composition, the differentially expressed genes were significantly enriched in MHC protein complex, cell surface, and vacuole; in terms of biological processes, the differentially expressed genes were significantly enriched in response to host immune response, response to cytokine, toll-like receptor signaling pathway, immune response-activating cell surface receptor signaling pathway, macrophage activation, antigen processing and presentation, regulation of MAPK cascade, and cellular protein modification process. It is suggested that upon administration of Danhong injection, the processes of RNA processing in cells, intracellular antigen presentation, MAPK cascade reaction, etc., are affected.

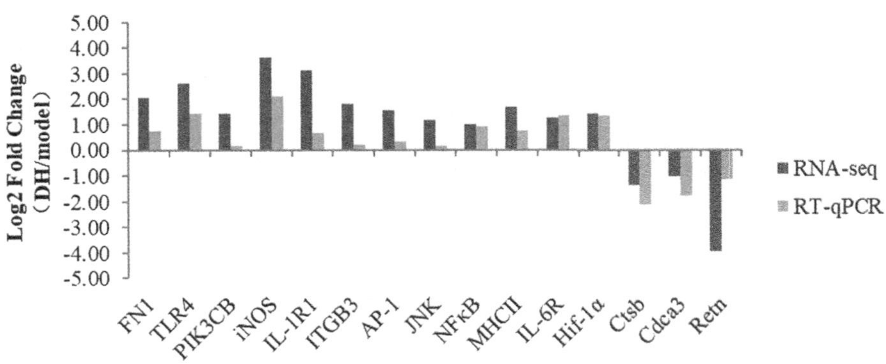

Fig. 9.8 qPCR-verified transcriptome sequencing results

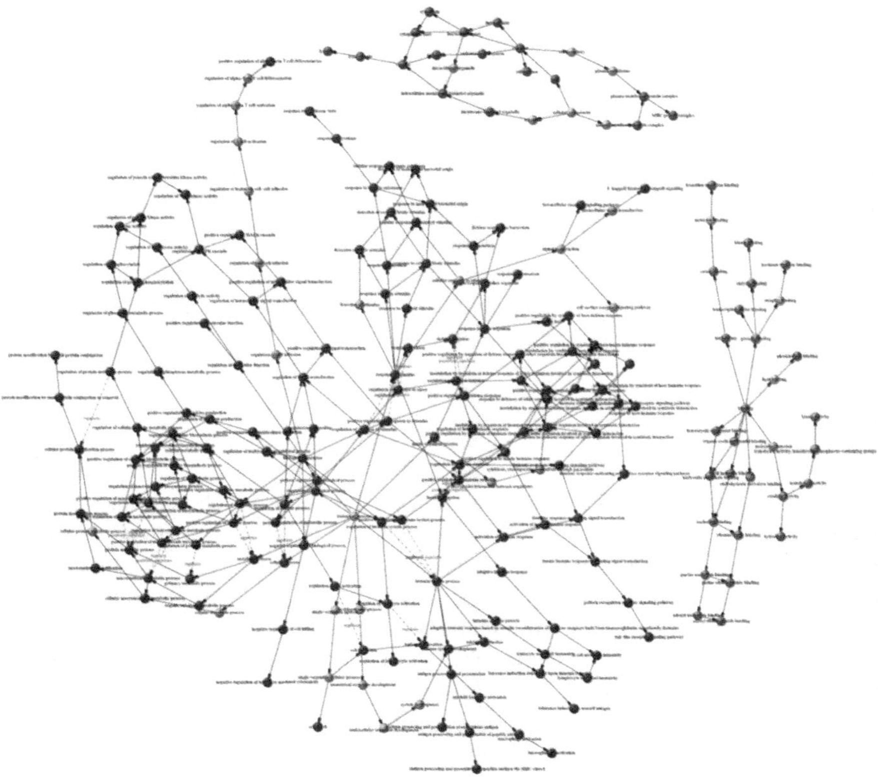

Fig. 9.9 GO Term network relationship diagram of Model group vs. Danhong group (Model-VS-DHI)

Enrichment analysis of KEGG signaling pathway: KEGG signal pathway enrichment analysis was conducted for differentially expressed genes, and the results of signal pathways with significant enrichment of differential genes among groups are as shown in Tables 9.7 and 9.8. The results demonstrate that the key pathways involved in the pharmacodynamic effect of Danhong injection are immune inflammation-related pathways such as antigen processing and presentation, platelet activation, T cell receptor signaling pathway, Fc epsilon RI signaling pathway, leukocyte transendothelial migration, chemokine signaling pathway, cell community pathway such as focal adhesion and regulation of actin cytoskeleton, and signal transduction pathways such as TNF signaling pathway, PI3K-Akt signaling pathway, MAPK signaling pathway, and Jak-STAT signaling.

Association Analysis Between Differentially Expressed Genes and Prediction Targets

By comparing and analyzing the obtained target predicted by network pharmacology with the differentially expressed genes in transcriptomics, it was found that in the

Table 9.7 Enrichment results of differentially expressed gene signaling pathways in blank group vs. model group (Control-VS-Model)

Pathway	Control-VS-Model (297)	All-gene (15026)	*P* value	*Q* value	Level 1	Level 2
Antigen processing and presentation	16	134	9.06E-09	2.39E-07	Organismal systems	Immune system
Fluid shear stress and atherosclerosis	13	214	0.000341	3.56E-03	Human diseases	Cardiovascular diseases
TNF signaling pathway	9	138	0.00169	1.35E-02	Environmental information processing	Signal transduction
Chemokine signaling pathway	11	212	0.003351	2.37E-02	Organismal systems	Immune system
Focal adhesion	12	265	0.006594	3.96E-02	Cellular processes	Cellular community
PI3K-Akt signaling pathway	15	386	0.010052	5.88E-02	Environmental information processing	Signal transduction

component-target-pathway network of the under-construction Danhong injection, 25.1% (118/470) of the targets were verified by transcriptomics (as shown in Fig. 9.10). The signaling pathways enriched by verified targets (as shown in Table 9.9) mainly involve biological processes such as cell signal transduction, inflammation and immunity, cytoskeleton morphological adhesion, and cell apoptosis. The components that have interaction with the verified targets are mentioned below according to the number of associated targets (numbers in brackets), from high to low: Salvianolic acid A (19), Salvianolic acid I (18), Salvianolic acid B (17), Salvianolic acid H (16), Lithospermic acid (16), Salvianolic acid K (16), Monomethyl lithospermate (15), Salvianolic acid E (15), Salvianolic acid G (14), Salvianolic acid D (11), Rosmarinic acid (10), Ethyl lithospermate (9), Salvianolic acid C (9), and Kaempferol-O-rutinoside (8).

9.2.2.2 Effect of Danhong Injection on Biochemical Indexes in Rats with Acute Blood Stasis

Animal Model

The SD rats were randomly divided into eight groups: blank control group, acute blood stasis model group, positive drug low molecular weight heparin calcium group (50μL/kg/d), positive drug aspirin group (10 mg/kg/d), Danhong injection low-dose

Table 9.8 Enrichment results of differentially expressed gene signaling pathways in model group vs. Danhong group (Model-VS-DHI)

Pathway	Model-VS-DHI_high (1541)	All-gene (15026)	*P* value	*Q* value	Level 1	Level 2
Antigen processing and presentation	47	134	8.26E-15	1.28E-12	Organismal systems	Immune system
TNF signaling pathway	42	138	4.47E-11	9.93E-10	Environmental information processing	Signal transduction
NF-kappa B signaling pathway	30	100	3.75E-08	5.08E-07	Environmental information processing	Signal transduction
Toll-like receptor signaling pathway	33	117	4.24E-08	5.49E-07	Organismal systems	Immune system
B cell receptor signaling pathway	27	87	8.18E-08	1.02E-06	Organismal systems	Immune system
Chemokine signaling pathway	46	212	6.46E-07	7.17E-06	Organismal systems	Immune system
Apoptosis	44	207	2.02E-06	2.09E-05	Cellular processes	Cell growth and death
MAPK signaling pathway	52	284	2.39E-05	2.07E-04	Environmental information processing	Signal transduction
Platelet activation	33	168	0.000184	1.33E-03	Organismal systems	Immune system
Jak-STAT signaling pathway	35	184	0.00023	1.62E-03	Environmental information processing	Signal transduction
Regulation of actin cytoskeleton	45	277	0.00124	7.71E-03	Cellular processes	Cell motility
Focal adhesion	43	265	0.001608	9.75E-03	Cellular processes	Cellular community
T cell receptor signaling pathway	24	124	0.001629	9.75E-03	Organismal systems	Immune system
Fc epsilon RI signaling pathway	17	81	0.003098	1.69E-02	Organismal systems	Immune system

Leukocyte transendothelial migration	29	167	0.003221	1.73E-02	Organismal systems	Immune system
Fluid shear stress and atherosclerosis	34	214	0.006504	3.16E-02	Human diseases	Cardiovascular diseases
HIF-1 signaling pathway	22	126	0.008884	3.84E-02	Environmental information processing	Signal transduction
PI3K-Akt signaling pathway	53	386	0.016814	6.41E-02	Environmental information processing	Signal transduction

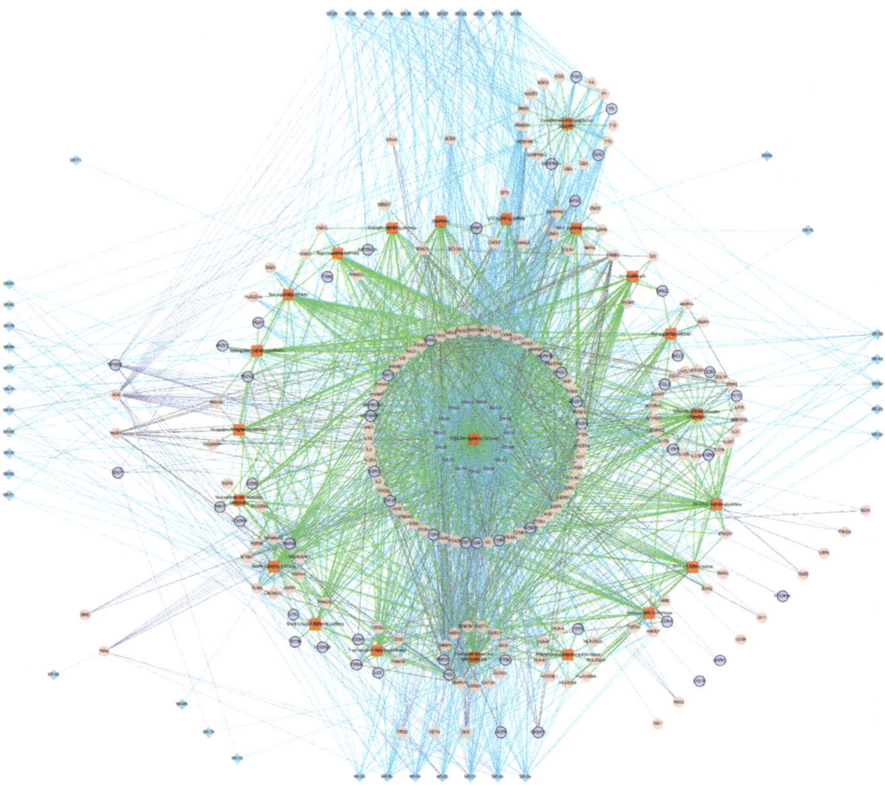

Fig. 9.10 Target verified by transcriptome in component-target-pathway network of Danhong injection (marked in purple)

group (0.75 mL/kg/d) (Clinical dose), medium dose group (1.5 mL/kg/d), and high-dose group (3 mL/kg/d), with ten rats in each group. Aspirin was given by gavage and Danhong injection was given intramuscularly. The blank control group and model group were intramuscularly injected with the same volume of normal saline once a day for ten consecutive days. After the last administration for 30 min, except for the blank control group, acute blood stasis modeling was performed on all rats in all the other groups, using the same method as mentioned in Sect. 6.2.2. After treatment, animals were put on fasting for 12 h and then administered once with DHI or normal saline, respectively; 15 min later, they were anesthetized with an intraperitoneal injection of 10% chloral hydrate 0.35 mL/100 g, and blood was taken from the heart, and they were sacrificed.

The collected rat whole blood was tested with a coagulation analyzer, blood rheometer, dynamic erythrocyte sedimentation rate tester, and platelet aggregation meter, to detect related indexes of hemorheology and coagulation function. Automatic biochemical analyzer, colorimetric kit, and ELISA determination kit were used to detect glutamic-pyruvic transaminase (ALT), glutamic oxaloacetic transaminase

Table 9.9 Signaling pathways enriched by verified targets

Enrichment pathway	Number of enriched targets	Biological process
PI3K-Akt signaling pathway	15	Cell signal transduction
Jak-STAT signaling pathway	7	
Ras signaling pathway	7	
HIF-1 signaling pathway	6	
TNF signaling pathway	6	
Cytokine-cytokine receptor interaction	8	Signal molecular interaction
B cell receptor signaling pathway	8	Inflammation and immunity
Natural killer cell mediated cytotoxicity	8	
Fc gamma R-mediated phagocytosis	7	
Antigen processing and presentation	6	
Focal adhesion	7	Cell community
Regulation of actin cytoskeleton	8	Cytoskeleton morphology
Apoptosis	4	Cell apoptosis

(AST), alkaline phosphatase (ALP), total protein (TP), creatinine (Cr), uric acid (UA), lactate dehydrogenase (LDH), creatine kinase isoenzymes (CK-MB), α-hydroxybutyrate dehydrogenase (α-HBDH), superoxide dismutase (SOD), malondialdehyde (MDA), myeloperoxidase (MPO), nitric oxide (NO), platelet activating factor (PAF), hypersensitive C-reactive protein (hs-CRP), interleukin1β (IL-1β), interleukin-6 (IL-6), interleukin-8 (IL-8), tumor necrosis factor-α (TNF-α), immunoglobulin A (IgA), immunoglobulin G (IgG), and immunoglobulin M (IgM). The measurement data obtained are all expressed as mean ± standard deviation. SPSS version 18.0 was used to analyze the data using One-Way ANOVA and T testing methods. P values <0.05 and P values <0.01 are considered statistically different.

Detection Results of Multiple Biochemical Indexes

In acute blood stasis rats, obvious abnormalities were found in inflammation and immune response, vascular endothelial function, oxidative stress, platelet aggregation, myocardial energy metabolism, and liver and kidney function. Danhong injection was significantly effective for 19 indexes of IgM, IgA, IgG, IL-1β, TNF-α, IL-6, IL-8, LDH, CK-MB, PAF, SOD, MDA, MPO, hs-CRP, NO, TP, ALP, Cr, and UA, indicating that Danhong injection can inhibit the inflammatory response in rats with acute blood stasis, improve immune function, protect cardiomyocytes, reduce body peroxidation damage, protect liver and kidney function, inhibit platelet aggregation, and improve vascular function (as shown in Table 9.10).

Most of the pharmacodynamic indicators investigated are representative indicators in the pathological process. The signal pathways where these indicators are

Table 9.10 Effects of Danhong injection on several biochemical indexes in rats

Efficacy	Index	Effect of Danhong injection
Hemorheology	Whole blood viscosity	↓
	Erythrocyte aggregation, electrophoresis, rigidity index	↓
	Maximum platelet aggregation rate	↓
	PAF	↓
Immune response	IgG	↓
	IgM	↓
	IgA	↓
Inflammatory response	IL-1β	↓
	TNF-α	↓
	IL-6	↓
	IL-8	↓
Myocardial enzyme spectrum	LDH	↓
	CK-MB	↓
Oxidative stress	MDA	↓
Endothelial function	NO	↑
Liver function	TP	↑
	ALP	↓
Renal function	Cr	↓
	UA	↑

located were fairly consistent with the predicted targets and the signal pathways enriched in transcriptomics, differentially expressed the genes. For example, Danhong injection can regulate the expression of pro-inflammatory factors by activating the TNF signaling pathway; The fluid shear stress and atherosclerosis pathway regulate the expression of eNOS, thereby affecting the production of NO and endothelial function.

9.2.3 Analysis of Regulatory Network of Danhong Injection in the Treatment of Cardiovascular Diseases

The regulatory network of Danhong injection in the treatment of cardiovascular diseases was analyzed after integrating target prediction, transcriptome detection, and measurement results of multiple biochemical indexes in rats with acute blood stasis (as shown in Fig. 9.11). The mechanism mainly involves the following aspects:

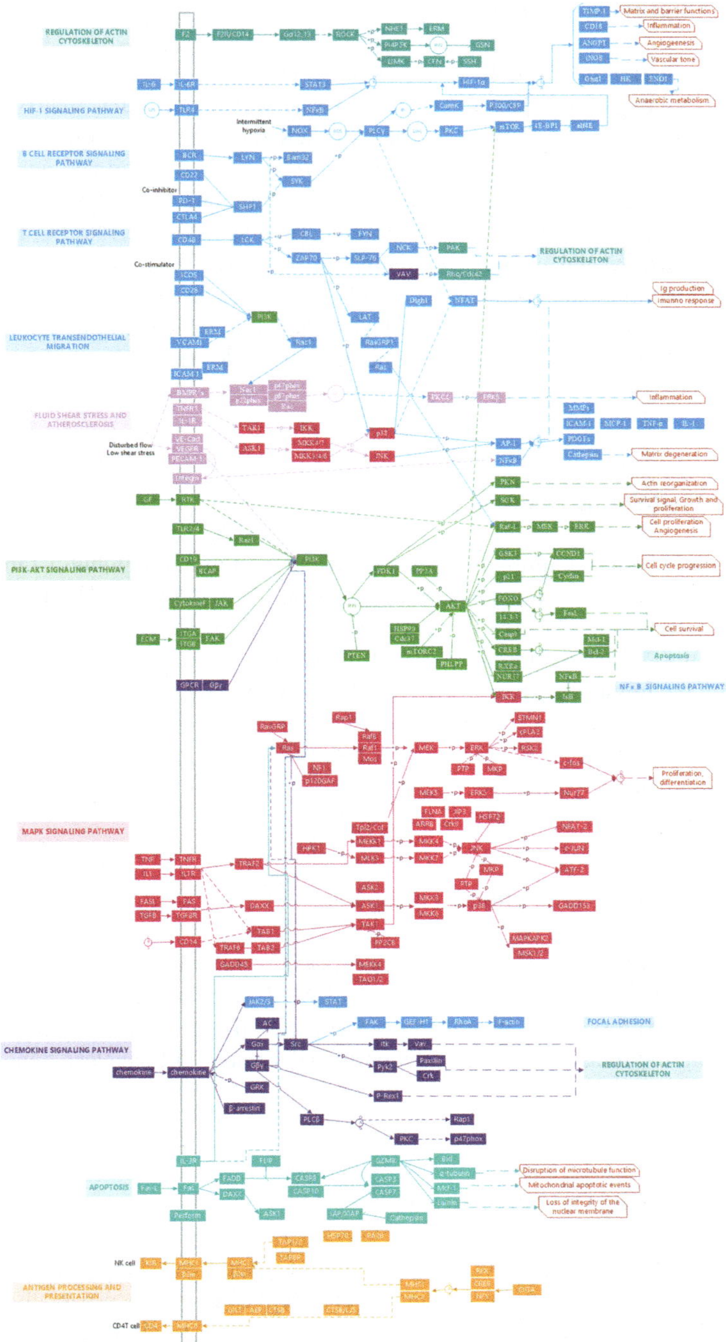

Fig. 9.11 Molecular mechanism of Danhong injection based on network pharmacology and transcriptomics

9.2.3.1 Improving Hemorheology

Danhong injection can bind to F2R receptors, chemokine receptors, and integrins through F2 (coagulation factor II), chemokines, and extracellular matrix, respectively, to activate the regulation of actin cytoskeleton, adhesion plaques, and PI3K-Akt signaling pathway, which plays a role in reducing red blood cell aggregation, electrophoresis, rigidity index, whole blood viscosity, and platelet aggregation. At the same time, chemokine receptors and integrins can also activate the PI3K-Akt signaling pathway and mediate inflammation response. Inflammation response is closely related to platelet activation and atherosclerotic disease progression. Therefore, Danhong injection inhibits platelet activation and reduces whole blood viscosity, which may be related to the regulation of PI3K-Akt pathway-related gene expression.

9.2.3.2 Modulating Immune Response

Danhong injection can inhibit the abnormal increase of immunoglobulin. On the one hand, its mechanism may regulate the expression of MHCI and MHCII on the cell surface by regulating the related genes in the antigen processing and presentation pathway, thus affecting the B cell and T cell receptor signaling pathways and regulating the immune response. On the other hand, it may also affect the activation of MAPK cascade reaction and the transcriptional regulation of immunoglobulin by NFAT through the TNFR1 receptor in the TNF signaling pathway, in order to regulate the immune response.

9.2.3.3 Inhibiting Inflammatory Response

The action target of Danhong injection is closely related to the TNF signaling pathway, PI3K-Akt signaling pathway, and MAPK signaling pathway, and can regulate the expression of inflammatory cytokines IL-1β, TNF-α, IL-6, and IL-8 by affecting the transcriptional regulation of AP-1 and NFκB nuclear transcription factors.

9.2.3.4 Reducing Oxidative Stress

Danhong injection can regulate the expression of related genes in the HIF-1 signaling pathway and fluid shear stress and atherosclerosis pathway, especially the key gene NOX. NOX is a key source of reactive oxygen species in the body, thus, regulating its expression can regulate the degree of oxidative stress in the body, affecting the expression of SOD, MDA, and other efficacy indicators. In addition, inflammatory factors such as IL-1β and TNF-α can activate NOX, therefore, a decrease in inflammatory levels also reduces oxidative stress levels.

9.2.3.5 Protecting Endothelial Function

Similar to the effect of oxidative stress, the mechanism of Danhong injection in protecting and improving endothelial function may be related to the regulation of HIF-1 signaling pathway and fluid shear stress and the expression of related genes in the atherosclerotic pathway. Among them, NOX can reduce the degradation of eNOS and reduce the level of NO in cells, while NO can in turn inhibit the activity of NOX, alleviating oxidative stress and vascular endothelial damage from the source [10]. NO has been proven to protect endothelial cells, improve endothelial cell function, and at the same time promote angiogenesis, and plays an important protective role in ischemic injury. In addition, Danhong injection may induce the production of HIF-1α by activating the PI3K or MAPK pathway. HIF-1α can activate the transcription of eNOS in endothelial cells, thereby promoting the production of NO. The biochemical index test results also show that the level of NO increases correspondingly after the administration of Danhong injection.

9.2.3.6 Protecting Myocardial, Liver, and Kidney Function

Danhong injection is closely related to PI3K-Akt signaling pathway and cell apoptosis pathway. These pathways not only regulate cell apoptosis, proliferation, and differentiation, but also participate in the regulation of oxidative stress and inflammatory response. Therefore, the protective effect of Danhong injection on myocardium, liver, kidney, and other organs may be related to the reduction of cell apoptosis, the alleviation of inflammation, and tissue damage caused by oxidative stress.

To sum up, this section adopts the network pharmacology method to establish the composition-target-pathway network of Danhong injection, and further experimentally verifies the prediction results through transcriptomics analysis and multiple biochemical indicator tests, and comprehensively analyzes and clarifies the molecular mechanism and regulatory network of Danhong injection.

Due to the complexity of components and functions of TCM, the limitations of technology in the past added to the lack of overall understanding of the mechanism of its action led to an unclear direction for in-depth research as well as lack of pertinence. Network pharmacology, which has developed strongly in recent years, aims to study complex issues from the holistic perspective and internal relevance. It coincides with the core ideas of Chinese medicine and has become a new strategy [11] for scientifically explaining the effectiveness of Chinese medicine. This chapter introduces the common methods of network pharmacology in the TCM research by taking Exocarpium Citri Grandis and Danhong injection as examples. It mainly includes the construction of component and target data, the prediction and analysis of active components and potential action targets, as well as the comprehensive analysis of the relationship between components, targets, pathways, and efficacy, in order to explore the overall complex mechanism of action of TCM. The development of network pharmacology research will provide an important basis for guiding the in-depth research and development and clinical application of Chinese medicine. With the development of network pharmacology and its integration with new technologies, network analysis methods will also have broader application prospects in Chinese medicine research.

References

1. Chen Y, Wu H, Nie YC, et al. Mucoactive effects of naringin in lipopolysaccharide-induced acute lung injury mice and beagle dogs. Environ Toxicol Pharmacol. 2014;38(1):279–87.
2. Liu Y, Wu H, Nie YC, et al. Naringin attenuates acute lung injury in LPS-treated mice by inhibiting NF-kappa B pathway. Int Immunopharmacol. 2011;11(10):1606–12.
3. Nie YC, Wu H, Li PB, et al. Anti-inflammatory effects of naringin in chronic pulmonary neutrophilic inflammation in cigarette smoke-exposed rats. J Med Food. 2012;15(10):894–900.
4. Liu MH, Zou W, Yang CP, et al. Metabolism and excretion studies of oral administered naringin, a putative antitussive, in rats and dogs. Biopharm Drug Dispos. 2012;33:123–34.
5. Huang DW, Sherman BT, Lempicki RA. Systematic and integrative analysis of large gene lists using DAVID bioinformatics resources. Nat Protoc. 2009;4(1):44–57.
6. Huang DW, Sherman BT, Lempicki RA. Bioinformatics enrichment tools: paths toward the comprehensive functional analysis of large gene lists. Nucleic Acids Res. 2009;37(1):1–13.
7. Ransom RF, Lam NG, Hallett MA, et al. Glucocorticoids protect and enhance recovery of cultured murine podocytes via actin filament stabilization. Kidney Int. 2005;68(6):2473–83.
8. Zhang H, Ma SF, Feng ZW, et al. Cardiovascular disease chemogenomics knowledgebase-guided target identification and drug synergy mechanism study of an herbal formula. Sci Rep. 2016;6:33963.
9. Liu H, Zhang WJ, Long CF, et al. Protective effects of traditional Chinese herbal formula compound xueshuantong capsule (CXC) on rats with blood circulation disorders. Biotechnol Biotechnol Equip. 2017;31(4):1–9.
10. Dusting GJ, Selemidis S, Jiang F. Mechanisms for suppressing NADPH oxidase in the vascular wall. Mem Inst Oswaldo Cruz. 2005;100(1):97.
11. Li S. Mapping ancient remedies: applying a network approach to traditional Chinese medicine. Science. 2015;350:S72–4.

Afterword

With the advent of biomedical big data and the artificial intelligence era, network pharmacology has huge growth potential and extensive application prospects in drug research and development, elucidation of disease mechanism, efficacy evaluation, precision medicine, and other aspects. Network pharmacology has dynamic interdisciplinary characteristics, involving systems biology, bioinformatics, network science, multi-direction pharmacology, systems pharmacology, and other related disciplines. Individuals engaged or interested in network pharmacology research also come from different fields, and there are varied opinions and viewpoints. This book systematically introduces the theory, method, and application of network pharmacology, focusing on the originality of the theory, the systematic methodology, and the intersection of application cases. Using a large number of cases, this paper introduces the details of the network pharmacology analysis process in detail, guides readers in quickly understanding the practice of network pharmacology, and strives to make readers from different fields gain new insights.

Each chapter of this book is drafted by experts and scholars with distinct professional backgrounds. The research groups involved in each chapter have distinct characteristics. Different groups are skilled in software, experiments, calculations, Western medicine, and Traditional Chinese Medicine. Attentive readers may ascertain the nuance during their perusal of each chapter. In the end, we did not format the content of each chapter, rather retained the characteristic features of each chapter. We don't avoid shortcomings when we develop our strengths, since this is the appeal of network pharmacology. As an interdisciplinary approach, we hope that experts and scholars from different backgrounds and fields can showcase their talents, as in the real world of network pharmacology, one can learn from others, thereby effectuating mutual development.

In fact, it is relatively rudimentary to render suggestions to incorporate calculations to chapters that focus on experiments, or to incorporate experiments to chapters that focus on calculations. However, network pharmacology is considerably young, and in the process of continuous development. The rapid growth of research has taken place in a span of 10–20 years; with a considerable number of results presented

S. Li (ed.), *Network Pharmacology*, https://doi.org/10.1007/978-981-16-0753-0

every year, or every month. We hope that readers will acknowledge the notable particulars of each chapter, and that in the future these points will make up for the ineffectual particulars. That being the case, we have taken the unusual step of revealing the true face of this newly written book first to readers. It is a book of the moment. It is a book that reflects the real world of pharmacological research on the network.

At the editorial meeting, everyone was enthusiastically and unanimously opposed to the "routinization" of network pharmacological analysis. Scientific research only seeks truth, and scientific methods are highly crucial, however, everything revolves around problems that need to be resolved through research, therefore problem orientation (clinical problems, scientific research issues, industrial issues, discipline development issues, etc.) is critical. At present, network pharmacological research evidently has varying challenges and therefore it is necessary to establish appropriate guidelines and norms. We have also attached to this book the first international standard *Network Pharmacology Evaluation Method Guide* (see Appendix A) in the field of network pharmacology of the World Federation of Chinese Medicine Societies, for our readers' reference.

We welcome interested research groups to join the book and make collective efforts to collaboratively publish the second and the third edition in the future, and to also co-compile a textbook when the network pharmacological research comes of age.

Editorial Committee

Appendix A: Network Pharmacology Evaluation Method Guide

Network pharmacology is an interdisciplinary discipline newly developed in the systematic research of drugs based on artificial intelligence and Big Data. It stresses the holistic system-level and biological networks when analyzing the molecular association laws between drugs and treatment objects. Focusing on studying drugs, it provides new ideas, especially for Chinese medicine research, which is based on a complex system. It is also widely applied to explore the active compounds of drugs and Chinese medicine, explain the overall action mechanisms, and analyze the compatibility regularity of drug pairs and formulas. It has provided new scientific and technological support for the rational clinical use of drugs and drug development.

With an increasing influence and application in the Big Data era, network pharmacology now faces great development opportunities and challenges in terms of theoretical analyses, algorithm development, and applications. The issue of integrating massive clinical and experimental data and combining scientific verification to reveal the regulation mechanisms of network pharmacology to carry out its research more effectively has become the main concern of researchers. In addition, there are multiple problems in the current network pharmacology studies, such as uneven research quality, lack of data standardization, and insufficient scientific verification. Establishing a rigorous, scientific, and unified standard for evaluating network pharmacology studies is urgently required to ensure this emerging discipline's healthy development.

Therefore, a normative evaluation standard of network pharmacology has been established to build association between drugs and diseases in biomolecular networks based on the "network target," the main theory of network pharmacology, and forms a "network target-system regulation"-based research mode and method that provides a new way to understand and explain the interactions between drugs and biological systems. The standard aims to make the "network target-system regulation"-based research mode, a new generation of drug research paradigm which is more rigorous and scientific and is widely recognized and promotes the standardized application of network pharmacology in drug analysis and experiment,

S. Li (ed.), *Network Pharmacology*, https://doi.org/10.1007/978-981-16-0753-0

and clinical pharmacological studies, thus promoting the rapid, healthy, and orderly development of the discipline. The network pharmacology standard is as follows:

Li S. Network pharmacology evaluation method guidance-Draft. World J Tradit Chin Med. 2021;7(1):146–154 (https://www.wjtcm.net/aheadofprint.asp)

Appendix B: The Pioneering Contribution of Chinese Medicine in the Origin and Development of Network Pharmacology

1. Evaluation of the original theory, method, and application of "Network target":

   (a) **Academician of Chinese Academy of Engineering, Yong-yan Wang wrote**: "Network pharmacology represents a new research concept and method in line with the overall characteristics of traditional Chinese medicine... It is expected to make the research of traditional Chinese medicine prescriptions join the forefront of contemporary science and technology and provide strong support for source innovation." (Journal of Traditional Chinese Medical Sciences 2019, 6:195–200)

   (b) **Academician of the Chinese Academy of Engineering, Bo-li Zhang spoke highly in*Twenty Years of Modernization of Traditional Chinese Medicine***: "In 2007, Shao Li of Tsinghua University first proposed the research framework of traditional Chinese medicine prescriptions based on biological network. By means of constructing the key technology platform of network pharmacology, it has broken through the key technologies of network-based disease gene and traditional Chinese medicine target prediction, traditional Chinese medicine discovery and compatibility screening, and biological network construction and analysis of disease and syndrome prescriptions." (Shanghai Science and Technology Press, 2016, p. 62)

   (c) **Academician of the Chinese Academy of Engineering, Chang-xiao Liu wrote:** "Network pharmacology arises at a historic moment based on the modern research of Chinese medicine... and has made great contributions to the interpretation of the connotation of traditional Chinese medicine, promoting the research of new traditional Chinese medicine drugs, and enhancing the achievements of modern research of traditional Chinese medicine." (Drug Evaluation Research 2018; 41:709–715). Innovative ideas of network targets and network analysis methods have opened a new avenue for the research of traditional Chinese medicine (CHM 2015; 7:3–17, CHM 2015; 7:27–38).

   (d) **Academician of Chinese Academy of Sciences, Ke-ji Chen wrote:** "The network target method is 'a significant change in drug discovery research,'

S. Li (ed.), *Network Pharmacology*, https://doi.org/10.1007/978-981-16-0753-0

and the above network analysis method is a 'systematic approach' to drug research, a potentially more effective strategy." (Chin J Integr Med 2012; 18:883–890)

(e) The review article written by **Pei-gen Xiao et. al, Academicians of The Institute of Medicinal Plant Development,** cited the Network Pharmacology research results of Liuwei Dihuang prescription, Qingluo Decoction, and Gegen Qinlian Decoction by Shao Li's research group, and believed that the Network Pharmacology research of traditional Chinese medicine has the potential to bridge the gap between traditional and modern medicine (Drug Development Research 2014; 75:299–312).

(f) In the cover article of Nature Reviews Genetics, **the founder of network biology and Academician of European Academy of Sciences, Barabási** evaluated the representative algorithm based on network target theory as "a network pharmacology method that in fact goes deep into the field of drug research." (Nature Rev Genet 2011;12:56–68)

(g) **Director of the Department of Pharmaceutical Biology, University of Mainz, Germany, Phytomedicine Editor-in-Chief Professor Efferth T commented: "**Network pharmacology methods can bring about a revolution from single target–single drug to network target-multi-component regulation (Applying these methods will lead to a shift…)." (Dawood et al. Front Pharmacol. 2018; 9:143)

(h) A long review of ***Encyclopedia of Systems Biology*****published by Springer Press** holds that "representative algorithms based on network targets are perfect examples of the concept of Network Pharmacology." (Encyclopedia of Systems Biology. 2013: 2106–2108)

(i) **Chairman of the Advisory Committee of the Office of Alternative Medicine of the NIH in the United States, Berman B** used the network target method as a representative case of network pharmacology (Front Physiol 2015; 6:225).

(j) **Gerard Bodeker, Chairman of the Global Initiative for Traditional Health Systems, Editor-in-chief of*****WHO Global Atlas of Traditional, Complementary and Alternative Medicine*****and professor at Oxford University Medical School**, believes that Asia has instigated a new approach to traditional medicine research, that is, network pharmacology. This new direction of understanding the complexity of traditional medicine is based on the concept of "network target" and is employed to understand the pharmacological mechanism of Qingluo Decoction and Liuwei Dihuang prescription (NWFP update 2015).

2. The pioneering contribution of Chinese medicine in the field of network pharmacology:

   (a) **The expert group led by Academician Bo-li Zhang evaluated in the appraisal of scientific research results:** "The pioneering achievements of network pharmacology have accomplished a major innovation of independent core technology of traditional Chinese medicine, provided a new perspective and method for the modernization and internationalization of traditional Chinese medicine, significantly promoted the heritage and development of traditional Chinese medicine and industrial upgrade, provided a new mode for the study of the complex system of traditional Chinese medicine, and opened up a new international frontier in the key technology of traditional Chinese medicine. This is a landmark achievement of the original innovation of traditional Chinese medicine, and has been highlighted at the international level." (Scientific and Technological Achievements Report, No. 201911ZK3557)

(b) **Member of the Indian National Academy of Medical Sciences, Patwardhan, commented:** "Shao Li pioneered the use of network pharmacology in Chinese medicine research..." (Indian J Tradit Know 2015, 14 (4):574–580). "Shao Li pioneered this endeavor and proposed using the network to provide new ways to understand diseases and drug intervention..." (Innovative Approaches in Drug Discovery. 2017:127–164) The important contribution of TCM in the field of network pharmacology.

(c) **Master of traditional Chinese medicine, Zhong-ying Zhou wrote:** "From the perspective of "relationship-network-function," Shao Li et al. studied the new strategies of "information integration-computational modeling-generating hypothesis-experimental verification..." This kind of thinking and method will enlighten and promote the progressive and detailed research on the nature of syndromes in the future. The key is that its research is based on the level of basic pathogenesis." (中医杂志, 2014, 55(14): 1171–1175)

(d) **Master of traditional Chinese medicine Jia-xiang Liu wrote:** "Shao Li et al. studied 1,446 kinds of traditional Chinese medicine ingredients... It will show great development potential in the field of cancer prevention and treatment." (World Science and Technology-Modernization of Traditional Chinese Medicine, 2019, 21(5): 943–948)

(e) **Professor Xiao-ming Wu and Professor Chun-fu Wu, editor-in-chief of*Chinese Natural Medicines*and Vice-Chairman of the Chinese Pharmaceutical Association**, believe that "in the era of big data, Chinese scientists have led a new interdisciplinary frontier of great prominence—TCM network pharmacology," and evaluated Shao Li as a "Pioneer of TCM Network Pharmacology." (Chinese Journal of Natural Medicines 2015:13:1–2)

(f) **Dan Xi, an expert in the office of complementary and alternative medicine of NIH/NRI, and others** evaluated Shao Li as a "Pioneer and expert in the study of traditional Chinese medicine with systems biology in China." (International Journal of Functional Informatics and Personalized Medicine 2009; 2:244–247)

(g) **Dan Xi, Director of the Research Development and Support Program of the Office of Complementary and Alternative Medicine at NIH/NCI in the United States,** evaluated the related methods and applications of network pharmacology: "It helps immensely to comprehend the complex mechanism of action and transformation of natural products." (JNCI Monographs. 2017; 52: lgx003)

(h) **In the supplement of *Traditional Asian Medicine* published by Nature in 2011, Professor Greef from the Netherlands** evaluated the research on cold and heat syndromes based on biological networks (Li et al. IET Systems Biology 2007) as "the precedent-setting systematic biological research of traditional Chinese medicine" and "indicating that Chinese medicine can become the driving force of personalized medicine." (Greef. Nature 2011; 480:S87)

(i) The research results of research on biomolecular network of cold and heat syndromes evaluated by the national ***Progress Report on TCM Metrology and Its Modern Research*** as "For the first time, it provides an additional explanation and basis for the internal mechanism of TCM syndromes from the perspective of biological network, and provides a new perspective for the multi-target integration and regulation effect of TCM compound prescription." (*Progress Report on TCM Metrology and Its Modern Research* 2009:54)

The manufacturer's authorised representative in the EU is Springer Nature Customer Service Centre GmbH, Europaplatz 3, 69115 Heidelberg, Germany. If you have any concerns regarding our products, please contact ProductSafety@springernature.com

Printed and bound by CPI Group (UK) Ltd, Croydon, CR0 4YY
30/09/2026
02225330-0017